Hybridoma Technology in the Biosciences and Medicine

Hybridoma Technology in the Biosciences and Medicine

Edited by
TIMOTHY A. SPRINGER
Dana-Farber Cancer Institute
Harvard Medical School
Boston, Massachusetts

Plenum Press • New York and London

Library of Congress Cataloging in Publication Data

Main entry under title:

Hybridoma technology in the biosciences and medicine.

Includes bibliographies and index.
1. Hybridomas. 2. Antibodies, Monoclonal. I. Springer, Timothy A. [DNLM: 1. Antibodies, Monoclonal. 2. Hybridomas—immunology. 3. Immunologic Technics. QW 575 H992]
QR185.8.H93H925 1985 616.07′9 85-12083
ISBN 0-306-41996-3

A Division of Plenum Publishing Corporation
233 Spring Street, New York, N.Y. 10013

Printed in the United States of America

To my mentors Jack Strominger and Cesar Milstein; to my mentor
Baruj Benacerraf, who inspired me to do this book; to Aliza,
who arrived while the book was in gestation; and to Noah and Jeanie.

Contributors

Hector L. Aguila Department of Cell Biology, Albert Einstein College of Medicine, New York, New York 10461

Frederick W. Alt Department of Biochemistry and Institute for Cancer Research, Columbia University, College of Physicians and Surgeons, New York, New York 10032

Donald C. Anderson Department of Pediatrics Baylor College of Medicine, Houston, Texas 77050

Antonio Bargellesi Department of Biological Chemistry, University of Genoa, Italy

Colin J. Barnstable Laboratory of Neurobiology, Rockefeller University, New York, New York 10021

Robert C. Bast, Jr. Division of Tumor Immunology, Dana-Farber Cancer Institute, and Department of Medicine, Harvard Medical School, Boston, Massachusetts 02115

David I. Beller Department of Pathology, Harvard Medical School, Boston, Massachusetts 02115

Joseph P. Brown Oncogen, Seattle, Washington 98121

Steven J. Burakoff Division of Pediatric Oncology, Dana-Farber Cancer Institute, and Department of Pediatrics, Harvard Medical School, Boston, Massachusetts 02115

Charles B. Carpenter Brigham and Women's Hospital, Harvard Medical School, Boston, Massachusetts 02115

Lan Bo Chen Division of Cell Growth and Regulation, Dana-Farber Cancer Institute, and Harvard Medical School, Boston, Massachusetts 02115

Carol Clayberger Department of Pediatrics, Stanford University School of Medicine, Stanford, California 94305.

Man Sung Co Department of Pathology, Harvard Medical School, Boston, Massachusetts 02115

Susan P. C. Cole Department of Microbiology and Immunology, Queen's University, Kingston, Ontario, Canada K7L 3N6

Mary Crimmins Division of Pediatric Oncology, Dana-Farber Cancer Institute, Boston, Massachusetts 02115

Linda K. Curtiss Department of Immunology, Research Institute of Scripps Clinic, La Jolla, California 92037

Ronald W. Davis Department of Biochemistry, Stanford University School of Medicine, Stanford, California 94305

Zelig Eshhar Department of Chemical Immunology, Weizmann Institute of Science, Rehovot, Israel

Douglas T. Fearon Department of Medicine, Harvard Medical School, and Department of Rheumatology and Immunology, Brigham and Women's Hospital, Boston, Massachusetts 02115

Glen N. Gaulton Departments of Medicine and Pathology, Tufts University School of Medicine, Boston, Massachusetts 02111

Mark I. Greene Departments of Medicine and Pathology, Tufts University School of Medicine, Boston, Massachusetts 02111

Julia L. Greenstein Division of Pediatric Oncology, Dana-Farber Cancer Institute, and Department of Pathology, Harvard Medical School, Boston, Massachusetts 02115

Gillian M. Griffiths Laboratory of Molecular Biology, Medical Research Council, Cambridge CB2 2QH, England

Edgar Haber Cardiac Unit and Cellular and Molecular Research Laboratory, Massachusetts General Hospital, and Department of Medicine, Harvard Medical School, Boston, Massachusetts 02214

G. Hale Department of Pathology, Division of Immunology, New Addenbrookes Hospital, University of Cambridge, Cambridge CB2 2QQ, England

Susan M. Hochschwender Receptor Biology Laboratory, Salk Institute, San Diego, California 92138

Pauline Johnson MRC Cellular Immunology Unit, Sir William Dunn School of Pathology, University of Oxford, Oxford OX1 3RE England

Paula Kavathas Department of Genetics, School of Medicine, Stanford University, Stanford, California 94305

Jonathan Kaye Department of Biology, University of California, San Diego, La Jolla, California 92093.

Thomas J. Kipps Department of Genetics, Stanford University School of Medicine, Stanford, California 94305

Danuta Kozbor Department of Microbiology and Immunology, Queen's University, Kingston, Ontario, Canada K7L 3N6

Jan P. Kraus Department of Human Genetics, Yale University School of Medicine, New Haven, Connecticut 06510

Alan M. Krensky Department of Pediatrics, Stanford University School of Medicine, Stanford, California 94305

Lorene K. Langeberg Receptor Biology Laboratory, Salk Institute, San Diego, California 92138

Jon M. Lindstrom Receptor Biology Laboratory, Salk Institute, San Diego, California 92138

Andrew D. Luster Laboratory of Cellular Physiology and Immunology, Rockefeller University, New York, New York 10021

Noboru Matsuzaki Department of Pathology, Harvard Medical School, Boston, Massachusetts 02115

Steven J. Mentzer Division of Pediatric Oncology, Dana-Farber Cancer Insitute, and Department of Surgery, Harvard Medical School, Boston, Massachusetts 02115

Cesar Milstein Laboratory of Molecular Biology, Medical Research Council, Cambridge CB2 2QH, England

Diana G. Myles Department of Physiology, University of Connecticut School of Medicine, Farmington, Connecticut 06032

Gary J. Nabel Department of Medicine, Brigham and Women's Hospital, and Harvard Medical School, Boston, Massachusetts 02115

Markus Nabholz Genetics Unit, Swiss Institute for Experimental Cancer Research (ISREC), Epalinges, Switzerland

Karen K. Nadakavukaren Division of Cell Growth and Regulation, Dana-Farber Cancer Institute, and Harvard Medical School, Boston, Massachusetts 02115

Jiri Novotny Cellular and Molecular Research Laboratory, Massachusetts General Hospital, and Harvard Medical School, Boston, Massachusetts 02115

Peter Parham Department of Cell Biology, Stanford University School of Medicine, Stanford, California 94305

Gregory D. Plowman Oncogen, Seattle, Washington 98121

Roberta R. Pollock Department of Cell Biology, Albert Einstein College of Medicine, New York, New York 10461

Daniel A. Portnoy Laboratory of Cellular Physiology and Immunology, Rockefeller University, New York, New York 10021

Paul Primakoff Department of Physiology, University of Connecticut School of Medicine, Farmington, Connecticut 06032

Ellen Pure Laboratory of Cellular Physiology and Immunology, Rockefeller University, New York, New York 10021

Jerome Ritz Division of Tumor Immunology, Dana-Farber Cancer Institute, and Department of Medicine, Harvard Medical School, Boston, Massachusetts 02115

Kenneth L. Rock Department of Pathology, Harvard Medical School, Boston, Massachusetts 02115

John C. C. Roder Department of Microbiology and Immunology, Queen's University, Kingston, Ontario, Canada K7L 3N6

Timothy M. Rose Oncogen, Seattle, Washington 98121

Sharon Rosenberg Division of Cell Growth and Regulation, Dana-Farber Cancer Institute, New England Deaconess Hospital, and Harvard Medical School, Boston, Massachusetts 02115

Frank H. Ruddle Department of Biology and Human Genetics, Yale University, New Haven, Connecticut 06511

Stephen E. Sallan Division of Pediatric Oncology, Dana-Farber Cancer Institute, and Department of Pediatrics, Harvard Medical School, Boston, Massachusetts 02115

Brian S. Schaffhausen Department of Biochemistry and Pharmacology, Tufts University School of Medicine, Boston, Massachusetts 02111

Matthew D. Scharff Department of Cell Biology, Albert Einstein College of Medicine, New York, New York 10461

Stuart F. Schlossman Division of Tumor Immunology, Dana-Farber Cancer Institute, and Department of Medicine, Harvard Medical School, Boston, Massachusetts 02115

Douglas W. Schneider Receptor Biology Laboratory, Salk Institute, San Diego, California 92138

Elizabeth L. Shepherd Division of Cell Growth and Regulation, Dana-Farber Cancer Institute, and Harvard Medical School, Boston, Massachusetts 02115

John J. Skehel National Institute for Medical Research, London NW7 1AA, England

Sandra J. Smith-Gill Laboratory of Genetics, National Cancer Institute, National Institutes of Health, Bethesda, Maryland 20205, and Department of Zoology, University of Maryland, College Park, Maryland 20742

Michael Snyder Department of Biochemistry, Stanford University School of Medicine, Stanford, California 94305

Gad Spira Faculty of Medicine, Technion, Haifa, Israel

Timothy A. Springer Laboratory of Membrane Immunochemistry, Dana-Farber Cancer Institute and Department of Pathology, Harvard Medical School, Boston, Massachusetts 02115

Glenn D. Steele, Jr. New England Deaconess Hospital, and Harvard Medical School, Boston, Massachusetts 02115

Tak Takvorian Division of Medical Oncology, Dana-Farber Cancer Institute, and Department of Medicine, Harvard Medical School, Boston, Massachusetts 02115

Ian S. Trowbridge Department of Cancer Biology, Salk Institute for Biological Studies, San Diego, California 92138

Jay C. Unkeless Laboratory of Cellular Physiology and Immunology, Rockefeller University, New York, New York 10021

Herman Waldmann Department of Pathology Division of Immunology, New Addenbrookes Hospital, University of Cambridge, Cambridge CB2 2QQ, England

Elizabeth S. Walker Division of Cell Growth and Regulation, Dana-Farber Cancer Institute, New England Deaconess Hospital, and Harvard Medical School, Boston, Massachusetts 02115

Janis Jacks Weis Department of Medicine, Harvard Medical School, Boston, Massachusetts 02115

Donald C. Wiley Department of Biochemistry and Molecular Biology, Harvard University, Cambridge, Massachusetts 02138

Alan F. Williams MRC Cellular Immunology Unit, Sir William Dunn School of Pathology, University of Oxford, Oxford OX1 3RE, England

Gillian R. Woollett MRC Cellular Immunology Unit, Sir William Dunn School of Pathology, University of Oxford, Oxford OX1 3RE, England

Introduction and Overview

Antibodies have played an important role in basic research and in medicine ever since their discovery in immune serum in the 1890s. How antibodies are produced, however, did not begin to be understood until 1957 when Burnet proposed the clonal selection hypothesis, a modification of a previous theory by Jerne. By the 1960s it became well established that antibody diversity is a reflection of the diversification of lymphocyte clones, that an individual lymphocyte produces only a single type of antibody, and that even homogenous antigens induce a heterogenous antibody response because of the many different lymphocyte clones with appropriate specificity for antigen which are induced by antigen to proliferate and secrete antibody. The implications of this understanding were realized in 1975 by Köhler and Milstein, who immortalized the "one lymphocyte–one antibody" concept in the form of "hybridomas". Hybridomas are hybrids between myeloma tumor cells and antigen-stimulated lymphocytes which can be cloned, grown in large quantity and for indefinite periods of time, and secrete high concentrations of monoclonal, and hence monospecific, antibodies. Since monospecificity is achieved by cloning the hybridoma cell, rather than by purifying the antigen, highly complex antigens can be used for immunization.

On the tenth anniversary of its first publication, it is clear that the Köhler and Milstein technique has truly revolutionized the way in which antibodies are used in biology. It has allowed the extraordinary diversity and specificity of the antibody response to be tapped in ways which were never possible before. Soon after publication of the hybridoma technique in 1975, it was not widely appreciated what a dramatic impact it would have. Widespread use of monoclonal antibodies came first in the field where they were developed, immunology. In the last few years, however, their use has spread rapidly into all fields of biology, including cell biology, biochemistry, microbiology, virology, parasitology, physiology, genetics, and molecular biology, and into areas of medicine such as pathology, hematology, oncology, cardiology, and infectious disease. The drug and biotechnology industries have also widely adopted monoclonal antibodies for applications ranging from diagnosis and therapy to the purification of cloned gene products. The contributions of monoclonal antibodies to science and to human health were recognized by the award of the Nobel Prize in Physiology and Medicine in 1984 to Milstein, Köhler, and Jerne.

Many advances and discoveries in the last ten years have been possible only by the application of hybridoma technology. In this same period of time, several other advanced immunological technologies have sprung up. The first of these is immunization with synthetic peptides, which is an alternative method of obtaining antibodies to highly defined regions of proteins. The second is the use of antibodies, either polyclonal or monoclonal, as an aid in gene cloning. The third is the ability to establish T cell clones or hybridomas, and utilize their secreted products. The state of the art of these technologies is described here, and some of their unique contributions to research and medical advances are illustrated. The emphasis is on developments and techniques which are important and applicable to work in a wide range of fields. The book is divided into five sections.

The first section describes the production of monoclonal antibodies and their subsequent improvement or modification by genetic techniques. The large body of theoretical understanding and practical experience in rodent hybridoma production which has accumulated since 1975 is summarized in the chapter by Eshhar. Custom-tailored screening strategies are described which take advantage of the diversity of the immune response to select antibodies with desirable specificity, affinity, subclass, or other characteristics. The production of human monoclonal antibodies has been a highly important challenge, but one that has met with less technical success than for rodent monoclonals. The chapter by Cole *et al.* summarizes approaches such as Epstein–Barr virus tranformation and hybridization with improved cell lines that should soon lead to substantial progress in human monoclonal antibody production.

Although it is difficult to improve on nature's design, antibodies will be genetically modified in their variable and constant regions in the next decade in the hope of doing just that. A prerequisite to these attempts is an accurate understanding of how the three-dimensional structure of the antibody combining site determines its specificity and affinity for antigen. This is described in the chapter by Haber. It sometimes is not feasible to obtain a monoclonal antibody with all the desired characteristics of affinity, constant region isotype, etc. One solution to this problem is to select genetically variant hybridomas. Heavy chain subclass (isotype) switching and mutations in antibody constant and variable regions occur spontaneously in hybridoma cells at low frequencies. The chapters by Spira *et al.* and Kipps describe efficient methods for the selection of such variants. Another method of altering monoclonal antibodies is by genetic engineering. Griffiths and Milstein describe a rapid method for nucleic acid sequencing of hybridoma heavy and light chains variable regions which does not require DNA cloning. This has facilitated an understanding of antibody structural diversity, and how changes in antibody structure correlate with the increase in antibody affinity seen during maturation of an immune response. Sequence information is also important for many potential genetic engineering applications, e.g., for guiding the synthesis of artificial variable regions containing mouse hypervariable regions inserted between human framework regions, to produce human-like antibodies with mouse-like antigen specificity. In the final chapter in this section, Alt describes how DNA rearrangements and somatic mutation contribute to the generation of antibody diversity, and then describes recent progress in molecular cloning and gene transfer which has elucidated the elements controlling Ig gene rearrangement and expression. The introduction of cloned, immunoglobulin-expressing genes into cell lines and into the germ line of animals is discussed. This technology now offers the prospect of structurally manipulating and expressing Ig genes to produce Ig molecules modified in any manner desired.

The second section of the book is devoted to the immunochemistry of monoclonal antibodies, and their use in basic biomedical research. The studies on the HLA supergene family described in the chapter by Parham illustrate many of the principles of monoclonal antibody immunochemistry. Topics include the fragmentation of the different mouse Ig subclasses with papain and pepsin, the effects of monoclonal antibody valency on affinity for antigen on the cell surface or in solution, the marked differences between antibodies in association and dissociation rates, the basis for enhancement or competition between different monoclonal antibodies binding to the same antigen, the induction of changes in antigen conformation by antibody binding, and the complex serological relationships among HLA antigens. Monoclonal antibodies have transformed protein purification, particularly the purification of low abundance and membrane proteins, from a task that was at best arduous and at worst unfeasible, to one that is routine. In the chapter by Johnson *et al.*, the key factors in the use of monoclonal antibodies in affinity chromatography are described. Additionally, the use of antibodies reactive with highly stable antigenic determinants in the purification of a reduced and alkylated subunit and of a tryptic fragment from two different membrane proteins is described.

The study of cell surface receptor structure, function, and gene structure has been greatly advanced by monoclonal antibody probes. The chapter by Trowbridge describes studies on the transferrin receptor, including the receptor's transmembrane organization, its biosynthesis and posttranslational modification, endocytic uptake of iron and its inhibition by monoclonal antibodies which also inhibit cell growth, and gene transfer. The chapter by Springer and Anderson describes a family of leukocyte surface proteins identified by monoclonal antibodies which inhibit cell adhesion. These surface proteins are deficient in the first genetic disease to be defined by use of monoclonal antibodies. The adhesion defects of genetically deficient cells are similar to those of monoclonal antibody-treated normal cells, validating the use of monoclonal antibodies as probes of cell surface functions. The immunochemical dissection of multi-subunit protein family relationships by crossreacting and noncrossreacting monoclonal antibodies is also described. The chapter by Weis and Fearon describes the use of anti-receptor monoclonal antibodies, which do not interfere with ligand binding, to purify and immobilize receptors for studies of receptor function. The method is demonstrated with surface receptors for complement components and the Epstein–Barr virus. The chapter by Hochschwender reviews studies on the acetylcholine receptor subunit structure and its function, the induction of experimental autoimmune myasthenia gravis by monoclonal antibodies, and some technical aspects of rat monoclonal antibody production.

Three chapters concern the use of monoclonals in cell biology to study molecular architecture, morphogenesis, and their relation to function. Myles and Primakoff describe the localization of antigens into discrete cell surface domains, using the anterior and posterior domains of the sperm head and tail as a model system. Chen *et al.* summarize work on the molecular components of the cytoskeleton, and describe morphological studies on localization in fixed cells, and functional studies on cells microinjected with monoclonal antibodies. In his chapter on molecular probes of the nervous system, Barnstable discusses the use of monoclonal antibodies to define different subclasses of neural cells and their organization within the retina. Many insights into the nervous system are forthcoming, including the identification of molecular gradients which may be important in pattern formation.

Three chapters describe the use of antibodies in the study of protein structure and function. The chapter by Curtiss describes the plasma proteins which mediate lipid traffic *in vivo*, their immunoassay, and how monoclonal antibodies might be used therapeutically to trigger cholesterol degradation. Smith-Gill reviews the use of monoclonal antibodies in studies of enzyme active sites and catalysis, and regulatory and subunit interactions. Skehel and Wiley present three-dimensional mug shots of a molecular disguise and escape artist, the influenza virus hemagglutinin. The epitopes on this three-dimensional structure to which monoclonal antibodies bind have been mapped with great accuracy by *in vivo* selection of variants which escape from antibody neutralization, and by studies of the naturally selected antigenic variants responsible for successive pandemics. Finally, Co *et al.* describe the use of the idea that the antibody combining site specific for a ligand has an "internal image" of the receptor for that ligand, to produce anti-idiotype monoclonal antibodies which are reactive with cellular receptors for virus.

The third section of the book concerns the use of antibodies in recombinant DNA technology. Dr. Schaffhausen summarizes the extensive experience to date on the production of antibodies to synthetic peptides, and distills out the key factors in detemining peptide immunogenicity, and the most successful coupling and immunization techniques. Antibodies to synthetic peptides are powerful reagents which have the advantage of being specific for a defined portion of a protein. Their many applications, ranging from site-specific reagents to the identification of gene products predicted from nucleotide sequences, are discussed.

Other chapters in this section deal with the use of polyclonal and monoclonal antibodies in the isolation of DNA clones. In some of these applications the specificity of monoclonal antibodies for only a single determinant on a molecule can be disadvantageous; in this case, monoclonal antibodies can serve as adjuncts for the affinity purification of antigen for polyclonal antiserum production. Chapters by Ruddle and Kavathas review the use of antibodies and fluorescence-activated cell sorting to isolate cells surface-expressing the products of transfected genes. Several strategies for isolating the transferred genes, a method for amplifying transfected genes, and successes in recombinant DNA cloning of the transferrin receptor and the Lyt-2 molecule are described. The idea of probing for genes cloned in bacteria by immunodetection of their expressed products has come to fruition with the development of the λgt11 expression vector, described in the chapter by Snyder and Davis. Both cDNA and yeast genomic DNA clones have been successfully expressed and detected.

Before polypeptide chains are fully elongated and released by ribosomes, they begin to assume conformations which are reactive with antibody. This allows isolation of specific polysome mRNAs. Techniques which have recently been improved for isolation of low abundance mRNAs are detailed by Kraus for polyclonal antibodies and by Brown *et al.* for monoclonal antibodies. Translation of exogenous mRNAs in *Xenopus* oocytes has long been an important assay in molecular biology. However, it was only recently found that signals for secretion or translocation of proteins to the cell surface are followed with high fidelity in *Xenopus* oocytes. Thus, mRNAs of foreign membrane proteins may be assayed by the appearance of their products on the oocyte surface, as related in the chapter by Unkeless *et al.*

The fourth section of the book describes the important uses of monoclonal antibodies in the diagnosis and treatment of disease. The chapter by Haber reviews the uses of antibodies *in vivo* for modulating hormone or receptor activities, reversing drug overdoses, imaging myocardial infarcts, and detecting thrombi. Three chapters deal with different aspects of transplantation and treatment of leukemia. Hale and Waldmann discuss the merits of antibodies which fix human complement, particularly a rat IgM which recognizes lymphocytes and many myeloid cells but spares hematopoietic precursor cells. Basic research on methods for enhancing complement-mediated lysis, by anti-antibodies, synergy, or preparation of monovalent antibodies, is also reviewed. Ritz *et al.* describe work with an anti-common acute lymphoblastic leukemia antibody. Ritz *et al.* and Hale and Waldmann discuss results to date of their *in vitro* and *in vivo* treatments for leukemia and to prevent graft-versus-host responses. Carpenter reviews the cellular basis of allograft rejection, and the use of anti-T cell antibodies to suppress kidney graft rejection.

The fifth section of the book deals with T lymphocytes. The cloning of T cells and T cell hybridomas has had an impact on immunology similar to that of B lymphocyte hybridomas. The antigen receptors of T lymphocytes, their helper, suppressor, and cytolytic functions, and secreted lymphokines and hematopoietic factors have become amenable to study. As a result of combining the monoclonal antibody and T cell cloning/hybridoma technologies, the long elusive antigen receptor of T lymphocytes has been biochemically and functionally characterized. This development is reviewed in the Kaye chapter, which serves as the introduction to this section. The ability of anti-receptor monoclonal antibodies to act as agonists or antagonists, depending on valency, is also described. The chapter by Rock provides a thorough review of T cell hybridomas, including parental cell lines, immunization, fusion, and screening methods, and applications for analysis of T cell function, products, and molecular biology. Nabholz describes the mechanisms which control the proliferation and activity of cytolytic T-lymphocytes, and their study with T cell hybridomas. One type of CTL hybridoma has the interesting property of growing independently of interleukin 2, but requires both interleukins 1 and 2 for induction of cytolytic activity. The chapter by Krensky *et al.* reviews the cloning of cytolytic T lymphocytes, and the functionally important molecules on the surface of these cells which have been defined by monoclonal antibodies. Nabel describes procedures for cloning different T lymphocytes subsets, the patterns of gene activation in these cells, and the derivation of a cloned gene for interleukin 3 from a cloned line. Finally, the interactions between T lymphocytes and macrophages, and the importance of interleukin 1 and gamma interferon in this regulatory circuit are reviewed by Beller.

Contents

Part V. T-CELL CLONES AND THEIR PRODUCTS

Part I

The Production and Improvement through Genetic Engineering of Monoclonal Antibodies

Chapter 1

Monoclonal Antibody Strategy and Techniques

ZELIG ESHHAR

1. Introduction

The novel approach of immortalizing specific antibody-forming cells by their fusion with myeloma cells was first introduced by Köhler and Milstein[1] in 1975. Since then it has been widely adopted as the method of choice for the preparation of monoclonal antibodies (MAbs) to a large spectrum of antigens, and today MAbs find application in almost all facets of the life sciences. The thousands of research articles published every year that report the use of MAb as the key reagent and the tens of biotechnology companies that are involved in MAb production exemplify only part of the revolutionary impact of monoclonal antibodies.

The "one-cell, one-antibody" axiom,[2] a direct outgrowth of Burnet's clonal selection theory,[3] provides the conceptual basis for the practical advantage offered by the MAb technique. Each clone of lymphocytes produces a single antibody specificity. Nevertheless, the immune response to most antigens is polyclonal; it involves hundreds of clones of lymphocytes, each secreting a different antibody. These antibodies are markedly heterogeneous. They usually consist of antibodies directed at different antigenic determinants, and even those that recognize the same defined determinant (or epitope) can utilize different combining sites and different constant regions. Hybridization of antibody-forming cells with malignant myeloma cells results in hybridomas in which the virtues of specific antibody secretion and continuous growth are combined. Further selection and cloning of the hybrid cells allows the derivation of monoclonal antibodies of predefined specificity and desired activity.

The main advantages of monoclonal antibodies produced by hybridomas over the polyclonal antibodies obtained by "conventional" immunization are reflected in the defined specificity, homogeneity, ability to obtain practically unlimited quantities of the same antibody in a reproducible manner, and the ability to immortalize the production of such monospecific reagents by freezing

ZELIG ESHHAR • Department of Chemical Immunology, Weizmann Institute of Science, Rehovot, Israel.

the hybridomas for unlimited periods. Probably the most exciting advantage provided by the B-cell hybridoma approach is that it enables the generation and selection of MAbs to almost any antigenic determinants, even minor impurities in a complex mixture, provided that specific assays can be designed that will allow the detection and selection of the desired antibody-forming hybrid clone. A controlled screening assay can also serve for the selection of a desired antibody displaying a certain immunoglobulin class or properties such as high avidity, binding of complement, protein A, or binding to Fc receptors.

When compared with "conventional" serology, however, there are some unusual properties resulting from the homogeneity and fine specificity of MAbs that must be recognized and considered. Monoclonal antibodies usually do not give precipitin reactions with antigens that do not contain repeating determinants. They are poor agglutinators and fail to direct complement-mediated lysis of cells expressing low density of the relevant antigen. The effect of some chemical modifications of the antibody molecule can be more dramatic on certain MAbs, and alterations of the environment or the antigenic determinant itself (due to modification, genetic polymorphism, or assay conditions) can give false negative and inconsistent results. In addition, cross-reactivity can be indicated by individual MAbs when similar antigenic determinants[4,5] such as short sequences, carbohydrate moieties, or some structural features can be recognized on different molecules by MAbs. These limitations are not manifested usually in polyclonal sera, which are composed of thousands of different antibodies, among which the odd MAb is a minority. Taken together, these drawbacks should always prompt us to evaluate the method of choice for selection of MAb in the light of the desired properties of the end product.

The method of establishing permanent cell lines capable of producing antibodies directed to predefined immunogen is based on the fusion of immune lymphocytes (usually spleen cells from mice or rats previously immunized with antigen) with myeloma cells adapted for growth in tissue culture conditions. The most common fusion agent is polyethylene glycol (PEG),[6] which replaced the Sendai virus that was used in the first fusion experiments.[1] A schematic illustration of the protocol usually employed for fusion, selection, cloning, and growth of hybridomas is depicted in Fig. 1. The selection for growth of hybrid cells is based only on the facts that (1) spleen cells die in tissue culture medium, and (2) the myeloma lines that serve for fusion are mutants lacking either the enzyme hypoxanthine-guanine phosphoribosyltransferase (HGPRT) (azaguanine-resistant) or thymidine kinase (bromodeoxyuridine-resistant). Such mutants die in the presence of aminopterin, which blocks the main pathway of DNA synthesis, because they cannot use the salvage pathway.[7] Only the hybrid cells between the spleen cells and the myeloma will survive in the presence of aminopterin, but for their growth they require hypoxanthine and thymidine that are utilized by the salvage pathway. The hybrid cells growing in hypoxanthine, aminopterin, and thymidine (HAT)[7] are then screened for their ability to produce and secrete the desired antibody. The positive hybridomas obtained after cloning are the source for monoclonal antibodies. Such cells can be cryo-

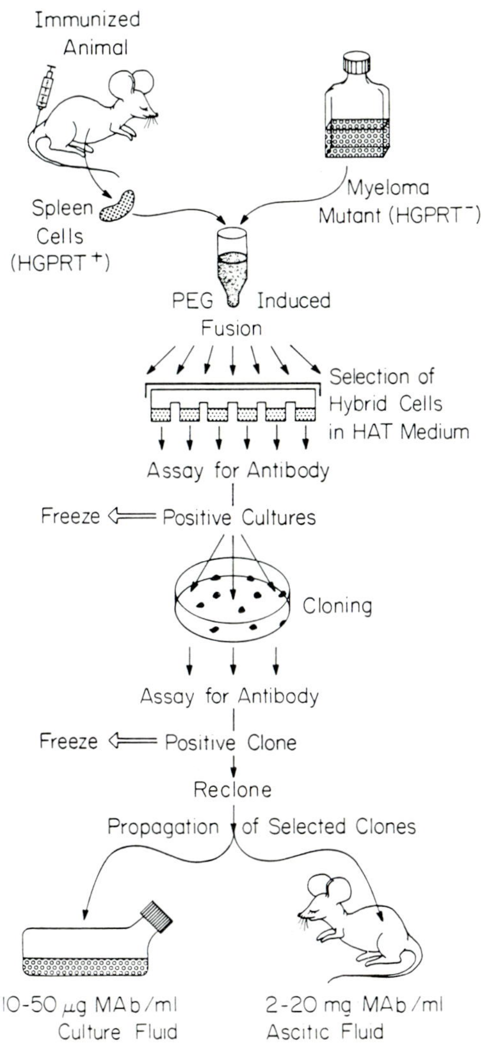

Figure 1. Protocol for generation of hybrid cells producing monoclonal antibodies.

preserved and for the production of large amounts of MAb they can be grown in mass cultures, where they secrete 10–50 μg antibody/ml, or propagated as ascites tumor, where they usually produce 1–10 mg/ml of MAb into the ascitic fluid.

The methodology involved in the derivation of monoclonal antibodies appears simple and does not require sophisticated procedures or expensive equipment. However, there are some crucial steps, especially in the screening and selection of positive hybridomas, that require preplanned, sensitive, simple, and fast assays. In addition, severe precautions and devotion have to be practiced with regard to the tissue culture conditions, especially during the first phase of the hybridoma's establishment. Although there is a large selection of literature describing the hybridoma technology and the procedures for preparation and characterization of MAbs, I have endeavored in this chapter to provide the reader, especially one who has not experienced the hybridoma–MAb technology before, with some useful background information and "state of the art" practical guidelines that will assist in embarking upon this laborious but rewarding adventure. Although hybridomas were originally introduced by immunochemists[8,9] for resolving basic questions in molecular immunology, the use of MAbs is becoming of great value in almost all biological disciplines. Therefore, in the next sections I will share my experience in the preparation of many MAbs to a diverse spectrum of antigens (ranging from synthetic antigens[10,11] and biologically active molecules[12–14] to complex cell surface antigens and receptors[15–17]), in order to acquaint the reader with the variables to be considered in connection with individual needs. Because of space limitations, I include only selected techniques that have proven helpful in our hands. Similar procedures and others either related to MAbs[18–26] or to antibodies in general[27–30] are readily available.

2. Factors That Control Immunogenicity

Immunogenicity is operationally dependent on the interplay between the chemistry of the antigen and the physiological state of the host.[31] Understanding the mechanism that determines the fate of a certain antigen after its introduction into a host and how it triggers a specific immune response will give us means to control and direct such responses. However, in spite of the immense progress made in recent years on the molecular and genetic mechanisms responsible for antibody diversity and on the pathways of B-cell differentiation and maturation, most of the factors that control the immunogenicity of a given molecule are still poorly understood.

2.1. The Effect of Antigen on B-Cell Differentiation and Proliferation

The specificity and affinity of the antibody molecule resides in the antibody combining site, which is encoded by the Ig variable-region set of genes, and determined in early stages of the B-cell differentiation by rearrangement events that assemble together first the functional heavy chain gene and later the functional light chain gene. Because these rearrangements join together genetic segments (V, D, and J) in a random way, much antibody diversity is generated during the differentiation of B cells.[32,33] The effector functions of the antibody are carried out by the constant region set of the heavy chain genes and are determined in a late stage of B-cell maturation by a process known as class switching.[34] The antigenic stimulus influences both parts of the antibody molecule, thus affecting both the specificity and class of the antibody. Most likely the first effect of the antigen is on competent B cells that express surface

IgM and IgD ($B\mu+\delta$ cell).[35] Each $B\mu+\delta$ cell displays only a single type of antigen-binding site. This binding site is present on both types of membrane-bound antibodies that serve as receptors for antigen. Upon antigenic stimulation, the B cells that bind the antigen start to proliferate and differentiate in several directions. These processes are triggered by antigen and mediated with the help of T cells. One line of differentiation leads to plasma cells that secrete IgM, whereas a second line of differentiation leads to B cells that can produce and secrete other classes of antibody (isotypes) with the same combining site (idiotype). In molecular terms, class switching results from a second kind of DNA rearrangement that joins the V gene in front of different constant genes.[36,37] However, the cellular events that are involved in class switching are not yet well defined, and it is not yet known whether this process is internally programmed or externally induced.

Some of the B cells (before and after class switching) do not differentiate into the terminal stage of antibody-secreting plasma cells. Such cells cease to divide and become memory cells. Upon secondary triggering with antigen, memory cells give rise to a larger secondary response. Usually in the secondary response there are fewer antibodies of the IgM class and the appearance of the other isotypes is more rapid.

Finally, persistence of antigen over long periods (hyperimmunization) can select for somatic mutants that occur from point mutations[38] in the variable region genes. If the mutation affects properties such as higher affinity, these variants can be selected by low concentrations of antigen and become a substantial part of the population.

2.2. Parameters That Support Strong Immunogenicity

A single antigen can elicit hundreds and thousands of different antibodies, and the immune response is usually very heterogeneous with respect to antibody specificity. This heterogeneity is due to the multiplicity of antigenic determinants and to the fact that each determinant can activate several B-cell clones with similar, but not identical, specificity.

In addition, quantitative differences with respect to the strength of the immune response also exist. We do not yet fully understand the mechanism that controls the intensity of response to a certain protein, or even to a certain antigenic determinant on the same molecule. Nevertheless, we know that genetic factors, the primary chemical composition, and the configuration and physical status of a molecule, as well as nonspecific substances (such as adjuvants) play important roles in influencing the immunogenicity of a given antigen. As a general rule, the following factors contribute to strong immunogenicity:

1. Greater phylogenetic distance between immunogen and recipient favors stronger response.

2. The larger the molecule, the better is the immunogen. Short peptides and small molecules are not immunogenic and have to be conjugated to macromolecules that act as carriers.
3. Repeating antigenic determinants within a molecule or aggregates of a molecule are more immunogenic.
4. Particulate antigens are stronger immunogens than water-soluble ones.
5. Exposed hydrophilic regions on the surface of protein, as well as exposed proteins on a cell, stimulate more antibodies.
6. Adjuvants improve and increase immunogenicity in a nonspecific manner.
7. Molecules that cannot be processed by mammalian enzymes (some polymers of D-amino acids or bacterial cell components) are often poor immunogens.

2.3. Regulation of Antibody Class

The physical form and the amount of the antigen, the choice of adjuvant, and the regimen of immunization influence the properties of the antibodies. For example, IgM antibodies are the first and major antibody class produced after primary immunization with most antigens. In certain cases, e.g. after immunization with weak immunogens or low amounts of antigens that contain repeating identical determinants (usually bacterial cell wall components and polysaccharides), IgM predominates after secondary immunization as well. Serum IgM antibodies are pentamers composed of five monomeric IgM units (each consisting of two heavy and two light chains) of 180 kD that are held together by a disulfide bond to a polypeptide called the J chain (15 kD). Because they are multivalent, IgM antibodies are better cross-linkers and agglutinators, and since they bind complement, they are very effective in complement-mediated cytolysis.

The major antibodies obtained after repeated immunization are the IgG antibodies of 150 kD, which are composed of four isotypes: IgG_1, IgG_2, IgG_3, IgG_4 in humans; IgG_1, IgG_{2a}, IgG_{2b}, and IgG_3 in mice; and IgG_1, IgG_{2a}, IgG_{2b}, and IgG_{2c} in rats. These antibodies are the major immunoglobulins in the serum, and generally have higher average affinity than IgM. The IgG isotypes differ with respect to their concentration in the serum, and their ability to bind complement, *Staphylococcus aureus* protein A, and Fc_γ receptors present on many cell types.

IgE antibodies of 190 kD, the rarest class of antibodies, appear in the serum in minute amounts (0.3 μg/ml), and are responsible for the allergic reactions mediated by binding to specific Fc_ϵ receptors on mast cells. There is good evidence that immunization with microgram amounts of antigen in the presence of aluminum hydroxide gel as adjuvant preferentially stimulates IgE responses,[39] while immunization with complete Freund's adjuvant suppresses IgE production in some cases.[40]

Finally, the IgA class of immunoglobulin is the major class of secretory antibody in the external secretions, such as saliva, colostrum, and gastrointestinal tract mucosa. The preferential production of IgA can be induced by oral administration of bacterial cell wall antigens.[41] The B cells found in the Peyer's patches of the intestines make primarily IgA antibodies in response to ingested antigens. In the serum, IgA is found in both monomeric and polymeric form and in secretory fluids mainly in dimeric form. The latter form contains a J piece, which attaches to the Fc portion of IgA,[42] and a secretory[43] piece, which is involved in the transport of IgA into the secretory fluids[44] and stabilizes it from proteolytic digestion in the gut.[45] IgA does not bind complement, but in its polymeric form is effective in neutralizing viruses and bacteria.

3. Strategy and Tactics for the Preparation of Monoclonal Antibodies

What are the factors to be considered before undertaking the fusion experiment? It is important that at the earliest stage the investigator, having defined the purpose of the studies and the target to be probed with MAb, should define the specificity and the desired properties of the antibody. Accordingly, one can decide about the optimal preparation of antigen to be used, what animal species to select, the best immunization protocol, which myeloma cells to use for fusion, and which screening procedures to adopt for fast and reliable selection of the desired MAb.

In this section, I have listed some rules and key elements that I believe contribute significantly to successful results. Of course, there are usually more alternatives than one, and several practical approaches that can be selected according to the individual's needs.

3.1. Purity and Form of Immunogen

1. The purity of the antigen to be used as immunogen is not crucial for generation of MAbs (in contrast with conventional antibodies).
2. Molecules of low molecular weight (<1000) are poor immunogens and have to be coupled to larger immunogenic molecules (carriers).
3. Aggregated and particulate antigens elicit stronger responses.
4. Antigen in its denatured form (including peptides) will not necessarily evoke antibodies that will react with its native form.

3.2. Immunization

1. Mice are usually preferred to rats. The latter are the species of choice to exhibit antibodies against mouse antigens and for the production of large amounts of ascites.
2. Adjuvant always helps to achieve stronger responses.

3. The mode of immunization and selection of adjuvant affect the relative proportion of different isotypes.
4. Amounts of protein antigen within the range of 1–100 μg and of 2×10^6–5×10^7 cells are sufficient to elicit good responses in mice.
5. Small amounts of antigen will stimulate the production of antibodies of higher affinity.
6. One should always boost with antigen in aqueous solution 2–4 days before fusion via intravenous (iv) or intraperitoneal (ip) routes.

3.3. Necessary Conditions for Proceeding to Fusion

Set for fusion only if:
1. You can detect antibody activity in serum from a test bleed diluted more than 1:50.
2. You have grown the myeloma cells in optimal conditions for at least 1 week.
3. You have checked the medium components for sterility and maximal support of growth.
4. You set up sensitive and fast screening assays.
5. You are ready to commit yourself to 3–4 weeks of continuous work.

3.4. The Fusion Process

Fusion protocols are simple and easy to follow and usually successful, if one sticks to one of them.
1. There is a direct relation between the ability of increasing PEG concentrations (>30% w/v) to induce cell fusion and toxicity.
2. The higher the concentration of PEG used, the shorter should be its incubation time with the cells.
3. The PEG should be carefully and slowly diluted out after the fusion.

3.5. Hybrid Cell Growth and Selection

1. Feedings and filler cells are optional.
2. Try to avoid growth of many clones per well by using low seeding density.
3. Do not allow dense growth! Dilute and transfer the hybridomas to fresh wells when required.
4. Aminopterin can be omitted 7–10 days after fusion. Phase out HAT with several changes of HT medium over a period of at least 10 days.
5. Freeze positive hybridomas as soon as possible.
6. Clone positive hybridomas as soon as possible.
7. Always repeat subcloning of positive clones.

4. Procedures for the Production of Monoclonal Antibodies

Many steps are involved in the production of MAbs, and there are certainly more ways than one to carry them out. In the following sections, I will indicate important variables in each step, and will describe in more detail the protocols of procedures that are being used in my laboratory. A broader selection of methods for monoclonal antibody production and their comprehensive analysis can be found in the recent book by Goding.[26]

4.1. Immunization

The degree of immunization of the animal that serves as spleen cell donor for fusion is of prime significance in determining the fate of the experiment. As a rule, production of detectable antibodies in the animal is a prerequisite for successful fusion. The main factors to be considered in designing the priming of spleen cells for fusion are the choice of immunogen, the choice of animal, and the regimen of immunization.

4.1.1. Choice of Immunogen

As stated in the previous section, the purity of the immunogen is not important (in any case, we "contaminate" it with adjuvant), providing that an assay system is available to detect the specific antibodies. This reflects one of the major advantages offered by the MAb approach. Although it is reasonable to assume that the frequency of the relevant hybridomas will increase in direct proportion to the increase of the relevant amount of antigen in the mixture used for immunization, laborious and excessive purification steps that usually result in loss of material and even denaturation can be avoided. As a rule, the antigen used for immunization should present the target antigenic determinants in a configuration as close as possible to that with which the desired MAbs are expected to interact. Many antibodies prepared by immunization with denatured proteins or peptides fail to react with the native proteins, and vice versa. For example, MAbs that were prepared against intact IgE and inhibit its binding to mast cell receptors[46] fail to bind to the isolated ϵ heavy chains. On the other hand, MAbs raised against the isolated variable region of heavy chain (V_H)[47] reacted with a hidden determinant that was not exposed on the native Ig. Similarly, MAbs that eventually will serve for staining of cell surfaces or react with functional receptors are better elicited by the injection of intact cells. On the other hand, antibodies that will be used to study fixed cells, such as antibodies to cytoskeletal elements, to the transmembrane, or cytoplasmatic regions of receptors, are best generated by the injection of purified molecules. A very useful practice is to raise the first set of monoclonal antibodies to a rare antigen by immunizing with crude or enriched preparations. These antibodies can be used to affinity purify the antigen, which can then serve to raise a second set of MAbs directed at different antigenic determinants.[12–14,48] Monoclonal an-

Table I. Cell Lines Available for Fusion

Cell line	Ig Class	Derived from	Ref.
Mouse			
X63-Ag8	IgG1, κ	MOPC-21	1
NS1-Ag4/1	κ, intracellular	X63	64
X63-Ag8.653	None	X63-Ag8	65
Sp2/0-Ag14	None	X63-Ag8 × BALB/c	66
NSO/1	None	NS1-Ag4/1	24
FO	None	Clone of SP2/0	20
S194/5XXO B4.1	None	S-194	67
MPC11-45.GTG 1.7	IgG2b, κ	MPC-11	68
FOX-NY	None	NS1	69
Rat			
Y3-Ag1·2·3	κ	LOU/C	70
YB2/0	None	(LOU × AO) F_1	71
IR983F	None	LOU/C	72

tibodies that are to be used with polypeptide chains still bound to polysomes or those produced in *in vitro* translation systems, or to detect mammalian gene expression products in bacteria, will serve their purpose if they recognize antigenic determinants that are not dependent on native structure and on processing events such as glycosylation. The best immunogens for such antibodies are the proteins purified from the aforementioned systems, or denatured proteins separated by polyacrylamide gel electrophoresis.[49,50] Such proteins can elicit antibodies when injected with the gel or when eluted from it. Small molecules, such as short peptides, hormones, nucleosides, or drugs, can be coupled to larger immunogenic proteins. The most common "carriers" are albumins, keyhole limpet hemocyanin, fowl gamma globulin, or synthetic polypeptides. The coupling method depends on the reactive groups available on the molecule.[51,52] A helpful method to increase the immugenicity of nonimmunogenic peptides is by aggregation using various cross-linkers.[53]

4.1.2. Choice of Animal Species

The choice of animal species and strain as immune spleen donor for fusion is largely dependent on the myeloma cell available (Table I) and the origin of the immunogen. Here I discuss only the mouse and rat myeloma lines that are readily available. The human myeloma cells are described in chapter 2 of this book. Mice are the most common species used for immunization, primarily because there are more murine myeloma cell lines available. In addition, mice are easier to breed and handle, and in general they respond better than rats. The BALB/c strain of mice is preferred, since all the murine myelomas competent for fusion were derived from this strain. Because of variation in the ability of different strains of mice to respond to certain antigens, low response in BALB/c should prompt the use of other inbred strains, and then the hybridomas should be propagated in the respective F_1 hybrid.

Rats are recommended for the large production of ascites and when MAbs against murine-specific antigens are being sought. The LOU/C strain of rats, from which the rat myeloma cells were derived,[54] should be used. The LOU/M strain, which is easier to breed and which accepts the LOU/C myeloma, can be used as well. For reasons as yet unclear, the efficiency of successful rat × rat hybridomas is lower in most laboratories than mouse × mouse. Therefore, many groups have fused rat spleen cells with mouse myeloma cells. These rat × mouse hybridomas appear to be stable producers of MAbs in tissue culture. They can also propagate and form ascites in nude or irradiated mice (500 R).

4.1.3. Immunization Procedure

For most proteins, a dose of 1–50 μg per injection per mouse or rat is sufficient to evoke a strong antibody response if the injection is repeated two or three times. If we consider five mice per injected group, it appears that any amount between 15 and 750 μg of pure protein is sufficient for immunization. Weak antigens will need to be injected more times. For soluble antigens, the first injections (one or two) are given in the presence of adjuvant and the next ones in aqueous solutions. The injected dose of intact cells is from 2×10^6 to 5×10^7 per mouse or rat. When cells serve as immunogen, adjuvant is not usually required.

Since dividing plasma cell blasts are probably the cells whose fusion with the myeloma cells yields the antibody-forming hybridoma,[55] it is necessary to challenge the mice with ip or iv injection of antigen in aqueous solution and to remove the spleen that contains the stimulated B cells at their optimal stage 3–4 days later. Some researchers recommend two ip injections at days −4 and −3, followed by an iv boost at day −2 before fusion.[56]

As discussed in the previous sections, the choice of adjuvant and regimen of immunization is dependent on the property and class of the desired antibody. For IgE antibodies, for example, 1–2 μg of allergen in alum is recommended.[39,57] For IgM antibodies that are advantageous for complement-mediated lysis, agglutination, or precipitation of polymeric antigens, primary responses are preferable. In this case, a single injection of 10–50 μg of soluble antigen is given intravenously, and 3–4 days later the spleen cells are taken for fusion.[58]

Primary responses to particulate antigens (red cells or viruses)[59] and secondary responses to soluble antigens can also be elicited *in vitro*.[60–62] In this case, normal spleen cells or immune spleen cells are incubated with the antigen for 4–6 days, and then are used for fusion. Most groups use T-cell-conditioned medium to support and facilitate the stimulation of the antibody-forming cells. Although it has been claimed that *in vitro* immunization requires less antigen and is more efficient, it has not yet justified itself as replacement for the *in vivo* immunization, and might be tried as a method to boost B cells when weak response is observed in the immunized animals.[63] The *in vitro* stimulation of peripheral blood lymphocytes by antigen and/or mitogen is the only method of obtaining human lymphocytes for fusion, because of ethical considerations.

Another manipulation that has proven helpful for enriching antibody-forming cells before the fusion is the adoptive transfer procedure.[57] In this procedure, the spleen cells from immunized mice are transferred into lethally irradiated (750 R) recipient mice, together with the antigen. The donor spleen cells home into the recipient spleen, where they proliferate and repopulate it. The antigenic stimulation drives the antigen-specific spleen cells to faster proliferation, and the lymphoblast population derived 4–6 days after transfer contains a high proportion of the antigen-specific antibody-forming cells. We also use this procedure to repopulate new mice with antigen-specific immunocompetent cells from unique mice, in order to continue and preserve the immunity to scarce antigens.

4.1.3a. Preparation of Antigen in Freund's Adjuvant

Antigen: About 3 mg/ml for protein antigens in phosphate-buffered saline (PBS).

Adjuvant: Complete Freund's adjuvant (CFA), Difco Laboratories. (Shake well before use!)

Preparation of emulsion: Into a glass syringe with a Luer lock put one volume of antigen in aqueous solution. Into a second, similar syringe, put 1.0–1.5 volumes of complete Freund's adjuvant. Remove excess air and use a special connector to connect the two syringes. The connector can be made of two welded no. 18 gauge Luer lock stainless steel needles, or can be a plastic version available from Hamilton, Inc. Reno, Nevada. A three-way plastic stopcock is another viable alternative. A water-in-oil emulsion is made by first pushing the aqueous phase into the oil and then rapidly pushing the emulsion from one syringe to the other until a test drop laid on water fails to disperse. With this procedure, all the antigen is recovered in the emulsion. The emulsion can be kept in the syringe for weeks at 4°C.

Note: Be careful while handling Freund's adjuvant, since it can cause an adverse reaction if accidently injected into one's hand. Syringes are cleaned with acetone before the usual detergent wash.

4.1.3b. Immunization Protocol. For most common antigens, groups of 5–10 animals are sufficient. Two- to 3-month-old mice or rats are the best recipients. The immunization regimen routinely used in our laboratory is as follows: about 50 μl of the antigen–CFA emulsion (50 μg) is injected intradermally into each rat or mouse (25 μl into each of hind footpads) using 27 gauge hypodermic needles. Two to 3 weeks later the same amount of the emulsion is injected subcutaneously or intradermally at multiple sites at both sides and back of the mouse. Ten to 14 days later individual animals are bled and the titer of the relevant antibodies is determined. The same assay as will be used later for screening the hybridoma supernatants is recommended for use at this point, and it provides an opportunity to evaluate the feasibility of the assay system. Animals that show the highest antibody titers are selected, and at least 3–4 weeks after the last boost they are injected ip with 20–100 μg of soluble antigen on the first day, and injected iv with the same dose on the following day. Three days after the intravenous boost, spleens are removed from two or three animals and their cells are used for fusion.

Several points need be emphasized:

1. If, after the two injections with CFA, the titer of antibody in the test bleeding is low (<1:100), additional injections can be given with antigen emulsified in incomplete Freund's adjuvant (lacking the mycobacteria), or with the antigen in aqueous solution. It is not uncommon to boost many times for a long period when only minute amounts of antigen are available or when weak immunogen is used. Sometimes it is good practice to boost the primed mice intraperitoneally with alum-precipitated antigen with or without 2×10^9 killed *Bordatella pertussis* organisms.
2. The rest period of at least 3 weeks between immunization and the prefusion challenge is also required for optimal B-cell stimulation. In the search to increase chances of production of high-affinity antibodies, we have found that it helps to prolong this rest period and to challenge with lower doses (2–10 μg) of antigen.
3. For cellular antigens, 2×10^7 cells are injected intraperitoneally in 2- to 3-week intervals in the same schedule as described above for the soluble antigen.
   If a virulent tumor is being used, we prefer to irradiate it (3000 R), at least before the first immunization.

4.2. Parental Cell Lines Available for Fusion

4.2.1. Choice of Myeloma

Table I presents a list of the most common mouse and rat myeloma lines that are serving as parental cells for the generation of B-cell hybridomas.

In choosing the myeloma line, one should consider both the species and the myeloma's own immunoglobulin (Ig) composition according to the desired end product. Rats are advantageous for large production of ascitic fluid, but their ability to respond to some antigens is lower than that of mice. In addition, only the IgG_{2c} class of rat Ig binds protein A, while all the IgG subclasses of the mouse bind it. The hybridomas derived from immune lymphocytes and myeloma cells producing either both heavy and light chains or light chain alone usually will continue to produce all the Ig chains originated from both parental cells. These chains can be assembled in different combinations and the resulting hybrid antibody often loses one or both of its binding sites. Therefore, for most purposes the nonproducing myelomas are preferred, since all of the antibodies produced and secreted will be dictated only by the immune cell.

Other properties of myeloma lines are related to their performance, such as growth rate, dependence on feeder cells, cloning efficiency, and tendency to fuse. In our laboratory, the NS1, X63-Ag8.653, and NSO/1 yielded similar high frequencies of hybridomas. Since NS1 produces k light chain and the cloning efficiency of X63-Ag8.653 without feeders is low, we routinely use the NSO/1 myeloma cell line. Another widely used cell line is the Sp2/0-Ag14 (abbreviated as Sp2), which was originated from a hybridoma that lost its ability to produce Ig.[66] A fast-grower variant of Sp2, the FO cell line, was selected for high fusion and high cloning efficiency.[20] Recently, another cell line was derived from the NS1 myeloma, the FOX-NY line.[69] This variant is deficient not only in HGPRT, but also in the enzyme adenosine phosphoribosyltransferase (APRT), which is encoded by chromosome 8. This allows an alternative selection system using adenosine, aminopterin, and thymidine. The advantage of this cell is that it enables the survival of hybridomas that have lost their x chromosome (which codes for HGPRT) during the HAT selection. The introduction of the Robertsonian 8·12 chromosome translocation into hydridomas made with the FOX-NY line ensures the survival of Ig producers during the selection process.[69]

Most of the plasmacytoma cell lines are available from the American Type Culture Collection (ATCC), 12301 Parklawn Drive, Rockville, Maryland 20852, or the Institute for Medical Research, NIGMS Cell Repository, Capewood and David Streets, Camden, New Jersey 08103.

4.2.2. Growth of Myeloma Cell Lines

The myeloma cells are generally grown in Dulbecco's modified Eagle's medium (DMEM) with high glucose (4.5 g/liter), or in RPMI, both supplemented with glutamine (2 mM final concentration), antibiotics (usually 100 U/ml penicillin and 10 μg/ml streptomycin), and 10% fetal calf serum (FCS) or 15% horse serum (HS). For practical reasons it is advisable to standardize with one medium for all cultures grown in a given laboratory. Cells are maintained at 37°C in a humid atmosphere of 7–10% CO_2 (DMEM) or 5% CO_2 (RPMI). In stationary suspension most myeloma cultures reach a concentration of 5×10^5 to 2×10^6 cells/ml. Spinner cultures are recommended for growth of large amounts of cells in logarithmic phase. This is an essential requirement for the rat line Y3.Ag1.2.3, which tends to adhere to the walls of the culture flask. The optimum conditions of a culture to be used for fusion are high viability and logarithmic growth for at least 1 week before fusion (do not exceed 3–8 $\times$ 10^5 cells/ml). To avoid revertants it is recommended not to keep the same culture for a long time, and to start new growth from frozen samples. If substantial cell death is observed in a myeloma culture held for 1 day or more in stationary phase (as can happen over long weekends), replace the old culture with a freshly thawed one. A good practice is occasionally to grow the cells in the presence of 8-azaguanine (30 μg/ml) and to check whether they all die in HAT. A routine check for mycoplasma is also advisable.

4.3. Tissue Culture Conditions for Growth and Selection of Hybridomas

The establishment and growth of hybridomas requires special attention and a high degree of commitment because it involves the growth of very low cell densities that are very vulnerable, and also because long-term cultures must be continuously monitored and nursed. Helpful background on tissue culture conditions in general can be found in the book *Cell Cultures for Biochemists*.[73] Here I will comment on some important specifics for the growth of hybridomas, and describe our group's recipes.

4.3.1. Quality and Sterility Control

All preparations are done with tissue-culture-grade, deionized and distilled water. All glassware is thoroughly cleaned by soaking in tissue-culture-grade detergent and rinsing with distilled water. For reproducible results and avoidance of unexpected crises, use a standard supplier and check new ingredients for their reactivity and sterility. We ensure the quality of the culture media by preparing them from concentrated stock solutions and powder that can be kept for longer periods than the ready-to-use media. Media are always kept in the dark at 4°C and every stock bottle is checked for sterility by removing a sample medium and incubating it with Nutrient-Broth (Difco) for 48 hr at 37°C. To avoid contamination we routinely add penicillin, streptomycin, and fungizone to the medium. Gentamicin is reserved to control outbreaks of penicillin–streptomycin-resistant bacteria.

4.3.2. Choice of Serum

We use heat-inactivated (56°C; 30 min) horse serum (HS) (virus- and mycoplasma-free) as the only serum source in the growth media for myeloma lines and hybridomas. Horse serum is cheaper than FCS and can effectively support the growth of hybridomas if selected for it. However, horse serum might interfere with some assay systems used for screening antibody activitity in hybridoma supernatants. Especially in cases when ^{125}I-protein A is being used, horse serum can increase the background. FCS does not usually contain Ig that binds to protein A and it is more useful in procedures that employ protein A or DEAE chromatography for purification of MAbs from spent medium.

We usually employ 20% HS in the culture medium for the first 2 weeks following fusion; then we gradually switch to 15% HS, the usual concentration. Cells will also grow in a 10% or lower concentration of HS, but at slower rates. FCS can be used at 10–15% final concentration.

Serum-free media that support the growth of the main myeloma lines used for fusion and their hybridoma products have been recently described[74,75] and are commercially available (Hana Media, Inc., Berkeley, California). We do not see any advantage of using such media in the establishment phase or in the initial growth phase of hybridomas. These media should be considered when the desired MAbs are directed against a serum component and when growth of hybridomas in serum-free conditions are advantageous for the purification of MAbs.

4.3.3. Selection of Serum

Although there has been significant improvement in recent years with regard to the quality of the sera for tissue culture supplied by most manufacturers, we still feel that it is a useful practice to select for good batches of serum. We routinely do this by comparing the ability of different concentrations of a few serum batches to support the growth of hybridoma cells. Several hybrid cells (preferably from a recent fusion) are serially diluted in 10, 15, and 20% of the tested sera in a microculture plate. Following 48–96 hr of incubation, wells are inspected for live dividing cells. The ability of the sera to support the growth of crowded cultures as well as lack of toxicity and ability to enable the growth of low concentrations of cells (down to one cell/well) are evaluated in comparison to a good batch of known serum. Large batches of serum can be kept frozen at −20°C for a long time (1–2 years) until used.

In the absence of hybridoma cells, the testing of sera can be carried out on the parental myeloma cells. For inexperienced investigators, an excellent prescreened fetal calf serum is available from HyClone Laboratories, Logan, Utah.

4.3.4. Preparation of Media and Solutions for Fusion

1. *DMEM*: Complete DMEM medium *without* serum:
   a. 500 ml Dulbecco's modified Eagle's medium, high glucose, pyruvate-free
   b. 5 ml Sodium pyruvate, ×100 stock = 100 mM; stored at 4°C
   c. 10 ml *L*-glutamine, ×100 stock = 200 mM; stored frozen, thawed at 56°C
   d. 5 ml Penicillin–streptomycin solution ×100 stock = 10,000 U/ml; keep frozen
   e. 2 ml Fungizone (optional), stock solution 250 μg/ml; store at 4°C
2. *DMEM-HS*: DMEM supplemented with 15% heat-inactivated (56°C, 30 min) horse serum. The complete medium can be stored at 4°C in the dark for up to 6 weeks.
3. *HAT Medium*: DMEM-HS supplemented with 1 ml of each of the following components a–c per 100 ml medium:
   a. Hypoxanthine 10^{-4} M, stock ×100 = 136 mg/100 ml H_2O (note: dissolve hypoxanthanine at 60–70°C)
   b. Aminopterin 4×10^{-7} M, stock × 100 = 1.76 mg/100 ml H_2O (note: to dissolve aminopterin, add 25 ml H_2O, 0.5 ml of 5 N NaOH, then neutralize with 5 N HCl; adjust to final volume with H_2O; sterilize by filtration through 0.2 μ Millipore filter; store at −20°C protected from light)
   c. Thymidine 1.6×10^{-5} M, Stock × 100 = 38.7 mg/100 ml H_2O

4. *HT Medium*: DMEM-HS supplemented with hypoxanthine and thymidine without aminopterin.
5. *Polyethylene glycol (PEG)*: To make 41% (w/v), add 4.2 ml of DMEM to 3 g of PEG 1500 (molecular weight 1300–1600), and dissolve in a well-capped vial at 56–60°C. Sterilize by filtration through 0.45 μ filter while warm. Alternatively, sterilize 20 g of PEG in a 100-ml flask in autoclave for 15–20 min; cool to 50°C and add 28 ml of DMEM, swirl to mix, and store at room temperature.

Both HAT components and PEG can now be obtained from a few companies that select and prepare ready to use stock solutions. Otherwise, we found that the individual HAT components from Sigma and PEG (molecular weight 1500) from Serva, Merck, BDH, or Baker give satisfactory results.

4.4. Fusion of Mouse Cells with Polyethylene Glycol

The fusion protocol we use has been adopted, with minor modifications, from the protocol originally described by Galfrè *et al.*[6] Although the membrane fusion efficiency increases with increasing PEG concentration, time of exposure, and temperature, the viability of the cells drops sharply when PEG concentrations above 30 and 50% are employed for more than 10 and 2 min, respectively. Thus, all fusion protocols operate within this range. Other important factors are the slightly basic pH (7.8–8.2) of the fusion solution, and the need to dilute out PEG slowly at the termination of the fusion. Although it has been reported that the addition of 15% dimethylsulfoxide to 42% PEG improves the fusion,[76] we and others[80] do not find it a necessary condition.

4.4.1. Preparation of Cells for Fusion

4.4.1a. Spleen Cells. Boost hyperimmune mice at days 4 and 3 before fusion by ip and iv injection, respectively.

Proceed to the next step only after the preparation of all media, PEG, and at least three pairs of fine operation scissors, four fine-tip, curved forceps, Petri dishes, and microplates.

Exsanguinate mice just before fusion and keep the serum.

Remove spleens from at least two mice under sterile conditions:

1. Spray mice with 70% alcohol.
2. Cut the superficial skin at the left side of the abdomen and pull aside the skin to reveal the spleen under the abdominal wall.
3. Spray the abdominal wall with 70% alcohol, let it dry, and incise it with scissors, just above the spleen.
4. Pull out the spleen carefully with forceps, and release it from the mesentery using fine forceps.
5. Transfer the spleen into DMEM in a Petri dish. Clean extra connective tissue and transfer into a new Petri dish with 5–10 ml DMEM.

6. Tease spleen apart by gentle pressing with sterile curved forceps.
7. Resuspend cells with a Pasteur pipette and transfer cell suspension into 12-ml capped conical plastic tube. Leave in a vertical position on ice for 10 min, letting large pieces of tissue settle.
8. Remove single-cell suspension with a Pasteur pipette to a new 10-ml conical tube, spin cells at 1000 rpm (200 × g) for 5 min at room temperature (RT). Resuspend in 10 ml DMEM, remove aliquot for cell counting (dilute 1:10 in 0.1% trypan blue for counting), spin cells again, and resuspend to the same volume of DMEM.

4.4.1b. Myeloma Cells

1. NSO cells (in logarithmic phase of growth) are removed from a flask into a 50-ml conical tube. Take sample for counting (dilute 1:1 with trypan blue).
2. Spin at 1000 rpm for 10 min. Resuspend cells in DMEM to 10×10^6/ml.

4.4.2. Procedure of Cell Fusion (Adopted from Galfrè *et al.*[6])

1. Put about 3 ml PEG, 50 ml DMEM, and 50 ml DMEM-HAT in a 37°C bath next to the hood.
2. Mix spleen lymphocytes and myeloma cells at a ratio of 5:1 in a 50-ml tube (not more than 10^8 spleen cells). Add DMEM to 40 ml. Centrifuge and remove *all* supernatant by careful aspiration. Flick tube gently to loosen the cell pellet.
3. Add 2.0 ml of prewarmed (37°C) PEG dropwise with a wide-opening pipette. Resuspend the cell pellet gently for 1 min. Do not destroy small aggregates. Incubate for additional 1 min at 37°C.
4. Add prewarmed DMEM (without serum!) dropwise to dilute PEG. The addition has to be done slowly with gentle mixing of cells. Add 5 ml in the first 5 min, then 10 ml in the next 5 min, and an additional 15–20 ml of DMEM in the last 5 min.
5. Centrifuge and remove supernatant. Add 5 ml of prewarmed DMEM-HAT and resuspend cells *very carefully*. Avoid pipetting too much, since this will break the fused cells apart. Add 10 ml DMEM-HAT and count viable cells. Try to count the number of viable NSO cells, which appear larger than most of the spleen cells.
6. Suspend fused cells to a concentration of $(1–5) \times 10^5$ viable NSO cells/ml in DMEM-HAT and distribute 0.1-ml aliquots in the wells of 96-well flat-bottom microculture plates (two drops from 5-ml pipette/well).
7. Incubate at 37°C in 8% CO_2 in a humid incubator.
8. After 4–5 days, add 0.1 ml of DMEM-HAT (prewarmed) to each well.
9. Seven to 9 days following fusion, feed the cultures by aspirating about half of the culture fluid, and replace it with prewarmed, fresh DMEM-HAT medium.

10. Inspect cultures for hybrid cell growth. When vigorous growth and change of color to yellow are observed, usually 10–14 days following fusion, supernatants can be removed (by sterile means) for screening of antibody activity. Wells are refilled with HT medium.
11. Ten to 14 days after fusion, HAT medium is replaced by HT medium, and 10 days later, by regular DMEM-HS medium. We usually duplicate the positive cultures and wean only one of them out of HAT.
12. Positive wells are transferred into cups of 24-well plates, and then to small (25 cm^2) culture flasks. Grow positive cultures at least in duplicates.
13. Follow expansion of cultures by repeated determinations for activity. Introduce controls and assays for specificity if needed. Hybrid cells secreting the desired antibodies should be frozen in liquid N_2 as early as possible (the content of two 1-ml cups is sufficient).
14. Clone the positive hybrid cultures.

4.4.3. Procedure of Cell Fusion (Adopted from Gefter *et al.*[77])

A slightly different but widely used fusion procedure is the method reported by Gefter *et al.*,[77] which employs lower PEG concentrations (32–38%) for longer periods of time. A typical protocol involves the following steps:

1,2. As in the Galfrè procedure (Section 4.4.2).
3. Resuspend cell pellet in 1 ml of 38% PEG 1500 at room temperature.
4. Centrifuge for 6 min (exactly!) at 1100 rpm.
5. Carefully aspirate PEG from pellet, loosen it by tapping, add 5 ml DMEM (no protein), and resuspend cells very gently with Pasteur pipette.
6. Centrifuge 1000 rpm for 5 min.
7. Resuspend pellet in HAT medium, count, and continue as in steps 6–14, described above.

4.4.4. Maintenance of Hybridomas after the Fusion

1. After fusion, cells can be distributed in either 24- or 96-well plates. In order to avoid growth of more than one hybrid per well, it is recommended to dilute the inoculum to less than 5×10^4 cells/well.
2. Some protocols recommend the seeding of cells after fusion in medium and serum for 24 hr, and then adding the HAT medium. It might slightly improve the rate of hybrid cell growth and the fusion efficiency; however, we found it to be an unnecessary step.
3. Hybrid cells can be cloned right after fusion. It is recommended to leave the cells for 24 hr following fusion in a 50-ml tissue culture flask in regular DMEM-HS, and then to clone them on soft agar containing HAT, as will be described below.
4. With regard to *feeding*, at least one replacement of medium is recommended about 1 week after onset of fusion. This serves to remove an-

tibodies secreted by the immune lymphocytes and to replenish nutrients. Afterward, the frequency of feeding is determined according to cell growth. When extensive growth is observed in the microplates, it is necessary to dilute the cell number or to transfer them into 24-well cluster plates.

5. Addition of *feeder cells* usually improves the cloning efficiency of the hybrid cells.[20] Feeders are usually thymocytes,[19,78] peritoneal macrophages,[59] or normal cells.[24] About 10^4 cells are added per microplate well. It is recommended that the macrophages and fibroblasts be irradiated before their addition. We add normal spleen cells as feeders [(1–5) $\times$ 10^4/well] only when unsatisfactory growth is observed, such as in the weaning period from HAT and HT (see below).
6. Sometimes the hybridomas do not look "happy" after the replacement of HT with normal growth medium. Likely explanations for this condition can be either residual amounts of aminopterin, which is a very effective inhibitor, or slow recovery of the activity of the relevant enzymes. In both cases, prolonged growth in HT and gradual weaning off it might be helpful. Sometimes crisis in this phase reflects mycoplasma infection (which was otherwise suppressed by aminopterin), in which case the appropriate measures must be taken. See details about mycoplasma detection and suggestions for its elimination in Goding's book.[26]
7. Removal of supernatants for screening should be attempted when there is substantial growth (50% or more of the bottom of the well is crowded by hybridomas) in most of the wells in a plate. This allows about 48 hr before dilution or transfer of hybridoma must be done, a period that should be sufficient for most screening assays. Do not feed for at least 48 hr before the removal of supernatants for screening, in order to allow accumulation of MAbs. Remove supernatants under sterile conditions (a multichannel pipette with sterile tips is very helpful for this purpose). Do not keep the plates out of the incubator for long periods.

4.5. Cloning of Hybrid Cells

Cloning and recloning of hybrid cells is essential to ensure the monoclonality of the antibodies and to get rid of nonproducer cells. Nonproducer hybridomas may exist in the original culture as well as in the later phases of growth. When decline in the production of MAb is observed, it is usually due to accumulation of nonproducer variants (a result of chromosome loss). These nonproducers have some metabolic advantage over the producer hybridomas and can overgrow and dominate the culture.

Two main methods of cloning are widely used: cloning in soft agar and cloning by limiting dilution. In the first method, cells are spread in soft agar and colonies that develop from single cells are randomly picked and transferred into liquid culture, where they are screened for MAb activity. In the second method, cells are diluted to less than one cell/well in microculture plates and the positive wells are selected. The advantage of the soft agar cloning is that it ensures clonality. It is, however, somewhat more complex, and is a longer procedure. In addition, some myeloma cell lines (X63.653, for example) result in hybridomas whose cloning efficiency in agar is very low. Cloning in agar is very convenient when the antigen is either red cells or other cells that can be lysed in the presence of antibodies and complement (or soluble antigens that can easily be coupled to red cells). In this technique (used by Köhler and Milstein in their original experiment),[1] the hybridoma colonies in agar are overlaid with agar that contains red cells and complement. Areas of lysis will appear around colonies that secrete IgM anti-red cell antibodies. Such colonies can easily be picked and further propagated. By the inclusion in the top agar of rabbit antibodies directed to various mouse isotypes it becomes possible also to identify anti-red cell MAbs of other classes.

Another technique that is based on cloning of hybridoma cells in agar is the replica method.[70] This method enables the detection of specific clones directly on the agar plate. Cellulose nitrate filters or plastic sheets that have been coated with the specific antigen are placed on top of the agar layer covering hybridoma colonies that have been seeded on soft agar. Specific antibodies secreted by the hybrid clones, which diffuse through the agar and react with the antigen on the filter, are detected with the aid of enzyme-conjugated or radioiodinated second antibodies. The antibody-forming clones are then identified using ELISA or autoradiography, respectively.

As mentioned before, cloning in agar in the presence of HAT can be attempted right after fusion. According to our experience, the method is of advantage only if a screening assay that will allow the detection of the clones directly on the agar is available. Neither assay method, the hemolytic focus nor the replica, is as sensitive as other screening methods that detect MAbs in the culture supernatant.

Another cloning system is based on the presence of immunoglobulins with antibody activity on the surface of some hybridoma cells. Using fluoresceinated antigen or antigen bound to flouresceinated microbeads,[80] it is possible specifically to stain these cells, which then can be detected and separated by the fluorescence activated cell sorter (FACS). The need for highly fluoresceinated antigens and the fact that not all hybridomas contain surface antibodies are considerable limitations of this technique.

4.5.1. Soft Agar Cloning

Reagents:

1. 2% Agar (Difco) in double-distilled H_2O; sterilize by autoclaving
2. DMEM $\times 2$ without serum; made from $\times 10$ stock or powder
3. Horse serum or FCS, heat-inactivated
4. Complete DMEM without serum (see Section 4.3.4)

Procedure:

1. Melt the 2% agar by heating carefully (over boiling water or in a microwave oven) and leave it in a 46°C water bath. Warm up DMEM ×2, DMEM, and serum in 46°C water bath.
2. Mix (for six 9-cm Petri dishes)
   25 ml DMEM ×2
   30 ml DMEM
   20 ml serum
   25 ml 2% agar
   Be careful to keep the mixture at 46°C.
3. Put 15 ml of the mixture in each Petri dish on a clean, leveled surface. Let the agar solidify for 15 min at RT outside the hood. *Put back* leftover agar to 46°C.
4. Prepare cells at 10^3, 5×10^3, 10^4 cells/ml in DMEM + serum. Warm to 37°C.
5. Put 1.2 ml of agar-DMEM into prewarmed sterile tubes, add 0.8 ml of the cell suspension, mix well, and immediately—
6. Add the 2 ml of the cell–agar mixture to the bottom agar layer and spread it (swirl) to cover the whole area. Let it solidify for 15 min outside the hood. Avoid shaking.
7. Incubate for about 10 days in a well-humidified incubator (8% CO_2 in air, 37°C).
8. Pick colonies by capillary Pasteur pipettes, and transfer into 0.1-ml complete growth medium in microculture plates.
9. Screen for specific antibody activity.

Notes:

1. Feeder cells can improve the cloning efficiency. Add 2×10^5 peritoneal macrophages or primary fibroblasts to each Petri dish and let them adhere to the plastic 6–18 hr before cloning.
2. Hybrid cells can be cloned directly after fusion or 24 hr later. In each case, HAT components should be added to the agar-DMEM.

4.5.2. Cloning under Conditions of Limiting Dilution

Cloning under limiting dilution conditions is preferred when the fraction of specific antibody-secreting hybridoma is lower than one in 10^3, and when the hybrid cells demonstrate low cloning efficiency on soft agar due to density-dependent growth early after fusion. The dependence on a certain density is overcome by the addition of 10^5 spleen cells or 10^6 thymocytes (rat or mouse) per well.

One way of cloning under limiting dilutions is to dilute the hybrid cells to less than one cell/well and to add 10^6 thymocytes/well to a microculture plate. When the cloning efficiency is not known, it is recommended to make serial dilutions by the serial transfer of 50 μl of cell suspension into 150 μl of medium using a multichannel pipette. Then 50 μl of feeder cells is added.

Watch for cell growth and check antibodies in supernatants of wells that received high dilutions of cells. At least 24–36 wells/dilution per cell should be placed. According to a Poisson distribution,[81] it is assumed that where 63% (or less) of the wells show cell growth, they most likely contain a single clone per well. Usually within 2 weeks, the "one-clone" wells reach cell density that allows screening for MAb. To ensure monoclonality, the cloning procedure has to be repeated for a few cycles until all the subclones detected appear to secrete the specific antibody.

4.6. Cryopreservation of Cells

Hybridomas can be kept frozen in liquid nitrogen for many years. Because hybridomas are vulnerable in the first weeks after their establishment and can easily be lost, it is a safe practice to freeze a few vials of cells right after the identification of the desired hybridomas. After the isolation of an active clone, grow a large batch of cells and freeze aliquots in a few dozen vials. These will serve as a safety stock.

Freezing of cells. Freezing medium: DMEM + 25–50% serum + 10% dimethylsulfoxide (DMSO) sterilized by filtration. Keep cold at 4°C.

1. Harvest cells and remove supernatant.
2. Resuspend cells in freezing medium to approximately 10^7/ml. Aliquot 1 ml per sterile 2-ml tube with screw cap (38 × 12.5) (Nunc no. 1078). Close cap tightly.
3. Freeze cells slowly, either by using a special apparatus designed for controlled freezing that fits the Union Carbide liquid N_2 containers, or by wrapping the vials in gauze and placing them in a polystyrene foam box that is then left for 12 hr in a deep freeze (−80°C). Tubes can then be transferred into liquid nitrogen, where they can be kept for a long time.

Thawing of cells:

1. Thaw frozen cells quickly at 37°C in a water bath.
2. Clean the tube with 70% alcohol.
3. *Immediately* when thawed, transfer cells on top of 10-ml cold growth medium.
4. Centrifuge cells, resuspend pellet in fresh growth medium (10 ml), and culture in two flasks.

4.7. Large-Scale Production of Monoclonal Antibodies

For large-scale production, hybridomas can be grown either in tissue culture, where they secrete up to 100 μg MAb/ml (usually 10–50 μg/ml), or *in vivo*, as tumors in the peritoneal cavity, where they produce up to 40 mg MAb ml (usually 2–10 mg/ml). The main advantage of tissue culture growth is that the hybridoma antibody is the only murine antibody in the tissue culture medium, and the major protein if serum-free medium is being used. The advantage of *in vivo* large-scale production has been large quantity and cheaper operation. However, recent developments by the rapidly growing biotechnical industry have made the *in vitro* large-scale production of MAbs the method of choice for commercial end products.

4.7.1. Growth under Tissue Culture Conditions

Because of economic as well as purification considerations, it is of benefit to grow the hybridomas in low serum concentrations and, if possible, in serum-free conditions. It is possible to adapt hybridomas for growth in low serum concentrations by transferring the culture in a few steps from 20% serum to 3–5%. Growth for 2–3 days in each concentration is enough. Recently, a few serum-free preparations have been suggested to support the growth of various hybridomas.[74,75] Since different conditions are required for the growth of various hybridomas and myelomas, preliminary trials are required in each combination in order to establish the optimal conditions. A useful practice is to grow the hybridomas in their regular medium, harvest them, and then resuspend in serum-free medium in a cell concentration of $(1–2) \times 10^6$/ml for 24 hr or more.

For large-scale growth, spinner bottles or roller bottles are useful. For maximal yield of monoclonal antibodies, harvest the supernatant at least 1 day after cells have reached the stationary phase of growth.

All the aforementioned procedures will prove adequate for the research laboratory setting. For scaling up to massive hybridoma cultures some new technologies have been developed, but their details are beyond the scope of this chapter.

4.7.2. Growth of Hybridomas in Animals

For large-scale production of MAbs, hybridomas can be grown in animals either as solid tumors, where the MAbs are harvested from the serum, or as ascites (single-cell peritoneal tumor), where the MAbs are secreted into the ascitic fluid. The amount of serum is limited; thus it is usually preferred to propagate the hybrid cells as ascites.

4.7.2a. Choice of Animal. Histocompatible strains and species are always preferable recipients for the growth of hybridomas. All murine myelomas adequate for fusion were derived from BALB/c mice, and if the immune cell parent was also of BALB/c mice, the resulting hybridomas should be inoculated into BALB/c or (BALB/c × DBA/2) F_1 mice, which are stronger animals than BALB/c and of the same H-2 type. If parental cells were obtained from another strain, say C57BL/6, the (BALB/c × C57BL/6) F_1 should be used for raising ascites.

Similarly, with rat × rat hybridomas, LOU/c rats, the parental strain of Y3 myeloma, or the histocompatible LOU/M strain should be used.

In the case of interspecies hybridoma such as mouse × rat, one should use immunosuppressed hosts, either nu/nu or irradiated (600–800 R) mice. It helps in the last case to inject the cells into the peritoneal cavity of irradiated mice in a large volume (~5 ml) of growth medium.

4.7.2b. Preparation of Ascites. About 2 weeks or more before inoculating the hybrid cells, the recipient mice and rats are injected ip with 0.5 ml (mice), or 1 ml (rats) of pristane (2,6,10,14-tetramethylpentadecane; Aldrich Chemical Co.). About (5–10) × 10^6 hybrid cells in 1 ml DMEM are then injected intraperitoneally. After about 10–14 days, but sometimes longer, enough ascitic fluid accumulates (noticed by the swelling of the belly of mice). It is removed by tapping (insertion of a no. 16 hypodermic needle into the lower part of the abdomen). The milky-appearing suspension is collected in a tube and further processed. The tapping can be repeated several times at 3- to 5-day intervals. Usually the titer of antibodies in the first tapping is lower. For further growth, 0.5 ml of ascites taken just after collection (before clot is formed) is injected into each pristane-treated fresh mouse.

Cells and fibrin clots are sedimented by centrifugation and the clear ascitic fluid is then stored frozen at −20°C.

It is a good practice to monitor the quantity and quality of the MAbs produced by hybrid cells that were growing continuously for a prolonged period either in culture or by serial transfers in mice. The simplest way is to titrate the level of specific antibodies periodically and to compare late and early samples. If a drop in activity is noticed, it is advisable to start a new growth from frozen samples, or to reclone the declining hybridomas and select the potent subclones for further propagation.

5. Screening Assays for Monoclonal Antibody Activity

5.1. Introduction

The immunoassay used for the screening of antibody activity in the hybridoma culture supernatant is a key factor that determines success in obtaining the desired MAbs. The screening procedure, a crucial step of the process, takes the greatest amount of time. It is therefore mandatory to work out the optimal conditions for the screening assay already before fusion. Serum from immunized animals can serve as an adequate source of antibodies. Practicing the screening procedure on an early bleeding may also help to select the best spleen donor candidate. The concentration of antibodies in the hybrid culture supernatants at the early phase of fusion is usually in the range of a few μg/ml and less, therefore it is good practice to design an assay procedure that will be sensitive to detecting antibodies in immune serum diluted 1:100 and more. Because the initial screenings are usually performed with hundreds and even thousands of assay samples that contain low amounts of antibodies, the main factors to be considered are sensitivity, simplicity, ability to test many samples, speed, and reliability. Exact quantitation of the antibody level is not important at this stage, and controls for specificity using various antigens (related and unrelated) can be done in the next phase after selecting the positive wells. In practice, any procedure in which antibodies can be detected can be used, provided that it satisfies the factors mentioned above.

Culture supernatants have been assayed for antibody activity in a variety of tests, such as standard or solid phase radioimmunoassay (RIA) and enzyme-linked immunosorbent assay (ELISA), that will be described in detail in the following sections. Other methods that are less frequently used are immunoflourescence, immunoprecipitation, neutralization of biological activity mediated by the antigen, complement-mediated lysis of target cells or coated red cells, hemagglutination, and others. These are described in detail elsewhere.[24–30]

It helps to adjust the screening assay according to the class and properties required from the desired MAbs. For example, if antibodies that bind protein A or complement are desired, they should be screened with protein A binding[21,82] and cytotoxic assays,[83] respectively. By the use of class- and subclass-specific second-step antibodies, one can select for MAbs of a given class. To select for antihapten-specific IgE antibodies, we used passive cutaneous anaphylaxis as the screening assay system.[57] If one seeks MAbs directed at an active site of a biologically active molecule such as an enzyme, receptor, hormone, or other antibody, antibodies should be selected that inhibit the given activity[84] or block specific ligand binding.[85] Note that in some cases, antibodies to cell receptors prove to mimic the hormone activity.[16] Neutralization of viral infectivity[86] is a helpful assay technique to select for a protecting MAb that will be discussed in more detail in Chapter 19 of this book. By using an adequate screening procedure, it is possible to select for MAbs that not only will display the desired specificity, but will also satisfy the functional objective. For example, to select for high-affinity antibodies destined to serve in immunodiagnostic tests, a low concentration of antigen should be used in the screening assay.[87–89] Similarly, for MAbs intended to serve for affinity purification of antigens from complex mixtures, it is helpful to select for a MAb that binds the antigenic molecule and can dissociate from it under conditions that will retain the activity of both the antigen and antibody. We have designed and used such screening procedures for the derivation of MAbs to human interferons.[12–14]

Other factors that determine the design of the screening procedure are related to the purity, accessibility, and physical form of the antigen. For highly purified, soluble, high-molecular-weight antigens that are available in large amounts, any of the solid phase assays can be used (see below). If the antigen is of small molecular weight, such as hormones, they can be coupled to a carrier molecule (other than that used for immunization!) and serve in the solid phase assays. Alternatively, the standard radioimmunoassay[90] can be employed using precipitation of the radioactive antigen by the MAb. For highly purified antigens that can be radiolabeled but are available in limited quantities (micrograms), the reverse solid phase radioimmunoassay that we developed[91] (see below) can be used successfully for the screening of MAbs. Insoluble and complex antigens can also be immobilized by binding to a solid matrix (via polylysine, for example), or the antigen–antibody complex can be recovered by centrifugation or filtration.

When the antigen preparation available is impure, one cannot use direct binding assays alone for the selection of specific MAbs. Usually such antibodies are selected on the basis of discriminatory analysis using proper negative controls that express all the unrelated components except the desired antigen. This approach is common practice when screening for monoclonal antibodies toward cellular or tissue antigens.[92] Screening by the immunofluorescence technique[93,94] is very useful when the antigenic preparation is composed of heterogeneous cells. Cytohistochemical staining by the immunoperoxidase method[95–97] is usually employed when the screening procedure is carried out on fixed tissue sections.

Another approach to sort for MAbs to functional antigens in a complex mixture is to select antibodies that will neutralize,[84,98–100] modify,[101] or precipitate[12–14] the activity mediated by the antigenic molecule.

Finally, if the screening assay procedure is complicated and cannot process many samples in a short time, one can consider performing the screening in two steps. The first step involves a fast but nonspecific assay that will reduce the number of hybrid cultures. The cultures obtained thereby can then be subjected to the specific but difficult assays. Such nonspecific first-phase screening can be the selection of hybridomas secreting antibodies by testing for the presence of mouse immunoglobulins.[102,103] Another practice is first to collect all hybridomas secreting antibodies reacting with a given cell, and then to select from them the desired antibodies, using more sophisticated and time consuming procedures.[16,98,104]

Using one assay or another, one has always to be aware of the problem that MAbs sometimes tend to be highly assay-specific. In other words, they may perform excellently in one assay, but give mediocre or even completely negative results in another.[105] This phenomenon is most likely due to the different preparative techniques (used in the various assays), which influence the expression of various epitopes. The changes are a reflection of the strict specificity of MAbs. To avoid such unpleasantness, especially in designing MAbs for immunodiagnostic use, it is recommended to employ the same conditions in the screening phase as will be used in the final assay.

5.2. Solid Phase Immunoassays

In the following sections, I will describe in detail screening procedures that are based on solid phase immunoassays[106] that have been routinely practiced in our laboratory. These assays satisfy the requisites put forward above, that is, they are sensitive, fast, and very simple. The assay is based on the fact that proteins adhere strongly to polyvinylchloride (PVC). Thus, each well of a

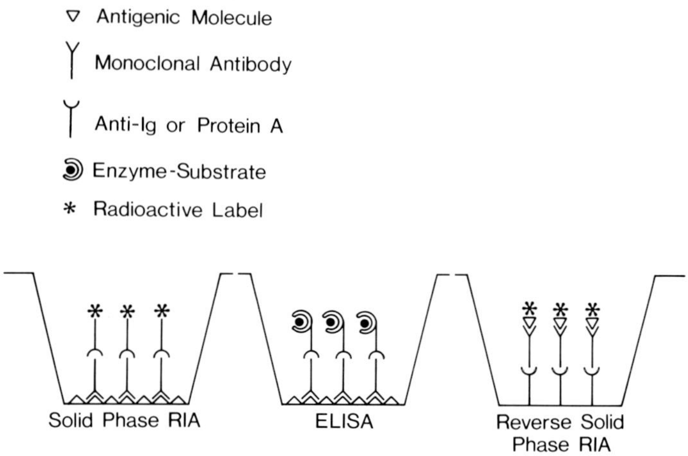

Figure 2. Solid phase immunoassays for screening for monoclonal antibodies.

PVC microtiter plate can absorb nanogram amounts of most proteins. The antibodies from hybridoma supernatants that were added to the antigen-coated plates will react with the bound antigen and, after washes, will be revealed by tagged anti-mouse Ig antibodies. The main advantage of this technique is that it does not require complex operations such as centrifugation or filtration to separate the nonbound antibody from the antigen–antibody complex. In addition, it is very convenient to transfer aliquots of supernatants from the hybridoma microculture plate to the assay microtiter plates. Multichannel pipettes (Titertek, Flow Laboratories) are useful for this purpose. Figure 2 describes the configuration of the three solid phase immunoassays that are detailed below.

5.2.1. Solid Phase Radioimmunoassay for Soluble Protein Antigens

This assay is a modification of the procedure described by Klinman.[107,108]

Materials:

1. Protein antigen (1–50 μg/ml in PBS)
2. ^{125}I-Labeled anti-mouse-Fab antibodies, or
3. ^{125}I-protein A
4. PVC microtiter plates (flexible polyvinylchloride, V-shape, Dynatech Laboratories)
5. 5% Fetal calf serum in PBS + 0.1% NaN_3 (FCS-PBS) or 1% bovine serum albumin in PBS + 0.1% NaN_3 (BSA-PBS)
6. 0.05% Tween 20 in PBS + 0.1% NaN_3 (Tween-PBS)

Procedure:

1. Add 50 μl of antigen solution into each well of a microtiter plate. Cover the plate and let incubate for 1–2 hr at room temperature (plates can also be kept for longer periods in a humid chamber at 4°C).

2. Remove antigen (can be kept for further coatings); wash once by filling the wells with PBS-FCS or PBS-BSA and flicking the fluid into a sink. Then refill the wells with PBS-FCS for 1 hr at RT to block the remaining protein-binding sites on the plastic. Wash an additional time. The wells can be filled at this stage with PBS-NaN_3 and kept for weeks at 4°C before use.
3. Transfer 50 μl supernatant from the hybridoma microculture plate into each well of the antigen-coated assay plate, using multichannel pipette and sterile tips. Incubate for 1–2 hr at RT or for longer periods at 4°C. Suck out supernatants and wash three times by dipping the plate into a tray filled with 0.05% Tween-20.
4. Add 50 μl of ^{125}I-anti-mouse-Fab′ or ^{125}I-protein A (approximately 100,000 cpm/well). Incubate for 1–2 hr at RT or for 4–16 hr at 4°C. Remove supernatant by suction into a special vacuum trap (*Radioactive*!!), wash ×4 with Tween-PBS.
5. Dry the plate under a lamp. Cut the walls using either a hot wire (should be done in a chemical hood to avoid toxic fumes) or pointed scissors. Count each well in a gamma counter. Alternatively, the plate can be autoradiographed by exposure over X-ray film and an intensifier screen.[109]

Notes:
1. Not all protein antigens bind with the same capacity to the PVC plastic. Optimal conditions have to be established using mouse antibodies. Nonprotein antigens can be coupled to carrier proteins and then serve for coating. Precoating of PVC with poly-DL-lysine (see below) can improve antigen binding capacity.
2. The protein or serum used to saturate the PVC and block nonspecific binding sites has to be adjusted to the antigenic system under study.
3. Because more than 90% of the murine antibodies contain the κ light chain, it is helpful to use anti-κ antibodies as the revealing radiolabeled antibodies. This reagent (or anti-Fab′) will react with most of the antibodies in the hybridoma's supernatant.
4. If protein A is serving for the detection of antibody binding, note that it binds better to murine IgG_{2a}, IgG_{2b}, and IgG_3 than to IgG_1.[21,82,110] IgM and IgE usually fail to bind protein A. Avoid protein A when using Ig as antigen. When protein A is being used, do not use serum to block nonspecific sites.
5. As controls for negative binding, use either medium, culture fluid or irrelevant hybridoma or 1:100 dilution of normal mouse serum. Negative wells should have less than 2000 cpm. Always include positive control of known concentration of immune serum that should have more than 10,000 cpm (if pure antigen is used).
6. Positive hybridomas are usually those that give a signal that is more than ×3 over background. Since some MAbs (especially of the IgM class) tend to stick nonspecifically, one should confirm the specificity

of the selected positive cultures by comparing the degree of binding of their antibodies to relevant and nonrelated antigen or just PBS-BSA.

5.2.2. Solid Phase Radioimmunoassay for Cellular Antigens

The principle of this assay[111] is similar to that described for the soluble antigen. Cells can be used unattached to the wells, they can be immobilized or fixed, and, when intracellular antigens are under study, cells can be permeabilized. In each case, the antigenic system studied will dictate the preferable method. When the assay is performed with unfixed cells, it should be carried out in the cold and in the presence of sodium azide to avoid antibody-inducing capping and shedding of surface antigens.

To analyze free cells, the 96-well plates are centrifuged in a refrigerated centrifuge for 5 min at 1000 rpm using special holders. The supernatants are removed either by suction or by gentle flicking, and cells are resuspended using a vortexer or microshaker. To avoid centrifugations, which are time-consuming, it is preferable to immobilize the cells in the PVC wells. The cell layer can be used as a solid phase target for the immunoassay.

The following procedure utilizes poly-L-lysine (PLL) as an anchor to attach cells to the wells. Viruses and crude membrane preparations can be absorbed as well to the PLL-coated wells.

Materials:

1. Poly-L-lysine (Miles, molecular weight 70,000–120,000), 1 mg/ml in saline-NaN_3
2. Cells, washed $\times 3$ with Hank's balanced salt solution and resuspended to 5×10^6/ml in cold PBS-NaN_3
3. ^{125}I-Anti-mouse Ig's, $(Fab')_2$ fragment, or ^{125}I-protein A
4. 5% Fetal calf serum in PBS + 0.1% NaN_3 (PBS-FCS)
5. V-Shape flexible microtiter plates

Procedure:

1. Coat wells with PLL by adding 50 μl of 1 mg/ml PLL to each well and leave for 15–30 min at RT. Remove PLL by suction and keep it for repeated use.
2. Add 25 μl of cell suspension to each well. Leave for 10 min, then centrifuge the plates using special holders for 5 min at 1000 rpm at 4°C. Remove supernatants by gentle flicking, fill the wells with PBS-FCS, and leave for 1 hr at 4°C or on ice to saturate the protein binding sites on the plastic and PLL.
3. Remove PBS-FCS; add 50 μl of hybridoma supernatant. Incubate for 1–4 hr in the cold. Remove supernatant, wash $\times 3$ with PBS-FCS by gentle flicking of the supernatant.
4. Add radioiodinated antibody or protein A, 25 μl to each well (approximately 10^5 cpm/well). Leave for 2–4 hr in the cold. Remove radioactive material by suction into special trap, then wash $\times 4$ in PBS-FCS.

5. Dry the plates under a lamp. Cut the wells into tubes and count in a gamma counter. Alternatively, the plates can be autoradiographed by exposure to X-ray film using an intensifer.[109]

Notes:

1. Another means for "anchoring" cells to PVC is to use specific antibodies or lectins to coat the wells before the addition of cells.
2. If the antigenic system is not influenced by fixation, the cells can be fixed to the plastic or PLL with freshly prepared 0.25% glutaraldehyde solution in PBS.[112] After 5–7 min at RT, glutaraldehyde is removed, and wells are washed ×3 with PBS and overlaid with 3% BSA in PBS for 1 hr at RT to saturate protein binding sites. Fixed cells can be kept for weeks at 4°C with PBS-NaN_3.
3. If intracellular antigens are studied, the immobilized cells should be permeabilized with cold (−20°C) ethyl alcohol.
4. If the cells under study carry Fc receptors, it is preferable to use ^{125}I-protein A or the $(Fab')_2$ fragment of the radiolabeled anti-mouse Ig antibody in order to avoid redistribution and pinocytosis of antigen–antibody complexes.[113]

5.2.3. Reverse Solid Phase Radioimmunoassay

We have developed this assay[91] for situations where the amounts of purified antigen are limited and not sufficient for the solid phase RIA or ELISA. The assay includes all the components of the solid phase RIA, but in reverse order (Fig. 2). It is based on the immobilization of the anti-mouse antibodies to the microtiter plate in the first step, followed by the addition of hybridoma supernatants containing the antibodies to be tested. After the removal of unbound material, radiolabeled antigen is added and allowed to react with the specific antibody. This procedure is very sensitive, gives a very low background, and is as fast and simple to perform as the other solid phase assays. It is important to use a purified or highly enriched preparation of anti-mouse Ig for the first coating, because an excess of irrelevant proteins will compete for absorption onto the plastic. Affinity purification of anti-mouse Fab′ on a mouse Ig column yields a very efficient preparation.

As radiolabeled antigen, one can use ^{125}I-iodinated proteins, small molecules such as hormones or haptens coupled to iodinated carrier protein, or any molecule that can be radiolabeled without destroying its antigenicity.

This procedure can also be employed with partially purified, radiolabeled antigen and *in vitro*-translated proteins labeled with ^{35}S-methionine. In these cases, the wells where antigen binding is apparent can be treated with SDS and the dissociated labeled antigen can be further analyzed by polyacrylamide gel electrophoresis. If the antigen has a defined activity, it is possible to dissociate the bound antigen from the assay well and analyze for its activity. Finally, the reverse solid phase RIA is recommended to select for MAbs with high affinity, because by labeling to high specific activity, low concentrations of antigen can be employed.

Materials:

1. Flexible polyvinylchloride, V-shaped, 96-well microtiter plates
2. Affinity-purified anti-mouse Fab′ antibodies 50 μg/ml in PBS-azide
3. ^{125}I-Antigen (approximately 1–10 μg/μCi) diluted to about 5×10^5 cpm/ml in PBS-BSA
4. 1% BSA in PBS + 0.1% NaN_3 (PBS-BSA)

Procedure:

1. To coat the wells of a 96-well PVC microtiter plate, add 50 μl of affinity-purified anti-mouse Ig antibodies (50 μg/ml). Incubate for 1 hr at RT.
2. Remove the antibodies (can be kept at 4°C for repeated usage). Wash ×2 with PBS-BSA.
3. Add to each well 50 μl of hybrid culture supernatant. Incubate for 1–2 hr at RT. Remove supernatants by suction and wash ×3 with PBS-BSA.
4. Add 50 μl of ^{125}I-antigen (about 25,000 cpm). Incubate for 1–2 hr at RT or 4–16 hr at 4°C.
5. Remove unbound radioactive material by suction into a trap. Wash ×4 with PBS, dry, cut wells, and count.

Notes:

1. Purified anti-class-specific antibodies or protein A can be used to coat the wells in the first stage if antibodies of a certain class are desired.
2. This procedure *is not* adequate to measure specific antibodies in immune sera, since the excess of serum immunoglobulin will compete with the binding of the specific antibodies to the anti-mouse Ig-coated wells.

5.2.4. Enzyme-Linked Immunosorbent Assay (ELISA) for Soluble and Cellular Antigens

The main principle of the ELISA technique is that in the final step of the assay, the anti-immunoglobulin or protein A is enzyme-labeled instead of radioiodinated. The degree of antibody binding is evaluated by color development that follows the addition of substrate to the system. The amount of color developed is proportional to the level of enzyme-bound antibody present.[114–116]

Although ELISA is somewhat less sensitive than RIA, the handling of samples and color development and its measurement are faster, especially with the automatic scanners that enable the reading, typing, and computing of the results of 96 wells within 1–2 min. Another practical advantage of ELISA, especially for the screening procedure, is that it allows fast evaluation of results and selection of positive wells based on visual observation.

Here we describe in more detail the procedure of ELISA using peroxidase-conjugated anti-Ig, although other enzyme conjugates, such as alkaline-phosphatase and β-galactosidase, are available.

Materials:
1. Antigen 2–10 μg/ml in PBS
2. Plates, ELISA-grade, flat-bottom or V-shape, nonsterile microtiter plates
3. Antibodies, hybridoma culture supernatant
4. PBS/T, PBS containing 0.05% Tween-20
5. Enzyme conjugate, peroxidase conjugated to IgG fraction of anti-mouse Ig (commercially available) diluted in PBS + 0.1%BSA + 0.05% Tween 20
6. Substrate, 2,2′-azinodi(3-ethylbenzthiazoline sulfonic acid) diammonium salt (ATBS), Sigma A-1888.
7. Substrate solution, ATBS 1 mg/ml plus H_2O_2 0.003%, in citrate–phosphate buffer freshly prepared by the mixing of 28 ml of 0.1 M citric acid + 22 ml of 0.2 M Na_2HPO_4 + 50 ml H_2O + 100 mg ABTS + 10 μl of 30% H_2O_2
8. Stop solution, 0.2 M citric acid (may be kept at 4°C)

Procedure:
1. Add 100 μl of antigen solution to each well.
2. Leave plate (covered) for 1–3 hr at RT.
3. Remove unbound antigen and wash wells ×3 with PBS/T.
4. Add 50–100 μl of each antibody dilution or supernatant to each well and incubate at 37°C for 30 min or 1–2 hr at RT.
5. Wash plate three times with PBS/T.
6. Add to each well 200 μl of the anti-Ig–peroxidase conjugate diluted freshly in PBS/T. Use conjugate dilutions that are recommended by the manufacturer, or determine the dilution in preliminary titration.
7. Incubate at 37°C for 30 min or 1–2 hr at RT.
8. Wash plate ×4 with PBS/T.
9. Add 100 μl of freshly made substrate solution, incubate at RT, and watch color development (usually within 30 min).
10. Add 100 μl of 0.2M citric acid to each well, to stop the reaction.
11. Read results in the automatic microelisa reader, using 630-nm filter.

Notes:
1. Avoid use of NaN_3 after step 4, since it inhibits peroxidase activity.
2. Some cells contain high endogenous levels of enzymes, which might result in high background; for example, B lymphocytes contain alkaline phosphatase[117] and macrophages contain peroxidase,[118]; therefore, if these cells are serving as target antigen, it is preferable to use another enzyme, such as β-galactosidase[112,119] or urease.[120]
3. For accurate reading, avoid scratches on the plate bottoms.
4. Some automatic scanners (the Dynatech Multiscan, for example) can accurately monitor the cheaper, flexible U- or V-shape PVC microtiter plates.
5. Nunc (Denmark) has developed a very helpful system (Nunc TSP) in which the microtiter plate lid has 96 sterile plastic prongs that fit the wells of the microculture plate. These can be sterilely coated with an-

tigen, dipped into the hybrid culture plate, left to let the antibody bind, removed, washed, and processed for ELISA in the assay plate.

ACKNOWLEDGMENTS. I am indebted to Tova Waks for her continuous assistance in establishing the procedures described herein. The skills of Bonda Lewis and Gary Burget in preparing the manuscript, and the support of DNAX Research Institute for Molecular and Cellular Biology, are gratefully acknowledged.

References

1. Köhler, G., and Milstein, C., 1974, Continuous cultures of fused cells secreting antibody of predefined specificity, *Nature* **256:**495–497.
2. Nossal G. J. V., and Lederberg, J., 1958, Antibody production by single cells, *Nature* **181:**1419–1421.
3. Burnet, F. M., 1957, A modification of Jerne's theory of antibody production using the concept of clonal selection, *Austr. J. Sci.* **20:**67–69.
4. Lane, D., and Koprowski, H., 1982, Molecular recognition and the future of monoclonal antibodies, *Nature* **296:**200–202.
5. Pillemer, E., and Weissman, I. L., 1981, A monoclonal antibody that detects a Vk-TEPC-15 idiotypic determinant cross reactive with a Thy-1 determinant, *J. Exp. Med.* **153:**1068–1079.
6. Galfrè, G., Howe, S., Milstein, C., Butcher, G. W., and Howard, J., 1977, Antibodies to major histocompatibility antigens produced by hybrid cell lines, *Nature* **266:**550–552.
7. Littlefield, J. W., 1964, Selection of hybrids from matings of fibroblasts *in vitro* and their presumed recombinants, *Science* **145:**709–710.
8. Cotton, R. G. H., and Milstein, C., 1973, Fusion of two immunoglobulin-producing myeloma cells, *Nature* **244:**42–43.
9. Kelly, T., Scharff, M. D., Cieplinski, W., Dharmgrongartama, B., Gefter, M. L., and Morrison, S. L., 1977, Regulation of immunoglobulin expression in mouse myeloma cells, *Cold Spring Harbor Symp. Quant. Biol.* **41:**781–791.
10. Parhami-Seren, B., Eshhar, Z., and Mozes, E., 1983, Fine specificity and idiotypic expression of monoclonal antibodies directed against (T,G)-A–L and its ordered analog (T,T,G,G)-A–L, *Immunology* **49:**6–16.
11. Bahr, G. M., Eshhar, Z., Ben Itzhak, R., Modabar, F. Z., Arnon, R., Sela, M., and Chedid, L., 1983, Monoclonal antibodies to the synthetic adjuvant muramyl dipeptide: Characterization and specificity, *J. Mol. Immunol.* **20:**745–752.
12. Novick, D., Eshhar, Z., and Rubinstein, M., 1982, Monoclonal antibodies to human interferon and their use for affinity chromatography, *J. Immunol.* **129:**2244–2248.
13. Novick, D., Eshhar, Z., Gigi, O., Marks, Z., Revel, M., and Rubinstein, M., 1983, Affinity chromatography of human fibroblast interferon (IFN-β_1), by monoclonal antibody columns, *J. Gen. Virol.* **64:**905–910.
14. Novick, D., Eshhar, Z., Fischer, D. G., Friedlander, J., and Rubinstein, M., 1983, Monoclonal antibody to human interferon-γ: Production, affinity purification and radioimmunoassay, *EMBO J.* **2:**1527–1530.
15. Moshly-Rosen, D., Fuchs, S., and Eshhar, Z., 1979, Monoclonal antibodies against defined determinants of acetylcholine receptor, *FEBS Lett.* **106:**389–393.
16. Schreiber, A. B., Lax, I., Yarden, Y., Eshhar, Z., and Schlessinger, J., 1981, Monoclonal antibodies against the receptor for epidermal growth factor induce early and delayed effects of epidermal growth factors, *Proc. Natl. Acad. Sci. USA* **78:**7535–7540.
17. Hadas, E., Hurwitz, E., and Eshhar, Z., 1984, Identification of a surface antigen common to murine lung and Lewis lung carcinoma by monoclonal antibodies, *Int. J. Cancer* **33:**369–376.
18. Melchers, F., Potter, M., and Warner, N. L. (eds.), 1978, *Current Topics in Microbiology and Immunology*, Volume 81, Springer-Verlag, New York.

19. Oi, V. T., and Herzenberg, L. A., 1980, Immunoglobulin-producing hybridoma cell lines, in: *Selected Methods in Cellular Immunology* (B. B. Mishell and S. M. Shiigii, eds.), Freeman, San Francisco, pp. 351–372.
20. Fazekas de St. Groth, S., and Scheidegger, D., 1980, Production of monoclonal antibodies: Strategy and tactics, *J. Immunol. Meth.* **35**:1–21.
21. Goding, J. W., 1980, Antibody production in hybridomas, *J. Immunol. Meth.* **39**:289–308.
22. Kennett, R. H., McKearn, T. J., and Bechtol, K. B. (eds.), 1980, *Monoclonal Antibodies and Hybridomas: A New Dimension in Biological Analyses*, Plenum Press, New York.
23. Hämmerling, G. J., Hammerling, U., and Kearney, J. F. (eds.), 1981, *Monoclonal Antibodies and T Cell Hybridomas, Perspectives and Technical Advances*, Elsevier/North-Holland, New York.
24. Galfrè, G., and Milstein, C., 1981, Preparation of monoclonal antibodies: Strategies and procedures, *Meth. Enzymol.* **73**:3–46.
25. Köhler, G., 1981, The technique of hybridoma production, in: *Immunological Methods*, Volume 2 (I. Lefkovits and B. Pernis, eds.), Academic Press, New York, pp. 285–298.
26. Goding, J. W., 1983, *Monoclonal Antibodies: Principles and Practice*, Academic Press, New York.
27. Weir, D. M. (ed.), 1978, *Handbook of Experimental Immunology*, 3rd ed. Academic Press, New York.
28. Williams, C. A., and Chase, M. W. (eds.), 1967–1976 *Methods in Immunology and Immunochemistry*, Volumes 1–5, Academic Press, New York.
29. Lefkovits, I., and Pernis, B. (eds.), 1981, *Immunological Methods*, Volumes 1 and 2, Academic Press, New York.
30. Langone, J., and Van Vunakis, H. (eds.), 1980–1981, Immunological techniques (Parts A, B, and C), in: *Methods in Enzymology*, Volumes 70, 73, 74, Academic Press, New York.
31. Crumpton, M. J., 1974, Protein antigens: The molecular bases of antigenicity and immunogenicity, in: *The Antigens*, Volume 2 (M. Sela, ed.), Academic Press, New York, pp. 1–78.
32. Leder, P., 1982, The genetics of antibody diversity, *Sci. Am.* **246**:102–113.
33. Tonegawa, S., 1983, Somatic generation of antibody diversity, *Nature* **302**:575–580.
34. Honjo, T., 1983, Immunoglobulin genes, *Annu. Rev. Immunol.* **1**:499–528.
35. Coffman, R. L., and Cohn, M., 1977, The class of surface immunoglobulin on virgin and memory B lymphocytes, *J. Immunol.* **118**:1806–1815.
36. Davis, M. M., Kim, S. K., and Hood, L., 1980, Immunoglobulin class switching developmentally regulated DNA rearrangement during differentiation, *Cell* **22**:1–2.
37. Marcu, K. B., Lang, R. B., Stanton, W. L., and Harris, L. J., 1982, A model for the molecular requirements of immunoglobulin heavy chain class switching, *Nature* **298**:87–92.
38. Gearhart, P., and Bogenhagen, D., 1983, Clusters of point mutations are found exclusively around rearranged antibody variable region genes, *Proc. Natl. Acad. Sci USA* **80**:3439–3444.
39. Levine, B. B., and Vaz, N. M., 1970, Effect of combination of inbred strain, antigen and antigen dose on immune responsiveness and reagin production in the mouse, *Int. Arch. Allergy Appl. Immunol.* **30**:156–163.
40. Tung, A. S., Chiorazzi, N., and Katz, D. H., 1978, Regulation of IgE antibody production by serum molecules. I. Serum from complete Freund's adjuvant-immune donors suppresses irradiation-enhanced IgE production in low responder mouse strains, *J. Immunol.* **120**:2050–2059.
41. Morisaki, I, Michalek, S. M., Harmon, C. C., Torii, S., and McGhee, J. R., 1983, Effective immunity to dental caries: Enhancement of salivary anti-*Streptococcus mutans* antibody responses with oral adjuvants, *Infect. Immunol.* **40**:577–584.
42. Koshland, M. E., 1975, Structure and function of the J chain, *Adv. Immunol.* **20**:41–69.
43. Tomase, T. B., and Grey, H. M., 1972, Structure and function of immunoglobulin A, *Prog. Allergy* **16**:81–185.
44. Kuhn, L. C., and Kraehenbuhl, J.-P., 1981, The membrane receptor for polymeric immunoglobulin is structurally related to secretory component, *J. Biol. Chem.* **250**:12490–12495.

45. Underdown, B. J., and Dorrington, K. J., 1974, Studies on the structural and conformational basis for the relative resistance of serum and secretory immunoglobulin-A to proteolysis, *J. Immunol.* **112**:949–959.
46. Baniash, M., and Eshhar, Z., 1984, Inhibition of IgE binding to mast cells and basophils by monoclonal antibodies to murine IgE, *Eur. J. Immunol.* **14**:799–807.
47. Eshhar, Z., Gigi, O., Givol, D., and Ben-Neriah, Y., 1983, Monoclonal anti-V_H antibodies recognize a common V_H determinant expressed on immunoglobulin heavy chains from various species, *Eur. J. Immunol.* **13**:533–540.
48. Springer, T. A., 1981, Monoclonal antibody analysis of complex biological systems: Combination of cell hybridization and immunoadsorbents in a novel cascade procedure and its application to the macrophage cell surface, *J. Biol. Chem.* **256**:3833–3840.
49. Springer, T. A., Kaufman, J. F., Siddoway, L. A., Mann, D. L., and Strominger, J. L., 1977, Purification of HL-A linked B lymphocyte alloantigens in immunologically active form by preparative sodium dodecyl sulfate–gel electrophoresis and studies on their subunit association, *J. Biol. Chem.* **252**:6201–6207.
50. Boulard, C., and Lecroisey, A., 1982, Specific antisera produced by direct immunization with slices of polyacrylamide gel containing small amounts of protein, *J. Immunol.* **50**:221–226.
51. Erlanger, B. F., 1980, The preparation of antigenic hapten–carrier conjugates: A survey, *Meth. Enzymol.* **70**:85–104.
52. Bauminger, S., and Wilcheck, M., 1980, The use of carbodiimides in the preparation of immunizing conjugates, *Meth. Enzymol.* **70**:151–159.
53. Reichlin, M., 1980, Use of glutaraldehyde as a coupling agent for proteins and peptides, *Meth. Enzymol.* **70**:159–165.
54. Bazin, H., Backers, A., Deckers, C., and Moriame, M., 1973, Transplantable immunoglobulin-secreting tumors in rats. V. Monoclonal immunoglobulins secreted by 250 ileocecal immunocytomas in LOU/W_sI rats, *J. Natl. Cancer Inst.* **51**:1359–1361.
55. Anderson, J., and Melchers, F., 1978, The antibody repertoire of hybrid cell lines obtained by fusion of ×63-Ag8 myeloma cells with mitogen-activated B cell blasts, *Curr. Top. Microbiol. Immunol.* **81**:130–139.
56. Stähli, C., Staehelin, T., Miggiano, V., Schmidt, J., and Haring, P., 1980, High frequencies of antigen specific hybridomas: Dependence on immunization parameters and prediction by spleen cell analysis, *J. Immunol. Meth.* **32**:297–304.
57. Eshhar, Z., Ofarim, M., and Waks, T., 1980, Generation of hybridomas secreting murine reaginic antibodies of anti-DNP specificity, *J. Immunol.* **124**:775–780.
58. Trucco, M. M., Stocker J. W., and Ceppellini, R., 1978, Monoclonal antibodies against human lymphocyte antigens, *Nature* **273**:666–668.
59. Hengartner, H., Luzzati, A., and Schreier, M., 1978, Fusion of *in vitro* immunized lymphoid cells with ×63Ag8, *Curr. Top. Microbiol. Immunol.* **81**:92–99.
60. Reading, C. L., 1982, *In vitro* immunization for the production of monoclonal antibodies, *J. Immunol. Meth.* **53**:261–291.
61. Luben, R., Bohlen, P., and Guillemin, R., 1982, Monoclonal antibodies to hypothalamic growth hormone releasing factor with picomoles of antigens, *Science* **218**:887–889.
62. Pardue, R. L., Brady, R. C., Perry, G. W., and Dedman, J. R., 1983, Production of monoclonal antibodies against calmodulin by *in vitro* immunization of spleen cells, *J. Cell Biol.* **96**:1149–1154.
63. Kozbor, D., and Roder, J., 1984, *In vitro* stimulated lymphocytes as a source of human hybridomas, *Eur. J. Immunol.* **14**:23–27.
64. Köhler, G., and Milstein, G., 1976, Derivation of specific antibody-producing tissue culture and tumor lines by cell fusion, *Eur. J. Immunol.* **6**:511–519.
65. Kearney, J. F., Radbruch, A., Liesegang, B., and Rajewsky, K., 1979, A new mouse myeloma cell line which has lost immunoglobulin expression but permits the construction of antibody secreting hybrid cell lines, *J. Immunol.* **123**:1548–1550.
66. Shulman, M., Wilde, C. D., and Köhler, G., 1978, A better cell line for making hybridomas secreting specific antibodies, *Nature* **276**:269–270.

67. Trowbridge, I. S., 1978, Interspecies spleen myeloma hybrid producing monoclonal antibodies against mouse lymphocyte surface glycoprotein T200, *J. Exp. Med.* **148:**313–323.
68. Margulies, D. H., Kuehl, W. M., and Scharff, M. D., 1976, Somatic cell hybridization of mouse myeloma cells, *Cell* **8:**405–415.
69. Taggart, R. T., and Samloff, I. M., 1983, Stable antibody producing murine hybridomas, *Science* **219:**1228–1230.
70. Galfrè, G., Milstein, C., and Wright, B., 1979, Rat × rat hybrid myelomas and a monoclonal anti-Fd portion of mouse IgG, *Nature* **277:**131–133.
71. Kilmartin, J. V., Wright, B., and Milstein, C., 1982, Rat monoclonal antitubulin antibodies derived by using a new nonsecreting rat cell line, *J. Cell Biol.* **93:**576–582.
72. Bazin, H., 1982, Production of rat monoclonal antibodies with the LOU rat nonsecreting IR983F myeloma cell line, in *Protides of the Biological Fluids* (H. Peeters, ed.), Pergamon Press, Oxford, pp. 615–618.
73. Adams, R. L. P., 1980, *Cell Culture for Biochemists*, Elsevier/North-Holland, Amsterdam.
74. Cleveland, W. L., Erlanger, B. F., 1983, Routine large-scale production of monoclonal antibodies in a protein free culture medium, *J. Immunol. Meth.* **56:**221–234.
75. Kovar, J., and Franek, F., 1984, Serum-free medium for hybridoma and parental myeloma cell cultivation—A novel composition of growth-supporting substances, *Immunol. Lett.* **7:**339–345.
76. Norwood, T. H., Zeigler, C. J., and Martin, G. M., 1976, Dimethyl sulfoxide enhances polyethylene glycol mediated cell fusion, *Somat. Cell Genet.* **2:**263–270.
77. Gefter, M. L., Margulies, D. H., and Scharff, M. D., 1977, A simple method for polyethylene glycol promoted hybridization of mouse myeloma cells, *Somat. Cell Genet.* **3:**231–236.
78. Lernhardt, W., Anderson, J., Coutinho, A., and Melchers, F., 1978, Cloning of murine transformed cell lines in suspension culture with efficiencies near 100%, *Exp. Cell Res.* **111:**309–316.
79. Sharon, J., Morrison, S. L., and Kabat, E. A., 1979, Detection of specific hybridoma clones by replica immunoadsorption of their secreted antibodies, *Proc. Natl. Acad. Sci. USA* **76:**1420–1424.
80. Parks, D. R., Bryan, V. M., Oi, V. T., and Herzenberg, L. A., 1979, Antigen specific identification and cloning of hybridomas with a fluorescence-activated cell sorter, *Proc. Natl. Acad. Sci. USA* **76:**1962–1966.
81. Lefkovitz, I., 1979, Limiting dilution analysis, in: *Immunological Methods*, Volume 1 (I. Lefkovits and B. Pernis, eds.), Academic Press, New York, pp. 355–370.
82. Goding, J. W., 1978, Staphylococcal protein A as an immunological reagent, *J. Immunol. Meth.* **20:**241–253.
83. Marshak-Rothstein, A., Fink, P., Gridley, T., Taulet, D. H., Bevan, M. J., Gefter, M. L., Properties and applications of monoclonal antibodies directed against determinants of the Thy-1 locus, *J. Immunol.* **122:**2491–2497.
84. Secher, D. S., and Burke, D. C., 1980, A monoclonal antibody for large scale purification of human leucocyte interferon, *Nature* **285:**446–450.
85. Moshley-Rosen, D., and Fuchs, S., 1981, Monoclonal anti-acetylcholine receptor antibodies directed against the cholinergic binding site, *Biochemistry* **20:**5920–5924.
86. Burstin, S. J., Spriggs, D. R., and Fields, B. N., 1982, Evidence for functional domains on the Reovirus type 3 hemagglutinin, *Virology* **117:**146–155.
87. Eshhar, Z., Kim, J. B., Bernard, G., Collins, W. P., Gilad, S., Lindner, H. R., and Kohen, F., 1981, Use of monoclonal antibodies to pregnandiol-3-glucoronide for the development of a solid-phase chemiluminescence immunoassay, *Steroids* **38:**89–106.
88. Kim, J. B., Bernard, G. J., Collins, W. P., Kohen, F., Lindner, H. R., and Eshhar, Z., 1982, Measurement of plasma estradiol-17 by solid-phase chemiluminescence immunoassay, *Clin. Chem.* **28:**1120–1124.
89. Kohen, F., Lichter, S., Eshhar, Z., and Lindner, H. R., 1982, Preparation of monoclonal antibodies able to discriminate between testosterone and 5α-dihydrotestosterone, *Steroids* **39:**453–459.

90. Yalow, R., 1978, Radioimmunoassay: A probe for the fine structure of biologic systems, *Science* **200:**1236–1245.
91. Eshhar, Z., Ben-Izhak, R., Ariel, N., and Arnon, R., 1983, Differences among individual CEA preparations and carcinomas of different origin as detected by monoclonal anti-CEA antibodies, in: *Protides of the Biological Fluids*, Volume 31 (H. Peeters, ed.), Pergamon Press, pp. 929–932.
92. Moller, B. (ed.), 1983, Functional T cell subsets defined by monoclonal antibodies, *Immunol. Rev.* **74:**1–160.
93. Ledbetter, J. A., and Herzenberg, L. A., 1979, Xenogeneic monoclonal antibodies to mouse lymphoid differentiation antigens, *Immunol. Rev.* **47:**63–90.
94. Reinherz, E. L., Kung, P. C., Golstein, G., and Schlossman, S. F., 1979, Separation of functional subsets of human T cells by monoclonal antibody, *Proc. Natl. Acad. Sci. USA* **76:**4061–4065.
95. Guesdon, J.-R., Ternynck, T., and Avrameas, S., 1979, The use of avidin–biotin interaction in immunoenzymatic techniques, *J. Histochem. Cytochem.* **27:**1131–1139.
96. Hsu, S.-M., Raine, L., and Fanger, H., 1981, The use of avidin–biotin peroxidase complex (ABC) in immunoperoxidase techniques, *J. Histochem. Cytochem.* **29:**577–596.
97. Yachi, A., Imai, K., Fujita, H., Horiya, Y., Tanda, M., Endo, T., Tsujisakai, M., and Kawaharada, M., 1984, Immunohistochemical distribution of the antigenic determinants detected by monoclonal antibodies to carcinoembryonic antigen, *J. Immunol.* **132:**2998–3004.
98. Meuer, S. C., Fitzgerald, K. A., Hussey, R. E., Hodgdon, J. C., Schlossman, S. F., and Reinherz, E. L., 1983, Clonotypic structures involved in antigen-specific human T cell function, *J. Exp. Med.* **157:**705–719.
99. Haskins, K., Kubo, R., White, J., Pigeon, M., Kappler, J., and Marrack, P., 1983, The major histocompatibility complex—Restricted antigen receptor on T cells. I. Isolation with a monoclonal antibody, *J. Exp. Med.* **157:**1149–1169.
100. Staerz, U., Pasternack, M. S., Klein, J. R., Benedetto, J. D., and Bevan, M. J., 1984, Monoclonal antibodies specific for a murine cytotoxic T lymphocyte clone, *Proc. Natl. Acad. Sci. USA* **81:**1799–1804.
101. Frackelton, A. R., and Rotman, B., 1980, Functional diversity of antibodies elicited by bacterial β-D-galactosidase, *J. Biol. Chem.* **255:**5286–5290.
102. Eshhar, Z., Blatt, C., Bergman, Y., and Haimovich, J., 1979, Induction of secretion of IgM from cells of the B cell line 38C-13 by somatic cell hybridization, *J. Immunol.* **122:**2430–2434.
103. Springer, T. A., 1983, Quantitation of hybridoma immunoglobulin and selection of myeloma or specific light chain loss variants, *Meth. Enzymol.* **92:**147–160.
104. Allison, J. P., McIntyre, B. W., and Bloch, D., 1982, Tumor specific antigen of murine T lymphoma defined with monoclonal antibody, *J. Immunol.* **129:**2293–2296.
105. Haaijman, J. J., Deen, C., Krose, C. J. M., Zijlstra, J. J., Coden, J., and Radl, J., 1984, A jungle full of pitfalls, *Immunol. Today* **5:**56–58.
106. Catt, K. J., and Tregear, G., 1967, Solid phase radioimmunoassay in antibody coated tubes, *Science* **158:**1570–1572.
107. Pierce, S. K., and Klinman, N. R., 1976, Allogeneic carrier specific enhancement of hapten-specific secondary B cell responses, *J. Exp. Med.* **144:**1254–1262.
108. Tsu, T. T., and Herzenberg, L. A., 1980, Solid phase radioimmunoassays, in: *Selected Methods in Cellular Immunology* (B. B. Mishel and S. M. Shiigi, eds.) Freeman, San Francisco, pp. 373–397.
109. Nowinski, R. C., Lostrum, M. E., Tam, M. R., Stone, M. R., and Burnette, W. N., 1979, The isolation of hybrid cell lines producing monoclonal antibodies against the p15(E) protein of ectotropic murine leukemia virus, *Virology* **93:**111–126.
110. Cy, P. L., Prowse, S. J., and Jenkin, C. R., 1970, Isolation of pure IgG1, IgG2a, and IgG2b immunoglobulins from mouse serum using protein A-Sepharose, *Immunochemistry* **15:**429–436.
111. Mason, D. W., and Williams, A. F., 1980, The kinetics of antibody binding to membrane antigens in solution and at the cell surface, *Biochem. J.* **187:**1–20.
112. Kincade, P. W., Lee, G., Sun, L., and Watanabe, T., 1981, Monoclonal rat antibodies to murine IgM determinants, *J. Immunol. Meth.* **42:**17–26.

113. Taylor, R. B., Duffus, W. P. H., Raff, M., and de Petris, S., 1971, Redistribution and pinocytosis of lymphocyte surface immunoglobulin molecules by anti-immunoglobulin antibodies, *Nature* **233**:225–229.
114. Engvall, E., and Pesce, A. J. (eds.), 1978, Quantitative enzyme immunoassay, *Scand. J. Immunol.* **8**(Suppl. 7) Blackwell Scientific Publishers, Oxford.
115. Engvall, E., 1980, Enzyme immunoassay ELISA and EMIT, *Meth. Enzymol.* **70**:419–438.
116. Maggio, E. T., 1980, *Enzyme Immunoassay*, CRC Press, Boca Raton, Florida.
117. Calvener, J. G., Harris, A. W., Mandel, T. E., Whitelaw, A., and Ferber, E., 1981, Alkaline phosphatase in hematopoietic tumor cell lines of the mouse: High activity in cells of the B lymphoid lineage, *J. Immunol.* **126**:1974–1977.
118. Williams, W. J., Beutler, E., Ersler, A. J., and Rundles, R. W., 1977, *Hematology*, 2nd ed., McGraw-Hill, New York.
119. O'Sullivan, M. J., Gremmi, E., Simmonds, A. D., Chiefegotti, G., Heyderman, E., Bridges, J. W., and Marks, V., 1979, A comparison of the ability of β-galactosidases and horseradish peroxidase enzyme–antibody conjugates to detect specific antibodies, *J. Immunol. Meth.* **31**:247–250.
120. Chandler, H. M., Cox, J. C., Healey, K., MacGregor, A., Premier, R. R., and Hurrell, J. G. R., 1982, An investigation of the use of urease-antibody conjugates in enzyme immunoassays, *J. Immunol. Meth.* **53**:187–198.

Chapter 2

Strategies for Production of Human Monoclonal Antibodies

SUSAN P. C. COLE, DANUTA KOZBOR, and JOHN C. C. RODER

1. Introduction

The potential of monoclonal antibodies (MAbs) as therapeutic agents has now been firmly established.[1] While the technology for the production of murine hybridoma MAbs has been refined enormously since it was introduced in 1975,[2,3] the technology for generating human MAbs initially lagged behind. However, recent advances now make it reasonable to suggest that it will soon be possible to generate human antibodies with as much success as murine antibodies are presently being produced. In this chapter, current strategies for the production of human MAbs are described.

2. Human versus Mouse Monoclonal Antibodies

Human MAbs will likely offer several therapeutic advantages over their murine counterparts in terms of toxicity and effectiveness. For example, many of the cancer patients that have been treated with murine MAbs[4–10] have developed a significant antibody response to the mouse immunoglobulin, which neutralized the therapeutic effect of the MAb. The immunogenicity of mouse antibody would also be expected in all chronic MAb therapies, thereby limiting its effectiveness. Human MAbs may be expected to stimulate a response to allotypic or idiotypic sites, but the incidence would be much less.

In addition, human MAbs could potentially provide a standard source of specific human immunoglobulins, such as Rh-immune globulin. The advantages of using human MAbs over the present method of obtaining antisera from Rh-negative donors either voluntarily immunized with Rh-positive blood or naturally sensitized during pregnancy are obvious. The use of purified human MAbs as opposed to human donor serum would preclude the possibility of

SUSAN P. C. COLE, DANUTA KOZBOR, and JOHN C. C. RODER • Department of Microbiology and Immunology, Queen's University, Kingston, Ontario, Canada K7L 3N6.

contamination by hepatitis virus and cytomegalovirus as well as HTLV-III, the infectious agent believed responsible for acquired immune deficiency syndrome.

Finally, from a basic science point of view, human MAbs are desirable for the study of human immune responses. In terms of understanding the human B-cell specificity repertoire, only human MAbs will yield new information. If the human antigen of interest is an autoantigen, then it is possible that low-level autoimmune responses may exist. Thus MAbs of unique specificities that would not be available in the mouse could be obtained if the autoreactive clones were "rescued" using human hybridoma techniques. These autoantigens would not likely be immunodominant, and therefore mice immunized with human tissue would express most of their antibody specificity repertoire against the other dominant antigens (species antigens, HLA, etc.). Furthermore, the development of human antiidiotypic antibodies could be very useful in triggering immune responses in the absence of antigen, especially in cases where poorly understood complex antigenic components are involved.

3. Epstein–Barr Virus

Epstein–Barr virus (EBV) was originally isolated in 1964 from a cultured cell line derived from an African Burkitt lymphoma biopsy[11] and shown to be the etiologic agent of infectious mononucleosis.[12] In infectious mononucleosis there is a pronounced increase in antibody of polyclonal specificity, including autoantibodies.[13] This observation suggested that EBV infection could lead to polyclonal activation of the infected lymphocytes. This idea was first confirmed experimentally by Rosen *et al.*,[14] who demonstrated that direct *in vitro* infection of purified human blood lymphocytes with EBV stimulated polyclonal secretion of immunoglobulin. EBV-induced immunoglobulin production in B lymphocytes is T-lymphocyte independent, although activated T lymphocytes can serve as modulators of this response.[15]

EBV is able to infect only those cells bearing EBV receptors that are closely associated with C3 receptors (Refs. 16 and 17 and Weis and Fearon, this volume, Chapter 12). In addition, small resting B lymphocytes are the most susceptible to infection.[18] The infection *in vitro* of B lymphocytes leads to permanent stimulation of cell growth, a phenomenon termed "transformation" or "immortalization." This "immortalization" preserves the characteristics of the original B cells, including EBV receptors, complement receptors, surface immunoglobulin, and secretory immunoglobulin. Those cells that grow out *in vitro* are termed lymphoblastoid cell lines (LCL).

Thus, *in vitro* transformation with EBV may be employed to obtain LCLs secreting antibodies to selected antigens. In fact, this method has been exploited successfully in numerous laboratories since the first report of Steinitz *et al.*,[19] who established anti-hapten antibody-producing human cell lines after preselection for hapten binding. LCLs secreting specific human MAbs against streptococcal carbohydrate A,[20] Rhesus antigen D,[21–23] and tetanus toxoid,[24] to mention but a few, have been established in this way.

An alternative strategy involves the EBV transformation of the total B-cell population (i.e., no preselection) followed by cloning and testing for specific antibody-producing cultures. This method has been used to isolate LCLs producing MAbs against diptheria toxoid,[25] acetylcholine receptor,[26] tetanus toxoid,[27,28] phosphorylcholine,[29] melanoma antigens,[30,31] and bacterial[32] and viral[33,34] antigens as well as many other antigens.

A major disadvantage of the EBV immortalization technique is that bulk cultures of EBV-transformed lines frequently lose their ability to produce specific antibody after long-term culture.[24,33] The reason for this instability is not clear, but may be due, at least in part, to the overgrowth of nonproducing cells within the culture.[33] Thus, in some cases, early cloning by limiting dilution has been reported to result in a stable antibody-producing cell line.[22,32,33] Several investigators have reported varying successes in cloning EBV-transformed cell lines. This variation is largely unexplained, but may be influenced by the immune status of the donor and the tissue from which the lymphocytes were derived, as well as the source of feeder layer cells used in cloning.[22,35,36] However, more complex intracellular events likely also play a role in the stabilization of specific antibody production, since cloning does not always stabilize the lymphoblastoid cell lines.[24,36] In addition to the instability of specific antibody production, a second limitation of the EBV immortalization technique is that low quantities of antibody (<1 μg/ml) are generally produced. As an alternative to EBV immmortalization, cell fusion (hybridoma) techniques may be employed for the production of human MAbs.

4. Human Hybridomas. Fusion Partners

4.1. Interspecies Hybrids

Murine MAbs are obtained by the fusion of murine myeloma cells with specific antibody-forming B lymphocytes from the spleens of immunized mice. The myeloma cell confers immortality onto the antibody-producing B lymphocyte and allows it to grow in culture and as a tumor in mice, whereas the B lymphocyte determines the specificity of the antibody produced by the hybridoma. In 1975, Schwaber[37] noted that some hybrids of mouse myeloma cells and normal human peripheral blood lymphocytes secreted human immunoglobulin. Thus, before the availability of human myeloma fusion partners, it appeared feasible to generate human MAbs by fusing human lymphocytes with murine myeloma cells, i.e., interspecies hybrids.[38] In fact, mouse × human hybrids have been described that secrete human antibody against tetanus toxoid,[39,40] human tumor-associated antigens,[41–43] multiple endocrine organs,[44] as well as others.

A limitation of interspecies hybrids lies in their preferential segregation of human chromosomes, and thus stable hybrids secreting specific human an-

Table I. Commonly Used Human Fusion Partners

Parent cell line	Fusion partner (HAT-sensitive derivative)	Ref.
RPMI 8226	8226-8AzR	70,71
U-266	SKO-007 (U-266AR_1)	72,73
	U-266 ($8Az^R$)	71
	FU-266	55
ARH-77	LICR-LON-HMy-2	41,74,75
GM-1500	GM-1500-6TG	48
	KR-4	58,59
WI-L2	UC 729-6	76,77
	LTR 228	78
	H35.1.1	79

tibodies are generally difficult to obtain. However, stable production of human antitetanus antibody from an interspecies hybrid for more than 8 months after fusion has been reported at least in one case.[40] On the other hand, loss of immunoglobulin production after 8–10 weeks in culture has been noted by others.[41,42]

Loss of human chromosomes from mouse × human hybrids does not appear random; human chromosomes 14 (heavy chain) and 22 (light chain λ) are preferentially retained, whereas chromosome 2 (light chain κ) is preferentially lost.[45,46] The stability of the chromosomal constitution is much greater in hybrids derived from parental cells of the same species; thus, to produce stable human × human hybridomas, establishment of fusion partners of human origin became necessary.

4.2. Human × Human Hybrids

Much of the work published on human × human hybridomas has used human LCLs as fusion partners (for a recent review, see Ref. 47). This is not surprising, considering there are a large number of human lymphoblastoid lines available, whereas there are only two widely available human myeloma cell lines, RPMI 8226 and U-266 (Table I). Human myeloma cell lines have proven difficult to establish and grow, whereas LCLs are considerably easier to establish, often arising spontaneously from lymphocytes of patients exposed to EBV as in the case of infectious mononucleosis. The most commonly used LCLs include derivatives of GM-1500, WI-L2, and ARH-77 (Table I).

One of the first studies of human × human hybrids of potential clinical interest was that of Croce *et al.*[48] Using peripheral blood lymphocytes from a patient with subacute sclerosing panencephalitis with very high titers of antibodies to measles virus, they obtained two hybridomas secreting antibody to measles virus nucleocapsid polypeptide. This group also fused peripheral blood lymphocytes from a patient with type I diabetes mellitus and isolated a hybridoma that produced antibodies to pancreatic islet cells.[49]

Using cells from a patient with idiopathic thrombocytopenic purpura and peripheral blood lymphocytes from patients with a variety of autoimmune diseases, including systemic lupus erythematosus, Schoenfeld *et al.*[50] obtained hybridomas secreting antibody to various nucleic acids, cold agglutinins, and platelets. Satoh *et al.*[44] generated hybridomas with lymphocytes from patients with a variety of autoimmune diseases, including insulin-requiring diabetes mellitus. Several MAbs obtained reacted with antigens in multiple endocrine organs, suggesting that such autoantibodies may explain, at least in part, multiple organ autoimmunity. Dwyer *et al.*[51] used lymphocytes from a patient with myasthenia gravis and produced a hybridoma that secreted a monoclonal anti-idiotypic antibody that reacted with a murine MAb to the nicotinic acetylcholine receptor. These types of studies have obvious important therapeutic potential in terms of diagnosis and treatment of autoimmune diseases.

Human × human hybridoma MAbs against tumor cells have also been generated using lymphocytes from several tissue sources from patients with malignant disease. In one case a hybrid was obtained that secreted antibody that bound to glioma surface components and not to normal brain cells[52] and, after intravenous injection of radiolabeled antibody, localized in the area of a recurrent cystic glioma.[53] An LCL has also been fused with lymph node lymphocytes from patients with malignant melanoma.[54] Several of the hybrids obtained secreted antibody that showed some specificity of binding to melanoma cell lines, but had a low growth rate, were relatively unstable, and produced low amounts of immunoglobulin.

4.3. Hybrid Fusion Partners

Mouse × human hybrid myelomas ("heteromyelomas") have been constructed in attempts to obtain a better fusion partner for human MAb production.[55,56] It was anticipated that a heteromyeloma would retain the superior fusion characteristics of the mouse myeloma cells and be better able to support stable human antibody production because of the presence of human chromosomes. Whether these heteromyelomas will truly prove to be better fusion partners remains to be determined, but the potential is promising.[56,57]

In our attempts to develop a better fusion partner, we have hybridized the human myeloma RPMI 8226 with our LCL KR-4 in the hopes that a hybrid fusion partner could be obtained that would support immunoglobulin synthesis in amounts comparable to myeloma cells but have a growth rate similar to an LCL. Two hybrid fusion partners (KR-12 and KR-22) have been obtained which fuse efficiently but do not appear to offer any significant advantages, at least in experiments to date, over the KR-4 LCL fusion partner (D. Kozbor, C. M. Croce, and J. C. C. Roder, unpublished results).

5. Epstein–Barr Virus Hybridoma Technique

Human MAbs may also be generated using the EBV hybridoma technique, an approach combining the advantages of both the EBV immortalization method and conventional human × human hybridoma technology, while overcoming some of their limitations.[47] This method was first described by us[58] and involves fusing EBV-immortalized antibody-producing cells with a human LCL. In this system both parental cells are immortal and therefore it was necessary to have a fusion partner with appropriate drug markers to counterselect against the parental cells. Thus thioguanine-resistant GM-1500 lymphoblastoid cells were rendered ouabain-resistant and the resulting line was designated KR-4. In our first study,[58] KR-4 was fused with an EBV-transformed, anti-tetanus toxoid-producing clone, B6, and hybrids selected in HAT:ouabain-containing medium. The hybridomas produced fourfold to eightfold more anti-tetanus toxoid antibody and cloned far more efficiently than the parental B6 line. Furthermore, specific antibody production has remained stable for more than 2 years.

In a second study[59] we have established EBV-immortalized cell lines from lymphocytes derived from peripheral blood, tumor-draining lymph nodes, bone marrow aspirates, tumors, and pericardial effusions from lung cancer patients. Clones from a number of these lines were screened for tumor-specific antibody production, but none were positive, suggesting that B lymphocytes specific for tumor antigens are rare in lung cancer patients. The EBV lines were then fused with KR-4 in an attempt to rescue low frequency B cell precursors (Fig. 1). More than 8% of hybridomas screened showed significant levels of activity, although most were not tumor cell specific, since they also reacted with EBV-infected cells from the lymphocyte donor. Two hybridomas showed apparent specific binding early after fusion, but this activity was lost upon continued growth, although, in general, hybrids continued to secrete high levels (up to 50 μg/ml) of IgM, in some cases beyond 18 months in culture. Thus the EBV hybridoma system should be useful for rescuing low frequency tumor-reactive B-cell precursors.

We have also constructed human hybridomas that produce antibodies against a number of antigen preparations of *Mycobacterium leprae*.[60] EBV-transformed cell lines from lepromatous leprosy patients were fused with KR-4 and hybrids screened for antibodies against three antigen preparations of armadillo-derived *M. leprae*, including (1) a soluble sonicate antigen, (2) a detergent extract of insoluble sonicated *M. leprae*, and (3) a phenolic glycolipid antigen. A number of reactive MAbs were obtained, which were further screened for specificity on a panel of antigens from four other mycobacteria. A total of nine cloned stable hybrids have been obtained with specificity for *M. leprae*. In comparison, 10,000 EBV-transformed lymphocyte clones from lepromatous leprosy patients were screened for anti-*M. leprae* antibody production and all the 42 clones that were initially positive lost their ability to produce antibodies within 6 weeks in culture. These results suggest that the EBV hybridoma system may be the optimal method for producing human MAbs from leprosy patients.

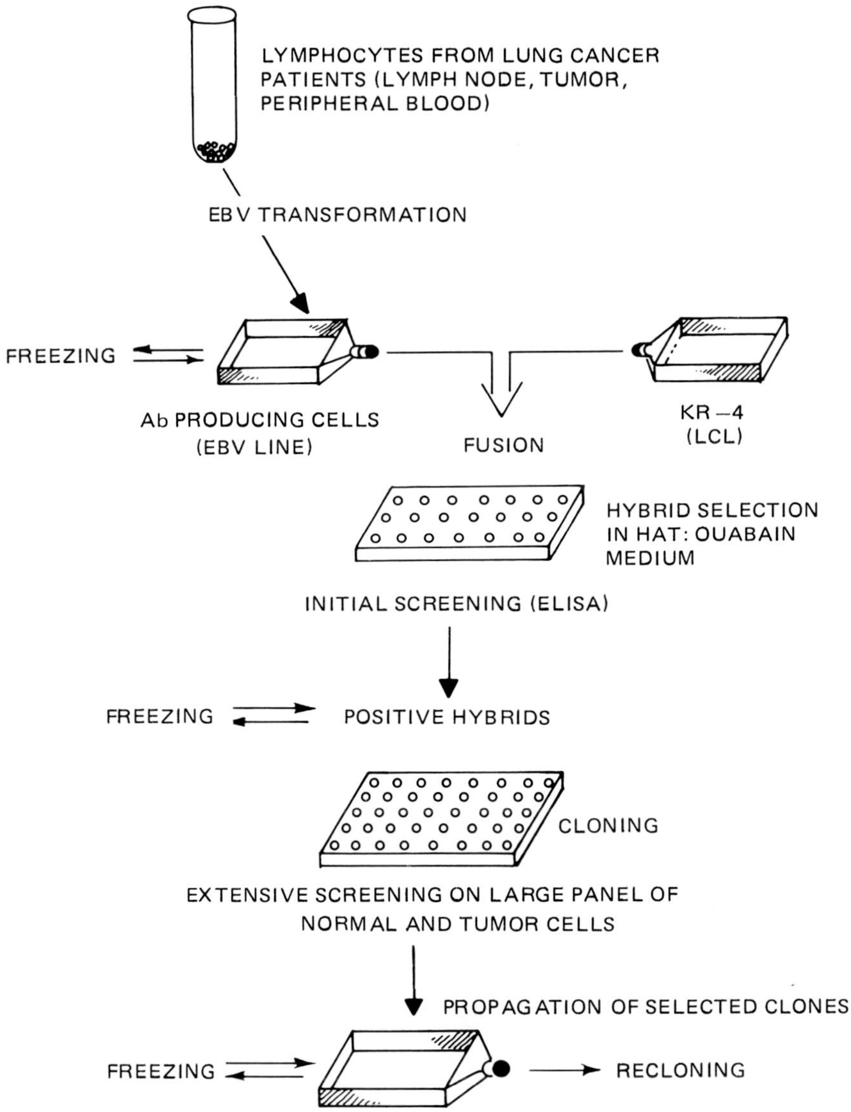

Figure 1. Strategy for production of human monoclonal antibodies specific for lung tumor antigens.

6. Large-Scale Production of Human Monoclonal Antibodies

6.1. Ascites Production

One of the problems remaining in human MAb technology is that of bulk production. Mouse hybridomas may be grown as ascites tumors in mice, increasing the yield of antibody up to 1000-fold. With human hybridomas, the use of immunodeficient mice is required to avoid xenograft rejection. Abrams *et al.*[61] have reported that murine × human hybridomas secreting human immunoglobulin grow readily in doubly pristane-primed nude mice. In our hands, this approach is not successful with human × human hybridomas. Instead, we and others[62] have found it necessary to passage the hybridoma in nude mice as a subcutaneous solid tumor, followed by *in vitro* culture, before intraperitoneal inoculation of the cells to grow as ascites.[47] In our studies, the appearance of ascites was not significantly affected by pristane-pretreatment of mice nor by depletion of natural killer cells with anti-asialo GM_1. On the other hand, irradiation of the mice enhanced production, as did the use of implanted β-estradiol pellets. Using these methods, it has been possible to obtain ascites fluid containing over 1.0 mg/ml human immunoglobulin. Unfortunately, the volume of fluid per mouse is usually small (<2 ml) and the fraction of animals developing ascites that are inoculated with human × human hybridoma cells is only about one-third. Thus current techniques are, in general, still unsatisfactory for routine production of large quantities of human antibodies.

6.2. Serum-Free Culture

As an alternative to ascites production, hybridomas may be grown in large-scale tissue culture systems. However, to be practical and economically feasible, a serum-free culture system is essential. Furthermore, elimination of serum would facilitate rapid purification of human immunoglobulins. Several systems have been described for growing human lymphocytes under serum-free conditions[63,64] but not human × human hybridomas. We have adapted several human hybrids to grow in serum-free RPMI 1640 medium in a stepwise fashion.[80] The hybrids did not grow well when the percentage of fetal bovine serum (FBS) was decreased to less than 5%, and essentially failed to thrive at 1% FBS. However, the cells readily adapted to growth in RPMI 1640 medium supplemented with 0.5% bovine serum albumin, transferrin (10 μg/ml), and 2-mercaptoethanol (5×10^{-5} M). Attempts to grow human hybrids in completely protein-free culture medium are in progress and include adaptation of hybrids to grow in a 1:1 mixture of Ham's F-12 medium and high-glucose Dulbecco's modified Eagle's medium (DMEM) supplemented with transferrin (5 μg/ml) and HEPES buffer (10 mM), pH 7.2. Thus it appears entirely feasible to grow human hybrids in serum-free culture and it is possible that this may become the method of choice for large-scale production of human MAbs.

7. Possible Limitations and Future Developments

While much effort has been directed toward finding the optimal fusion partner, little is known about how the status of donor lymphocytes influences fusibility and immunoglobulin production beyond the fact that mitogen-, antigen-, or EBV-stimulated lymphocytes fuse with higher frequencies. It is apparent that peripheral blood lymphocytes from humans offer the only readily available source of lymphocytes for fusion, although such lymphocytes are not necessarily the most ideal.[59] It has been our experience[59] and that of others (J. Gardner, Ontario Cancer Foundation, London Clinic, personal communication) that, using the EBV hybridoma technique, the number of human immunoglobulin-producing hybrids and the isotype of immunoglobulin secreted varies greatly but reproducibly with the EBV cell line fused.

The chances of success in obtaining specific human MAbs still depends largely on either (1) the prior deliberate immunization of human subjects to enrich antigen-specific B-cell precursors (which is not always possible or ethically feasible), or (2) the presence of autoantibodies such as in autoimmune diseases. *In vitro* immunization has been used with some success in human systems,[65,66] but this technique is not yet developed for routine application. Advances in this area will likely be necessary before the use of human MAb technology becomes widespread.

Concern has often been expressed regarding the presence of either EBV or retroviruses in MAb preparations intended for human use. Xenotropic retroviruses are released from many murine hybridomas or fusion partners and are known to be infectious for human cells.[67] This knowledge, however, has not prevented the experimental use of murine MAbs in man. The EBV used for the generation of human MAbs is derived from the B95-8 marmoset cell line.[68] This virus transforms human B lymphocytes *in vitro* and the EBV nuclear antigen, EBNA, is expressed but the viral cycle is not completed. Therefore, infectious virus is not released, although the possibility of contaminating cell supernatants with transforming viral DNA does exist at least in theory. However, virus and viral DNA may be inactivated or removed from MAb preparations,[69] which can be monitored by sensitive DNA hybridization techniques[57] or other methods. Of considerable interest is the recent report[57] that a number of hybrids generated from an EBV-transformed human B-cell line and a heteromyeloma did not retain the EBV genome, as determined by EBV–DNA hybridization methods and immunofluorescence tests for EBNA. Thus it would seem possible, once specific hybrids are obtained, to select variants that do not carry viral DNA.

ACKNOWLEDGMENTS. We wish to thank E. Vreeken and I. Louwman for excellent technical assistance. We also thank P. Pritchard for her help in preparing this manuscript.

D. Kozbor is a Research Fellow of the National Cancer Institute of Canada. This work was supported by grants from the Terry Fox Special Initiatives Program of the National Cancer Institute, the Medical Research Council, the World Health Organization, and the Natural Sciences and Engineering Research Council.

References

1. Levy, R. L., and Miller, R. A., 1983, Biological and clinical implications of lymphocyte hybridomas: Tumor therapy with monoclonal antibodies, *Annu. Rev. Med.* **34:**107–116.
2. Köhler, G., and Milstein, C., 1975, Continuous cultures of fused cells secreting antibody of predefined specificity, *Nature* **256:**495–497.
3. Langone, J. J., and Van Vunakis (eds.), 1983, *Methods in Enzymology*, Volume 92, Part E, Academic Press, New York.
4. Miller, R. A., and Levy, R., 1981, Response of cutaneous T-cell lymphoma to therapy with hybridoma monoclonal antibody, *Lancet* **ii:**226–230.
5. Miller, R. A., Maloney, D. G., Warnke, R., and Levy, R., 1982, Treatment of B-cell lymphoma with monoclonal anti-idiotype antibody, *N. Engl. J. Med.* **306:**517–522.
6. Miller, R. A., Maloney, D. G., McKillop, J., and Levy, R., 1981, *In vivo* effects of murine hybridoma monoclonal antibody in a patient with T-cell leukemia, *Blood* **58:**78–86.
7. Ritz, J., Pesando, J. M., Sallan, S. E., Clavell, L. A., Notis-McConarty, J., Rosenthal, P., and Schlossman, S. F., 1981, Serotherapy of acute lymphoblastic leukemia with monoclonal antibody, *Blood* **58:**141–151.
8. Sears, H. R., Atkinson, B., Herlyn, D., Ernst, C., Matteis, J., Steplewski, Z., and Koprowski, H., 1982, Phase I clinical trial of monoclonal antibody in treatment of gastrointestinal tumours, *Lancet* **i:**762–765.
9. Nader, L. M., Stashenko, P., Hardy, R., Kaplan, W. D., Button, L. N., Kufe, D. W., Antman, K. H., and Schlossman, S. F., 1980, Serotherapy of a patient with a monoclonal antibody directed against a human lymphoma-associated antigen, *Cancer Res.* **40:**3147–3154.
10. Dillman, R. O., Shawler, D. L., Sobol, R. E., Collins, H. A., Beauregard, J. C., Wormsley, S. B., and Royston, I., 1982, Murine monoclonal antibody therapy in two patients with chronic lymphocytic leukemia, *Blood,* **59:**1036–1045.
11. Epstein, M. A., Achong, B. G., and Barr, Y. M., 1964, Virus particles in cultured lymphoblasts from Burkitt's lymphoma, *Lancet* **i:**702–703.
12. Henle, G., Henle, W., and Diehl, V., 1968, Relation of Burkitt's tumor-associated Herpes-type virus to infectious mononucleosis, *Proc. Natl. Acad. Sci. USA* **59:**94–107.
13. Wollheim, F. A., and Williams, R. C., 1966, Studies on the macroglobulins of human serum. I. Polyclonal immunoglobulin class M (IgM) increase in infectious mononucleosis, *N. Engl. J. Med.* **274:**61–67.
14. Rosen, A., Britton, S., Gergely, P., Jondal, M., and Klein, G., 1977, Polyclonal Ig production after Epstein–Barr virus infection of human lymphocytes, *Nature* **267:**52–54.
15. Bird, A. G., and Britton, S., 1979, A new approach to the study of human B lymphocyte function using an indirect plaque assay and a direct B cell activator, *Immunol. Rev.* **45:**41–67.
16. Jondal, M., Klein G., Oldstone, M. B. A., Bokish, V., and Yefenof, E., 1976, Surface markers on human B and T lymphocytes. VIII. Association between complement and Epstein–Barr virus receptors on human lymphoid cells, *Scand. J. Immunol.* **5:**401–410.
17. Yefenof, E. and Klein, G., 1977, Membrane receptor stripping confirms the association between EBV receptors and complement receptors on the surface of human B lymphoma lines, *Int. J. Cancer* **20:**347–352.
18. Aman, P., Ehlin-Henriksson, B., and Klein, G., 1984, Epstein–Barr virus susceptibility of normal human B lymphocyte populations, *J. Exp. Med.* **159:**208–220.
19. Steinitz, M., Klein, G., Koskimies, S., and Makela, O., 1977, EB virus-induced B lymphocyte cell lines producing specific antibody, *Nature* **269:**420–422.
20. Steinitz, M., Seppala, F., Eichman, K., and Klein, G., 1979, Establishment of a human lymphoblastoid cell line with the specific antibody production against group A streptococcal carbohydrate, *Immunobiology* **156:**41–47.
21. Boylston, A. W., Gardner, B., Anderson, R. L., and Hughes-Jones, N. C., 1980, Production of human IgM anti-D in tissue culture by EB-virus transformed lymphocytes, *Scand. J. Immunol.* **12:**355–358.

22. Crawford, D. H., Barlow, M. J., Harrison, J. F., Winger, L., and Huehns, E. R., 1983, Production of human monoclonal antibody to Rhesus D antigen, *Lancet* **i**:386–388.
23. Koskimies, S., 1979, A human lymphoblastoid cell line producing specific antibody against Rh-antigen D, *Scand. J. Immunol.* **10**:371 (abstract).
24. Kozbor, D., and Roder, J. C., 1981, Requirements for the establishment of high titered human monoclonal antibodies against tetanus toxoid using the Epstein–Barr virus technique, *J. Immunol.* **127**:1275–1280.
25. Tsuchiya, S., Yokoyama, S., Yoshie, O., and Ono, Y., 1980, Production of diptheria antitoxin antibody in Epstein–Barr virus-induced lymphoblastoid cell lines, *J. Immunol.* **124**:1970–1976.
26. Kamo, I., Furukawa, S., Tada, A., Mano, Y., Iwasaki, Y., and Furuse, T., 1982, Monoclonal antibody to acetylcholine receptor: Cell line established from thymus of patient with myasthenia gravis, *Science* **215**:995–997.
27. Zurawski, V. R., Haber, Jr., E., and Black, P. M., 1978, Production of antibody to tetanus toxoid by continuous human lymphoblastoid lines, *Science* **199**:1439–1441.
28. Zurawski, V. R., Spedden, Jr., S. E. Black, P., and Haber, E., 1978, Clones of human lymphoblastoid cell lines producing antibody to tetanus toxoid, *Curr. Top. Microbiol. Immunol.* **81**:152–155.
29. Yoshie, O., and Ono, Y., 1980, Anti-phosphorylcholine antibody producing cells in human lymphoblastoid cell lines established by transformation with Epstein–Barr virus, *Cell. Immunol.* **56**:305–315.
30. Irie, R. F., Sze, L. L., and Saxton, R. E., 1982, Human antibody to OFA-1, a tumor antigen, produced *in vitro* by Epstein–Barr virus-transformed human B-lymphoid cell lines, *Proc. Natl. Acad. Sci. USA* **79**:5666–5670.
31. Watson, D. B., Burns, G. F., and MacKay, I. R., 1983, *In vitro* growth of B lymphocytes infiltrating human melanoma tissue by transformation with EBV: Evidence for secretion of anti-melanoma antibodies by some transformed cells, *J. Immunol.* **130**:2442–2447.
32. Rosen, A., Persson, K., and Klein, G., 1983, Human monoclonal antibodies to a genus-specific chlamydial antigen, produced by EBV-transformed B cells, *J. Immunol.* **130**:2899–2902.
33. Crawford, D. H., Callard, R. E., Muggeridge, M. I., Mitchell, D. M., Zanders, E. D., and Beverley, P. C. L., 1983, Production of human monoclonal antibody to X31 influenza virus nucleoprotein, *J. Gen. Virol.* **64**:697–700.
34. Seigneurin, J. M., Desgranges, C., Seigneurin, D., Paire, J., Renversez, J. C., Jacquemont, B., and Micouin, C., 1983, Herpes simplex virus glycoprotein D: Human monoclonal antibody produced by bone marrow cell line, *Science* **221**:173–175.
35. Stein, L. D., Ledgley, C. J., and Sigal, N. H., 1983, Patterns of isotype commitment in human B cells: Limiting dilution analysis of Epstein–Barr virus-infected cells, *J. Immunol.* **130**:1640–1645.
36. Winger, L., Winger, C., Shastry, P., Russell, A., and Longenecker, M., 1983, Efficient generation *in vitro*, from human peripheral blood cells, of monoclonal Epstein–Barr virus transformants producing specific antibody to a variety of antigens without prior deliberate immunization, *Proc. Natl. Acad. Sci. USA* **80**:4484–4488.
37. Schwaber, J., 1975, Immunoglobulin production by a human–mouse somatic cell hybrid, *Exp. Cell. Res.* **93**:343–354.
38. Levy, R., Dilley, J., Brown, S., and Bergman, Y., 1980, in: *Monoclonal Antibodies. Hybridomas: A New Dimension in Biological Analysis* (R. H. Kennett, T. J. McKearn, and K. B. Bechtol, eds.), Plenum Press, New York, pp. 137–153.
39. Kozbor, D., Roder, J. C., Chang, T. H., Steplewski, Z., and Koprowski, H., 1982, Human anti-tetanus toxoid monoclonal antibody secreted by EBV-transformed human B cells fused with a murine myeloma, *Hybridoma* **1**:323–328.
40. Gigliotti, F., and Insel, R. A., 1982, Protective human hybridoma antibody to tetanus toxin, *J. Clin. Invest.* **70**:1306–1309.
41. Sikora, K., and Wright, R., 1981, Human monoclonal antibodies to lung-cancer antigens, *Br. J. Cancer* **43**:696–700.
42. Sikora, K., and Phillips, J., 1981, Human monoclonal antibodies to glioma cells, *Br. J. Cancer* **43**:105–107.

43. Schlom, J., Wunderlich, D., and Teramoto, Y. A., 1980, Generation of human monoclonal antibodies reactive with human mammary carcinoma cells, *Proc. Natl. Acad. Sci. USA* **77**:6841–6845.
44. Satoh, J., Prabhakar, B. S., Haspel, M. V., Ginsberg-Feblner, F., and Notkins, A. L., 1983, Human monoclonal autoantibodies that react with multiple endocrine organs, *N. Engl. J. Med.* **309**:217–220.
45. Croce, C. M., Shander, M., Martinis, J., Circurel, L., D'Ancoma, G. G., and Koprowski, H., 1980, Preferential retention of human chromosome 14 in mouse × human B cell hybrids, *Eur. J. Immunol.* **10**:486–488.
46. Erikson, J., Martinis, J., and Croce, C. M., 1981, Assignment of the genes for human λ immunoglobulin chains to chromosome 22, *Nature* **294**:173–175.
47. Cole, S. P. C., Campling, B. G., Atlaw, T., Kozbor, D., and Roder, J. C., 1984, Human monoclonal antibodies, *Mol. Cell. Biochem.* **62**:109–120.
48. Croce, C. M., Linnenbach, A., Hall, W., Steplewski, Z., and Koprowski, H., 1980, Production of human hybridomas secreting antibodies to measles virus, *Nature* **288**:488–491.
49. Eisenbarth, G. S., Linnenbach, A., Jackson, R., Scearce, R., and Croce, C. M., 1982, Human hybridomas secreting anti-islet autoantibodies, *Nature* **300**:264–267.
50. Schoenfeld, Y., Rauch, J., Massicotte, H., Datta, S. K., Andre-Schwartz, J., Stollar, B. D., and Schwartz, R. S., 1983, Polyspecificity of monoclonal lupus autoantibodies produced by human–human hybridomas, *N. Engl. J. Med.* **308**:414–420.
51. Dwyer, D. S., Bradley, R. J., Urquhart, C. K., and Kearney, J. F., 1983, Naturally occurring anti-idiotypic antibodies to myasthenia gravis patients, *Nature* **301**:611–614.
52. Sikora, K., Alderson, T., Phillips, J., and Watson, J. V., 1982, Human hybridomas from malignant gliomas, *Lancet* **i**:11–14.
53. Phillips, J., Sikora, K., and Watson, J. V., 1982, Localisation of glioma by human monoclonal antibody, *Lancet* **ii**:1214–1215.
54. Warenius, H. M., Taylor, J. W., Durack, B. E., and Cross, P. A., 1983, The production of human hybridomas from patients with malignant melanoma. The effect of pre-stimulation of lymphocytes with pokeweed mitogen, *Eur. J. Cancer Clin. Oncol.* **19**:347–355.
55. Teng, N. N. H., Lam, K. S., Riera, F. C., and Kaplan, H. S., 1983, Construction and testing of mouse–human heteromyelomas for human monoclonal antibody production, *Proc. Natl. Acad. Sci. USA* **80**:7308–7312.
56. Foung, S. K. H., Perkins, S., Raubitschek, A., Larrick, J., Lizak, G., Fishwild, D., Engelman, E. G., and Grumet, F. C., 1984, Rescue of human monoclonal antibody production from an EBV-transformed B cell line by fusion to a human–mouse hybridoma, *J. Immunol. Meth.* **70**:83–90.
57. Bron, D., Feinberg, M. B., Teng, N. N. H., and Kaplan, H. S., 1984, Production of human monoclonal IgG antibodies against Rhesus (D) antigen, *Proc. Natl. Acad. Sci USA* **81**:3214–3217.
58. Kozbor, D., Lagarde, A., and Roder, J. C., 1982, Human hybridomas constructed with antigen-specific, EBV-transformed cell lines, *Proc. Natl. Acad. Sci. USA* **79**:6651–6655.
59. Cole, S. P. C., Campling, B. G., Louwman, I. H., Kozbor, D., and Roder, J. C., 1984, A strategy for the production of human monoclonal antibodies reactive with lung tumor cell lines, *Cancer Res.* **44**:2750–2753.
60. Atlaw, T., 1983, Human monoclonal antibodies against *Mycolbacterium leprae*. M. Sc. Thesis. Queen's University at Kingston, Ontario.
61. Abrams, P. G., Ochs, J. J., Giardina, S. L., Morgan, A. C., Wilburn, S. B., Wilt, A. R., Oldham, R. K., and Foon, K. A., 1984, Production of large quantities of human immunoglobulin in the ascites of athymic mice: Implications for the development of anti-human idiotype monoclonal antibodies, *J. Immunol.* **132**:1611–1613.
62. Truitt, K. E., Larrick, J. W., Raubitschek, A. A., Buck, D. W., and Jacobson, S. W., 1984, Production of human monoclonal antibody in mouse ascites, *Hybridoma* **3**:195–199.
63. Sharath, M. D., Rinderknecht, S. B., and Weiter, J. M., 1984, Human immunoglobulin synthesis in a serum-free medium, *J. Lab. Clin. Med.* **103**:739–748.
64. Farrant, J., Newton, C. A., North, M. E., Weyman, C., and Brenner, M. K., 1984, Production of antibody by human B cells under serum-free conditions, *J. Immunol.* **68**:25–34.

65. Kozbor, D., and Roder, J. C., 1984, *In vitro* stimulated lymphocytes as a source of human hybridomas, *Eur. J. Immunol.* **14**:23–27.
66. Strike, L. E., Devens, B. H., and Lundak, R. L., 1984, Production of human–human hybridomas secreting antibody to sheep erythrocytes after *in vitro* immunization, *J. Immunol.* **132**:1798–1803.
67. Weiss, R. A., 1982, Hybridomas produce viruses as well as antibodies, *Immunol. Today* **3**:292–294.
68. Miller, G., and Lipman, M., 1973, Release of infectious Epstein–Barr virus by transformed marmoset leukocytes, *Proc. Natl. Acad. Sci. USA* **70**:190–194.
69. Crawford, D. H., Huehns, E. R., and Epstein, M. A., 1983, Therapeutic use of human monoclonal antibodies, *Lancet* **i**:1040 (letter).
70. Matsuoka, Y., Moore, G. E., Yagi, Y., and Pressman, D., 1967, Production of free light chains of immunoglobulin by a hematopoietic cell line derived from a patient with multiple myeloma, *Proc. Soc. Exp. Biol. Med.* **125**:1246–1250.
71. Abrams, P. G., Knost, J. A., Clarke, G., Wilburn, S., Oldham, R. K., and Foon, K. A., 1983, Determination of the optimal human cell lines for development of human hybridomas, *J. Immunol.* **131**:1201–1204.
72. Nilsson, K., Bennich, H., Johansson, S. G. O., and Ponten, J., 1970, Established immunoglobulin producing myeloma (IgE) and lymphoblastoid (IgG) cell lines from an IgE myeloma patient, *Clin. Exp. Immunol.* **7**:477–489.
73. Olsson, L., and Kaplan, H. S., 1980, Human–human hybridomas producing monoclonal antibodies of predefined antigenic specificity, *Proc. Natl. Acad. Sci. USA* **77**:5429–5431.
74. Burk, K. H., Drewinko, B., Trejillo, J. M., and Ahearn, M. J., 1978, Establishment of a plasma cell line *in vitro, Cancer Res.* **38**:2508–2513.
75. Edwards, P. A. W., Smith, C. M., Neville, A. M., and O'Hare, M. J., 1982, A human–human hybridoma system based on a fast growing mutant of the ARH-77 plasma cell leukemia-derived line, *Eur. J. Immunol.* **12**:641–648.
76. Levy, J. A., Viroloinen, V., and Defendi, V., 1968, Human lymphoblastoid lines from lymph node and spleen, *Cancer* **22**:517–524.
77. Glassy, M. C., Handley, H. H., Hagiwara, H., and Royston, I., 1983, UC 729-6, a human lymphoblastoid B-cell line useful for generating antibody-secreting human–human hybridomas, *Proc. Natl. Acad. Sci. USA* **80**:6327–6331.
78. Larrick, J. W., Truitt, K. E., Raubitschek, A. A., Senyk, G., and Wang, J. C. N., 1983, Characterization of human hybridomas secreting antibody to tetanus toxoid, *Proc. Natl. Acad. Sci. USA* **80**:6376–6380.
79. Chiorrazzi, N., Wasserman, R. L., and Kunkel, H. G., 1982, Use of Epstein–Barr virus-transformed B cell lines for the generation of immunoglobulin-producing human B cell hybridomas, *J. Exp. Med.* **156**:930–935.
80. Cole, S. P. C., Vreeken, E. H., and Roder, J. C., 1985, Antibody production by human × human hybridomas in serum-free medium, *J. Immunol. Meth.*, in press.

Chapter 3

The Antibody Combining Site

EDGAR HABER and JIŘÍ NOVOTNÝ

1. Introduction

Antibodies are characterized by regions of conserved as well as variable amino acid sequence. Small portions of each molecule, highly variable in structure (the complementarity-determining regions), are arranged to form the surface that binds antigen. The amino acid sequences of the polypeptide chain segments that fold to form this region (approximately 60 amino acid residues) determine the nature of the antigen recognized. Three segments of the heavy and three of the light chain participate in forming the site.

How is the incredible sequence variability that characterizes the complementarity site determined? A number of mechanisms have been invoked. First, different heavy and light chains may assort, possibly in random permutations and combinations. Second, sequence variability is determined by several mechanisms. The variable region of the light chain, making up approximately its amino-terminal half, is the product of two genes: V_L, which occurs in several hundred copies, and J_L, four copies of which have been identified.[1–4] V_L and J_L may occur in any combination, providing a source of considerable variability. In addition, the region at their junction is subject to variation by virtue of nonhomologous somatic recombination. The heavy chain variable region is the product of three genes: V_H, in several hundred copies; D, in ten or more copies; and J_H, in four copies.[5,6] As in the light chain, any permutation and/or combination of these genes may occur and two sites of somatic recombination are present. These mechanisms alone can account for 10^7 different complementarity-determining regions (see Tonegawa[7] for review). In addition, somatic point mutation[8] has been shown to occur at high frequency in V, D, and J segments. Recently, Clarke *et al.*[9] have demonstrated that gene conversion among sets of related variable region genes is also a likely mechanism for generating diversity. Thus, the number of possible antibodies may well exceed 10^{10}.

EDGAR HABER • Cardiac Unit and Cellular and Molecular Research Laboratory, Massachusetts General Hospital, and Department of Medicine, Harvard Medical School, Boston, Massachusetts 02114. JIŘÍ NOVOTNÝ • Cellular and Molecular Research Laboratory, Massachusetts General Hospital, and Harvard Medical School, Boston, Massachusetts 02114.

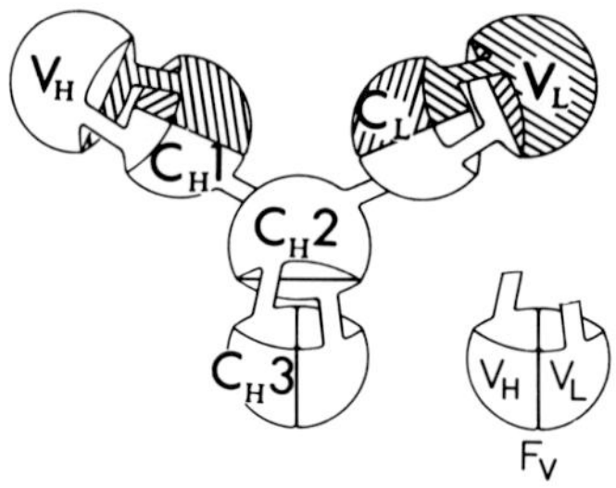

Figure 1. A low-resolution structure of Fab fragment NEW. (Modified from Ref. 54.)

In this chapter we address two rather important questions concerning the antibody combining site. First, what is its three-dimensional structure and how is it suited to binding a specific ligand; and second, how may the primary structure of the combining site, which of course determines tertiary structure, be related to the selectivity and affinity for a particular ligand bound by that site?

Antibodies are signal molecules in the sense that they not only recognize antigens, but, perhaps more importantly, convey an information that non-self structures are present in the organism. When antibodies complex with antigens, the complement system is activated and the signal is transmitted. In keeping with the signal function, immunoglobulins are rather large molecules with parts of the molecule specialized for antigen binding and other parts of the molecule specialized for signal transfer. For our purposes, however, only the antigen-binding function is important, and we will accordingly limit ourselves to that small part of immunoglobulin structure that is involved in antigen recognition.

2. Structure of the Antibody Combining Site

It is significant that immunoglobulin structure has a modular design.[10–12] Both the light chains (molecular weight 25,000) and the heavy chains (molecular weight 50,000) are composed of several domains, each of which consists approximately of 110 amino acid residues (Fig. 1). The antigen-binding function is concentrated in the NH_2 terminal, so-called variable domains of both the light and heavy chains.[13,14] It has been demonstrated experimentally that the isolated variable domains can refold without the rest of the polypeptide chain,[15] and this fact justifies our discussion of the antigen-combining function without paying attention to the rest of the molecule.

On the primary structural level, the light and heavy chain variable domains (V_L and V_H) contain segments conspicuous by their different lengths and amino acid sequences when various chains from the same organism are compared. There are three such segments in both V_L and V_H and their positions within the V_L and V_H amino acid sequence are homologous. It has been hypothesized that these "hypervariable loops," designated L1, L2, L3, H1, H2, and H3, are responsible for antibody specificity and that they actually form the antigen-binding site.[16] Accordingly, they are also known as complementarity determining regions. X-ray crystallographic structures of three Fab fragments

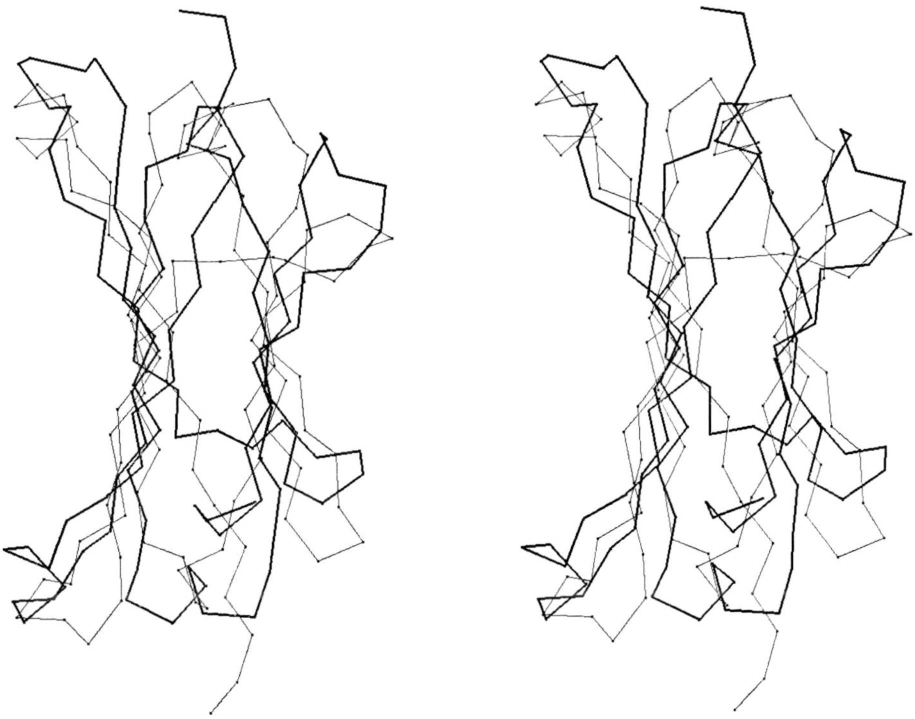

Figure 2. A stereo α-carbon tracing of the polypeptide backbone of mouse (heavy line) and human (light line) light chain constant domains. The picture emphasizes a strong structural homology between the two domains that contrasts with a much lower amino acid sequence homology. The bilayer structure of the domains is clearly visible. Note that the two β-sheets are close-packed in the middle but splay apart at the ends where the regular β-strands are connected by reverse loops. Immunoglobulin molecule arises by a close-packing of the concave domain surfaces that gives rise to domain dimers. The dimers can be viewed as two β-sheet bilayers, or sandwiches, stacked onto each other, forming a four-layered, close-packed structural unit. (Stereo drawings are best viewed with a stereoviewer, an instrument produced by Abrams Instruments, Lansing, Michigan. To view the stereo drawings with the unaided eye, one must view the two images with eyes decoupled, i.e., focused to "infinity." For further information on viewing stereo drawings, see Ref. 55.)

(human KOL[17] and NEW[18]; mouse MCPC 603[19]) and two V_L–V_L dimers from Bence-Jones proteins REI[20] and MCG[21] indeed confirmed that, by noncovalent association of the V_L and V_H domains, all six loops come into close contact and form a contiguous area on the surface of the V_L–V_H dimer from which the binding site is constructed. There are low-resolution crystallographic data available for antigens complexed with the Fab fragments NEW[22] and MCPC 603.[19] Both the antigens (menadione in the case of NEW, and phosphorylcholine in the case of MCPC 603) are located in a groove, or cavity, surrounded by the hypervariable regions.

Given the crystallographic data, it is possible to discuss antibody specificity and its modulation in structural terms. Antibody domains share the same architectural motif, two antiparallel β-sheets close-packed face to face[23,24] (Fig.

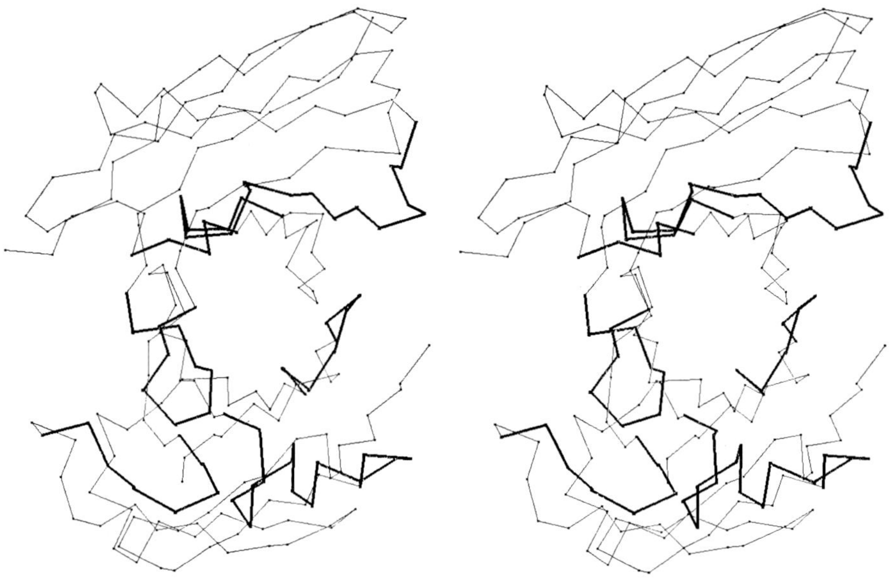

Figure 3. A schematic stereo view (α-carbon tracing) of the MCPC 603 V_L–V_H domain dimer. Dimerization can be considered as a pseudo-twofold symmetry operation (the V_L and V_H domains are roughly superimposable) and the dimer (or Fv fragment) is oriented in such a way that the pseudo-twofold symmetry axis is approximately perpendicular to the plane of the paper. The axis also serves as an axis of the binding site (i.e., V_L–V_H interface). The hypervariable loops are emphasized and it can be seen that they come close together in space, forming a contiguous area (the binding site) at the "top" of the V_L–V_H interface.

2). The basic building blocks of immunoglobulin domains are therefore β-strand segments and reverse loops connecting these strands. The domains are linked together by rather extended "hinge" or "switch" peptides, long enough to permit relative movements of domains with respect to each other.

Domains from different chains associate together by noncovalent forces to form domain heterodimers. Each domain can be viewed as having two β-sheet surfaces and in the complete immunoglobulin molecule one of the β-sheets faces the solvent, whereas the other mediates a contact with the other domain of the pair. The principal difference between a V_L–V_H type of dimerization and the constant–constant domain pairs lies in the fact that the β-sheets involved in the domain interface are different in the two domain types.[25]

In further discussion we limit ourselves to the V_L–V_H type of domain dimers. The variable domains usually consist of eight or nine β-strands, as opposed to the constant domains, which are seven-stranded. Lesk and Chothia[24] described the "immunoglobulin fold" as a consecutive sequence of β-strands A–G, with side-by-side topology of the two β-sheets A-B-D-E and C-F-G. In the variable domains, then, there is an additional β-strand subsequent to the C strand and the topology of the second β-sheet can be schematically described as C′-C-F-G. The V_L and V_H domains associate by their C′-C-F-G β-sheets in a

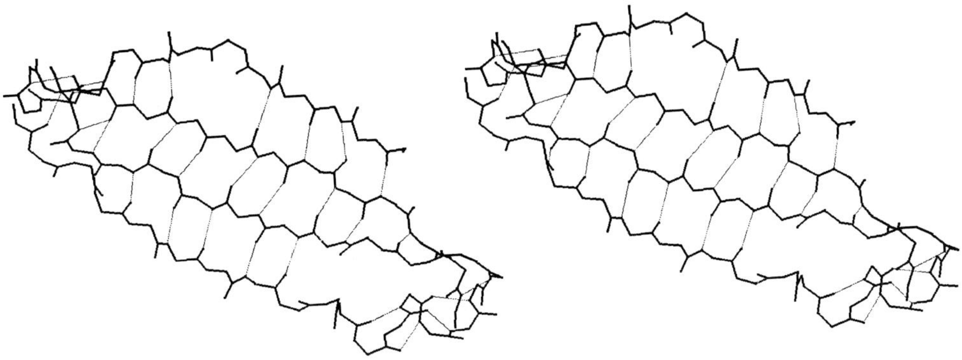

Figure 4. A detailed stereo schematic view of the polypeptide chain backbone of one of the β-sheets from the heavy chain constant domain CH3. Light lines denote hydrogen bonds typical for the antiparallel β-sheet. Note the twist of individual β-strands and the curvature of the whole sheet.

very specific way and it is their association that gives rise to the antigen-combining site (Fig. 3).

It has been known that β-sheets are not flat, as originally suggested by Pauling and Corey,[26] but twisted[27] (Fig. 4). The V_L–V_H contact β-sheets are not only twisted but also strongly curved (coiled), giving an impression of being wrapped counterclockwise around a cylindrical surface. This peculiar feature

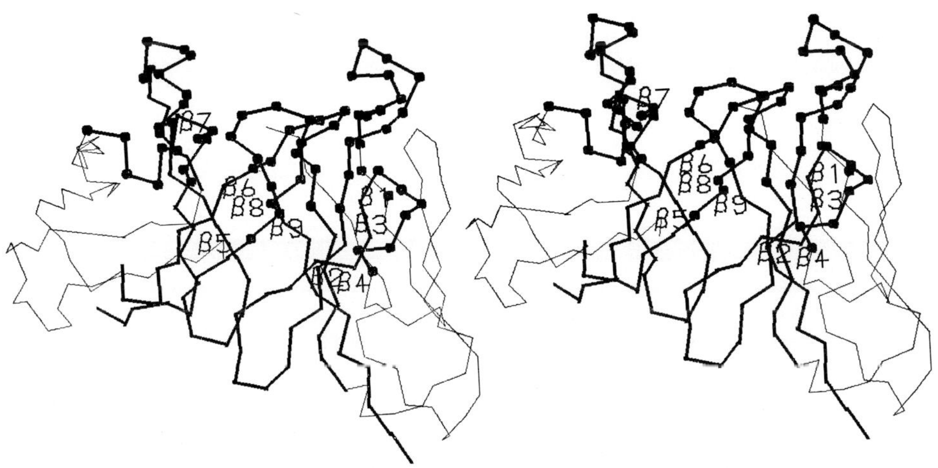

Figure 5. Antibody binding region. A stereo α-carbon drawing of V_L–V_H domain dimer of a mouse Fab fragment MCPC 603.[19] V_L domain is at right; V_H domain is at left. The interface β-sheets, represented by heavy lines are highly curved and their noncovalent contact forms a nearly perfect cylindrical barrel the upper surface of which constitutes the antigen combining site. The Cα atoms of hypervariable residues are represented as heavy dots. The nine β-strands that form the V_L–V_H interface are numbered β1–β9 in correspondence with Fig. 6. (Reprinted from Ref. 28 by permission.)

```
                25  27a b c       28  30        35          40          45         50        55        60
KOL S1       S C S G T|S S N I - - - - G S D|S V N W Y Q Q|L P G M A P|K L L I Y|R D A M R P S G V P D R
NEW S1       S C T G S|S S N I - - - G A G N|H V K W Y Q Q|L P G T A P|K L L I F|- - - - - - - H N N A R
MCPC603 S1   S C K S S|Q S L L N S G N Q K N|F L A W Y Q Q|K P G Q P P|K L L I Y|G A S T R E S G V P D R
                      |-------- L1 ---------|      β1                    β2     |---- L2 ----|

                   85          90        95  97a b 98 100
KOL S2           S D Y Y C A S|W N N S D N A Y|V F G T G T K V
NEW S2           A D Y Y C Q S|Y D R S - - L R|V F G G G T K L
MCPC603 S2       A V Y Y C Q N|D H S Y P L - -|T F G A G T K L
                      β3      |----- L3 -----|      β4

              30      35          40          45        50  52a b c 53 55       60       65
KOL S3       F S S Y|A M Y W V R Q|A P G K G|L E W V A|I I W D D G S - -|D Q H Y|A D S V K G R
NEW S3       F D D Y|Y S T W V R Q|P P G R G|L E W I G|Y V F Y H G - - -|T S D T|D T P L R S R
MCPC603 S3   F S D F|Y M E W V R Q|P P G K R|L E W I A|A S R N K G N K Y|T T E Y|S A S V K G R
              |H1|        β5                   β6    |------ H2 -------|  β7

                       90             95    100a b c d e f g h 101        105
KOL S4             T|G V Y F C A R D|G G H G F C S S A S C F G P|D Y W G Q G T P V
NEW S4             T|A V Y Y C A R D|L I A G - - - - - - - - C I|D V W G Q G S L V
MCPC603 S4         T|A I Y Y C A R N|Y Y G S T W - - - - - - Y F|D V W G A G T T V
                           β8       |------------ H3 -----------|       β9
```

Figure 6. Polypeptide-chain segments that constitute the binding region and V_L–V_H interface. Homologous segments from different structures are aligned to maximize amino acid homology. Boldface letters indicate hypervariable loops. Boxes denote β-sheet strands. Hypervariable loops are denoted by horizontal bars. The first two sets of sequences are parts of the light chain variable domain; the last two sets of sequences are parts of the heavy chain variable domain. The numbering system is that of Ref. 56. Amino acids are given in the one-letter code.[57] (Reprinted from Ref. 28 by permission.)

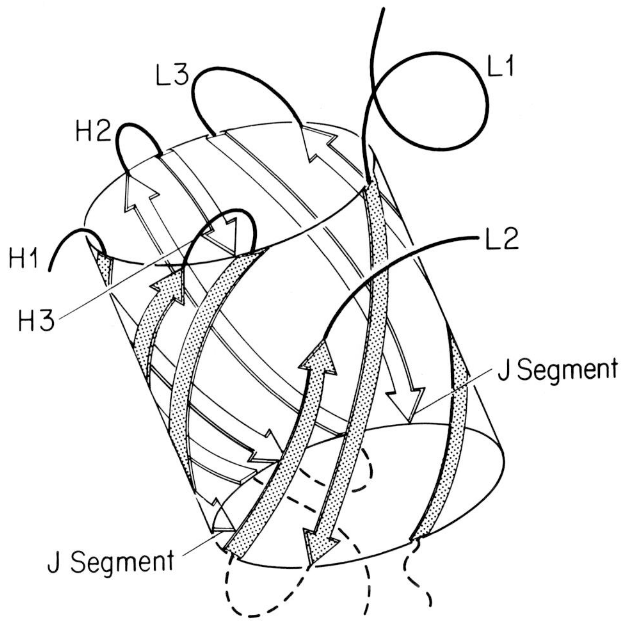

Figure 7. Topology of the binding site barrel. Four hairpin segments organize themselves along a cylindrical surface. The two segments on the right are parts of the light chain. The two segments on the left are parts of the heavy chain. The shapes of the hypervariable loops are indicated schematically, and only their most general features are given. In all three structures studied, the domain–domain interface is closely packed, leaving no free space between the two β-sheets. (Reprinted from Ref. 28 by permission.)

seems to be characteristic of the V_L–V_H interface and gives rise to a paradoxical existence of a third "β-barrel" formed by walls of the two interacting β-barrels of V_L and V_H domains[23] (Fig. 5).

The unique geometry of the antibody-binding site barrel has been studied quantitatively by measuring its dimensions and by least-squares fitting of well-defined mathematical surfaces into the polypeptide backbones that form the β-barrel.[28] It is found that the V_L–V_H interface has an elliptical, or rather prismatic, cross section with the major and minor semiaxes of about 1 and 0.7 nm, respectively, and its top-to-bottom twist of 210°. This geometry seems to be very well conserved, since all the crystallographic structures studied so far give virtually identical geometrical parameters.

Conservation of the geometry of the interface is in strong contrast with variability of the hypervariable loops that provide connections between the β-strands of the interface barrel. The underlying amino acid sequences are displayed in Fig. 6 and a schematic picture of the binding region is shown in Fig. 7. It is interesting to note that one of the β-strands in each of the domains corresponds to the so-called J piece, i.e., it is coded for by the "J" gene segment separate from the rest of the variable region gene by an intron.[5,29,30] The region of V gene–J gene junction maps into the L3 and H3 hypervariable loops and it is evident that a substantial part of amino acid sequence variability is generated by various ways of splicing the two gene segments together. In the heavy chain genes, there is a third short gene segment, D, that becomes inserted in between the V–J junction[2,31]; the D segment corresponds exactly to the H3 loop.

A picture that emerges from the structural analysis is that of a conserved structural scaffold (the V_L–V_H interface β-barrel) on which the hypervariable regions are attached. While it is obvious that amino acid sequence variations in the hypervariable loops change the shape of the outer parts of the binding site, it is more difficult to account for that part of antibody specificity modulation that is mediated by hypervariable residues participating in formation of the bottom of the binding site.[32,33] A number of hypervariable positions are, in fact, buried from the solvent, being part of the β-strands and mediating the V_L–V_H contacts. The total contact surfaces between V_L and V_H domains are 17.56 nm^2 in the Fab fragment KOL, 19.39 nm^2 in the Fab fragment MCPC 603, and 17.09 nm^2 in the Fab fragment NEW. Thus, the average interface area of a single variable domain is 9 nm^2, 36% of which consists of polar residues. The hypervariable loops contribute about half of the total contact surface (47% in KOL, 53% in MCPC 603, and 42% in NEW[28]).

When the effect of amino acid substitutions on antibody specificity is studied, it can be seen that single-residue exchanges at the bottom of the binding site and inaccessible to solvent or antigen have a dramatic effect on antibody specificity. In particular, side chains of residues Leu-L96, Glu-H35, and Asp-H101, known to be indispensable for the specificity of phosphorylcholine-binding myelomas,[34–36] are either totally or partially buried in the V_L–V_H interface. Other hypervariable residues, such as carboxy-terminal parts of L1 and H1 or amino-terminal parts of J gene segments, also form part of the V_L–V_H contact surface. One is therefore left with an interesting conclusion that the domain–domain contact surface, even though it is not accessible in the free antibody structure, is directly involved in antibody specificity. It is possible that, due to the close packing at the interface, changes in volumes of buried side chains may induce changes in the bottom surface of the binding site. Such a result would be consistent with the structural variability found in hemoglobins and the core of immunoglobulin domains. Alternatively, structural changes induced by antigen binding could expose some of these buried residues. It has indeed been observed by direct X-ray crystallography that conformation of amino acid side chains at the binding site of the V_L–V_L dimer MCG rearranges when large aromatic ligands are introduced.[37]

3. Digoxin-Specific Monoclonal Antibodies

A detailed crystallographic study of a set of immunoglobulins binding the same antigen is not yet available. Thus, detailed variations in the three-dimensional structure of the site in terms of specific antigen recognition cannot yet be examined. Much can be learned, however, by studying the variation in

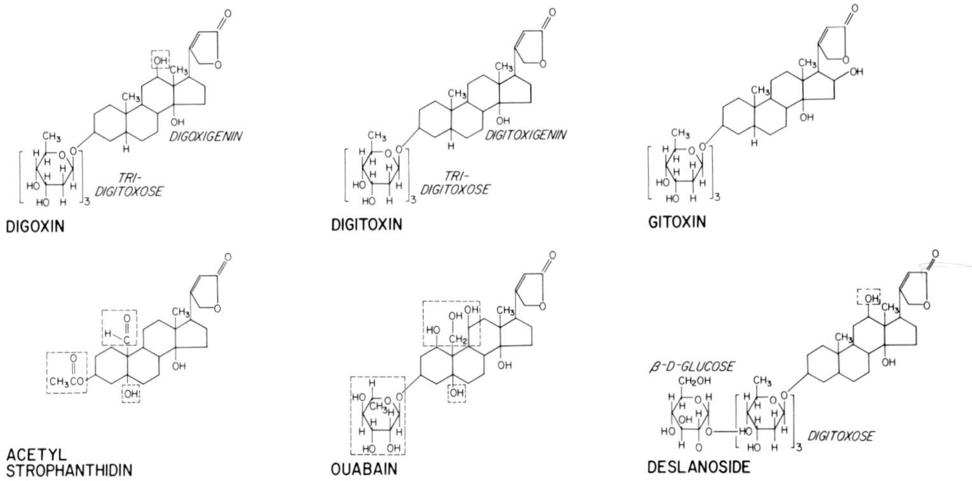

Figure 8. Structures of digoxin and related cardiac glycosides. Differences in steroid ring substitutions are indicated by broken lines. (Reprinted from Ref. 58.)

amino acid sequence within the combining site in relation to antigen binding specificity. We have elected to study a set of monoclonal antibodies specific for digoxin, because this provides an opportunity to examine fine specificity of binding in a high-affinity system with a very large ligand, the crystallographic coordinates of which are fully available.

Digoxin, in contrast to other haptens, is a relatively large organic molecule (Fig. 8), measuring 31 × 8 × 9 Å, which allows it to occupy nearly completely a typical antibody combining site, 34 × 12 × 7 Å.[38] Its molecular structure[39] and that of five analogues have been determined by X-ray crystallography. The molecule consists of a steroid backbone, a lactone ring, and three digitoxose sugars (Fig. 8). Of particular interest in immunologic studies is the rigidity of the steroid ring, which does not allow major conformational changes when functional groups are substituted. There are 64 available structural analogues that differ in substitutions on the steroid ring and in the number and identity of sugar residues, permitting an examination of fine antibody specificity.[40]

3.1. Production of Digoxin-Specific Monoclonal Antibodies

The immunizing antigen was synthesized by covalently coupling digoxin through its terminal digitoxose moiety to human serum albumin, utilizing periodate oxidation of the terminal digitoxose sugar.[41] Four strains of mice were examined, BALB/c, SWR/J, RF/J and A/J, but only A/J mice gave a significant positive primary response to digoxin.[42] The frequency of digoxin-specific precursor B cells in adult A/J mice was determined to be 1/35,000. The A/J mice were thus selected as the strain used in subsequent fusion experiments.

Immunizations were carried out intraperitoneally utilizing complete Freund's adjuvant followed by intravenous boosting. Somatic cell fusion was carried out by the general approach of Köhler and Milstein,[43] utilizing secreting cell lines in early experiments. Later, the nonsecreting line Sp2/0-Ag1431 was used exclusively in order to avoid the problem of mixed-chain molecules for affinity and structure studies. The RIA used for screening culture media from fusion wells for antidigoxin antibody is based on that reported by Klinman *et al.*,[44] using digoxin-hemocyanin as antigen. The hybridoma cultures were amplified in the ascites of BALB/c × A/J mice.

3.2. Characterization of Digoxin-Specific Monoclonal Antibodies

Digoxin-specific hybridoma proteins were purified from ascites by ion-exchange chromatography on DEAE-cellulose, or affinity chromatography on digoxin-BSA-Sepharose or ouabain-amine-Sepharose. The average intrinsic affinity constant K_0 was determined for each subcloned antidigoxin hybridoma present in the culture media or after purification from ascites. An RIA utilizing ^{3}H-digoxin and dextran-coated charcoal to separate free ^{3}H-digoxin from antibody-bound digoxin was used. This method has been shown previously to yield affinity data comparable to those obtained by equilibrium dialysis using rabbit antiouabain antisera.[45] The specificity of each antidigoxin antibody for related cardiac glycosides was assessed by the inhibition of binding of antibody in the dextran-charcoal RIA.[45] Each of the compounds in Table I, in addition to digoxin, was tested with this method to determine the amount of the compound required to achieve 50% inhibition relative to that required for unlabeled digoxin. Amino acid sequence analysis of heavy and light chains and peptide fragments were done by Edman degradation in a modified Beckman spinning cup sequencer,[46,47] and Pth-amino acids were analyzed by high pressure liquid chromatography.[48,49]

More than 20 subcloned digoxin-specific monoclonal antibodies are now available for study. Of these, 12 have been examined in detail with respect to affinity, specificity, and partial amino acid sequence. The isotype and affinity of each monoclonal antibody are shown in Table II. All but three of the proteins are IgG1 in isotype, and the others are either IgG2a or IgG2b. The affinity for digoxin of all of the antibodies is very high, ranging from 1.1×10^9 to 1.7×10^{12}.

Figure 8 details the structures of the cardiac glycosides and aglycones used in fine specificity analysis. Structural differences that proved to have significant consequences with respect to antigenic recognition include: the presence or absence of sugar moieties (e.g., digitoxin vs. digitoxigenin); substitutions on the A and B rings (digoxin vs. ouabain or acetylstrophanthidin); a substitution on the C ring (12-OH) that differentiates digoxin from digitoxin; or substitution on the D ring (16-OH) that differentiates gitoxin from digitoxin. The two typical sets of binding curves shown in Fig. 9 compare the binding of selected compounds to two different monoclonal antibodies. For hybridoma 40-160, note

Table I. Concentration of Inhibitor Relative to Digoxin Giving 50% Inhibition of ^{3}H-Digoxin Binding, Grouped by Inhibition Sets[a]

	Antibody	Digoxigenin	Digitoxin	Digitoxigenin	Deslanoside	Gitoxin	Ouabain	Acetylstrophanthidin
A	26-10	1.1	1.2	3.5	0.93	3.5	66	1.5
A_1	45-20	2.4	1.6	17.1	n.d.	24	10.6	12.8
B	35-20	0.85	3.0	2.5	0.88	20	350	110
C	40-160	3.7	1.1	10	0.91	29	140	32
D_1	40-020	7.7	95	>1000	0.91	(29)	>1000	>100
	40-090	9.6	80	>1000	0.98	40	>1000	>1000
	40-100	9.1	94	>1000	0.99	34	>1000	>1000
D_2	40-060	16	120	>1000	0.99	44	>1000	>1000
E_1	40-040	13	2.6	49	1.1	23	>1000	>100
	40-140	13	1.2	21	1.0	34	>1000	>100
E_2	40-10	20	1.4	120	1.0	27	>1000	440
F	45-10	16	9.1	196	n.d.	47	>1000	>1000

[a] Reprinted from Ref. 58. n.d., Not determined.

Table II. Binding Affinities of Antidigoxin Hybridomas[a]

Antidigoxin antibody	Isotype	K_0
Dig 26-10	$IgG2_a$, κ	6.9×10^9
Dig 35-20	IgG1, κ	1.9×10^9
Dig 40-020	IgG1, κ	1.7×10^9
Dig 40-040	IgG1, κ	3.0×10^{11}
Dig 40-060	IgG1, κ	6.2×10^9
Dig 40-090	IgG1, κ	3.8×10^{10}
Dig 40-100	IgG1, κ	6.4×10^9
Dig 40-120	$IgG2_a$, κ	2.6×10^{11}
Dig 40-140	IgG1, κ	1.1×10^9
Dig 40-160	IgG1, κ	2.6×10^{11}
Dig 45-20	$IgG2_a$, λ	1.7×10^{12}

[a] From Ref. 58.

that the binding of digoxin, digitoxin, and deslanoside are indistinguishable. Thus, the presence or absence of 12-OH or the addition of D-glucose to the third digitoxose sugar appears to have no influence. Digoxigenin and digitoxigenin bind less well, indicating significant participation of the digitoxose sugars. Acetylstrophanthidin, ouabain, and gitoxin bind still less well. While several changes characterize the difference between digoxin and acetylstrophanthidin

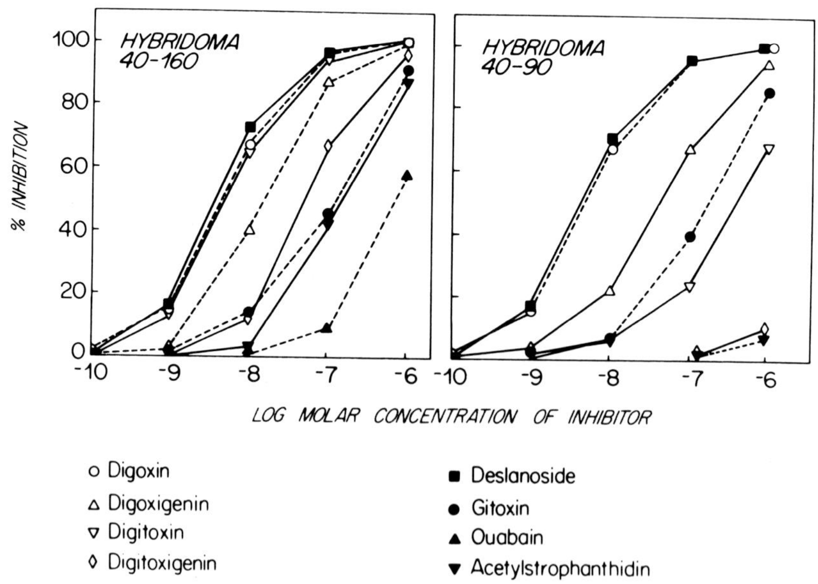

Figure 9. Inhibition of binding of two monoclonal antibodies (40-160; 40-090) to ^3H-digoxin by various cardiac glycosides, using a dextran-coated charcoal radioimmunoassay. (Reprinted from Ref. 58.)

and ouabain (these include both alterations in the sugars and changes in substitutions on the A and B rings), gitoxin differs from digitoxin only in the absence of 12-OH and the presence of 16-OH. Since 12-OH is not involved in antigen recognition (no difference between digoxin and digitoxin), a structure on the D ring, 16-OH, interferes with binding. Thus, in the case of antibody 40-160, it is likely that the antibody combining site is in contact with both the digitoxose sugars and the D ring of the steroid, two rather distant parts of the molecule, without being significantly influenced by structures in between.

The inhibition profile of hybridoma 40-090 in Fig. 9 is quite different from that of 40-160. Here, only deslanoside binds with equal affinity to digoxin, indicating that the terminal glucose sugar does not participate in antigen binding. In contrast to 40-160, removal of 12-OH causes a profound diminution in binding. As in 40-060, removal of the digitoxose sugars or addition of substitutions on the A, B, and C rings significantly affects binding. Thus, for antibody 40-090, the A, B, and C rings of the steroid, as well as at least the first digitoxose sugar, are in contact with the antibody combining site.

Similar studies were carried out with each of 12 monoclonal antibodies; the results are summarized in Table I. The table lists the concentrations of unlabeled inhibitor (as a multiple of the concentration of digoxin = 1.0) required to effect 50% inhibition of binding of ^{3}H-digoxin. The 12 monoclonal antibodies can be divided into nine sets by virtue of a similar specificity profile; for example, 45-20 and 26-10, shown at the top, recognize all of the compounds with very similar affinities. Minor differences between these include a lesser binding of ouabain by 26-10 and diminished binding of digitoxigenin and gitoxin by 45-020. Antibody 35-20 differs from 26-10 in that it recognizes all compounds tested equally except ouabain and acetylstrophanthidin. Hybridoma 26-10 does not differentiate among any of the compounds except ouabain. The difference in structure between ouabain and acetylstrophanthidin is the presence of substitutions on the β surface of the ring in the former, but not present in the latter. Thus, binding to one surface of the steroid A and B rings, as opposed to the other, differentiates the two specificities. In groups D1 and D2, the presence of the 12-OH and the presence of the digitoxose sugars are both important, as shown by the significant reduction of binding when either digitoxin or digoxigenin is compared to digoxin. In groups E1 and E2, neither 12-OH nor the sugars are of importance, although substitutions of any kind on the A and B rings eliminate measurable binding. Group F is similar, although there is somewhat more influence of sugars and 12-OH.

3.3. Amino Acid Sequence Studies

Partial amino acid sequence data from both the heavy and the light chains of the 12 monoclonal antibodies are shown in Figs. 10 and 11. Both light and heavy chains can be divided into at least five and six homology groups, respectively. Thus, because of several repeats in some of these sets, a limited number of V_H and/or V_L region genes may be selected among digoxin-specific

```
          1       10        20        30   35a   40        50 52a      60
26-10     EVQLQQSGPELVKPGASVRMSCKSSGYIFTDFYMN·WVRQSHGKSLDYIGYISPYSGVTGYNQLF

40-120    DVQLQESGPGLVKPSQSLSLTCTVTGYSITSDYAWSWIRQFPGNKLEWMGYIT.YNGY
40-040    -------------------------------------- --------------.----
40-140    --------------------------------------------R--------
40-160    -------------------------------Y--------
35-20     ----------------------------F--E---N----------------S.-S-S

40-020    EVHLVESGGGLVKPGGSLKLSCVASGFTFSSYAM·SWVRQTPEKRLEWVGGIS·SGDGYTYYPDTVKGRFTI
40-060    ------------------------------T---·------------------·------
40-090    ----------------------------------·------ -- --------·---
40-100    ----------------------------------·---------------

45-020    EVQLVESGGDLVEPGGSLKLSCAA GFISNNYAM·EW  Q PG

40-150    DVKLVESGGGLVKPGGSLKLSCAASGFTFRSYYM.AWVRQIPDKRLEWVATIS.ISDIYTYYPDNV

40-050    Blocked
```

Figure 10. Partial amino acid sequences of antidigoxin hybridoma heavy chains. A one-letter code is used.[57] Numbering is according to Kabat *et al.*[56] The sequences are arbitrarily divided into six homology sets. In each set the sequences are compared to the topmost member of the set. Lines indicate identity with the sequence above. (Reprinted from Ref. 58.)

antibodies (although this conclusion must be confirmed when fusion products from additional individual animals can be examined, since eight of the 12 antibodies derive from the same fusion). It is of great interest that similar light chains can be associated with different heavy chains; 26-10, which has a unique heavy chain not homologous with any in this set, has a light chain similar to those utilized in antibodies 40-060, 40-090, and 40-100, confirming the hypothesis that permutations of light and heavy chains may play a role in the generation of antibody diversity. On the other hand, another homology group of heavy chains, 40-120, 40-040, 40-140, 40-160, and 35-20, are each associated with the same group of light chains that are very closely related to one another. This set of light chains differs from six other antidigoxin light chains sequenced, in that they are five residues shorter in CDR1. Of the third homology group of heavy chains in Fig. 10, three members, 40-090, 40-060, and 40-100, share the same homology group of light chains (sequence data are unavailable for 40-020). Thus, the majority of heavy chain sets (possibly representing V_H gene families or even somatic mutants of the same V_H gene) associate with the same light chain set, although exceptions occur. These findings can be compared to observations made with a set of phosphorylcholine-specific hybridomas[50] in which a single V_H gene product appears to be associated with one of three $V\kappa$ gene products. A second V_H gene product is only occasionally used.

V_H region gene sets do not appear to determine antigen-binding specificity. Within each set, varied fine specificities for hapten are found. Even the second homology set of heavy chains in Fig. 10 (40-120, etc.) that is associated with

```
               1       10        20     27abcde 30        40        50        60
26-10          DVVMTQTPLSLPVSLGDQASISCRSSQSLVHSNGNTYLNWYLQKAGQSPKLLIYKVSNRFSGVPD
40-060         -------------------------------------- -----P----------
40-090         ---------------------F---------------- -----P-----
40-100         ---------------------F---------------- -----P-------- -

40-150         DVVMTQT LQL   IGQPASISCKSSQ LLNSDGQ Y

40-040         DIKMTQSPSSMYASLGERVTITCKASQ·····DINSYLSWFQQKPGKSPKTLIY TK LVDG
40-160         -- --------------------- --·····------- -  ----
40-140         ---------------------------·····-------------     ----
40-120         ---L---------------I-------·····--D--------------- ---R--R----
35-20          -----------F---------------·····------N-------R---I---RANR----

40-050         DIVLTQSPASLAVSLGQRATISCRASKSVST·SGYSHIHWYQQK

45-020         BLOCKED
```

Figure 11. Partial amino acid sequences of antidigoxin hybridoma light chains. The sequences are divided arbitrarily into five homology sets. For further details see legend to Fig. 10. (Reprinted from Ref. 58.)

a single homology set of light chains is characterized by at least four distinguishable sets of antigen-binding specificities (Table I). Of course, sequence analysis is as yet incomplete and these variable regions may well be associated with different D or J genes, or alternatively, somatic mutation may be decisive in altering specificity.

Each of these monoclonal antibodies, with the exception of 40-090 and 40-100, has been distinguished by possessing either a unique amino acid sequence, antigen specificity profile, or V_H gene based upon Southern blots of hybridoma DNA (R. Near, personal communication). While 26-10 and 45-020 have similar, although not identical specificities, they have very different V_H and V_L sequences (see Fig. 10). Although 40-040 and 40-140 have identical partial V_L and identical V_H sequences, save one substitution at position 44 in V_H, they utilize different V_H genes based on DNA Southern blots using a J probe (R. Near, personal communication). The pair of antibodies 40-040 and 40-120 have identical partial V_H sequences. Southern blots suggest that the same V_H and J_H gene is used for both. Their affinities for digoxin are identical within experimental error (3.0×10^{11} and 2.6×10^{11} in Table II) and they fall into similar specificity groups (E1 and E2 in Table I), differing only significantly in digitoxigenin binding. Yet, they differ at six amino acid residues out of 60 light chain positions sequenced.

It is now apparent that a further understanding of the determinants of fine specificity must await the determination of the complete sequence of a number of closely related antibodies. The complete variable domain sequence of antibody 26-10 has been determined (J. Novotný and M. N. Margolies, unpublished data) (Fig. 12). The heavy chain J region of 26-10 is unusual in that it is derived from the J_H4 gene by two somatic mutations (positions 111 and 113

H Chain

```
1                 10                    20                    30                    40
E V Q L Q Q S G P E L V K P G A S V R M S C K S S G Y I F T D F Y M N W V R Q S

                  50                    60                    70                    80
H G K S L D Y I G Y I S P Y S G V T G Y N Q K F K G K A T L T V D K S S S T A Y

                  90                    100                   110
M E L R S L T S E D S A V Y Y C A G S S G N K W A M D Y W G H G A S V T V S S
```

L Chain

```
1                 10                    20                    30
D V V M T A T P L S L P V S L G D Q A S I S C R S S Q S L V H S N G N T Y L N

40                    50                    60                    70
W Y L Q K A G Q S P K L L I Y K V S N R F S G V P D R F S G S G S G T D F T L

  80                    90                    100                   110
K I S R V E A E D L G I Y F C S Q T T H V P P T F G G G T K L E I K R
```

Figure 12. The complete variable domain amino acid sequence of the antidigoxin hybridoma 26-10 (J. Novotný and M. N. Margolies, unpublished data). Complementarity-determining regions are enclosed within boxes. Fab fragments of this hybridoma have been successfully crystallized.[51] (Reprinted from Ref. 58.)

in Fig. 12). The nearly complete variable region sequence of the unrelated antidigoxin antibody 35-20 (not shown) has also been determined. Antibody 35-20 utilizes an entirely different V_H and D gene. The remarkable differences that are apparent throughout the variable region indicate the convergence of two very different structural solutions for binding the same ligand.

A rigorous approach to understanding fine specificity is the construction of a three-dimensional model of the antibody combining site. Antibody 26-10 has now been crystallized with and without digoxin in the combining site.[51] We eagerly await the uncovering of structural details.

4. A Look into the Future

One might now ask whether the systematic exploration of variable region sequences of antibodies of defined specificity will ever lead to a detailed understanding of structure–function relationships in the antibody combining site. Some rather interesting insights have already been obtained from spontaneous mutants occurring in the phosphorylcholine system (see above). We have described here sequence variations in antidigoxin monoclonal antibodies that are likely responsible for alterations in antigen binding. These molecules, and those reported for the phosphorylcholine system, were selected for study by screening products of somatic cell fusion or mutant myelomas selected *in vitro*. Perhaps a more directed approach than waiting for the desired mutations to appear is required. As discussed above, the digoxin-specific antibody 26-10 of known amino acid sequence is presently being studied by X-ray crystallography,[51] and we shall soon know the precise relationship between the atoms of the ligand and the antibody combining site. Yet it is too much to expect that an entire set of digoxin-specific antibodies can be examined by X-ray crystallography, since this method depends primarily on luck to produce suitable crystals and their isomorphous derivatives, and secondarily, on long and arduous effort. Since it appears that a member of the V_H germ-line gene family of 35-20 is available, it may be possible to utilize it as a probe to isolate the rearranged gene from the hybridoma. The techniques for inserting such cloned germ-line genes into myeloma cell cultures and expressing the resulting immunoglobulin efficiently have now been developed.[52,53] It is only a short step to applying site-directed mutagenesis of the cloned gene. When this is accomplished, one can ask direct and critical questions concerning the role of each amino acid side chain in the antibody combining site or idiotope. It should also be possible to learn the rules for combining site construction, so that antibody specificity may be dictated and refined at will.

ACKNOWLEDGMENT. This work was supported by USPHS NIH grant #5 RO1 HL19259, Antibodies as Tools in Cardiovascular Research.

References

1. Brack, C., Hirama, M., Lenhard-Schuller, R., and Tonegawa, S., 1978, A complete immunoglobulin gene is created by somatic recombination, *Cell* **15**:1–14.
2. Sakano, H., Kurosawa, Y., Weigert, M., and Tonegawa, S., 1981, Identification and nucleotide sequence of a diversity DNA segment (D) of immunoglobulin heavy-chain genes, *Nature* **290**:562–565.
3. Seidman, J. G., Leder, A., Nau, M., Norman, B., and Leder, P., 1978, Antibody diversity: The structure of cloned immunoglobulin genes suggests a mechanism for generating new sequences, *Science* **202**:11–17.
4. Seidman, J. G., Max, E. E., and Leder, P., 1979, A kappa-immunoglobulin gene is formed by site-specific recombination without further somatic mutation, *Nature* **280**:370–375.
5. Early, P., Huang, H., Davis, M., Calame, K., and Hood, L., 1980, An immunoglobulin heavy chain variable region gene is generated from three segments of DNA: V_H, D, and J_H, *Cell* **19**:981–992.
6. Weigert, M., Gatmaitan, L., Loh, E., Schilling, J., and Hood, L., 1978, Rearrangement of genetic information may produce immunoglobulin diversity, *Nature* **276**:785–790.
7. Tonegawa, S., 1983, Somatic generation of antibody diversity, *Nature* **302**:575–581.

8. Gearhart P. J., 1983, Effect of somatic mutation on antibody affinity, *Ann. N.Y. Acad. Sci.* **418**:171–176.
9. Clarke, S. H., Claflin, J. L., and Rudikoff, S., 1982, Polymorphisms in immunoglobulin heavy chains suggesting gene conversion, *Proc. Natl. Acad. Sci. USA* **79**:3280–3284.
10. Singer, S. J., and Doolittle R. F., 1966, Antibody active sites and immunoglobulin chains, *Science* **153**:13–25.
11. Hill, R. L., Delaney, R., Fellows, R. E., and Lebovitz, H. E., 1966, The evolutionary origins of the immunoglobulins, *Proc. Natl. Acad. Sci. USA* **56**:1762–1769.
12. Edelman, G. M., 1970, The covalent structure of a human gamma G-immunoglobulin. XI. Functional implications, *Biochemistry* **9**:3197–3205.
13. Hilschmann, N., and Craig, L. C., 1965, Amino acid sequence studies with Bence-Jones proteins, *Proc. Natl. Acad. Sci. USA* **53**:1403–1409.
14. Titani, K., Whitely, E., Avogardo, L., Putnam, F. M., 1965, Immunoglobulin structure: Partial amino acid sequence of a Bence-Jones protein, *Science* **149**:1090–1092.
15. Hochman, J., Inbar, D., and Givol, D., 1973, An active antibody fragment (Fv) composed of the variable portions of heavy and light chains, *Biochemistry* **12**:1130–1135.
16. Wu, T. T., and Kabat, E. A., 1970, An analysis of the sequences of the variable regions of Bence-Jones proteins and myeloma light chains and their implications for antibody complementarity, *J. Exp. Med.* **132**:211–250.
17. Marquart, M., Deisenhofer, J., Huber, R., and Palm, W., 1980, Crystallographic refinement and atomic models of the intact immunoglobulin molecule Kol and its antigen-binding fragment at 3.0 Å and 1.0 Å resolution, *J. Mol. Biol.* **141**:369–391.
18. Saul, F. A., Amzel, L. M., and Poljak, R. J., 1978, Preliminary refinement and structural analysis of the Fab fragment from human immunoglobulin new at 2.0 Å resolution, *J. Biol. Chem.* **253**:585–595.
19. Segal, D. M., Padlan, E. A., Cohen, G. H., Rudikoff, S., Potter, M., and Davies, D. R., 1974, The three-dimensional structure of phosphorylcholine-binding mouse immunoglobulin Fab and the nature of the antigen binding site, *Proc. Natl. Acad. Sci. USA* **71**:4298–4302.
20. Epp, O., Colman, P., Feilhammer, H., Bode, W., Schiffer, M., and Huber, R., 1974, Crystal and molecular structure of a dimer composed of the variable portions of the Bence-Jones protein REI, *Eur. J. Biochem.* **45**:513–524.
21. Schiffer, M., Girling, R. I., Ely, K. R., and Edmundson, A. B., 1973, Structure of a lambda-type Bence-Jones protein at 3.5-Å resolution, *Biochemistry* **12**:1620–1631.
22. Amzel, L. M., Poljak, R. J., Saul, F., Varga, J. M., and Richards, F. F., 1974, The three dimensional structure of a combining region–ligand complex immunoglobulin NEW at 3.5-Å resolution, *Proc. Natl. Acad. Sci. USA* **71**:1427–1430.
23. Richardson, J. S., 1981, The anatomy and taxonomy of protein structure, *Adv. Protein Chem.* **34**:167–339.
24. Lesk, M. A., and Chothia, C., 1982, Evolution of proteins formed by beta-sheets. II. The core of the immunoglobulin domains, *J. Mol. Biol.* **160**:325–342.
25. Edmundson, A. B., Ely, K. R., Abola, E. E., Schiffer, M., and Panagiotopoulos, N., 1975, Rotational allomerism and divergent evolution of domains in immunoglobulin light chains, *Biochemistry* **14**:3953–3961.
26. Pauling, L., and Corey, R. B., 1951, Configurations of polypeptide chains with favored orientations around single bonds: Two new pleated sheets, *Proc. Natl. Acad. Sci. USA* **37**:729–740.
27. Chothia, C., 1973, Conformation of twisted beta-pleated sheets in proteins, *J. Mol. Biol.* **75**:295–302.
28. Novotný, J., Bruccoleri, R., Newell, J., Murphy, D., Haber, E., and Karplus, M., 1983, Molecular anatomy of the antibody combining site, *J. Biol. Chem.* **258**(23):14433–14437.
29. Bernard, O., and Gough, N. M., 1980, Nucleotide sequence of immunoglobulin heavy chain joining segments between translocated V_H and mu constant regions genes, *Proc. Natl. Acad. Sci. USA* **77**:3630–3634.
30. Newell, N., Richards, J. E., Tucker, P. W., and Blattner, F. R., 1980, J genes for heavy chain immunoglobulins of mouse, *Science* **209**:1128–1132.

31. Siebenlist, U., Ravetch J. V., Korsmeyer, S., Waldmann, T., and Leder, P., 1981, Human immunoglobulin D segments encoded in tandem multigenic families, *Nature* **294:**631–635.
32. Stevens, F. J., Westholm, F. A., Solomon, A., and Schiffer, M., 1980, Self-association of human immunoglobulin kappa I light chains: Role of the third hypervariable region, *Proc. Natl. Acad. Sci. USA* **77:**1144–1148.
33. Horne, C., Klein, M., Polidoulis, I., and Dorrington, K. J., 1982, Noncovalent association of heavy and light chains of human immunoglobulins. III. Specific interactions between VH and VL, *J. Immunol.* **129:**660–664.
34. Rudikoff, S., Satow, Y., Padlan, E., Davies, D., and Potter, M., 1981, Kappa chain structure from a crystallized murine Fab′: Role of joining segment in hapten binding, *J. Mol. Immunol.* **18:**705–711.
35. Cook, W. D., Rudikoff, S., Giusti, A., and Scharff, M. D., 1982, Somatic mutation in a cultured mouse myeloma cell affects antigen binding, *Proc. Natl. Acad. Sci. USA* **79:**1240–1244.
36. Rudikoff, S., Giusti, A. M., Cook, W. D., and Scharff, M. D., 1982, Single amino acid substitution altering antigen-binding specificity, *Proc. Natl. Acad. Sci. USA* **79:**1979–1983.
37. Edmundson, A. B., Ely, K. R., and Hurron, J. N., 1984, A search for site-filling ligands in the Mcg Bence-Jones dimer: Crystal binding studies of fluorescent compounds, *Mol. Immunol.* **21:**561–576.
38. Kabat, E. A., 1966, The nature of an antigenic determinant, *J. Immunol.* **97:**1–11.
39. Go, K., Kartha, G., and Chen, J. P., 1980, Structure of digoxin, *Acta Cryst. B* **36:**1811–1819.
40. Fieser, L. F., and Fieser, M., 1959, Cardiac-active principles, in: *Steroids*, Reinhold, New York, pp. 727–809.
41. Smith, T. W., Butler, V. P., and Haber, E., 1970, Characterization of antibodies of high affinity and specificity to the digitalis glycoside digoxin, *Biochemistry* **9:**331–337.
42. Mudgett-Hunter, M., Margolies, M. N., Ju, A., Haber, E., 1982, High-affinity monoclonal antibodies to the cardiac glycoside digoxin, *J. Immunol.* **129:**1165–1172.
43. Köhler, G., and Milstein, C., 1975, Continuous cultures of fused cells secreting antibody of predefined specificity, *Nature* **256:**495–497.
44. Klinman, N. R., Pickard, A. R., Sigal, N. H., Gearhart, P. J., Metcalf, E. S., and Pierce, S. K., 1976, Assessing B cell diversification by antigen receptor and precursor cell analysis, *Ann. Immunol. (Paris)* **127C:**489–502.
45. Smith, T. W., 1972, Ouabain specific antibodies and immunochemical properties and reversal of Na-K-ATPase inhibition, *J. Clin. Invest.* **51:**1583–1593.
46. Brauer, A. W., Margolies, M. N., and Haber, E., 1975, The application of 0.1 M Quadrol to the microsequence of proteins and the sequence of tryptic peptides, *Biochemistry* **14:**3029–3035.
47. Novotný, J., and Margolies, M. N., 1983, Amino acid sequence of light chain variable region from a mouse anti-digoxin hybridoma antibody, *Biochemistry* **22:**1153–1158.
48. Margolies, M. N., and Brauer, A. W., 1978, Protein microsequencing using high pressure liquid chromatography of phenylthiohydantoin amino acids, *J. Chromatogr.* **148:**429–439.
49. Margolies, M. N., Brauer, A. W., Oman, C. L., Klapper, D. G., and Horn, M. J., 1982, Improved automatic conversion for use with a liquid-phase sequencer, in: *Proceedings of IVth International Conference on Methods in Protein Sequence Analysis* (M. Elzinga, ed.), Humana Press, Clifton, New Jersey, pp. 189–203.
50. Clarke, S. H., Claflin, J. L., Potter, M., and Rudikoff, S., 1982, Polymorphisms in anti-phosphocholine antibodies reflecting evolution of immunoglobulin gene families, *J. Exp. Med.* **157:**98–113.
51. Rose, D. R., Seaton, B. A., Petsko, G. A., Novotný, J., Margolies, M. N., Locke, E., and Haber, E., 1983, Crystallization of the Fab fragment of a monoclonal anti-digoxin antibody and its complex with digoxin, *J. Mol. Biol.* **164:**203–206.
52. Alt, F. W., and Baltimore, D., 1982, Joining of immunoglobulin heavy chain gene segments: Implications from a chromosome with evidence of 3 D–J_H fusions, *Proc. Natl. Acad. Sci. USA* **79:**4118–4122.
53. Oi, V. T., Morrison, S. L., Herzenberg, L. A., and Berg, P., 1983, Immunoglobulin gene expression in transformed lymphoid cells, *Proc. Natl. Acad. Sci. USA* **80:**825–829.

54. Poljak, R. J., Amzel, L. M., Avey, H. P., Becka, L. N., and Nisonoff, A., 1972, Structure of Fab′ NEW at 6 Å resolution, *Nature New Biol.* **235**:137–140.
55. Dickerson, R. E., 1983, The DNA helix and how it is read, *Sci. Am.* **246**(6):94–111.
56. Kabat, E. A., Wu, T. T., and Bilofsky, H., 1979, Sequences in immunoglobulin chains: Tabulation and analyses of amino acid sequences of precursors, V-regions, C-regions, J-chains and BP microglobulins, NIH Publication, 80-2008.
57. IUPAC-IUB Commission on Biological Nomenclature, 1968, A one-letter notation for amino acid sequences. Tentative Rules, *J. Biol. Chem.* **243**:3557.
58. Haber, E., and Margolies, M. N., Combining site specificity and idiotypy: A study of antidigoxin and antiarsonate antibodies, in: *The Biology of Idiotypes* (M. I. Greene and A. Nisonoff, eds.), Plenum Press, New York, pp. 141–170.

Chapter 4

The Generation of Better Monoclonal Antibodies through Somatic Mutation

GAD SPIRA, ANTONIO BARGELLESI, ROBERTA R. POLLOCK, HECTOR L. AGUILA, and MATTHEW D. SCHARFF

1. Introduction

Hybridoma technology[1] and the monoclonal antibodies it provides have made it possible to apply serology to many new basic and clinical problems. Among the many benefits of hybridoma technology are the potential of obtaining pure antibodies from impure immunogens, the chemical homogeneity of monoclonal antibodies, making them reliable reagents, the large amounts of antibody that can be generated, and the ability to renew exactly the same antibody whenever it is needed.

The potential of generating a library of monoclonal antibodies specific for a particular antigen has prompted investigators to think more carefully about the kinds of antibodies needed for the specific tasks they hope to accomplish. They can then select the monoclonal that, based on its affinity, specificity, and effector functions, is best suited for that particular task. However, it is not always possible to generate such a library of monoclonal antibodies, either because the antigen of interest is weakly immunogenic or because it elicits antibodies of only one class or subclass.

The need for monoclonals of different classes and subclasses is due to the different properties of each class or subclass. For example, mouse IgM and IgG2 antibodies fix complement, while IgG1 does not and therefore cannot mediate complement-dependent cytotoxicity.[2] IgG3 monoclonals may be relatively insoluble and difficult to use.[3] IgM and IgA antibodies disappear quickly from the circulation, while IgG antibodies persist for longer periods of time. In addition, inherent properties of Ig molecules sometimes make them imperfect reagents. Their multivalency results in the formation of antigen–antibody complexes that can cause tissue damage. The Fc regions of many Ig molecules bind

GAD SPIRA • Faculty of Medicine, Technion, Haifa, Israel. ANTONIO BARGELLESI • Department of Biological Chemistry, University of Genoa, Italy. ROBERTA R. POLLOCK, HECTOR L. AGUILA, and MATTHEW D. SCHARFF • Department of Cell Biology, Albert Einstein College of Medicine, New York, New York 10461.

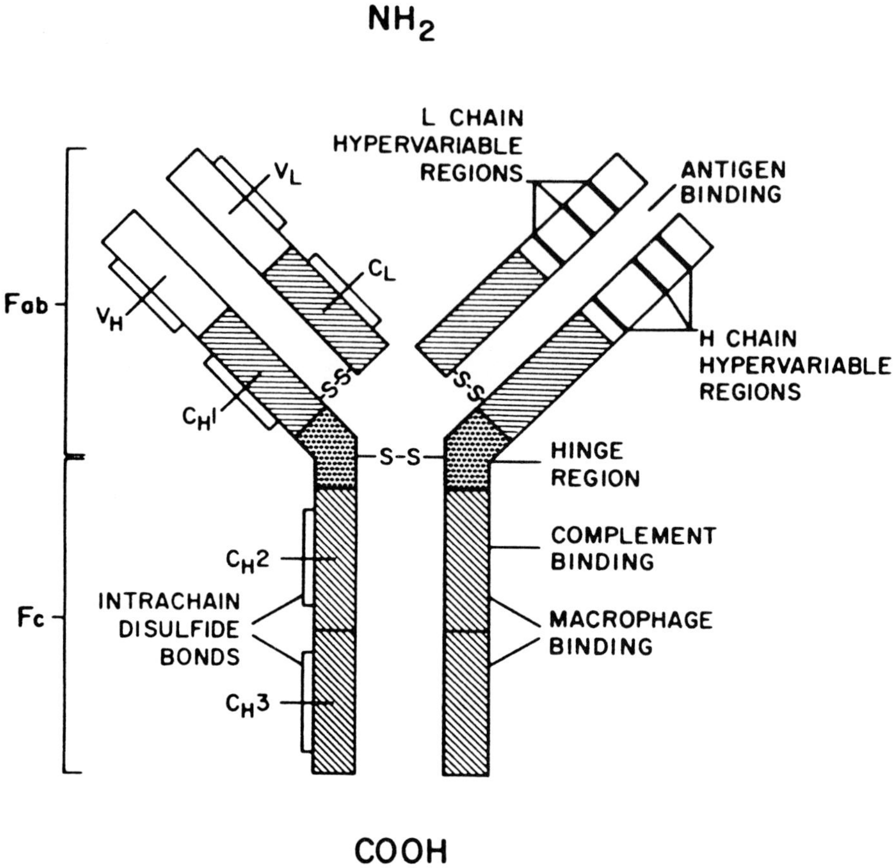

Figure 1. The structure of an IgG antibody molecule.

to receptors on macrophages and many other normal cells, with the result that radioactive monoclonals or monoclonals conjugated to cytotoxic agents will target normal cells as well as cells bearing the tumor or differentiation antigen.

One way to deal with some of these problems is to use enzymatic or chemical cleavage to produce Fab fragments (Fig. 1). Half (HL) molecules can also be generated by reduction of the inter-H-chain disulfide bonds. Such procedures have been used successfully and may be the best way to make monoclonals that will not form antigen–antibody complexes or bind to the Fc receptors. However, the yields of Fab fragments from some monoclonals are low and the intra- and extravascular metabolism of such fragments is quite different than from the intact molecule.

A potential alternative that would still provide homogeneous and reproducible reagents but overcome some of these problems is to isolate structural mutants of particularly useful monoclonals with the goal of further increasing their usefulness. Since hybridomas grow in culture, this may be done by iden-

Table I. Phenotypes of Somatic Mutants of Cultured Antibody-Producing Cells

Changes in Ig expression
Loss mutants (H^-L^+, H^+L^-, H^-L^-)
Quantitative mutants
Changes in Ig structure
Class and subclass switches
Deletions
Point mutations

tifying somatic mutants that have changes in their structure. Such mutants may ultimately be constructed using recombinant DNA technology, but we still need to know more about the structural basis of antibody functions before we can be certain where to introduce site-specific mutations or small deletions. We have therefore taken the approach of isolating somatic mutants in tissue culture and then determining the effect of these mutations on antibody functions.[4] Such studies could also provide valuable information on the molecular genetics of different parts of the Ig genes.

It is possible to isolate somatic mutants with changes in immunoglobulin structure, because of the instability of immunoglobulin genes in cultured myeloma and hybridoma cells.[5] Studies from many laboratories have shown that mutants with a variety of phenotypes occur (Table I). The spontaneous frequency of such mutants is often as high as 10^{-3}–10^{-4} and, where it has been examined, mutagenesis increases this frequency appreciably.[5] Mutations in other genes, such as those involved in drug resistance, arise at frequencies of 10^{-6}–10^{-7}, suggesting that the immunoglobulin genes are uniquely unstable in cultured antibody-forming cells.[5]

Mutants that have lost the ability to produce one or another of the Ig polypeptide chains or have increased immunoglobulin expression (Table I) are important in the hybridoma technology. Nonproducers may arise and take over a culture, causing the loss of a valuable monoclonal. On the other hand, mutants that have increased production make it possible to generate larger amounts of antibody in culture medium and ascitic fluid. These can sometimes be identified by overlaying clones in soft agar with antibody or antigen and recovering those few clones that are surrounded by the largest amounts of antigen–antibody precipitate.[6]

There are three sorts of structural mutants of particular interest in the hybridoma technology: (1) class and subclass switch variants; (2) mutants with deletions or point mutations in the constant region leading to changes in effector functions; and (3) mutants with changes in antigen binding. In the following sections we will discuss techniques for identifying such mutants and discuss examples of each of these phenotypes.

2. Class and Subclass Switch Variants

During normal B-cell development, B cells initially synthesize IgM antibodies and then, as a result of antigenic stimulation and the influence of accessory cells, often differentiate to produce antibodies of the IgG, IgE, and IgA classes.[7] Many years ago we observed that IgG2b-producing myeloma cells often switched to expressing IgG2a molecules, which contained the same variable region as the original cell line.[8] Switches between other IgG subclasses and classes occurred less frequently, but both Rajewsky and his colleagues[9] and Herzenberg and his colleagues[10] showed that such switch variants could be isolated using the fluorescence activated cell sorter. A variety of studies[9–12] led to the suggestion that the molecular mechanisms involved may be different[13] than those that occur *in vivo*.[14] However, since little is known about the molecular events in normal cells,[7,14] this is still an unresolved question. Birshtein and her colleagues[15] have shown that variants with constant regions containing sequences from two different IgG subclasses (hybrid heavy chains) also arise and it is not clear whether or not this happens *in vivo*.

Irrespective of whether the class and subclass switching that occurs in cultured antibody-forming cells is a reflection of normal mechanisms, switch variants can be very useful monoclonal antibodies. While it is clear that such variants can be obtained by cell sorting,[9,10] this technology is not available to all investigators. In addition, it requires that the switch variant express easily detectable amounts of surface Ig. Muller and Rajewsky[16] described an alternative approach based on the technique of sib selection described by Cavalli-Sforza and Lederberg in 1956.[17] We have used a similar approach, which exploits sib selection and an enzyme-linked immunoassay (ELISA).[18]

The general scheme for selecting IgG producers from an IgM-producing hybridoma is illustrated in Fig. 2. The particular hybridoma used in these studies was producing IgM κ antibody that bound phosphorylcholine. Using commercial reagents, we constructed an ELISA assay that would easily detect a small amount of IgG in the presence of a large excess of IgM. This was done by adsorbing affinity-purified anti-IgG to the wells of ELISA plates, incubating with medium containing a mixture of IgM and IgG, and then probing the plate with alkaline phosphatase conjugated to anti-IgG.[18]

Since the frequency of IgM to IgG switches is one in 10^6–10^7 cells and reconstruction experiments revealed that we could detect one IgG-producing cell among 1000 or more IgM-producing cells, we performed the initial sib selection by plating out 1000 cells/well in 20–30 96-well microtiter dishes (Fig. 2). By screening the medium from each well for IgG, we were able to identify rare IgG-producing clones among the approximately $(2–3) \times 10^6$ parental IgM-producing hybridomas.[18] Once a positive well was identified, the cells from that well were plated out at lower cell densities and wells containing IgG-producing cells identified as described above. These wells were considerably enriched for the switch variant and were cloned first by limiting dilution and then in soft agarose.[6,19] An illustrative sib selection of an IgM (PC140.4) to IgG1 (S31.G1) is presented in Fig. 3.

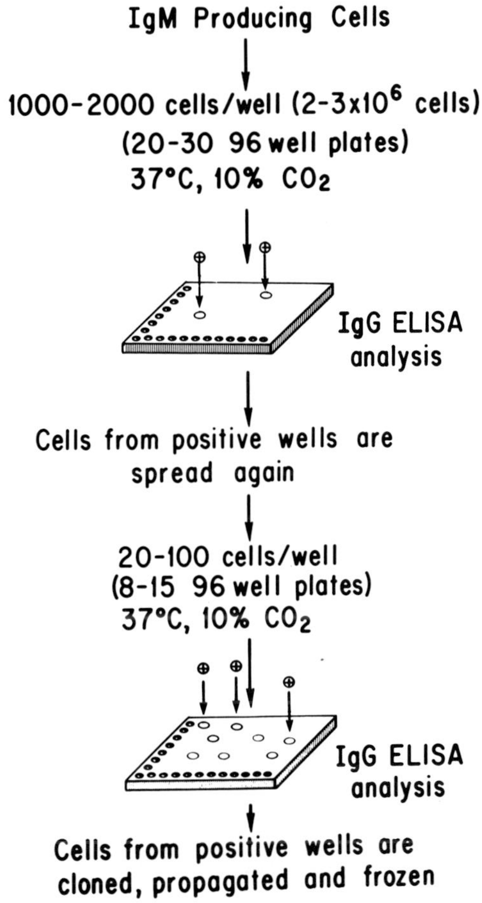

Figure 2. The isolation of IgM to IgG class switch variants.

The sib selection approach has several advantages over cell sorting. It can be used by any laboratory experienced in the hybridoma technology, uses commercially available reagents, and does not require special equipment. Further, one person can identify class and subclass switches even when they are rare and can screen for different Ig subclasses in the same experiment. Finally, switches that do not express membrane Ig are readily identified.

We have now done similar experiments with a number of independent IgM-producing hybridomas and with IgG-producing hybridomas where we wished to obtain a switch from one IgG subclass to another.[18,20,21] We have also obtained sequential switches from IgM to IgG1 and then to IgG2b or IgG2a. In each case it has been possible to obtain the desired switches. Some examples are presented in Table II. The crucial points are: (1) that all of the switches expressed a new constant region but retained the ability to bind the same antigen as the parental hybridoma; (2) irrespective of whether the parental hybridoma expressed surface Ig, both surface-positive and surface-negative switches could be obtained; and (3) most (but not all) of the switches identified

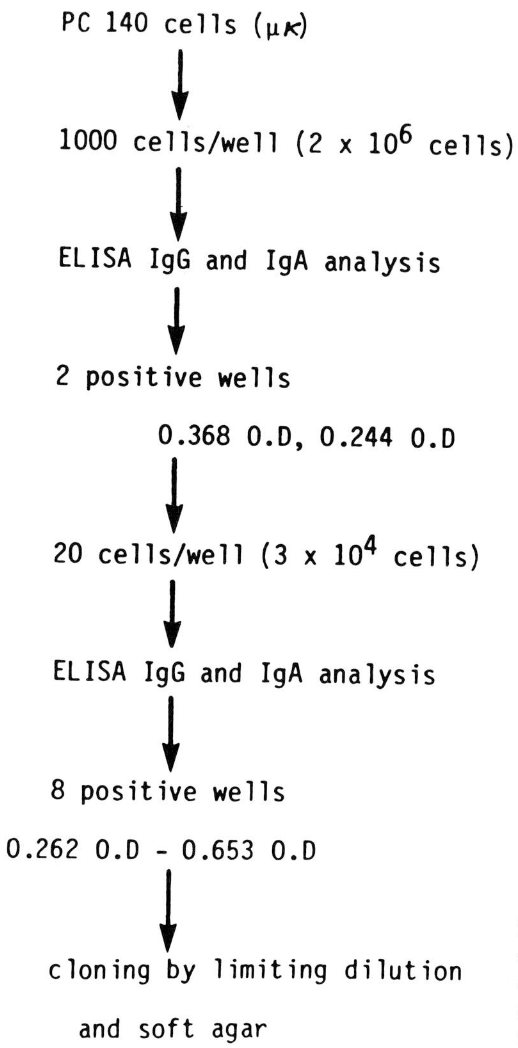

Figure 3. Sib selection of an IgM to IgG class switch variant. Progressive enrichment for the class switch variant was carried out as described in Figure 2. The O.D. of the ELISA reaction of the positive wells is presented.

produced more immunoglobulin than the parental cell. This is not surprising, since the wells containing the most IgG give the strongest signal and are routinely selected for propagation at each step in the sib selection.

Subclass switches obtained by Muller and Rajewsky[22] and by Parham *et al.*[2] were very useful. Likewise, some of the switches described in Table II solved important practical problems. Although many antiphosphorylcholine (PC) hybridomas have been generated in a large number of laboratories, we are only aware of two IgG2b-producing, PC-binding monoclonal antibodies of the T15 idiotype. One of these lacks some of the T15 idiotopes. Using the PC 140 and P223 IgM PC-binding T15 hybridomas, we have been able to generate IgG2b monoclonals either directly from IgM or by sequentially switching from IgM

Table II. Characteristics of Parental Lines and Derived Switches

Cell line				
Parental	Switches	Ig class[a]	Surface Ig	Antigen binding
PC 140.4	—	IgM	+	+[d]
	S31.G1	IgG1	+	+
	S31.G_b[b]	IgG2b	+	+
	S31.G_a[b]	IgG2a	±[c]	+
PC 140.4.1	—	IgM	+	+[d]
	S31.L1	IgG1	−	+
P223.B3	—	IgM	+	+[d]
	8A1.G_b	IgG2b	−	+
P223.B3.1	—	IgM	+	+[d]
	8A1.L1	IgG1	−	+
5/9	—	IgG3	+	+[e]
	1/12	IgG1	+	+
	6/12	IgG1	+	+
	7/7	IgG2b	+	+
	8/8	IgG2a	+	+

[a] All cell lines have κ light chain.
[b] Secondary switch from S31.G1.
[c] Less than 6% of the cells are surface Ig positive.
[d] Phosphorylcholine binding.
[e] Binds human T4 helper cells.

to IgG1 to IgG2b (Table II). We have also generated IgG2a T15 PC-binding switches which were previously unavailable.

The 5.9 monoclonal is an unusual reagent, which recognizes 5–15% of human T4 helper cells.[23] However, 5.9 is a cryoglobulin and precipitates irreversibly in the cold, making it difficult to store or ship. By switching its variable region from the relatively insoluble γ3 to the more soluble γ1 constant region, it was possible to greatly increase its solubility while maintaining its specificity, thus making it a more useful reagent.[20] We have also generated IgG1 to IgG2a switches with a monoclonal that recognizes an antigen on the surface of colonic cancer cells. The IgG2a antibody mediates antibody-dependent, macrophage-mediated cytotoxicity for the tumor cells.[21]

These examples reveal the potential usefulness of class and subclass switches and it is likely that this will become a standard adjunct to the hybridoma technology. The detailed analysis of the genetics and molecular biology of these events should provide insight into the mechanism by which class switching occurs in culture cells and may also be useful in studying regulatory aspects of the immunoglobulin class and subclass switches.

3. Deletion Mutants

A second major class of mutants that we have generated have deletions involving all or most of their C_H2 or C_H3 domains (see Fig. 1). In the example

Table III. Structural and Functional Characteristics of Ar13.4 Mutant Monoclonals

Cell line	H Chain size,[a] kD	Domain predominately affected	Assembly		Binding to Fc receptor	Fixation to complement[b]
			H_2L_2,%	HL, %		
Ar13.4	55	—	100	0	+	+
ArM1	39	C_H3	27	73	−	+
ArM2	41	C_H3	18	83	−	+
ArM16	39	C_H2	100	0	−	−
ArM20	39	C_H2	100	0	−	−

[a] The size of the heavy chains was measured on unglycosylated proteins synthesized in the presence of tunicamycin.
[b] Complement fixation was measured with H_2L_2 molecules of ArM1 and ArM2.

we will describe, we started with a hybridoma secreting an IgG2b κ antibody that binds azophenylarsonate (Ars). Because deletion mutants are relatively rare, the cells were mutagenized and then cloned in soft agarose and overlayed with antisera that reacted with determinants on the C_H3 or C_H2 domain. Unstained clones were marked and then the dishes were overlayed with an antiserum that reacted with determinants throughout the IgG2b molecule. Clones that were unstained with the first antibody and then became stained with the second were recovered. Approximately 0.05% of the clones were deletion mutants.[24]

The general characteristics of these mutants is described in Table III. All of the mutants have smaller H chains than the parent and indirect evidence suggests that they are lacking all or most of either the C_H2 or C_H3 domain. Mutants missing determinants in the C_H2 domain do not bind complement and are not glycosylated, as would be suggested from many other studies. However, they do assemble into H_2L_2 molecules.[24]

Mutants with deletions involving their C_H3 domains are partially blocked in assembly, confirming the importance of the C_H3 domain in the noncovalent association of heavy chains. The assembled molecules do fix complement.[24]

Neither type of mutant binds to the Fc receptors on macrophages or on B cells. However, another mutant, called M3.11, which lacks all of its C_H3 domain and has an asparagine instead of a lysine as the COOH-terminal residue of its C_H2 domain,[25] binds to macrophage but not to B-cell receptors.[26] The mutant M3.11 migrates slightly faster than M1 on SDS gels and the determination of the structural basis for this difference may provide insight into the sequences required for binding to macrophage Fc receptors.

The rate at which monoclonal antibodies disappear from the circulation will play a crucial role in their effectiveness in passive immunization and in targeting to tumors. For example, an antibody that persists for long periods of time will be a more effective agent in protecting against toxins or infectious agents, while one that disappears more rapidly may target tumors more specifically. While it is known that the Fc region determines the intravascular metabolism of immunoglobulins,[27,28] the exact location of the amino acid sequences that determine the serum half-life have not yet been determined. The importance of sequences or conformations in both the C_H2 and C_H3 domains was confirmed by the fact that mutants with deletions of either of these domains differ from the intact IgG2b molecule in their intravascular half-life. A larger portion of mutants with both sorts of deletions leaves the intravascular space during the first 24 hr after injection. In addition, the 10% or so of antibody that remain in the circulation decays with a slightly faster half-life than the parents.[29]

4. Antigen Binding Mutants

The third type of somatic mutants, which we believe will ultimately be very useful, are ones with single amino acid substitutions in their variable regions that have led to a change in antigen binding. Because many monoclonal antibodies have moderate or low affinities, it would obviously be useful to be able to select for somatic mutants in tissue culture with higher affinities. In principle this should be possible, since some of the monoclonal antibodies that differ by one or a few amino acid substitutions from the germ-line gene that codes for them have higher affinities than monoclonals with the germ-line sequence.[30,31] However, we are not aware of an example of a mutant monoclonal that has been generated in tissue culture and has a higher affinity, probably because such mutants will be difficult to identify. Rajewsky and his colleagues have identified somatic variants of monoclonal antibodies that have changes in their amino acid sequence.[32] We have identified similar mutants using a cultured mouse myeloma cell (S107).[4] This S107 myeloma cell line produces an IgA κ antibody that binds phosphorylcholine (PC), is of the T15 idiotype, and has the germ-line sequence in its heavy and light chain variable region. This is the same antibody that is made by BALB/c[33] and other mice in response to immunization with some bacterial polysaccharides.

By overlaying clones in agar with antigen, we have been able to detect mutants with decreases in antigen binding. Such mutants arise spontaneously in some clones at frequencies as high as 0.1%.[24] This decrease in antigen binding is due to single amino acid substitutions in the heavy chain variable region.[35,36] In one of these mutants, U4, the glutamic acid at residue 35 in the first hypervariable region has been replaced by an alanine.[36] This results in an almost complete loss of antigen binding, indicating the importance of Glu-35 in PC binding. Davies and Metzger[3] suggested that the Glu at 35 forms a hydrogen bond with the tyrosine at residue 94 in the light chain and is important in maintaining the conformation of the antigen-binding site. This is confirmed by the presence of glutamic acid at residue 35 in almost all PC-binding antibodies[38] and the fact that two other members of the T15 heavy-chain V-region family, which are not expressed in PC-binding antibodies, do not code for a glutamic acid at residue 35.[39] While the U4 mutant has greatly decreased binding for phosphorylcholine, it has acquired the ability to bind other phosphorylated compounds, such as dsDNA, phosphorylated protamine, and cardiolipin.[40] This suggests the interesting possibility that somatic mutants with increased binding to cross-reacting antigens can be generated.

The U1 mutant has substituted an alanine for the aspartic acid in the fifth residue of J. It has a decrease in antigen binding, but has not completely lost the ability to bind PC.[35] These studies show that somatic mutants that have single amino acid substitutions that cause changes in antigen binding can arise frequently and spontaneously in culture. It therefore seems likely that, if adequate assays can be developed, monoclonal antibodies with increases in binding can also be identified. In fact, starting with the U1 low-binding mutant, we have identified spontaneous revertants that have returned to wild-type binding.[34,41] The study of the frequency of antigen-binding mutants and of the molecular mechanisms responsible may also provide insights into the generation of antibody diversity.

5. Conclusion

Since hybridoma cells growing in culture undergo rearrangements and mutations in their immunoglobulin genes, it is possible to obtain somatic mutants that have changes in structure and are even more effective reagents than the parental monoclonal antibody. While the generation and use of such somatic mutants is only beginning to be developed and exploited, it offers the opportunity not only to generate more useful monoclonal antibodies, but also to learn more about the structural basis of antibody functions. Ultimately, such information will allow the routine generation of such antibodies through recombinant DNA technology.

Acknowledgments. R. R. Pollock is a postdoctoral fellow of the Arthritis Foundation. This work was supported by grants from the NIH (A15231 and AI10702), NSF (PCM 8316160), and ACS (IM-317C) and a Cancer Center Grant (3PO CA1330). Dr. Spira was supported by the Atrah Foundation.

References

1. Köhler, G., and Milstein, C., 1975, Continuous cultures of fused cells secreting antibody of predefined specificity, *Nature* **256:**495–497.
2. Parham, P., Kipps, T. J., Ward, F. E., and Herzenberg, L. A., 1983, Isolation of heavy chain class switch variants of a monoclonal anti-DC1 hybridoma cell line: Effective conversion of noncytotoxic IgG1 antibodies to cytotoxic IgG2 antibodies, *Hum. Immunol.* **8:**141–151.
3. Grey, H. M., Hirst, J. W., and Cohn, M., 1971, A new mouse immunoglobulin: IgG3, *J. Exp. Med.* **133:**289–304.
4. Teillaud, J. L., Desaymard, C., Giusti, A. M., Haseltine, B., Pollock, R. R., Yelton, D. E., Zack, D. J., and Scharff, M. D., 1983, Monoclonal antibodies reveal the structural basis of antibody diversity, *Science* **222:**721–726.
5. Morrison, S. L., and Scharff, M. D., 1981, Mutational events in mouse myeloma, *CRC Crit. Rev. Immunol.* **3:**1–22.

6. Coffino, P. R., Baumal, R., Laskov, R., and Scharff, M. D., 1972, Cloning of mouse myeloma cells and detection of rare variants, *J. Cell. Physiol.* **79**:429–439.
7. Cebra, J. J., Komisar, J. L., and Switzer, P. A., 1984, C_H isotype "switching" during normal B-lymphocytic development, *Annu. Rev. Immunol.* **2**:493–548.
8. Preud'homme, J.-L., Birshtein, B. K., and Scharff, M. D., 1975, Variants of a mouse myeloma cell line which synthesize immunoglobulin heavy chains having an altered serotype, *Proc. Natl. Acad. Sci. USA* **72**:1427–1430.
9. Liesegang, B., Radbruch, A., and Rajewsky, K., 1978, Isolation of myeloma variants with predefined variant surface immunoglobulin by cell sorting, *Proc. Natl. Acad. Sci. USA* **75**:3901–3905.
10. Dangl, J. L., and Herzenberg, L. A., 1982, Selection of hybridoma variants using the fluorescence activated cell sorter, *J. Immunol. Meth.* **52**:1–14.
11. Radbruch, A., Liesegang, B., and Rajewsky, K., 1980, Isolation of variants of mouse myeloma X63 that express changed immunoglobulin class. *Proc. Natl. Acad. Sci. USA* **77**:2909–2913.
12. Eckhardt, L. A., Tilley, S. A., Lang, R. B., Marcu, K. B., and Birshtein, B. K., 1983, DNA rearrangements in MPC-11 immunoglobulin heavy chain class switch variants, *Proc. Natl. Acad. Sci. USA* **79**:3006–3010.
13. Sablitzky, F., Radbruch, A., and Rajewsky, K., 1982, Spontaneous immunoglobulin class switching in myeloma and hybridoma cell lines differs from physiological class switching, *Immunol. Rev.* **67**:59–72.
14. Shimizu, A., and Honjo, T., 1984, Immunoglobulin class switching, *Cell* **36**:801–803.
15. Tilley, S. A., Eckhardt, L. A., Marcu, K. B., and Birshtein, B. K., 1983, Hybrid γ_{2b}–γ_{2a} genes expressed in myeloma variants: Evidence for homologous recombination, *Proc. Natl. Acad. Sci. USA* **80**:6967–6971.
16. Muller, C. E., and Rajewsky, K., 1983, Isolation of immunoglobulin class switch variants from hybridoma lines secreting anti-idiotope antibodies by sequential sublining, *J. Immunol.* **131**:877–881.
17. Cavalli-Sforza, L. L. and Lederberg, J., 1956, Isolation of pre-adaptive mutants in bacteria by sib selection, *Genetics* **41**:367–381.
18. Spira, G., Bargellesi, A., Teillaud, J.-L., and Scharff, M. D., 1984, The identification of monoclonal class switch variants by sib selection and an ELISA assay, *J. Immunol. Meth.* **74**:307–315.
19. Zack, D. J., and Scharff, M. D., 1984, The identification of somatic mutations in immunoglobulin expression and structure, in: *Single-Cell Mutation Monitoring Systems* (A. A. Aversari and F. J. deSerres, eds.), Plenum Press, New York, pp. 233–263.
20. Bargellesi, A., Spira, G., and Scharff, M. D., 1984, Loss of cryoprecipitability in anti-human T-cell monoclonal by subclass switching, Submitted for publication.
21. Staplewski, Z., Spira, G., and Scharff, M. D., Manuscript in preparation.
22. Muller, C. E., and Rajewsky, K., 1984, Idiotope regulation by isotype switch variants of two monoclonal anti-idiotope antibodies, *J. Exp. Med.* **159**:758–772.
23. Corte, G., Mingari, M. C., Moretta, A., Damiani, G., Moretta, L., and Bargellesi, A., 1982, Human T cell subpopulation defined by monoclonal antibody: I) A small subset is responsible for proliferation to allogeneic cells to soluble antigens and for helper B cell differentiation, *J. Immunol.* **128**:16–20.
24. Yelton, D. E., and Scharff, M. D., 1982, Mutant monoclonal antibodies with alterations in biological functions, *J. Exp. Med.* **156**:1131–1148.
25. Kenter, A. L., and Birshtein, B. K., 1979, Genetic mechanism accounting for precise immunoglobulin domain deletion in a variant of MPC-11 myeloma cells, *Science* **206**:1307–1309.
26. Teillaud, J.-L., Diamond, B., Pollock, R. R., Fajtova, V., and Scharff, M. D., 1984, Fc receptors on cultural myeloma and hybridoma cells, *J. Immun.* (in press).
27. Spiegelberg, H. L. and Fishkin, B. G., 1972, The metabolism of human γG immunoglobulins of different heavy chain subclass. III. The metabolism of heavy chain disease proteins and of Fc fragment of myeloma proteins, *Clin. Exp. Immunol.* **10**:599–607.

28. Yasmeen, D., Ellerson, J. R., Dorrington, K. J., and Painter, R. H., 1976, The structure and function of immunoglobulin domains. IV. The distribution of some effector functions among the Cγ2 and Cγ3 homology region of human immunoglobulin, *J. Immunol.* **116**:518–526.
29. Pollock, R. R., Metlay, J. P., Birshtein, B. K., and Scharff, M. D., 1984, Intravascular metabolism of normal and mutant monoclonal antibodies, *Fed. Proc.* **43**:1682 (abst.).
30. Rodwell, J. D., Gerhart, P. J., and Karush, F., 1983, Restriction in IgM expression. IV. Affinity analysis of monoclonal anti-phosphorylcholine antibodies, *J. Immunol.* **130**:313–322.
31. Rothstein, T. L., and Gefter, M., 1983, Affinity analysis of idiotype positive and idiotype-negative-ars-binding hybridoma proteins and ars-immune sera, *Mol. Immunol.* **20**:161–168.
32. Dildrop, R., Bruggeman, M., Radbruch, A., Rajewsky, K., and Beyrenther, K., 1982, Immunoglobulin V region variants in hybridoma cells. II. Recombination between V genes, *EMBO J.* **1**:635–640.
33. Kohler, H., 1975, The response to phosphorylcholine: Dissecting an immune response, *Transplant Rev.* **27**:24–56.
34. Cook, W. D., and Scharff, M. D., 1977, Antigen-binding mutants of mouse myeloma cells, *Proc. Natl. Acad. Sci. USA* **74**:5687–5691.
35. Cook, W. D., Rudikoff, S., Giusti, A. M., and Scharff, M. D., 1982. Somatic mutation in a cultured mouse myeloma cell affects antigen binding, *Proc. Natl. Acad. Sci. USA* **79**:1240–1244.
36. Rudikoff, S., Giusti, A. M., Cook, W. D., and Scharff, M. D., 1982, Single amino acid substitution altering antigen-binding specificity, *Proc. Natl. Acad. Sci. USA* **79**:1979–1983.
37. Davies, D. R., and Metzger, H., 1983, Structure basis of antibody function, *Annu. Rev. Immunol.* **1**:87–117.
38. Gerhart, P. J., Johnson, J. D., Douglas, R., and Hood, L., 1981, IgG antibodies to phosphorylcholine exhibit more diversity than their IgM counterparts, *Nature* **291**:39–44.
39. Crews, S., Griffin, J., Huang, H., Calame, K., and Hood, L., 1981, A single V_H gene segment encodes the immune response to phosphorylcholine: Somatic mutation is correlated with the class of the antibody, *Cell* **25**:59–66.
40. Diamond, B., and Scharff, M. D., 1984, Somatic mutation of the T15 heavy chain gives rise to an antibody with autoantibody specificity, *Proc. Natl. Acad. Sci. USA* **81**:5841–5844.
41. Zack, D., Rudikoff, S., Giusti, A. M., and Scharff, M. D., Revertants of antigen binding mutants of S107, Manuscript in preparation.

Chapter 5

Switching the Isotype of Monoclonal Antibodies

THOMAS J. KIPPS

1. Introduction

Isotype switch variant selection is an important adjunct to monoclonal antibody technology. Through the production of hybridomas, we can now harness the specificity of the humoral immune response to generate virtually unlimited amounts of monoclonal antibody of desired specificity. Unfortunately, a selected hybridoma may fail to secrete specific immunoglobulin with an isotype of desired functional activity. This problem may be alleviated through the selection of isotype switch variants that secrete antibody of a different immunoglobulin isotype but with preserved antigen-binding specificity. In addition, by selecting hybridomas that produce monoclonals differing from one another in isotype only, comparative studies can be performed on the functional activities of the different murine immunoglobulin isotypes. Such studies may increase our understanding of potential uses of monoclonal antibodies in cell biology and medicine.

This chapter will review current concepts of immunoglobulin isotype switching, discussing several advances that facilitate the selection of switch variant hybridomas.

2. Mouse Immunoglobulin Isotypes

The capacity to change the isotype of an existing murine monoclonal antibody may greatly enhance its utility. It has long been recognized that major differences exist in the biological activities of the different mouse immunoglobulin isotypes.[1] Pentameric IgM, for example, is particularly efficient in hemagglutination and in directing complement-mediated cytolysis. IgE, on the other hand, is unable to fix complement, but is extremely cytophilic for mast cells and basophils, providing for the specific triggering of anaphylaxis. Even among the subclasses of mouse IgG, namely IgG1, IgG2a, IgG2b, and IgG3, major

THOMAS J. KIPPS • Department of Genetics, Stanford University School of Medicine, Stanford, California 94305.

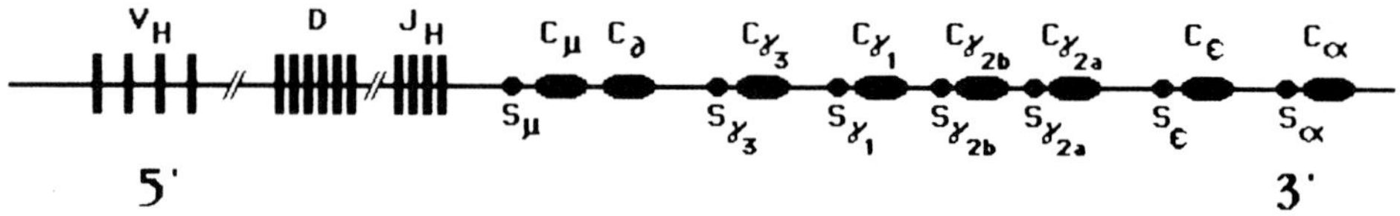

Figure 1. The murine heavy chain immunoglobulin gene complex. The distances between the constant region loci (C) are not drawn to scale, which in kilobases (kb) are: 5′-J_H-(6.5 kb)-$C\mu$-(4.5 kb)-C_δ-(55 kb)-$C\gamma_3$-(34 kb)-$C\gamma_1$-(21 kb)-$C\gamma_{2b}$-(15 kb)-$C\gamma_{2a}$-(14 kb)-C_ϵ-(12kb)-C_α.[27] (S, Switch region; V_H, variable region gene; D, diversity segment; J_H, joining segment.

differences exist. IgG2a and IgG2b fix complement through the conventional pathway, whereas most IgG1 and IgG3 do not.[1–3] Although IgG2a and IgG2b, but not IgG1, are capable of directing passive cutaneous anaphylactic (PCA) reactions in the guinea pig, only IgG1 is able to direct PCA in the mouse.[1–4] More recently, we have detected differences between these three classes of murine antibody in their capacities for directing antibody-dependent cell-mediated cytotoxicity (ADCC) by human K cells.[5] IgG2a functions best in human ADCC. IgG2b directs only intermediate levels of activity, but functions significantly better than IgG1. Furthermore, mouse immunoglobulin isotypes of antitumor antibodies apparently differ in their ability to influence tumor growth in experimental animals.[6–9] Thus, by defining the methodology for isotype switch variant selection, a hybridoma producing a monoclonal antibody of desired specificity may be modified to secrete antigen-specific immunoglobulin with an isotype of desired biological activity.

3. The Genetics of Immunoglobulin Isotype Expression

The immune system has evolved complex genetic machinery for immunoglobulin isotype expression, allowing it to link a usefully permuted variable region gene to any one of the different heavy chain constant region genes through the process of isotype switching. The immunoglobulin heavy chain isotypes are coded for by individual gene loci arranged in tandem along a chromosome region that is 200 kilobases long and 3′ of the variable region gene complex of mouse chromosome 12 (Fig. 1).[10–12] Prior to immunoglobulin gene expression, at least two DNA rearrangements are required to form a functional VDJ gene, composed of the variable (V_H), diversity (D), and joining (J_H) gene segments that together code for the variable region of the antibody heavy chain.[13,14] The VDJ gene is subsequently transcribed with one of the several heavy chain isotype genes to produce a single mRNA transcript that is translated to form the antibody heavy chain. Subsequent rearrangements apparently occur to produce an isotype "switch," allowing for the expression of the same VDJ gene with a different heavy chain isotype gene.

Several models have been proposed to describe the molecular events involved in the isotype switch. One theorizes that selective processing of a large RNA transcript may allow for translation of the variable region with different constant region isotypes.[15,16] This model may account for the coordinate expression of IgM and IgD.[17–19] A second model proposes that the genes on a single DNA strand internally recombine, deleting the gene coding for the formerly expressed isotype and bringing into juxtaposition the VDJ gene with the newly expressed isotype gene.[20,21] Another model theorizes that this type of DNA rearrangement results instead from unequal recombination between newly formed sister chromatids.[22–25]

Theories postulating that isotype switching results from rearrangement of the heavy chain constant region genes have received considerable support from the analysis of isotype genes in plasmacytomas.[10,13,18,20,24,26] These studies have demonstrated that the expressed heavy chain isotype gene is repositioned immediately downstream, or 3′, of the VDJ gene through DNA rearrangement(s) that delete intervening constant region exons. Rearrangement of the DNA is noted to occur at so-called "switch regions" (S), located 5′ of each heavy chain locus except delta (Fig. 1). These regions share short repetitive sequences [i.e., TGAGC and TGGG(G)],[27] which possibly allow for pairing of different switch region loci for S–S recombination. These regions also may act as binding sites for postulated switch recombinases that catalyze the DNA rearrangements necessary for isotype switching.

These features of the immunoglobulin gene complex have important implications for the design of an isotype switch variant selection. Analyses of the DNA from several hybridomas have demonstrated rearrangements of isotype genes similar to that noted in myelomas, with deletion of the genes coding for isotypes located 5′ of the expressed heavy chain isotype gene.[28,29] Such deletions make switching to these isotypes impossible, unless switch recombination could occur with the upstream isotype genes positioned on the nonexpressed homologous chromosome. Indeed, we have observed interchromosomal recombination between isotype genes in cultured hybridomas.[30] Variants have also been selected that express an upstream isotype gene[31,32]; however, this has been observed only when cloned switch variant cell populations were selected for "back-switch" variants producing antibody of the original parental isotype. As such, these examples of "back-switch" variants may not be representative of hybridomas obtained through a hybrid fusion. It should be noted that rearrangements and deletions of constant region genes frequently occur in the nonexpressed heavy chain gene complex.[24,28,33,34] Thus, before attempting to select variants expressing an isotype gene located 5′ of the originally expressed heavy chain gene, it is best to determine whether the gene coding for the desired isotype is still present in the hybridoma's genome.

4. Spontaneous Isotype Switching in Myelomas and Hybridomas

In vitro isotype switching was first observed in the IgG2b-secreting MPC 11 myeloma.[35] After mutagenesis with melphalan or ICR 191, approximately 0.5% of the cells cloned in soft agar expressed myeloma protein with altered heavy chains, a few of which reacted with antibodies specific for mouse IgG2a. Subsequent characterization of these variants confirmed that some of these clones had indeed undergone an isotype switch from IgG2b to IgG2a, while retaining expression of the same light chain genes and heavy chain VDJ rearrangement.[36–38] Although spontaneously occurring switch variants of MPC 11 were also noted, these were relatively rare and difficult to isolate by soft agar cloning techniques. Staining the myeloma cells with fluorescein-conjugated antibody specific for mouse IgG2a, however, Rajewsky and his associates demonstrated that these relatively rare spontaneous switch variant cells could be isolated from MPC 11 using the fluorescence activated cell sorter (FACS).[39] By selecting cells based on variant surface immunoglobulin expression, these investigators increased the efficiency of isolating variant myeloma cells two- to threefold over the previously employed technique of antibody–agar overlay.

Spontaneous isotype switching subsequently was observed in monoclonal antibody-producing hybridomas.[3,5,32,40–43] Switch variant hybridomas are detected at frequencies similar to those found in myeloma cell populations (see Section 6). Importantly, such hybridoma variants produce antibodies with idiotypic specificities, antigen-binding activities, and antibody light chains that are identical to that of the antibodies produced by the parent hybridoma.

In vitro isotype switching apparently results from DNA rearrangement(s) similar in many ways to those found in plasmacytomas.[29] The newly expressed heavy chain gene is found generally 3′ of the expressed VDJ gene, this resulting from excision of DNA coding for the formerly expressed isotype. Although the sites of recombination responsible for such rearrangement(s) may be outside the physiological switch regions (S), switch variants generally produce antibodies that are analogous to physiologically occurring antibodies of the same isotype in their molecular weight, glycosylation, and primary protein sequence.

5. Techniques of Switch Variant Selection

5.1. Cloning in Soft Agar

The first method used for selecting variant hybridomas involved cloning the cells in soft agar.[44] After discrete colonies are detected, heterologous isotype-specific antibody is added to the agar plates. Either the presence of a surrounding precipitin ring (positive selection) or lack thereof (negative selection) signals the presence of a variant clone. Since this method screens for alteration(s) in the secreted antibody, it can potentially be used to select variants from myelomas having little or no surface immunoglobulin. Although this technique has been used successfully to isolate a number of interesting variants of MPC 11,[35,36] it may be limited to selecting variants that arise at relatively high frequencies. This is because one can easily screen only a limited number of cells with this method, usually $(1-5) \times 10^4$.

A permutation on the soft agar cloning technique that may be useful in limited settings is that of clonal abortion. Köhler and Shulman used this method for selecting variants from a hybridoma-secreting IgM specific for the hapten trinitrophenol.[45] Hybridoma cells were conjugated with the hapten so as to make their secreted antibody self-reactive. The cells were then plated in soft agar to which guinea pig complement was added. Only variants producing antibody that could not fix complement or bind antigen would survive under such selective pressure. Although this group did not isolate isotype switch variants, they succeeded in selecting a variety of variant hybridomas secreting variant IgM molecules. It remains to be seen whether this method may be successful in selecting noncomplement-fixing isotype variants when the probability of isotype switching is higher, i.e., from IgG2a to IgE (see Section 6).

5.2. Sequential Sublining

A more recent method of switch variant selection is through sequential sublining[42] or sib selection (see Spira *et al.*, this volume, Chapter 4). Hybridomas are plated into microtiter plates at approximately 10^4 cells per well. After 3–4 days of culture, the supernates are harvested and assayed for the presence of variant isotype using a sensitive solid phase radioimmunoassay. Wells identified as possibly containing switch variant cells are grown up in culture and the cycle is repeated. Through several rounds of such sequential sublining, variant cells may become sufficiently enriched to allow cell cloning.

5.3. Fluorescence Activated Cell Sorting

A powerful way to isolate switch variant hybridomas is to use the fluorescence activated cell sorter (FACS). As mentioned previously, this method selects cells based on their expression of surface immunoglobulin, which for hybridomas is of the same isotype as the secreted antibody. Cells are stained with fluorochrome-labeled antibodies specific for the variant isotype and the most brightly fluorescent cells are selected. In less than 1 hr of sorting, one can easily screen 10^7 hybridomas, enriching them for switch variants more than a thousandfold. Of course, operational knowledge of the FACS is required. A detailed description of this is outside the scope of this chapter and the reader is referred to a recent review.[46]

Although selection of the first switch variants required many weeks with successive rounds of enrichment sorting,[39] several improvements have been made that significantly lessen the time and effort required for variant isolation. Currently, it is possible to detect, and in many cases clone, switch variant cells in only a single sort.[5,47] The following sections will describe several important measures either necessary or helpful for rapid detection of isotype switch variant hybridomas using the FACS.

5.3.1. Staining Reagents

Efficient variant selection is predicated on the quality of the fluorescent reagent(s) used to label variant cells. Close attention must be given to both the specificity and staining intensity of a given antibody preparation. The fluorescence conferred upon the variant cell by the staining reagent should be bright enough to allow for easy discrimination from cells having bright autofluorescence. Since the autofluorescence of individual cells within a given hybridoma population may vary over nearly an order of magnitude in brightness, staining reagents ideally should increase the mean fluorescence of cell populations bearing desired isotype(s) tenfold.

5.3.1a. Heterologous Antibody. Fluorescein-conjugated heterologous anti-isotype antibodies can serve as excellent selective reagents. These are generally prepared in the goat, since immunoglobulins of this animal tend not to be cytophilic for murine cells. Antibodies purified from the immune sera must be extensively absorbed with other mouse antibody isotypes to render them uniquely specific for the heavy chain isotype of interest prior to fluorescein conjugation.

Heterologous immunoglobulin preparations are composed of heterogeneous antibodies with many different binding affinities for mouse immunoglobulin. As such, the staining intensity may be quite sensitive to changes in antibody concentration.[3] Titrations with control hybridomas expressing the desired isotype should be performed at several different concentrations of antibody to determine not only the amount of antibody required for saturation staining of a given number of cells, but also the optimal antibody concentration for effective staining (usually 25–50 μg/ml). For selecting hybridoma variants present at 10^{-4}–10^{-7} within a hybridoma population, the same antibody concentration is used; however, the cell concentration is increased fivefold, so that only one-fifth the total amount of antibody required for saturation staining of positive control hybridomas is used.

Heterologous anti-isotype antibodies are commercially available. Many reputedly specific reagents unfortunately do not have the specificity required for rare cell sorting. Exceptions are the FITC-conjugated goat anti-isotype antibodies recently made available from Southern Biotechnology Associates (Birmingham, Alabama). We have tested several and found them well suited for selecting isotype switch variants.

5.3.1b. Monoclonal Antibody. Monoclonal antiallotypic antibodies may have several advantages over heterologous anti-isotype antibodies for selecting switch variants. Many are isotype-specific, thus obviating the need for absorption.[48,49] Most bind with high affinity, making staining intensity less sensitive to changes in antibody concentration. Also, by mixing two fluorescein-conjugated antiallotype antibodies that noncompetitively bind to different sites on immunoglobulins of a selected isotype, the staining intensity achieved with monoclonal antibodies may be comparable to that of heterologous antibody preparations.[50,51]

5.3.1c. Fluorochromes. Fluorescein isothiocyanate (FITC) is the most widely used fluorescent molecule for labeling specific antibody, partly because

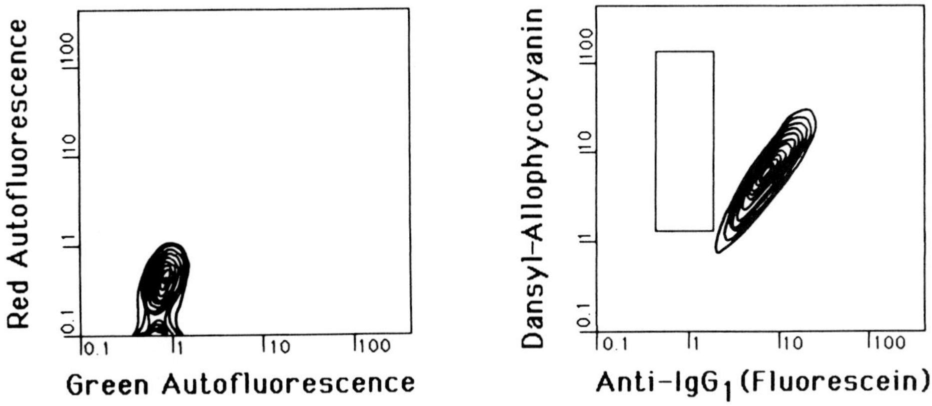

Figure 2. Fluorescence staining of IgG1 antidansyl-antibody-producing hybridomas. Hybridomas were stained with FITC–goat anti-mouse IgG1 and dansyl-allophycocyanin. Histograms depict fluorescence intensity of (right) stained and (left) unstained hybridomas when excited at 488 and 600 nm with a dual-laser FACS-II equipped with logarithmic amplifiers. The numbers on the ordinate and abscissa refer to the relative fluorescence intensity. Boxed area in the histogram on the right circumscribes the sorting gate used for switch variant selection.

it is so readily conjugated to proteins via the isothiocyanate moiety.[52] For variant sorting, however, it is important to monitor the average number of fluorescein molecules covalently attached to the isotype specific antibody. This fluorescein to protein ratio (F/P) can be calculated from the measured light absorption of the conjugated protein at 280 and 495 nm.[52] Antibodies with F/P ratios less than two may not stain cells with sufficient intensity for variant sorting. On the other hand, overconjugation may make the antibodies nonspecifically "sticky." Therefore, for variant sorting, antibodies with F/P ratios of three to four generally work best.

The advent of phycobiliproteins may allow for new dimensions in hybridoma variant selection.[53,54] These brightly fluorescent proteins may be coupled with haptens, allowing for specific staining of hybridomas producing antihapten antibodies. One can stain with a combination of one fluorochrome linked to antigen and a second linked to anti-isotype antibody, and carry out multiparameter analysis and sorting using a dual-laser FACS. Seen in Fig. 2, for example, are histograms of stained and unstained hybridomas producing IgG1 monoclonal antibody specific for the hapten dansyl (5-dimethylaminonaphthalene-1-sulfonyl). Staining for dansyl is achieved with the hapten conjugated to allophycocyanin, a phycobiliprotein with bright fluorescence at wavelengths between 640 and 680 nm when excited at 600 nm. By concommitantly staining with FITC–anti-IgG1, one can select for variants that have lost surface IgG1 expression but retain antigen-binding activity (boxed area of Fig. 2). Variants so selected are primarily isotype switch variants producing IgG2b antidansyl antibody.

5.3.2. Exclusion of Dead Cells

For efficient rare cell sorting, it is necessary to exclude dead and dying cells. Such cells increase the background fluorescence and decrease the staining reagent's effective concentration by nonspecifically absorbing the fluorescein-labeled antibody. Thus, cells should be greater than 90% viable prior to sorting. Even so, the proportion of dead cells usually will exceed that of switch variants. For this reason, we include propidium iodide at 1μg/ml in the antibody staining mixture. This dye labels dead and dying cells, making them brightly red fluorescent when excited by the argon dye laser at 488 nm. As such these cells can be electronically excluded from analysis and sorting.[46,51]

5.3.3. Paucipopulation Sorting

Enhanced sensitivity for detecting switch variant hybridomas can be achieved through paucipopulation sorting.[47] Even with the best of staining reagents and sorter conditions, the maximum enrichment that can be achieved with the FACS is on the order of 10^3–10^4. Thus, when sorting for cells present at frequencies of 10^{-6}–10^{-7}, the sorted sample will consist primarily of parent-type hybridomas. By sorting 5, 25, or 125 cells into individual wells of a 96-well microtiter plate, however, a limiting dilution of switch variant cells is achieved. After 1 week of culture, the supernates from the separate wells can be assayed for the variant isotype using a solid phase radioimmune assay (RIA). Using the Poisson distribution, the number of switch variant cells actually sorted can be calculated from the proportion of wells found positive for the desired isotype.

This method has several advantages. First, it permits direct determination of the proportion of variants found within a given population without the need for collating data from successive rounds of sorting. Second, it increases the speed at which variants can be isolated. For, after the first sort, paucipopulations of cells that are greatly enriched for variants can be identified. Thus, approximately 2 weeks after the initial sort, the switch variants in these populations can be cloned.

6. Kinetics of Isotype Switching

The analysis of the kinetics with which spontaneously arising switch variants emerge within a culture of hybridomas is basically a problem in population genetics. The proportion of variants within a given hybridoma population will depend on the intrinsic rate(s) of spontaneous isotype switching per cell division, the growth rate(s) of the hybridomas and their newly generated switch variant progeny, and the per generation rate(s) of subsequent switching in individual switch variant cells.

Luria and Delbruck formulated an analysis of the rate at which mutant-type cells emerge within a microbial population[55] that may apply to switch

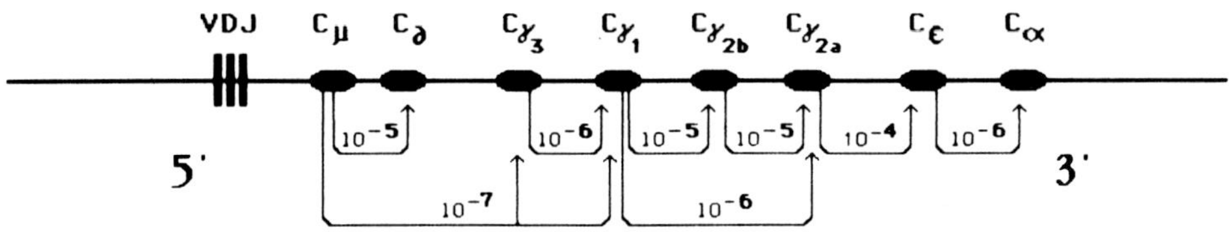

Figure 3. Approximate spontaneous isotype switch frequencies per cell division in cultured murine hybridomas. VDJ, Rearranged variable region gene complex; C, constant region loci.

variant hybridomas. For logarithmically growing cultures, they concluded that the proportion of mutants will increase linearly with time, provided that the mutation rate is low, backmutation is neglible, the growth rates of mutant and wild-type cells are equal, and the proportion of mutants to wild-type cells remains relatively small. Although exceptions are observed, these same conditions are met by many hybridoma switch variant families. Thus, for most hybridomas, the relative proportion of switch variants should increase with the number of generations spent in culture. This has been verified experimentally.[47]

Catcheside[56] derived a formula useful for calculating the actual mutation rate of cells within a logarithmically growing culture prior to achieving mutational equilibrium:

$$m = 2(\ln 2)\,\frac{M_2/N_2 - M_1/N_1}{G}$$

where m is the mutation rate per cell per generation, M_1 and M_2 are the numbers of mutants at times 1 and 2, N_1 and N_2 are the numbers of cells at these two time points, and G is the number of generations elapsed between times 1 and 2.

By determining the proportion of variants within a given hybridoma population at two separate times, one can use the above formula to obtain approximations of the switch variant frequency per cell per generation. Figure 3 depicts the generalized spontaneous isotype switch frequencies in cultured hybridomas (T. J. Kipps, unpublished observations). These frequencies may not apply to all hybridomas and are meant to serve only as approximations. Several points, however, are worth emphasizing. The rates of spontaneous isotype switching are comparable to conventional spontaneous mutation frequencies, these rates ranging from 10^{-4} to 10^{-7}. The probabilities of isotype switching vary, depending on the isotypes of both parent and switch variant hybridomas. Switch events occurring with the highest probability exchange the expression of one isotype gene to that of its nearest 3′ neighbor. Switching to isotypes located farther downstream apparently can occur directly, however. The probability of such spontaneous events is much greater than the product of probabilities for successive switching through an isotype variant intermediate. Spontaneous switching to isotype genes located 5′ of the heavy chain gene expressed by the hybridoma after fusion has not been detected.

7. Effects of Mutagens on the Rate of Isotype Switching

Several mutagens have been found to increase the number of antibody heavy chain variants. Cells generally are cultured for one cell cycle with a mutagen at concentrations that reduce the viability of the treated cells by 40%. At this dose, melphalan or ICR 191 significantly augments the number of antibody heavy chain variants of the MPC 11 myeloma.[35] Most of these, however, are not switch variants and secrete altered heavy chains of the parent isotype.[57] We have observed four- to eightfold increases in the number of isotype switch variants found in newly subcloned hybridomas so treated with hydroxyurea.[47] The relative increase in the proportion of variants found in drug-treated hybridoma populations that previously had been cultured for several weeks, however, is not as apparent, due to the accumulation of spontaneous variants within the culture, increasing the switch variant "background" of matched untreated controls. Recently, it has been reported that UV induces high rates of spontaneous isotype switching in a human lymphoblastoid cell line.[58] Whether this is also true for murine hybridomas remains to be tested.

Acknowledgments. The author is indebted to Dr. Leonard A. Herzenberg for his many stimulating discussions and his invaluable advice. T.J.K. is a special fellow of the Leukemia Society of America.

References

1. Nisonoff, A., Hopper, J. E., and Spring, S. B., 1975, Immunoglobulins of the rabbit, mouse, guinea pig, and horse, in: *The Antibody Molecule* (F. J. Dixon and H. G. Kunkel, eds.), Academic Press, New York, pp. 313–345.
2. Ey, P. L., Russell-Jones, G. J., and Jenkin, C. R., 1980, Isotypes of mouse IgG-I. Evidence for 'non-complement-fixing' IgG_1 antibodies and characterization of their capacity to interfere with IgG_2 sensitization of target red blood cells for lysis by complement, *Mol. Immunol.* **17**:699–710.
3. Parham, P., Kipps, T. J., Ward, F. E., and Herzenberg, L. A., 1983, Isolation of heavy chain class switch variants of a monoclonal anti-DC1 hybridoma cell line: Effective conversion of non-cytotoxic IgG1 antibodies to cytotoxic IgG2 antibodies, *Hum. Immunol.* **8**:141–151.
4. Ovary, Z., Fahey, J. L., and Barth, W. F., 1965, The immunoglobulins of mice. III. Skin sensitizing activity of mouse immunoglobulins, *J. Immunol.* **94**:410–415.
5. Kipps, T. J., Parham, P., Punt, J., and Herzenberg, L. A., 1985, Importance of isotype in human antibody dependent cell-mediated cytotoxicity directed by murine monoclonal antibodies, *J. Exp. Med.*, **161**:1–17.
6. Wright, P. W., and Bernstein, I. D., 1980, Serotherapy of malignant disease, *Prog. Exp. Tumor Res.* **25**:140–162.
7. Matthews, T. J., Collins, J. J., Roloson, G., Thiel, H.-J., and Bolognesi, D. P., 1981, Immunologic control of the ascites form of murine adenocarcinoma 755. IV. Characterization of the protective antibody in hyperimmune serum, *J. Immunol.* **126**:2332–2336.

8. Langlois, A. J., Matthews, T., Roloson, G. J., Thiel, H.-J., Collins, J. J., and Bolognesis, D. P., 1980, Immunologic control of the ascites form of murine adenocarcinoma 755. V. Antibody-directed macrophages mediate tumor cell destruction, *J. Immunol.* **126**:2337–2340.
9. Herlyn, D., and Koprowski, H., 1982, IgG_{2a} monoclonal antibodies inhibit human tumor growth through interaction with effector cells, *Proc. Natl. Acad. Sci. USA* **79**:4761–4765.
10. Honjo, T., and Kataoka, T., 1978, Organization of immunoglobulin heavy chain genes and allelic deletion model, *Proc. Natl. Acad. Sci. USA* **75**:2140–2145.
11. Adams, J. M., Kemp, D. J., Bernard, O., Gough, N., Webb, E., Tyler, B., Gerondakis, S., and Cory, S., 1981, Organization and expression of murine immunoglobulin genes, *Immunol. Rev.* **59**:5–32.
12. Shimizu, A., Takahasi, N., Yaoita, Y., and Honjo, T., 1982, Organization of the constant region gene family of mouse immunoglobulin heavy chain, *Cell* **28**:499–506.
13. Davis, M., Calame, K., Early, P., Livant, D., Joho, R., Weissman, I., and Hood, L., 1980, An immunologlobulin heavy chain gene is formed by at least two recombination events, *Nature* **283**:733–739.
14. Early, P., Rogers, J., Davis, M., Calame, K., and Hood, L., 1980, An immunoglobulin heavy chain variable region gene is generated from three segments of DNA: VH, D and JH, *Cell* **19**:981–992.
15. Wall, R., Choi, E., Kuehl, M., and Rodgers, J., 1981, RNA processing in immunoglobulin gene expression, *Cold Spring Harbor Symp. Quant. Biol.* **45**:879–885.
16. Yaoita, Y., Kumagai, Y., Okumura, K., and Honjo, T., 1982, Expression of lymphocyte surface IgE does not require switch recombination, *Nature* **297**:697–699.
17. Early, P., Rogers, J., Davis, M., Calame, K., Bond, M., Wall, R., and Hood, L., 1980, Two mRNAs produced from a single immunoglobulin mu gene by alternative RNA processing pathways, *Cell* **20**:313–319.
18. Maki, R., Roeder, W., Traunecker, A., Sidman, C., Wabl, M., Raschke, W., and Tonegawa, S., 1981, The role of DNA rearrangement and alternative RNA processing in the expression of immunoglobulin delta genes, *Cell* **24**:353–365.
19. Moore, K. W., Rogers, J., Hunkapiller, T., Early, P., Nottenburg, C., Weissman, I., Bazin, H., Wall, R., and Hood, L., 1981, Expression of IgD may use both DNA rearrangement and RNA splicing mechanisms, *Proc. Natl. Acad. Sci. USA* **78**:1800–1804.
20. Kataoka, T., Kawakam, T., Takahashi, N., and Honjo, T., 1980, Rearrangement of immunoglobulin gamma-1-chain gene and mechanism for heavy-chain class switch, *Proc. Natl. Acad. Sci. USA* **77**:919–923.
21. Dunnick, W., Rabbitts, T. H., and Milstein, C., 1980, An immunoglobulin deletion mutant with implications for the heavy-chain switch and RNA splicing, *Nature* **286**:669–675.
22. Sakano, H., Maki, R., Kurusawa, Y., Roeder, W., and Tonegawa, S., 1980, Two types of somatic recombination are necessary for the generation of complete immunoglobulin heavy-chain genes, *Nature* **286**:676–679.
23. Honjo, T., Nakai, S., Nishida, Y., Kataoka, T., Yamawaki-Kataoka, Y., Takahashi, N., Obata, M., Shimizu, A., Yaoita, Y., Nikaido, T., and Ishida, N., 1981, Rearrangements of immunoglobulin genes during differentiation and evolution, *Immunol. Rev.* **59**:33–68.
24. Cory, S., Webb, E., Gough, J., and Adams, J., 1981, Recombination events near the immunoglobulin C-mu gene join variable and constant region genes, switch heavy chain expression, or inactivate the locus, *Biochemistry* **20**:2662–2671.
25. Cory, S., and Adams, J. M., 1980, Deletions are associated with somatic rearrangement of immunoglobulin heavy chain genes, *Cell* **19**:37–43.
26. Coleclough, C., Cooper, D., and Perry, R. P., 1980, Rearrangement of immunoglobulin heavy chain during B lymphocyte development as revealed by studies of mouse plasmacytoma cells, *Proc. Natl. Acad. Sci. USA* **77**:1422–1426.
27. Kataoka, T., Miyata, T., and Honjo, T., 1981, Repetitive sequences in class-switch recombination regions of immunoglobulin heavy chain genes, *Cell* **23**:357–368.
28. Hurwitz, J. L., Coleclough, C., and Cebra, J. J., 1980, C_H gene rearrangements in IgM-bearing B cells and in the normal splenic DNA component of hybridomas making different isotypes of antibody, *Cell* **22**:349–359.

29. Sablitzky, F., Radbruch, A., and Rajewsky, K., 1982, Spontaneous immunoglobulin class switching in myeloma and hybridoma cell lines differs from physiological class switching, *Immunol. Rev.* **67**:59–72.
30. Kipps, T. J., and Herzenberg, L. A., 1984, Allotype switch variants: Demonstration of interchromosomal recombination in isotype switch of cultured monoclonal antibody-producing hybridomas, In preparation.
31. Radbruch, A., Liesegang, B., and Rajewsky, K., 1980, Isolation of variants of mouse myeloma X63 that express changed immunoglobulin class, *Proc. Natl. Acad. Sci. USA* **77**:2909–2913.
32. Dangl, J. L., Parks, D. R., Oi, V. T., and Herzenberg, L. A., 1982, Rapid isolation of cloned isotype switch variants using fluorescence activated cell sorting, *Cytometry* **2**:395–401.
33. Lang, R. B., Stanton, L. W., and Marcu, K. B., 1982, On immunoglobulin heavy chain switching: Two gamma 2b genes are rearranged via switch sequences in MPC-11 cells but only one is expressed, *Nucleic Acids Res.* **10**(2):611–630.
34. Cory, S., Adams, J. M., and Kemp, D. J., 1980, Somatic rearrangements forming active immunoglobulin mu genes in B and T lymphoid cell lines, *Proc. Natl. Acad. Sci. USA* **77**(8):4943–4947.
35. Preud'homme, J. L., Birshtein, B. K., and Scharff, M. D., 1975, Variants of a mouse myeloma cell line that synthesize immunoglobulin heavy chains having an altered serotype, *Proc. Natl. Acad. Sci. USA* **72**:1427–1430.
36. Francus, T., Dharmgrongartama, B., Campbell, R., Scharff, M. D., and Birshtein, B. K., 1978, IgG2a-producing variants of an IgG2b-producing mouse myeloma cell line, *J. Exp. Med.* **147**:1535–1550.
37. Francus, T., and Birshtein, B. K., 1978, An IgG_{2a}-producing variant of an IgG_{2b}-producing mouse myeloma cell line. Structural studies on the Fc region of parent and variant heavy chains, *Biochemistry* **17**(20):4324–4331.
38. Eckhardt, L. A., Tilley, S. A., Lang, R. B., Marcu, K. B., and Birshtein, B. K., 1982, DNA rearrangements in MPC-11 immunoglobulin heavy chain class-switch variants, *Proc. Natl. Acad. Sci. USA* **79**:3006–3010.
39. Liesegang, B., Radbruch, A., and Rajewsky, K., 1978, Isolation of myeloma variants with predefined variant surface immunoglobulin by cell sorting, *Proc. Natl. Acad. Sci. USA* **75**:3901–3905.
40. Neuberger, M. S., and Rajewsky, K., 1981, Switch from hapten-specific immunoglobulin M to immunoglobulin D secretion in a hybrid mouse cell line, *Proc. Natl. Acad. Sci. USA* **78**:1138–1142.
41. Baumhackel, H., Liesegang, B., Radbruch, B., Rajewsky, K., and Sablitzky, F., 1982, Switch from NIP specific IgG3 to IgG1 in the mouse hybridoma cell line S24/63/63, *J. Immunol.* **128**:1217–1220.
42. Muller, C. E., and Rajewsky, K., 1983, Isolation of immunoglobulin class switch variants from hybridoma lines secreting anti-idiotope antibodies by sequential sublining, *J. Immunol.* **131**:877–881.
43. Thammana, P., and Scharff, M. D., 1983, Immunoglobulin heavy chain class switch from IgM to IgG in hybridoma, *Eur. J. Immunol.* **13**:614–619.
44. Coffino, P., and Scharff, M. D., 1971, Rate of somatic mutation in immunoglobulin production by mouse myeloma cells, *Proc. Natl. Acad. Sci. USA* **68**:219–223.
45. Köhler, G., and Shulman, M. J., 1980, Immunoglobulin M mutants, *Eur. J. Immunol.* **10**:467–476.
46. Parks, D. R., and Herzenberg, L. A., 1984, Fluorescence activated cell sorting: Theory, experimental optimization and application in lymphoid cell biology, *Meth. Enzymol.* **108**:197–241.
47. Kipps, T. J., and Herzenberg, L. A., 1984, The fluorescence activated cell sorter: Complementary tools in immunodiagnosis and immunotherapy, in: *Rapid Methods in Immunology and Microbiology*, Springer-Verlag, Berlin, In press.
48. Huang, C., Parsons, M., Oi, V. T., Huang, H. S., and Herzenberg, L. A., 1983, Genetic characterization of mouse immunoglobulin allotypic determinants (allotypes) defined by monoclonal antibodies, *Immunogenetics* **18**:311–321.

49. Parsons, M., Oi, V. T., Huang, C. M., and Herzenberg, L. A., 1983, Structural characterization of mouse immunoglobulin allotypic determinants (allotypes) defined by monoclonal antibodies, *Immunogenetics* **18:**323–334.
50. Oi, V. T., and Herzenberg, L. A., 1979, Localization of murine Ig-1b and Ig-1a (IgG2a) allotypic determinants defined with monoclonal antibodies, *Mol. Immunol.* **16:**1005–1018.
51. Dangl, J. L., and Herzenberg, L. A., 1982, Selection of hybridomas and hybridoma variants using the fluorescence activated cell sorter, *J. Immunol. Meth.* **52:**1–14.
52. Goding, J. W., 1976, Conjugation of antibodies with fluorochromes: Modification of the standard methods, *J. Immunol. Meth.* **13:**215–236.
53. Oi, V. T., Glazer, A. N., and Stryer, L., 1982, Fluorescent phycobiliprotein conjugates for analysis of cells and molecules, *J. Cell Biol.* **93:**981–986.
54. Hardy, R. R., 1984, Purification and coupling of fluorescent proteins for use in flow cytometry, in: *Handbook of Experimental Immunology*, 4th ed. (D. M. Weir, C. C. Blackwell, L. A. Herzenberg, and L. A. Herzenberg, eds.), Blackwell, Edinburgh, In press.
55. Luria, S. E., and Delbruck, M., 1943, Mutation of bacteria from virus sensitivity to virus resistance, *Genetics* **28:**491–511.
56. Catcheside, D. G., 1949, in: *The Genetics of Micro-organisms*, Pitman, London, pp. 158–162.
57. Birshtein, B. K., Preud'homme, J.-L., and Scharff, M. D., 1974, Variants of mouse myeloma cells that produce short immunoglobulin heavy chains, *Proc. Natl. Acad. Sci. USA* **71:**3478–3482.
58. Rosen, A., and Klein, G., 1983, UV light-induced immunoglobulin heavy-chain class switch in a human lymphoblastoid cell line, *Nature* **306:**189–190.

Chapter 6

The Analysis of Structural Diversity in the Antibody Response

GILLIAN M. GRIFFITHS and CESAR MILSTEIN

1. Introduction

The heterogeneity of the antibody response presented a major problem to immunochemists wishing to study antibody structures. Such studies required large amounts of a single immunoglobulin molecule, which could not be obtained from normal immune sera. The discovery that multiple myelomas were tumors originating from a single clone of antibody-producing cells and hence gave rise to a homogeneous source of immunoglobulin was therefore extremely important and enabled the first structural studies of immunoglobulin molecules to be carried out.[1,2] Mouse plasmacytomas were particularly important because they provided homogeneous sources of antibodies that could be passaged and adapted to cell culture.[3,4] The use of myelomas provided a vast amount of information concerning immunoglobulin structure.[5–7] Myelomas also provided the early material to study the immunoglobulin gene organization of mouse and man. It was clear from these studies that a vast amount of structural diversity can be generated from a finite number of immunoglobulin genes (reviewed in Ref. 8). However, a detailed study of the structural diversity of the antibody response to a defined antigen was not possible, since myelomas do not originate from a response to a defined antigen. The most exciting aspect, namely the change during the maturation of the response, could not be defined at the molecular level.

The analysis of structural diversity in the antibody response to a defined antigen only became possible with the development of hybridoma technology.[9] Using this technique, it became possible to immunize animals and dissect the complexity of the response by generating hybridomas against the immunogen. The cloned hybridomas could then be used to produce unlimited supplies of a single antibody species with a defined antigenic specificity. Although hybridomas provided the reagents essential for addressing questions concerning the importance of structural diversity in the development of an antibody re-

GILLIAN M. GRIFFITHS and CESAR MILSTEIN • Laboratory of Molecular Biology, Medical Research Council, Cambridge CB2 2QH, England.

sponse, the analysis of the immunoglobulins produced often proved cumbersome in comparison with the production of the hybridomas themselves. To overcome this problem we have developed the technique of dideoxy sequencing of the mRNA encoding the immunoglobulin light and heavy chains that are produced at relatively high levels by these hybridomas. Using this technique, it is possible to analyze rapidly the degree of antibody diversity in an immune response at the more informative nucleic acid level. The technique has been simplified for use on a large scale and we have used it to analyze a large number of hybridomas produced at different stages of the antibody response to a defined antigen.

2. RNA Sequencing

The technique of dideoxy sequencing of mRNA is a modification of Sanger's dideoxy DNA sequencing[10] as first developed by Hamlyn *et al.*[11] A synthetic oligonucleotide is used to prime at a designed site on the mRNA template. cDNA synthesis can then be initiated by means of reverse transcriptase in the presence of all four dNTPs, one of which is labeled with ^{32}P. The cDNA synthesis can be terminated in a nucleotide-specific fashion by incorporation of each of the dideoxy nucleotide analogues. Since each cDNA transcript begins at the same 3′ site, as defined by the primer, gel fractionation can be used to fractionate the cDNAs according to size and hence reveal the sequence of nucleotides in the RNA template. This is illustrated in Fig. 1.

The sequencing of the MOPC-21 κ light chain using the dideoxy sequencing suggested that this technique would offer several advantages for a comparative study of immunoglobulin V regions:

1. Only a small number of primers designed to anneal to conserved regions of the immunoglobulin mRNA sequences would be required to sequence a large number of related V regions.
2. Extensive purification of the immunoglobulin mRNA would not be required, since the primer itself would constitute an important purification step, annealing only to the region of complementary sequence.
3. Furthermore, the method incorporated the rapid dideoxy, gel fractionation techniques developed for DNA sequencing, and should therefore provide a rapid analysis of V region expression at the nucleic acid level.

3. Analyzing Immunoglobulin Diversity by mRNA Sequencing

In order to realize the full potential of the dideoxy RNA sequencing for use in a large-scale analysis it was necessary to modify and develop certain aspects of the technique such that the method was simple and reliable.

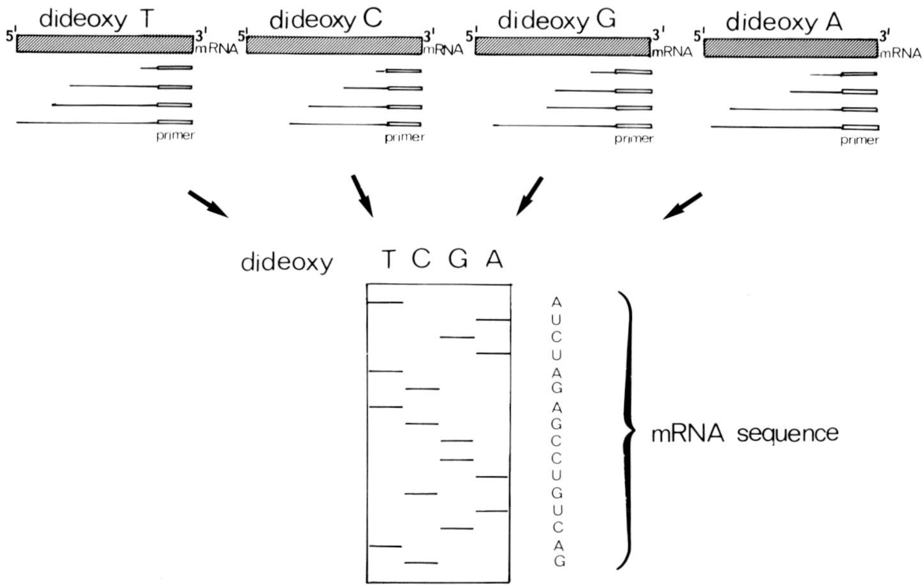

Figure 1. Diagrammatic representation of a sequencing reaction. Four cDNA reactions are carried out using the same mRNA and the same primer in the presence of all four deoxynucleotides and reverse transcriptase. Each reaction contains only one of the four dideoxynucleotides. Random incorporation of dideoxynucleotides produces a series of transcripts all corresponding to stops produced by the analogue. So, for example, incorporation with dideoxy-T produces transcripts all ending at points that correspond to an A in the mRNA.

3.1. RNA Preparation

The study of a large number of hybridomas requires a large number of mRNA preparations, which can also entail a great deal of tissue culture. It was therefore necessary to define a suitable method of RNA purification which minimized not only the amount of work involved, but also reliably gave good results. Early sequencing attempts demonstrated that mRNA encoding the immunoglobulin light chains could be sequenced successfully using a preparation of total cellular RNA,[12] without poly A^+ purification. Unfortunately, the results using primers for sequencing the heavy chains were less successful and the efficiency of priming to the heavy chain message was often inadequate. In order to obtain good sequences for both the light and the heavy chain, purification to the poly A^+ stage was essential.

The method of RNA purification finally adopted is based upon the direct isolation of poly A^+-containing species from a cytoplasmic cell fraction by direct binding of oligo-dT. The attraction of this method was that poly A^+-containing species were isolated in a one-step process.[13] This method is fully described in a later section, but can be summarized: Cells are lysed by NP40.

The cytoplasmic fraction, isolated by spinning out the nuclei, is treated with proteinase K to remove ribonucleases and other proteins. Poly A^+-containing species are then isolated directly from this fraction by addition of oligo-dT cellulose in 0.5 M NaCl. The oligo-dT cellulose can be spun out of a relatively large volume and transferred to a column from which the bound RNA can be eluted at low salt and 50°C. RNA prepared in this way is routinely used for sequencing both the light and heavy chain RNA templates.

There are several significant advantages to this method of RNA preparation. First, only a relatively small number of cells are required. As few as 2×10^8 cells have been used, yielding 50–100 μg of poly A^+ RNA. Cells were routinely grown in a 1-liter roller flask from which 800 ml of cells (4×10^8) could be harvested every other day. RNA could be isolated both from freshly harvested cells and from cells kept frozen at −70°C for long periods of time. In this way the tissue culture involved was minimized and it was possible to grow up many cell lines at once. In addition, the poly A^+-enriched RNA provided enough material for at least 50 sequencing reactions. Furthermore, the method was technically simple and very fast, involving only a few hours of work for each batch of RNA samples prepared. Two problems were encountered when initially using this technique. The first was inhibition of cDNA synthesis by the presence of SDS. Often SDS contamination would be seen by a slight cloudiness apparent in the redissolved pellet. By routinely washing the final RNA pellet with 3 × 500 μl of cold 80% ethanol the problem has been subsequently avoided. The second problem encountered was that of degradation during purification. RNA degradation was characterised by a low yield of RNA and the presence of only short transcripts after cDNA synthesis. This problem, presumably due to RNase activity during the isolation process, could be avoided by the addition of 10 mM vanadyl ribonucleoside complexes to the lysis buffer. These complexes have been found to bind many RNases and inhibit their activity.[14] In addition, the use of these inhibitors seemed to increase the average yield of RNA. It should be noted, however, that when isolating RNA from hybridomas the use of such inhibitors is not usually necessary.

3.2. Conditions for cDNA Synthesis

The direct sequencing of a mRNA molecule by the dideoxy approach described depends upon the accurate synthesis of a cDNA from the mRNA template. This reaction is catalyzed by the enzyme reverse transcriptase. The quality of the sequencing obtained thus depends upon the purity of the enzyme and the reaction conditions being optimal. A variety of studies carried out before 1978 suggested that a great many factors were involved in producing full-length transcripts of cDNA.[15] However, studies carried out with highly purified reverse transcriptase showed that many of these factors were in fact acting by inhibiting contaminating RNases in the preparation.[16,17] Optimal conditions were found to depend upon pH, temperature, and the concentrations of deoxyribonucleoside triphosphates, monovalent cations, and divalent cations. Retzel *et al.*[17] reported a dramatic increase in the length of cDNA synthesis by increasing the concentration of monovalent cations, and the optimal conditions proposed were 75 μM dNTP, 148 mM NaCl (or KCl), and 6 mM Mg^{2+}, buffered at pH 8.1, and incubated at 42°C. By these criteria, the original conditions used in RNA sequencing were not optimal.[18] In these reactions the concentrations used were 50 μM dNTP (1.5 μM labeling dNTP), 50 mM KCl, and 5 mM $MgCl_2$, buffered at pH 8.3, and incubated at 42°C. Clearly the concentrations of monovalent cations and the dNTPs used were likely to be limiting cDNA synthesis. The use of the high concentration of a monovalent cation during RNA sequencing was found to give marginally better incorporation of the labeled dNTP during cDNA synthesis without producing adverse side reactions (such as annealing of the primer at sequence-related sites on the RNA template, or the formation of secondary structures that might prevent cDNA synthesis or cause problems during gel electrophoresis).

Early sequencing gels also suggested that the low concentration of the labeling dNTP was a limiting factor in early sequencing reactions. A number of nonspecific chain terminations were observed that could be accounted for by the low concentration of labeling nucleotide in the reaction. In these cases a band occurred in all four tracks regardless of the dideoxynucleotide present, and the nucleotide at this position could not be determined. Analysis of the gels indicated that such terminations frequently occurred at the position immediately preceding incorporation of the labeled dNTP. Hence it appeared that when the growing cDNA chain reached the position preceding the point where the labeled dNTP should be incorporated it was not always able to continue. Consequently chains terminated prematurely at this position in all four dideoxy reactions, regardless of nucleotide specificity. In dideoxy DNA sequencing this problem was encountered and overcome by the addition of a high concentration of unlabeled dNTP corresponding to the labeling dNTP, midterm in the reaction,[10] allowing any prematurely terminated chains to proceed to completion.

A similar chase reaction, providing a high concentration of all four dNTPs (250 μM), was found to be effective in RNA sequencing only when carefully buffered to maintain a pH of 8.3 at 42°C. The pH of this mixture was found to be very important and the pH of all chase mixes at 42°C was checked immediately preceding addition. The effect of a chase is clearly demonstrated in Fig. 2. This gel shows two sequencing reactions using the same preparation of mRNA and the same primer. The only difference is the addition of a chase reaction to the four lanes (ddT, ddC, ddG, and ddA) on the right side. At two positions, marked with arrows, artifact bands running across all four tracks in the unchased reaction disappear with chasing. In addition, the background is much lower in the chased reaction, and the gel much easier to read. Even so, certain artifacts remain, depending on the deoxynucleotide being used to label the reactions. For this reason reactions are always carried out in duplicate, labeling with two different nucleotides (Fig. 3).

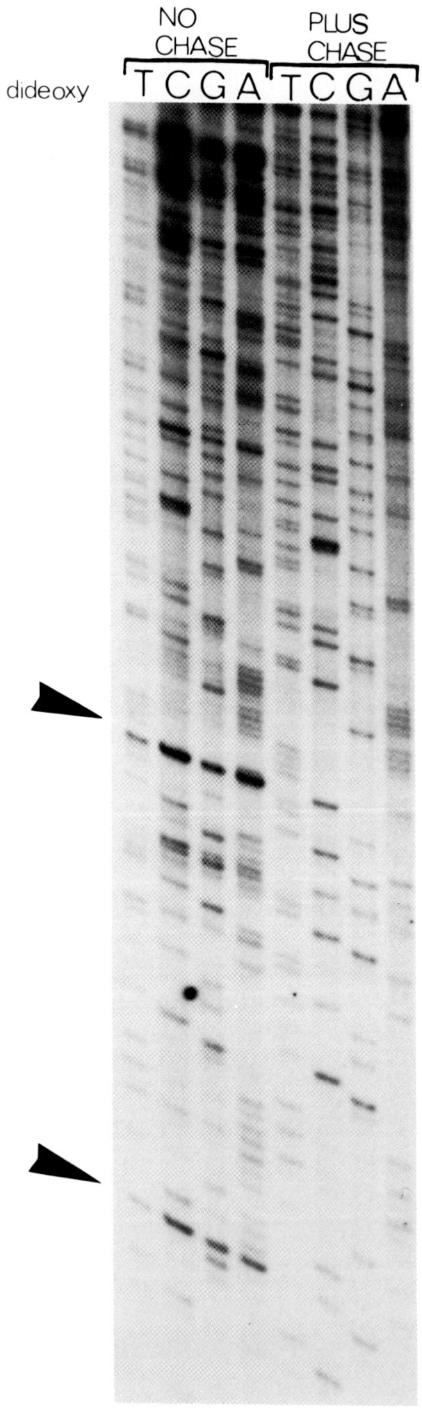

Figure 2. Two sequencing reactions using the same mRNA preparation and primer terminating reactions with dideoxys T, C, G, and A as shown. Both reactions were labeled by incorporation of [α,^{32}P]dATP. Fifteen minutes after the initial addition of enzyme a chase of all four dNTPs was added to the four lanes on the right. This removed artifact bands as indicated on the left with arrows.

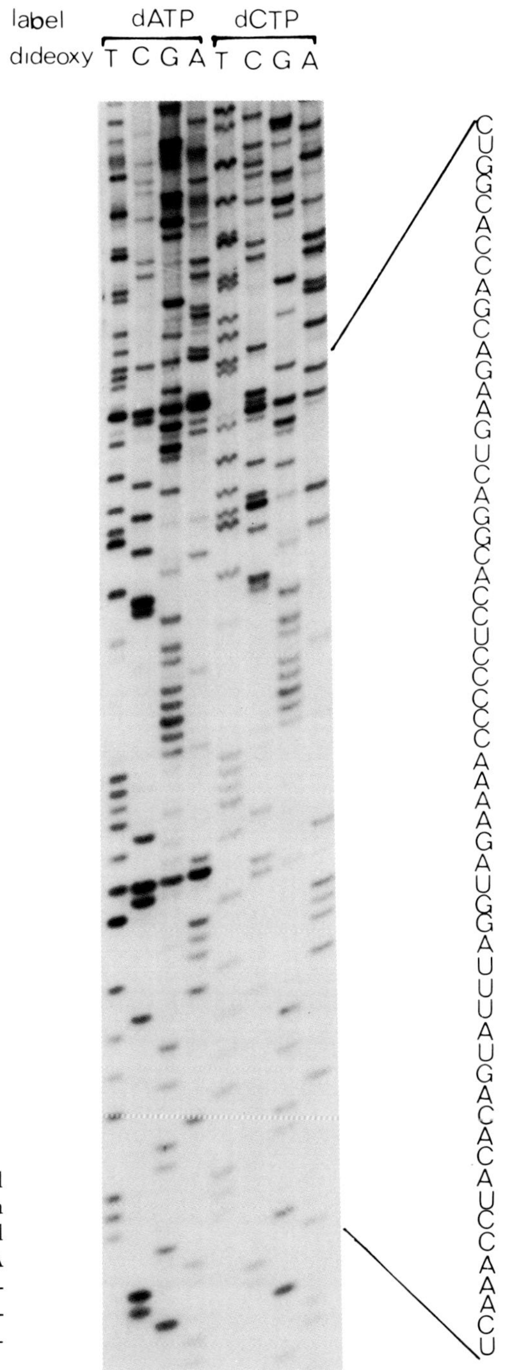

Figure 3. Two sequencing reactions are used to produce the final mRNA sequence, shown on the right. The same mRNA is sequenced using the same primer but labeling the cDNA transcripts with two different deoxynucleotides. In this case the reactions have been labeled with [α^{32}P]dATP and [α^{32}P]dCTP. ^{35}S-Labeled deoxynucleotides can also be used.

3.3. Choice of Primers

The choice of primers was not insignificant. All primers were designed against relatively conserved regions of the mRNA template by comparison with other immunoglobulin sequences, and were usually 15 bases in length. Sequences requiring G-rich primers were avoided, as were sequences that would produce complementarity within the primer. In the case of the κ and μ constant region primers, several different synthetic oligonucleotides were tested, priming at slightly different sites within these regions. The quality of sequencing did not appear to depend on the site of priming.

4. Protocol

4.1. Isolation of Poly A-Containing RNA from Cells

Typically 3×10^8 cells were used, yielding approximately 120 μg of poly A-containing RNA. Cells were washed in Earle's medium to remove traces of serum and either used immediately or frozen at −70°C. If frozen cells were used, care had to be taken to disperse clumps during thawing at 37°C.

Lysis was in 10 ml of LB per 10^8 cells (0.14 M NaCl, 1.5 mM $MgCl_2$, 10 mM Tris pH 8.6, 0.5% NP40). Cell nuclei were removed by centrifugation at 2800 rpm, 4°C, for 20 min.

The postnuclear supernatant was digested with proteinase K for 30 min at 37°C by addition of an equal volume of 2× PK buffer (200 mM Tris pH 7.5, 300 mM NaCl, 25 mM EDTA, 200 μg/ml proteinase K), which had been predigested for 15–20 min at 37°C. Proteinase K was subsequently denatured by heating for 3 min at 60–65°C. The mixture was cooled on ice and brought to a final concentration of 0.5 M NaCl.

Oligo-dT cellulose, prewashed first with 0.1 M NaOH and then with elution buffer (EB; 10 mM Tris pH 8, 5 mM EDTA, 0.5% SDS) at 50°C and equilibrated in binding buffer (BB; 500 mM NaCl, 10 mM Tris pH 8, 5 mM EDTA, 0.5% SDS), was added directly to the cytoplasmic RNA in PK buffer (approximately 0.1 g per 5×10^8 cells) and mixed at room temperature for 30 min. The oligo-dT was pelleted, transferred to a column, and washed with 3×1.5 column volumes of BB, 3× 1.5 column volumes of WB (100 mM NaCl, 10 mM Tris, 5 mM EDTA, 0.5% SDS) and eluted with 3× 1.5 column volumes of EB at 50°C.

RNA was precipitated with 0.3 M NaAc, 2.5 volumes of ethanol at −20°C for 12 hr.

4.2. RNA Sequencing

The following solutions were prepared:

1. Reverse transcriptase buffer:

a. 10× RT: 500 mM Tris pH 8.3, 1.5 M KCl, 100 mM $MgCl_2$
b. 200 mM Dithiothreitol (DTT) in H_2O
c. 5× RT was made fresh each time by diluting an equal volume of (a) and (b)

2. Stock solutions of nucleotide triphosphates:
   a. 1.0 mM stock solutions of dTTP, dGTP, dATP, dCTP in ddH_2O
   b. 100 μM stocks of ddTTP, ddCTP, ddGTP in ddH_2O
   c. 2 μM stock of ddATP
3. 5× dNTP-A mix: the following stock solutions were mixed:

dTTP 1.0 mM stock	400 μl
dGTP 1.0 mM stock	400 μl
dCTP 1.0 mM stock	400 μl
50 mM Tris pH 8, 1 mM EDTA	160 μl
ddH_2O	240 μl

4. Each ddNTP was diluted with a suitable quantity of dNTP-A. Ratios of 1:1 and 2:1 (deoxy:dideoxy) were tested, and the correct working mix determined empirically.
5. Chase mix: (a) stock solution of all four dNTPs at 2.5 mM in H_2O. (b) Working solution 250 μM dATP, dGTP, dCTP, dTTP, 100 mM Tris pH 8.3 at 42°C + approximately 1 U RT (enzyme) per reaction chased. *Note*: immediately prior to use the pH of the chase mix was checked (at 42°C) using pH indicator paper, and then the correct amount of RT added.
6. Formamide dyes 0.1% xylene cyanol FF, 0.1% bromophenol blue, 10 mM EDTA in deionized formamide.
7. Reverse transcriptase (RT) was supplied by Anglican Biotechnology, Colchester, England or Life Sciences, St. Petersburg, Florida.

4.3. Sequencing Reactions

1. Reactions were carried out in 1.5-ml Eppendorf vials, which as supplied were found to be free of ribonuclease activity. The use of these tubes simplified the whole procedure: additions could be made using a Gilson Pipetman or a Hamilton 1- or 2-μl dispensing syringe, and proper mixing of the reagents achieved by centrifugation. In this way eight sets of sequencing reactions could be handled simultaneously.
2. A quantity of 12.5 μl of [α^{32}P]dATP (400 Ci/mmole, 1 mCi/ml) was dried down in a siliconized, RNase-free glass tube and the following additions were made: 4 μl of 5× RT, 2–4 μg of poly A-enriched RNA, 30–120 ng of synthetic oligonucleotide primer (determined by titration for each primer) and ddH_2O to a final volume of 12 μl.
3. Three-microliter aliquots were made to four separate 1.5-ml capped Eppendorf tubes and deoxy/dideoxy mixes and enzyme added:

aliquot	3.0 μl	3.0 μl	3.0 μl	3 μl
deoxy/dideoxy				
ddTTP	2.0 μl			
ddCTP		2.0 μl		
ddGTP			2.0 μl	
ddATP				2.0 μl
RT (4 U/ml)	0.5 μl	0.5 μl	0.5 μl	0.5 μl

Note: Reverse transcriptase was diluted in ddH_2O immediately prior to use.

4. The reaction vials were sealed and the reagents mixed by centrifugation (15 sec in Eppendorf centrifuge 5413).
5. Reaction mixtures were incubated for 15 min at 42°C.
6. One microliter of chase mix (pH 8.3) was added to each reaction and mixed by centrifugation, and the incubation was continued for a further 15 min at 42°C.
7. Four microliters of formamide dyes was added to terminate each reaction and the mixtures heated to 100°C for 3 min prior to gel electrophoresis, using 6% gels.

5. Analyzing the Structural Diversity of the Antibody Response to Oxazolone

By combining hybridoma technology with that of dideoxy mRNA sequencing technology, a study of the structural diversity of the antibody response to the antigen 2-phenyloxazolone has been carried out in this laboratory. More than 50 different oxazolone-specific hybridomas have been generated from different stages of the response and the light and heavy chain V regions determined by mRNA sequencing.

The hapten 2-phenyl oxazolone (Ox) serves as a relatively simple antigen when conjugated to a carrier such as chicken serum albumin (CSA). Immunization of Ox–CSA elicits an antibody response of restricted heterogeneity in several strains of mice. Using such a simple system, it has been possible to define some of the genetic mechanisms that contribute to the diversity of the antibody response at different stages after immunization.

Hybridomas have been generated at 7 and 14 days after primary immunization and at 3 days after a secondary immunization with Ox–CSA. In order to obtain full V region sequences for these hybridomas five primers were designed which primed to relatively conserved regions within the immunoglobulin mRNA (Figure 4). The V_H and V_L regions of 26 hybridomas from the primary response revealed that 20 of these hybridomas used the same basic sequences—each of the V_H and the V_L region sequences, even in hybridomas derived from different mice. The frequent occurrence of identical sequences suggested that they were the result of expression of a single pair of germ-line genes which we named V_H-Ox_1 for the heavy chain and V_k-Ox_1 for the light

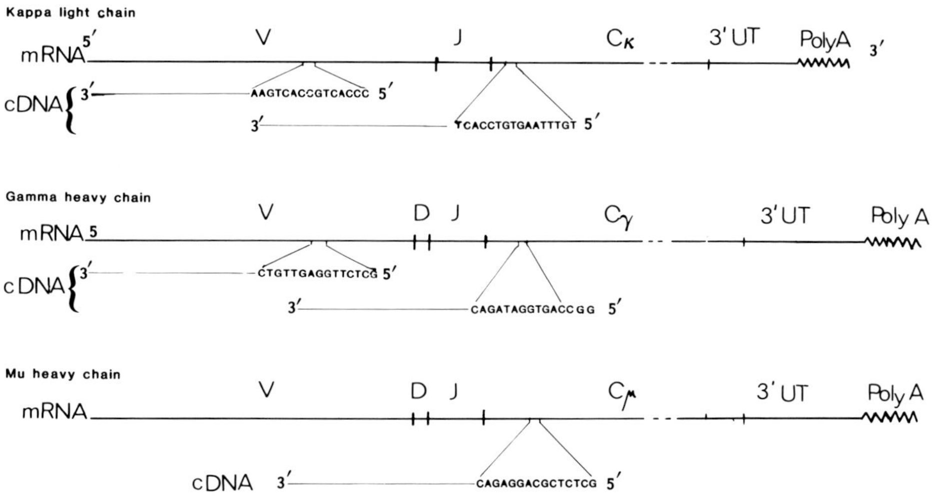

Figure 4. Diagram to illustrate the relative positions of primer used in sequencing on the various mRNA templates. The templates encoding the immunoglobulin mRNAs for the κ light chain, γ heavy chain, and μ heavy chains are illustrated indicating the regions encoding the variable (V), diversity (D), joining (J), constant (C), 3′ untranslated (3′UT), and poly A regions of the message. The sequences of the primers used are shown at the sites where they were complementary.

chain. The complete sequences of the V regions expressed by these hybridomas obtained by RNA sequencing provided a very detailed picture of the mechanisms that produced antibody diversity at the different stages of the response.

The primary response to oxazolone appears to be dominated by the expression of the two germ-line genes V_k-Ox_1 and V_H-Ox_1.[21] In contrast, the secondary response appears to be dominated by the expression of quite different germ-line genes.[22] The majority of hybridomas isolated from the primary response expressed both V_H-Ox_1 and V_k-Ox_1. Furthermore, the combinatorial and junctional mechanisms that could produce diversity either by the use of different D and J segments or by variation in the precise site of joining of these segments are highly restricted in the antibody response to oxazolone. For example in the heavy chain the V_H-Ox_1 sequence is consistently joined to D and J segments that are highly related in sequence and identical in length. In the light chain there is a strong preference for the use of J_5 and an absolute conservation of a leucine residue at position 96, a position where sequence variation is often introduced during V–J recombination. Even in the secondary response, when the majority of hybridomas were found to be expressing V genes from other families, those that expressed the Ox_1 genes demonstrate the same basic antibody structure. There is, however, a striking difference between the Ox_1 antibodies observed from the day 7 response and those observed from later stages of the response. At day 7 both V_H-Ox_1 and V_k-Ox_1 are expressed in an unmutated form.[23] However, at day 14 and in the secondary response, all hybridomas expressing these genes show a small number of nucleotide changes which predict amino acid changes in the antibody molecule (Fig. 5). Further-

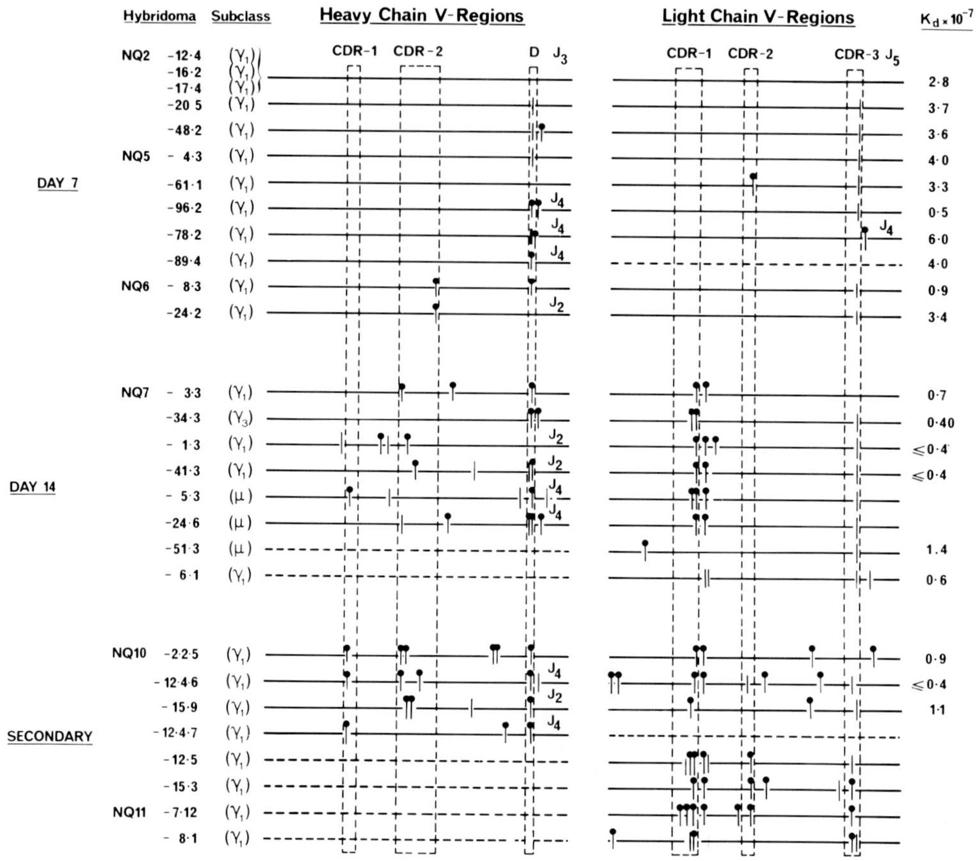

Figure 5. Diagrammatic comparison of the mRNA sequences from anti-2-phenyl oxazolone-secreting hybridomas derived at different stages after immunization with Ox–CSA.[21] The variable region sequences of each hybridoma have been compared with the sequences of V_H-Oxl and V_k-OXl, respectively. Unbroken horizontal lines denote sequence identity, broken lines represent extensive sequence differences. A vertical bar shows the relative position of codons containing differences. A black circle indicates that these changes predict an amino acid difference at this position. Complementarity-determining regions (CDR-1, -2, -3) have been marked, as have the D and J regions. Where different J segments are observed these are represented according to the numbering of Sakano *et al.*[23] Dissociation constants K_d are shown on the right.

more, these variant antibodies show a significantly higher affinity for oxazolone than do their germ-line counterparts. These changes are most likely to have arisen as a result of somatic point mutation and the results suggest that somatic point mutation followed by antigenic selection is important in the maturation of the antibody response to the antigen oxazolone. The importance of these results is that they demonstrate the structural changes that occur during the development of an antibody response to a defined antigen. By using mRNA sequencing it has been possible to define these changes at the nucleic acid level and identify the genetic mechanisms that contribute to the structural diversification of the antibody response.

References

1. *Antibodies*, 1967, Cold Spring Harbor Symposia on Quantitative Biology, Volume 32, Cold Spring Harbor, New York.
2. Cohen, S., and Milstein, C., 1967, Structure and biological properties of immunoglobulins, *Adv. Immunol.* **7**:1–89.
3. Potter, M., 1972, Immunoglobulin-producing tumors and myeloma proteins of mice, *Physiol. Rev.* **52**:631–670.
4. Horibata, K., and Harris, A. W., 1970, Mouse myelomas and lymphomas in culture, *Exp. Cell Res.* **60**:61–70.
5. Gally, J. A., and Edelman, G. M., 1972, The genetic control of immunoglobulin synthesis, *Annu. Rev. Genet.* **6**:1–30.
6. Pink, J. R. L., and Milstein, C., 1967, Disulphide bridges of immunoglobulin G1 heavy chains, *Nature* **214**:939–941.
7. Kabat, E. A., Wu, T. T., Bilofsky, M., Reid-Muller, M., and Perry, M., 1983, *Sequences of Proteins of Immunological Interest*, National Institutes of Health, Bethesda, Maryland.
8. Honjo, T., 1984, Immunoglobulin genes, *Annu. Rev. Immunol.* **1**:499–528.
9. Köhler, G., and Milstein, C., 1975, Continuous culture of fused cells secreting antibody of predefined specificity, *Nature* **256**:495–497.
10. Sanger, F., Nicklen, S., and Coulson, A. R., 1977, DNA sequencing with chain terminating inhibitors, *Proc. Natl. Acad. Sci. USA* **74**:5463–5467.
11. Hamlyn, P. H., Brownlee, G. G., Cheng, C. C., Gait, M. J., and Milstein, C., 1978, Complete sequence of constant and 3′ non-coding regions of an immunoglobulin mRNA using the dideoxynucleotide method of RNA sequencing, *Cell* **15**:1067–1075.
12. Auffray, C., and Rougeon, F., 1980, Purification of mouse immunoglobulin heavy chain messenger RNAs from total myeloma RNA, *Eur. J. Biochem.* **107**:303–314.
13. Favaloro, J., Treisman, R., and Kamen, R., 1980, *Meth. Enzymol.* **65**:718–729.
14. Berger, S. L., and Birkenmeier, C. S., 1979, Inhibition of intractable nucleases with ribonucleoside-vanadyl complexes: Isolation of mRNA from resting lymphocytes, *Biochemistry* **18**:5144–5149.
15. Williams, J. G., (ed.), 1981, *Genetic Engineering*, Volume 1, Academic Press, New York.
16. Buell, G. N., Wickens, M. P., Payvar, F., and Schimke, R. T., 1978, Full length cDNA synthesis from hen oviduct mRNAs, *J. Biol. Chem.* **253**:2471–2482.
17. Retzel, E. F., Collet, M. S., and Farus, A. J., 1980, Enzymatic synthesis of deoxyribonucleic acid by avian reverse transcriptase *in vitro*: Optimum conditions required for transcription of large ribonucleic acid templates, *Biochemistry* **19**:513–518.
18. Kaartinen, M., Griffiths, G. M., Hamlyn, P. H., Markham, A. F., Karjalainen, K., Pelkonen, J. L. T., Mäkelä, O., and Milstein, C., 1983, Anti-oxazolone light and heavy chain mRNA sequences, *J. Immunol.* **130**:937–945.
19. Mäkelä, O., Kaartinen, M., Pelkonen, J. L. T., and Karjalainen, K., 1978, Inheritance of antibody specificity V. Anti-2-phenyl oxazolone in the mouse, *J. Exp. Med.* **198**:1644.
20. Kaartinen, M., Griffiths, G. M., Markham, A. F., and Milstein, C., 1983, mRNA sequences define an unusually restricted IgG response to 2 phenyl-oxazolone and its early diversification, *Nature* **304**:320–324.
21. Griffiths, G. M., Berek, C., Kaartinen, M., and Milstein, C., 1984, Somatic mutation and the maturation of the immune response to 2-phenyl oxazolone, *Nature* **312**:271–275.
22. Berek, C., Griffiths, G. M., and Milstein, C., 1985, Manuscript in preparation.
23. Sakano, H., Maki, R., Kurosawa, Y., Roeder, W., and Tonegawa, S., 1980, Two types of somatic recombinations are necessary for the generation of immunoglobulin gene recombination, *Nature* **286**:670–683.

Chapter 7

Expression of Cloned Immunoglobulin Genes

FREDERICK W. ALT

1. Introduction

The variable region of immunoglobulin (Ig) heavy and light chain genes is encoded by multiple genetic elements. Over the past several years, intensive study has yielded remarkable new insights into both the mechanism by which these different elements are assembled to form the complete gene and the numerous types of diversification processes that occur during the assembly of these elements. In addition, this period has also witnessed the development of new technologies for isolating, expressing, and potentially even creating functional Ig genes. Among these are cell transformation procedures for expressing cloned genes in cell lines, germ-line introduction procedures for expressing cloned genes in the animal, and the development of cell lines that are active in immunoglobulin gene recombination processes and will assemble introduced immunoglobulin gene segments into complete genes. Together, these advances potentially offer many novel methods to produce natural or modified Ig gene products. In this context, the purpose of this chapter is to review what is known about the assembly and expression of endogenous and introduced Ig genes.

2. Mechanism of Immunoglobulin Gene Assembly

2.1. Immunoglobulin Gene Structure

The basic unit of a typical immunoglobulin molecule is composed of two identical heavy and two identical light polypeptide chains. The amino terminus of these chains contains a region of variable amino acid sequence (V region) in which reside the primary determinants of antigen-binding specificity. The remainder of each chain is comprised of a region of constant amino acid se-

FREDERICK W. ALT • Department of Biochemistry and Institute for Cancer Research, Columbia University, College of Physicians and Surgeons, New York, New York 10032.

quence, which for both heavy and light chains may be one of several types. The constant portion of the heavy chain has been implicated in a variety of effector functions, including complement fixation, Fc receptor binding, and others. It is now clear that the DNA sequences encoding both the heavy and light chain variable region are assembled from component gene segments upstream of the DNA sequences encoding the corresponding constant region sequences (for review see Ref. 1).

2.2. Assembly of the Heavy Chain Variable Region

In both the human and the mouse, the variable region of an immunoglobulin heavy chain is encoded by at least three separate germ-line DNA elements: the variable gene segment V_H, the diversity segment D, and the joining segment J_H (Fig. 1A).[2–4] In the genome of the mouse, these elements are encoded in three separate clusters: the four J_H segments lie within a 2-kb (kilobase) region approximately 5 kb 5′ to the nearest C_H gene (C_μ), and the 12 characterized D segments lie in a cluster from 1 to 80 kb 5′ to the J_H cluster.[1–5] Approximately 100–200 V_H segments lie at an as yet unknown distance 5′ to the D segments.[6,7] The organization of the human J_H region resembles that of the mouse,[4] but little is known about the structure and organization of human D and V_H gene segments.

Recombination between the various variable region gene segments is apparently mediated by a set of highly conserved recognition sequences that consist of a palindromic heptamer and a characteristic nonamer separated by a spacer region; these sequences may serve as targets for recombinases.[1–3,8] A complete recognition sequence starting with the heptamer lies flush with the 3′ side of each V_H and D segment and flush with the 5′ side of each D and J_H segment (Fig. 1B).[2,3,8] The spacer length for the D recognition sequence is 12 bp (base pairs), while for the V_H and J_H it is 23 bp. Recombination can apparently take place only between elements that are flanked, respectively, by recognition sequences containing 12- and 23-bp spacers.[1–3] Thus, assembly of a complete V_HDJ_H variable region gene is necessarily mediated by D to J_H and V_H to D recombination events. These joining events occur early in the pre-B stage of B-lymphocyte differentiation, and generally occur in a distinct order: a D segment is first joined to a J_H segment, and subsequently a V_H segment is added to the DJ_H complex (summarized in Fig. 1).[7]

The assembly of V gene elements has been proposed to result from a two-step, nonreciprocal recombination event (Fig. 1).[9] The first step involves a double-strand cleavage between the elements and their flanking recognition sequences accompanied by the precise fusion of the recognition heptamers—which results in the loss from the cell of both the fused sequences and the sequences between them—as a circle. The second step involves the imprecise fusion of the D and J_H (or V_H and DJ_H) in a process that can include the loss of bases from the potential coding sequence of one or both partners and the

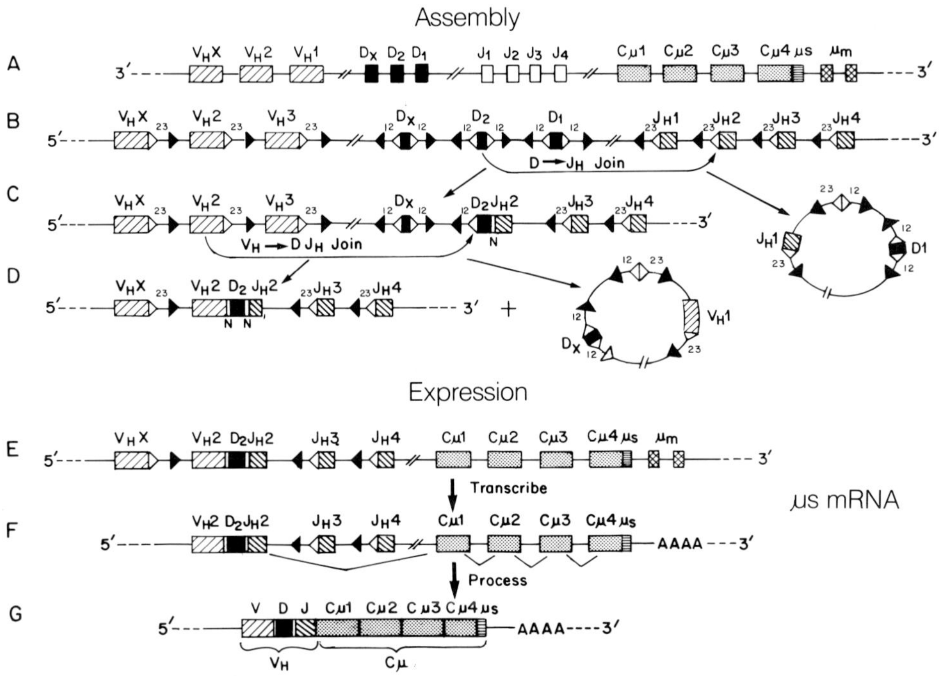

Figure 1. Assembly and expression of immunoglobulin heavy chain genes. Upper panels: Assembly (A) The organization of the germ-line heavy chain gene segments, shown schematically. (B–D) The intermediate structures and by-products of heavy-chain variable-region gene (V_HDJ_H) assembly. Variable (V_H), diversity (D), and joining (J_H) segments are indicated. Regions at the point of recombination where bases can be either lost or added (N regions) are indicated as N. The four major μ heavy-chain constant-region exons ($C_\mu 1$–4) as well as the secretion- (μ_s) and membrane-specific mini-exons (μ_m) are also indicated. (◁, ▷) 5′ and 3′ recognition heptamers, respectively; (◀, ▶) 5′ and 3′ recognition nonamers, respectively. The spacer length (in base pairs) between the heptamer and nonamer sequences is indicated as 12 or 23. Linear structures are within the chromosome and circular structures have been excised from the chromosome. For further details see Ref. 7 and the text. Lower panels: Expression. (E) An assembled μ heavy gene. (F) Its primary transcript. (G) Removal of intervening sequences from the primary transcript by RNA processing mechanisms, leading to the generation of the mature μ heavy mRNA. Only the generation of the secretion-specific form of the μ mRNA is indicated. The generation of the membrane-specific form is described in the text and reviewed in Ref. 48 and 49. For simplicity, a small intron that separates the 5′ leader sequence from the body of the variable region is not indicated.

addition of new bases at the point of recombination. Flexibility in this recombination point is an important source of antibody diversity.[1]

2.3. Assembly of Light-Chain Variable-Region Genes

For both the human and the mouse, light chains can be of either the κ or the λ type. The light chain variable region gene is composed of two gene segments; the variable gene segment V_L and the joining segment J_L.[10–12] The 3′

side of the V_L gene segments and the 5′ side of the J_L segments are directly flanked by conserved recognition sequences essentially identical to those flanking the V_H gene elements, but in this case, either the V_L or the J_L, respectively, contains the 12- or 23-bp spacers.[1,10–12] These elements are fused subsequent to the production of a complete heavy chain by the pre-B cell[13] via a two-step, nonreciprocal process similar to that outlined for heavy chain, except that no extra bases have been observed in V_LJ_L joints.[1]

2.4. Heavy Chain Class Switching

The class of an Ig molecule is determined by the constant region of its heavy chain. During the differentiation of a B cell to a plasma cell, the class of Ig produced by its progeny may change from IgM to a different class (i.e., IgG or IgA), while maintaining the same variable region specificity. This phenomenon, termed H chain class switching, allows a single clone of B cells to generate progeny that maintain the same antigen-binding (V_H) specificity linked to different C_H effector functions. This class switch process is effected by a recombination deletion mechanism distinct from that involved in variable region gene assembly.[14–16] The order of the C_H genes in the mouse has been determined to be 5′-(V_HDJ_H-C_μ-C_δ-$C_{\gamma3}$-$C_{\gamma1}$-$C_{\gamma2b}$-$C_{\gamma2a}$-C_ϵ-C_α)-3′.[17] Expression, for example, of γ_{2b} heavy chains results from juxtaposition of the $C_{\gamma2b}$ gene segment to the expressed V_HDJ_H complex by deletion of the intervening DNA sequence, including the C_μ C_δ $C_{\gamma3}$ and $C_{\gamma1}$ genes.[14,15] Unlike the V_HDJ_H assembly process, the switch recombination process takes place far from any coding regions of the gene and thus does not have an effect on the gene structure (reviewed in Ref. 18). This property allows for easy exchange of C_H regions in cloned and expressed genes, as described below.

3. Assembly of Transfected Genes

Recently, two different groups have demonstrated site-specific assembly of Ig variable region gene segments that were transfected into lymphoid cell lines.[19,20] Probably the key factor in these experiments was the derivation of lines that were in the active stages of Ig gene assembly. To date, all such lines have been derived by transformation of murine pre-B cells with the Abelson murine leukemia virus (A-MuLV).[7,13,21–24]

3.1. Assembly of Transfected V_H Gene Segments

Liver is the site of B-cell differentiation in the fetal mouse and is a rich source of very early B cells. Correspondingly, when early fetal liver is used as a source of transformants, nearly all of the transformants obtained represent the earliest defined stage of the B-cell pathway: a null cell with D to J_H rear-

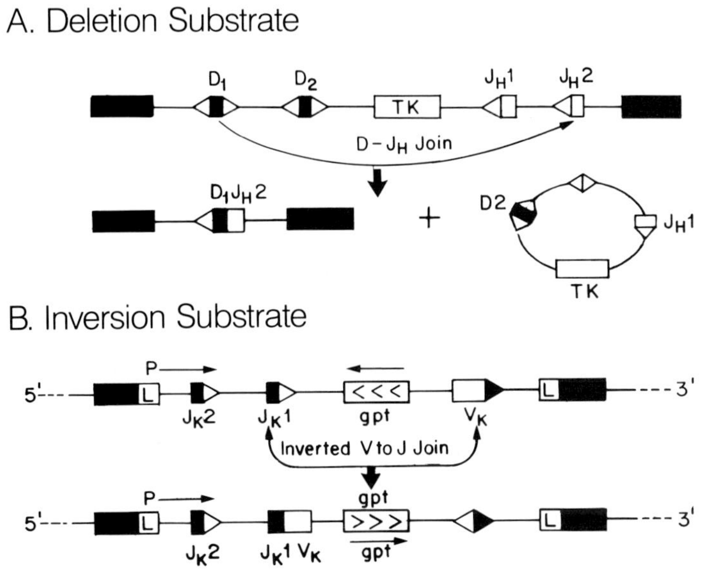

Figure 2. Variable region gene recombination substrates. (A) A deletion substrate. Excision of an intervening TK gene from the chromosome as a result of D to J_H recombination is indicated. The D segments, TK gene, and J_H segments are indicated. (◁, ▷) 5′ and 3′ recognition elements (nonamer–spacer-heptamer), respectively. Blackened areas indicate host chromosomal sequences. For further details see the text and Ref. 20. (B) A retrovirus-based inversion substrate. Activation of an intervening *gpt* gene by inverted joining between V_κ and J_κ segments is indicated. The *gpt* gene and 5′ and 3′ LTRs of the virus (L) are indicated. The transcriptional orientation of the *gpt* gene and a promotor (P) in the 5′ LTR are indicated by arrows. Other symbols above. See the text and Ref. 19 for further details.

rangements on both chromosomes and no light chain gene rearrangement.[7,13] Strikingly, when such cells are propagated in culture they actively append V_H segments to preexisting DJ_H complexes, indicating that they are active in the enzymatic processes leading to the construction of the complete heavy chain variable region gene.[7,23,24] To analyze the process of the heavy chain variable region gene construction, recombinant plasmids containing murine D and J_H segments separated by the herpes simplex virus thymidine kinase (TK) gene (Fig. 2A) were introduced into TK^- derivatives of fetal liver transformants by unlinked cotransformation with the pSV2-*neo* gene.[20] The latter gene is a dominant marker and confers resistance to growth in the presence of the antibiotic G418 (which is toxic to mammalian cells).[25] In such cotransformation protocols, the introduced construct and the second dominant marker gene integrate in close proximity into the genome of the host cell.[26] Once clones are derived that express both the TK and pSV-*neo* activities, one can select for site-specific recombinants between the D and J_H segments by selecting for cells that have lost the introduced TK gene [by growth in the presence of 5-bromodeoxyuridine (BrdU)], but which retain the bulk of the introduced DNA by maintaining a selection for retention of the cointroduced pSV2-*neo* gene.[20] Because introduced DNA is often unstable in the cells, the continued positive selection may be critical.[20,26] Analyses of many such BrdU-resistant transformants indicated that essentially all had lost the internal TK gene as a result of site-specific joining events between the D and J_H segments (Fig. 2A).[20] In fact, in some transformants, the rate of this joining process is so great that rearrangements accumulate to readily detectable levels in the population, even in the absence of any selection.[20,27] A number of these rearrangements have been molecularly cloned and the nature of the joints analyzed by DNA sequencing. In all cases the joints occurred within regions of the D and J_H segments found in physiological joints, but in each, the site of joining within either the D or J_H segment was unique.[20] Thus, the joining process in these lines appears to be a faithful replica of the endogenous joining process. Numerous independent integrations of this construct were found to be actively joined in these lines; thus, a precise chromosomal location of the variable region gene elements is not required for recognition and site-specific joining by the V_H recombinase.[20,27] Because there is no reason to believe that such lines would not also append V_H gene segments to DJ_H complexes to form complete variable region genes, this system offers a unique method for the generation of multiple V_H sequences that differ only by the presence of microheterogeneity in the V_HDJ_H joint, or even the generation of hybrid variable gene segments using segments from different species or different types of chains. Using techniques described below, such artificialy created V_H (or V_L) regions could be linked to C_H (or C_L) regions and expressed within complete heavy (or light) chains.

3.2. Assembly of Transfected Light Chain Gene Segments

Bone marrow is the site of B-cell differentiation in the adult mouse. When adult marrow cells are transformed by Abelson virus, the majority of transformants have already assembled and usually express a complete heavy chain gene.[13] However, some of these lines now assemble κ light chain variable regions when propagated in culture.[21] Such lines have been exploited for analyses of the assembly of introduced light chain variable region gene segments.[19] In these experiments, a different approach was taken from that used for heavy chains. The gene segments were introduced via a Moloney murine leukemia virus (M-MuLV)-derived retrovirus vector into a marrow-derived line that actively assembled κ genes during propagation in culture.[19] The scheme to select subclones that had site-specific joining was based upon inverted joining (diagrammed in Fig. 2B): the V_κ and J_κ segments were placed in the vector in opposite transcriptional orientations, with a selectable marker gene (*Eco-gpt*)[28] between them. The marker gene was also in the opposite orientation from the transcriptional promotor sequence contained in the long terminal repeats (LTRs) of the retrovirus. Thus, because the selectable marker gene did not contain its own promotor, it could only be activated if it was inverted and could then run off of the retrovirus promotor.[19] Such an inversion vector allows recovery of both the $V_\kappa J_\kappa$ joint as well as the reciprocal joint of the signal sequences. To form infective virions the construct was cotransfected with the pSV2-*neo* gene into the ψ_2 cell line,[29] which constitutively produces MuLV proteins but is unable to package the resident virus genome. G418-Resistant transformants were selected, which also transcribed the cotransfected retrovirus construct. The transcripts from the retrovirus vector were packaged (due to recognition of the long terminal repeats) by the ψ_2 cell, and the resultant virions could be used to infect actively rearranging marrow-derived transformed lines at high frequency. Subsequently, *gpt*-positive subclones were selected, and the rearranged constructs were molecularly cloned and analyzed.[19] These experiments unequivocally confirmed several aspects of the two-step joining model described above. A number of independent joints were analyzed and in each the joint occurred in different points within the potential V_κ and J_κ coding sequence. However, in all cases the involved recognition heptamers were precisely joined (Fig. 2B).[19]

Besides being much more efficient than DNA transformation procedures, the retrovirus vectors usually integrate at the edges of their LTRs, minimizing the possibility of constructs being interrupted by the integration event; such interrupted, integrated constructs occur at a significant level in the DNA transformation protocols. Because of these advantages, retrovirus vectors should also be the method of choice for expression of cloned Ig cDNA sequences (see below).

3.3. *In Vitro* Assembly of Variable Region Genes

Despite intensive efforts, to date there have been no reports of successful assembly of variable region gene segments *in vitro*. The most interesting approaches to identify recombinase activity have involved treatment of vectors containing V, D, or J segments with extracts from cells that manifest recombinase activity with respect to endogenous genes and subsequently assaying the treated vectors for double-stranded breaks in the vicinity of the recognition heptamers—the first step in the recombination model outlined above. Although such activity has been found, its nature has thus far been interpreted cautiously, due to lack of precise specificity in the cutting site and lack of tissue specificity.[30,31]

4. Control of Immunoglobulin Gene Expression

During B-lymphocyte differentiation there is a dramatic increase in the level of Ig gene expression. Mature plasma cells synthesize as much as 100- to 1000-fold more heavy and light chains as their pre-B or B-cell predecessors.[32] Comparison of the structure and expression of functionally rearranged immunoglobulin genes to that of their component gene segments has revealed multiple factors involved in the control of Ig gene expression.

4.1. Promotors

Each functional V_H or V_L segment contains 5′ flanking sequences that are involved in transcriptional initiation (promotor sequences). Based on various types of experiments, at least two separate sequences appear to be necessary for transcriptional regulation. The first is TATAA-box-like elements that lie upstream from and help to determine the transcriptional initiation site.[33,34] Such sequences appear to be a part of the promotor apparatus of most eukaryotic genes. A second sequence that appears to be necessary for active transcription is a highly conserved (across the different Ig gene families and across species) octonucleotide lying upstream of the $V\kappa$ promotor and in the inverse orientation at a similar position upstream of the V_H promotor.[35,36,37] Gene transfer experiments have suggested that the octonucleotide is essential for efficient κ gene transcription.[36]

4.2. Enhancer Elements

At least several of the hundreds of germ-line V_H gene segments are transcribed at a high level in the very early stages of B-cell differentiation.[37] However, the unrearranged light or heavy chain V gene segments do not appear to be transcribed significantly in mature B cells or plasma cells[37,38]; they are only transcribed at high levels in mature cells if rearrangement places them in association with the J_H or J_L region.[38] The physiological significance of the occurrence of germ-line V gene expression in the early B-cell differentiation stages or its cessation in the later stages is not currently understood. However, several studies of the regulatory regions 5′ to the V transcriptional initiation site indicated that these are not altered after rearrangement.[33,34] Thus, there must be additional regulatory regions downstream of the V segment that are involved with high level expression of the rearranged V gene segment in mature cells.

Several observations suggested that transcriptional regulatory regions might lie between the J_H (J_L) region and the C_μ (C_L) gene. First, both C_μ and C_κ gene segments are transcribed in the absence of V gene rearrangement,[39–41] and second, deletions in the J_H to C_μ intron were correlated with the *cis*-acting loss of heavy chain gene transcription in cultured A-MuLV cell lines.[42] The apparent properties of such a regulatory sequence were reminiscent of those ascribed to viral enhancer sequences—positive control elements for transcription that act relatively independently of orientation or distance with respect to the promotor (reviewed in Ref. 43). Gene transfer studies (see below) identified such an enhancer element in the J–C introns of both heavy and light chain genes.[34,44–47] Although the currently defined enhancer elements appear to be involved in the high-level, tissue-specific activation of Ig gene expression, the exact role of the enhancer elements, the various elements lying 5′ to the promotor, and perhaps other elements yet to be defined in the overall control of Ig gene transcription remains to be determined.

4.3. Splicing

Once assembled, transcription of a complete heavy or light chain gene is initiated 5′ to the V region and terminated 3′ to the downstream C region gene (Fig. 1). The primary transcript passes through several major introns: for both heavy and light chains there is one intron within the V segment, and another major intron separating the J region from the C region exon(s). Thus, the complete Ig V region gene is attached to the appropriate downstream constant region gene at the level of RNA processing (Figs. 1E–1G). Appropriate splice donor sequences occur just 3′ to each functional J_H and J_L segment, while splice acceptor sites occur immediately 5′ to each C gene. Only the J segment containing the appended V (D) segment is spliced to the C region, with the remaining, downstream J regions spliced out along with the rest of the intervening sequence (see Refs. 48 and 49 for review). The fact that the V and C portions of the Ig genes are encoded in independent exons offers a simple method for exchanging functional portions of biologically significant Ig molecules (see below).

While the light chain constant region genes are encoded by a single exon, the larger heavy chain genes are encoded by multiple exons, including two alternative 3′ mini-exons, which encode termini specific for the secreted or membrane-bound forms of the heavy chain protein.[50,51] Whether or not the primary transcript is polyadenylated at a site between the membrane and secretion-specific mini-exons (Figs. 1E–1G) appears to determine whether an mRNA encoding the membrane-bound or secreted form of the heavy chain is made.[48–52] In terminally differentiated cells of the B lineage or their derivative tumors (myelomas) the generation of the secreted form of μ heavy chain mRNA is highly predominant, while at earlier stages of the pathway both secreted and membrane forms are produced at more equal levels.[51,52] Thus, the secreted form of the protein is the predominant form made from complete genes transfected into myelomas.

5. Expression of Introduced Genes

There are two general strategies for the expression of cloned Ig genes in mammalian cells. One is the expression of a genomic clone that represents a functionally rearranged Ig gene, while the other involves the expression of a cDNA copy of the appropriate H or L chain mRNA. Currently, most efforts have been directed at the first method, for two reasons. First, it is usually much easier to clone a gene than to clone a full-length cDNA copy of the corresponding mRNA. Second, most such studies have focused on the control of Ig gene expression; such studies can only be accomplished by transfection of a complete gene that operates from its own promotor and contains the various other types of regulatory elements.

5.1. Expression of Introduced Genomic Clones

Expression of cloned Ig genes has been achieved either by methods to generate high-level transient expression or by methods for long-term (stable) expression. Transient expression is a technique usually employed to look rapidly at expression of transfected sequences (within 24–48 hr after transfection) that were introduced via vectors that can replicate to high copy numbers extrachromosomally.[46,47] This technique is invaluable for certain types of regulatory studies, but is less useful for long-term production of specific gene products. Therefore, this approach will not be considered further. Long-term expression of introduced Ig genes has been achieved by numerous investigators.[53–58] In general, however, these studies have had a common theme. The gene to be expressed was incorporated into a preexisting vector, which contained a selectable marker gene, and the resulting construct was introduced into the mammalian cells by one of three commonly used procedures (see below). Stable transformants, which were isolated based on a drug resistance conferred by the transferred marker gene, were then analyzed for expression of the introduced Ig gene. Such studies clearly indicated that Ig genes were expressed efficiently only when introduced into lymphoid cells, and additional analyses of this type indicated that the primary agent necessary for such tissue-specific expression was the Ig enhancer element.[34,44–47] In fact, attachment of an SV40 enhancer allowed expression of a murine Ig gene in a human carcinoma line.[59]

The vectors commonly used in these experiments are pSV2-*gpt* or pSV2-*neo*, which contain dominant genes conferring resistance of the recipient cells to growth in mycophenolic acid and G418, respectively.[25,28] Such vectors can theoretically accept large amounts of additional DNA. In one study[57] more than 20 kb of additional sequences (including complete heavy and light chain genes) was successfully transformed and expressed within a pSV2-*neo* vector. The thymidine kinase gene or other selectable genes can also be used if appropriate drug-resistant recipient lines exist. The various types of constructs have been introduced into lymphoid cells by one of three methods: calcium phosphate precipitation,[60,61] DEAE-dextran-mediated transformation,[34] or protoplast fusion.[62] Transformation efficiencies as high as 10^{-3} have been reported using protoplast fusion and the J558 myeloma.[54] Others have achieved efficiencies from 10^{-4} to 10^{-6} with various types of mature and immature lymphoid lines using the various transformation protocols.[34,53–57] In general most workers have found that the three methods give comparable levels of transformation, with perhaps some bias in favor of the protoplast fusion method (reviewed in Ref. 63). One study has found that nearly 1% of myeloma cells transformed by the DEAE-dextran protocol transiently express the transfected Ig gene.[34] However, the stable transformation frequency of this line is only 10^{-6}. Thus, the low frequency at which some lines are stably transformed does not appear to result solely from inefficient DNA uptake.[34]

A number of studies have documented the production of complete heavy or light chains from transfected Ig genes, often at levels approaching that of the endogenous chains of the transfected cell. One study has demonstrated the production of complete Ig from H and L chains transfected within the same construct.[57] In this study, the rearranged Ig μ heavy chain and κ light chain genes from a hybridoma producing 2,4,6-trinitrophenol (TNP)-specific IgM were cloned into the pSV2-*neo* vector and introduced into various myeloma or hybridoma cell lines (including nonproducer lines) by the protoplast fusion method and the transfected population selected for G418 resistance. Transformation efficiency ranged from 10^{-4} to 10^{-6}. Some transformants produced high (nearly normal) levels of complete IgM derived from the transfected genes, and this molecule had normal anti-TNP activity.[57] These experiments demonstrated that nonproducing plasmacytoma lines still have all of the necessary specialized functions for the assembly and secretion of complete Ig molecules.

Several studies have clearly demonstrated the feasibility of artificial class switching (exon exchange) via restriction fragment shuffling.[34,58] In one case,[34] the V_H gene segment was separated from the downstream δ constant region of a cDNA clone by digestion with an enzyme that cut specifically within the J_H2 region (J_H2 was utilized in the V_HDJ_H joint). The resulting fragment was attached to the appropriate site in the J_H2 segment of a germ-line clone that contained downstream the remainder of the J_H to C_μ intron and all of the C_μ exons. Transfection of this gene resulted in the expression of a functional μ chain containing the specific variable region.[34] In another study,[58] a productively rearranged V_H gene was attached to the C_κ gene and the construct introduced into a myeloma line. Significantly, the introduced gene was expressed and the resultant protein had a V_H region fused to a C_κ region. This experiment indicates that the J_H splice donor and C_κ splice acceptor sequences can mediate functional assembly of the hybrid mRNA.[58] Similar methods should allow exchange of constant regions between any cloned Ig genes; in fact, these methods should allow joining of human C regions to murine V regions of clinical importance.[75,76,77]

5.2. Expression of cDNA Copies of Ig mRNA

Because a cDNA copy of an mRNA does not have all of the sequences necessary to promote its own expression, such sequences must be provided from a heterologous source. During the past few years this problem has been facilitated by the development of a large variety of eukaryotic expression vectors.[64] In general, such vectors have utilized segments of the genomes of eukaryotic DNA or RNA tumor viruses to provide all of the necessary elements for efficient expression (transcriptional promotors, splice sites, polyadenylation sites, enhancer sequences) of sequences inserted into an expression site. Retrovirus-based expression vectors should be particularly useful, for the reasons outlined in Section 3.2. To date, there have been no reports of expressed Ig cDNA sequences in such vectors.

5.3. Expression of Complete Immunoglobulins in Bacteria

There have been several examples of low-level expression of modified forms of Ig molecules in bacteria, but few examples of high-level expression of complete Ig chains. In the most successful study,[65] the leader sequences were removed from cDNA clones of the μ heavy chain and λ light chains that make up 4-hydroxy-3-nitrophenol (NP)-specific IgM and the sequences were inserted into a bacterial expression plasmid in which they were transcribed from the bacterial tryptophan operon promotor. In appropriate host strains both proteins were produced as insoluble products. The λ protein accumulated to as much as 13% of the total *Escherichia coli* protein, and the μ chain was also produced in substantial levels (1%).[65] Oligonucleotide replacement mutagenesis to make the μ translation initiation codon more accessible was necessary to achieve high expression levels.[66] In addition, both μ and λ proteins were expressed from compatible plasmids in the same cell. Functional antibody could be generated by dialysis of extracts under conditions in which disulfide interchange occurs, although the efficiency was quite low.[65] Clearly, it seems that the limiting factor in using lower eukaryotes or prokaryotes for the production of large quantities of specific antibodies is the development of methods for the efficient reassociation of the chains.

6. Transgenic Mice

Cloned genes can be introduced into the mouse germ line by microinjection into fertilized mouse eggs.[67–71] This procedure introduces the cloned gene into every cell of the resultant mouse; the introduced genes are usually integrated in multiple, tandem copies (as many as 100 copies per cell). Such introduced genes are quite often expressed, and in some cases, notably Ig genes, they appear to be expressed almost exclusively in the same tissues in which the homologous endogenous genes are expressed.[67–71] This technology provides an unparalleled system for studying the control of immunoglobulin gene rearrangement and expression in a physiological setting. In addition, it potentially offers unique opportunities for the production of various types of useful Ig molecules.

6.1. Expression of Cloned Heavy Chain Genes

A functionally rearranged BALB/c V_H gene isolated from a γ2b-expressing hybridoma was fused approximately 2 kb upstream to the entire germ-line C_μ region, and the resulting construct was introduced into the germ line of C57/BL6 mice.[71] In the resultant transgenic mice, the introduced heavy chain gene was present in about 20–140 copies per diploid genome. The particular V_H gene employed was chosen because its heavy chain product produces an NP binding antibody when combined with a λ_1 light chain. Since there is but a single λ_1 V gene in the mouse, expression of the transfected gene could be monitored by the level of anti-NP in the serum. The response is strain-specific and therefore the response from the introduced BALB gene could be distinguished from the endogenous C57/BL6 response. There were a number of very significant conclusions from this study.[71] First, the introduced heavy chain showed a clearly tissue-specific pattern of expression, with high levels of expression in both B and T cells, but little or none in other tissues. The expression in T cells is consistent with the finding that these cells transcribe the unrearranged, endogenous heavy chain locus.[39,41] Thus, the lack of Ig production by T cells appears to be solely a result of the lack of complete rearrangement of this locus in this cell type. A second major finding was that the transgenic mice had up to 400-fold elevated levels of the NP-binding antibody, and the increased levels were clearly contributed by the introduced gene. Thus, it is possible to program a mouse to make antibodies that it otherwise could not make.

6.2. Expression of a κ Light Chain Gene

Transgenic mice have also been produced by the microinjection of a cloned κ light chain gene (V + C) that corresponds to that expressed by the MOPC-21 myeloma line.[69] The introduced κ gene was present in from 20 to 95 copies per diploid genome in the resultant transgenic mice. Six independent κ gene transgenic mice were analyzed and all were found to express the transgenic κ gene exclusively in B lymphocytes. In contrast to the heavy chain gene, little or no κ gene expression was found in T lymphocytes; this result is consistent with the absence of any form of κ gene expression in T cells, and further suggests that the heavy and light chain genes are subject to normal control processes.[70]

6.3. Conclusions

The relatively precise tissue-specific regulation of transgenic Ig gene expression and the lack of such tissue-specific expression in various other transfected cell types are postulated to be due to the presence of a sequence within the transfected Ig genes that interacts with lymphocyte-specific *trans*-acting factors that result in activation regardless of chromosomal position. It seems possible that this sequence is the *cis*-acting enhancer element that was present in both the heavy and light chain constructs and is also necessary for expression of Ig genes transfected in cultured lymphoid cells.[70,71] The tissue-specific expression of Ig genes suggests that it may also be possible to obtain tissue-specific rearrangement of transgenic Ig gene segments as occurs when such segments are transfected into appropriate cell lines. Due to the high copy number at which the transgenic genes are integrated, such introduced genes may in fact be rearranged with some preference to endogenous genes at early stages of development. Strong evidence exists to indicate that allelic and isotype exclusion of Ig heavy and light chain genes (expression of only one heavy and one light chain allele per cell) results from a feedback of the complete heavy chain gene, which shuts off any further heavy chain rearrangement,[7] and feedback from a complete Ig molecule (H + L), which shuts off further light chain gene rearrangement.[72] Thus, if appropriate, introduced Ig gene segments are preferentially rearranged and expressed (yielding multiple species due to joining diversification), they might shut off most endogenous gene rearrangements[73,74] and thereby contribute significantly to immune responses of the transgenic animal. Such a system might ultimately be exploited to produce specific human antibodies in rodents.

7. Summary

Rapid progress in the areas of molecular cloning and gene transfer have already contributed significantly to elucidating the various elements controlling Ig gene expression. This technology, in combination with recent advances in the area of site-directed mutagenesis, now offers the further prospect of manipulating the structure of expressed Ig genes to produce Ig molecules modified in any manner desired. Thus, it should be easily possible to produce antibodies with specific changes in variable region gene structure to examine or modify antigen-binding properties. Specific modulations of constant region sequences combined with *in vitro* exon shuffling should help elucidate the structural correlates of specific effector functions. On a more practical level, techniques such as exon shuffling might also prove clinically valuable if it is possible to functionally substitute human C regions onto murine V regions of useful specificity.[75,76,77]

References

1. Tonegawa, S., 1983, Somatic generation of antibody diversity, *Nature* **302**:575–581.
2. Early, P., Huang, H., Davis, M., Calame, K., and Hood, L., 1980, An immunoglobulin heavy chain variable region gene is generated from three segments of DNA: V_H, D and J_H, *Cell* **19**:981–992.
3. Sakano, H., Maki, R., Kurosawa, Y., Roeder, W., and Tonegawa, S., 1980, Two types of somatic recombination are necessary for the generation of complete immunoglobulin heavy chain genes, *Nature* **266**:676–683.
4. Ravetch, J. V., Siebenlist, U., Korsmeyer, S., Waldmann, T., and Leder, P., 1981, Structure of the human immunoglobulin μ locus: Characterization of embryonic and rearranged J and D genes, *Cell* **27**:583–591.
5. Wood, C., and Tonegawa, S., 1983, Diversity and joining segments of mouse immunoglobulin heavy chain genes are closely linked and in the same orientation: Implications for the joining mechanism, *Proc. Natl. Acad. Sci. USA* **80**:3030–3034.
6. Brodeur, P., and Riblet, R., 1984, The immunoglobulin heavy chain variable region (*Igh-V*) locus in the mouse, *Eur. J. Immunol.* **14**:922–930.
7. Alt, F. W., Yancopoulos, G. D., Blackwell, T. K., Wood, C., Thomas, E., Boss, M., Coffman, R., Rosenberg, N., Tonegawa, S., and Baltimore, D., 1984, Ordered rearrangement of immunoglobulin heavy chain variable region segments, *EMBO J.* **3**:1209–1219.

8. Kurosawa, Y., and Tonegawa, S., 1982, Organization, structure and assembly of immunoglobulin heavy chain diversity (D) DNA segments, *J. Exp. Med.* **155**:201–218.
9. Alt, F. W., and Baltimore, D., 1982, Joining of immunoglobulin heavy chain gene segments: Implications from a chromosome with evidence of three D–J_H fusions, *Proc. Natl. Acad. Sci. USA* **79**:4118–4122.
10. Brack, C., Hirama, M., Lenhard-Schuller, R., and Tonegawa, S., 1978, A complete immunoglobulin gene is created by somatic recombination, *Cell* **15**:1–14.
11. Sakano, H., Huppi, K., Heinrich, G., and Tonegawa, S., 1979, Sequences at the somatic recombination sites of immunoglobulin light chain genes, *Nature* **280**:288–294.
12. Max, E., Seidman, J., and Leder, P., 1979, Sequences of five potential recombination sites encoded close to an immunoglobulin K constant region gene, *Proc. Natl. Acad. Sci. USA* **76**:3450–3454.
13. Alt, F., Rosenberg, N., Lewis, S., Thomas, E., and Baltimore, D, 1981, Organization and reorganization of immunoglobulin genes in A-MuLV-transformed cells: Rearrangement of heavy but not light chain genes, *Cell* **27**:381–390.
14. Yaiota, Y., and Honjo, T., 1980, Deletion of immunoglobulin heavy chain genes from expressed allelic chromosome, *Nature* **286**:856–858.
15. Maki, R., Traunecker, A., Sakano, H., Roeder, W., and Tonegawa, S., 1980, Exon shuffling generates an immunoglobulin heavy chain gene, *Proc. Natl. Acad. Sci. USA* **77**:2138–2142.
16. Davis, M., Calame, K., Early, P., Livant, D., Joho, R., Weissman, I., and Hood, L., 1980, An immunoglobulin heavy-chain gene is formed by at least two recombinational events, *Nature* **283**:733–742.
17. Shimizu, A., Takahashi, N., Yaiota, Y., and Honjo, T., 1982, Organization of the constant-region gene family of the mouse immunoglobulin heavy chain, *Cell* **248**:499–506.
18. Shimizu, A., and Honjo, T., 1984, Immunogulin class switching, *Cell* **36**:801–803.
19. Lewis, S., Gifford, A., and Baltimore, D., 1984, Joining of V_K to J_K gene segments in a retroviral vector introduced into lymphoid cells, *Nature* **308**:425–428.
20. Blackwell, T. K., and Alt, F. W., 1984, Site-specific recombination between immunoglobulin D and J_H segments that were introduced into the genome of a murine pre-B cell line, *Cell* **37**:105–112.
21. Lewis, S., Rosenberg, N., Alt, F., and Baltimore, D., 1982, Continuing kappa-gene rearrangement in a cell line transformed by Abelson murine leukemia virus, *Cell* **30**:807–816.
22. Yaoita, Y., Matsuami, N., Choi, C. Y., Sugiyama, H., Kishimoto, T., and Honjo, T., 1983, The D–J_H complex is an intermediate to the complete immunoglobulin heavy-chain V-region gene, *Nucleic Acids Res.* **11**:7303–7315.
23. Yancopoulos, G. D., Desiderio, S. V., Paskind, M., Kearney, J. F., Baltimore, D., and Alt, F. W., 1984, Preferential utilization of the most J_H-proximal V_H gene segments in pre-B cell lines, *Nature* **311**:727–733.
24. Desiderio, S., Yancopoulos, G. D., Paskind, M., Thomas, E., Boss, M., Alt, F., and Baltimore, D., 1984, V_H gene assembly in cultured A-MuLV transformants, *Nature* **311**:752–755.
25. Southern, P., and Berg, P., 1982, Transformation of mammalian cells to antibiotic resistance with a bacterial gene under the control of the SV 40 early region promotor, *J. Mol. Appl. Genet.* **1**:327–341.
26. Robins, D. M., Ripley, S., Henderson, A. S., and Axel, R., 1981, Transforming DNA integrates into the host chromosome, *Cell* **23**:29–39.
27. Blackwell, T. K., Yancopoulos, G. D., and Alt, F. W., 1984, Joining of immunoglobulin heavy chain variable region gene segments *in vivo* and within a recombination substrate, in: *Molecular Biology of Development* UCLA Symposia on Molecular and Cell Biology, Volume 19, Alan R. Liss, New York, pp. 537–547.
28. Mulligan, R. C., and Berg, P., 1981, Selection for animal cells that express the *E. coli* gene coding for xanthine guanine phosphoribosyl transferase, *Proc. Natl. Acad. Sci. USA* **78**:2072–2076.
29. Mann, R., Mulligan, R., and Baltimore, D., 1983, Construction of a retrovirus packaging mutant and its use to produce helper-free defective retrovirus, *Cell* **33**:153–159.

30. Desiderio, S., and Baltimore, D., 1983, Double-stranded cleavage by cell extracts near recombinational signal sequences of immunoglobulin genes, *Nature* **308**:860–862.
31. Kataoka, T., Kondo, S., Nishi, M., Kodaira, M., and Honjo, T., 1984, Isolation and characterization of endonuclease J: A sequence-specific endonuclease cleaving immunoglobulin genes, *Nucleic Acids Res.* **12**:5995–6010.
32. Schibler, U., Marcu, K. B., and Perry, R. P., 1978, The synthesis and processing of mRNAs specifying heavy and light chain immunoglobulins in MPC-11, *Cell* **15**:1495–1509.
33. Clarke, C., Berenson, J., Goverman, J., Crews, S., Siu, G., Boyer, P., and Calame, K., 1982, An immunoglobulin promoter region is unaltered by DNA rearrangement and somatic mutation during B cell development, *Nucleic Acids Res.* **10**:7731–7749.
34. Neuberger, M. S., 1983, Expression and regulation of immunoglobulin heavy chain gene transfected in lymphoid cells, *EMBO J.* **2**:1373–1378.
35. Parslow, T. G., Blair, D. L., Murphy, W. J., and Granner, D. K., 1984, Structure of the 5′ ends of immunoglobulin genes: A novel conserved sequence, *Proc. Natl. Acad. Sci. USA* **81**:2650–2654.
36. Falkner, F. G., and Zachau, H. G., 1984, Correct transcription of an immunoglobulin kappa gene requires an upstream fragment containing conserved sequence elements, *Nature* **310**:71–74.
37. Yancopoulos, G., and Alt, F. W., 1985, Developmentally controlled and tissue-specific expression of unrearranged V_H gene segments, *Cell* **40**:269–279.
38. Mather, E. L., and Perry, R. P., 1981, Transcriptional regulation of immunoglobulin V genes, *Nucleic Acids Res.***9**:6855–6867.
39. Kemp, D., Harris, A., Cory, S., and Adams, J., 1980, Expression of the Ig C_μ gene in mouse T and B lymphoid and myeloid cell lines, *Proc. Natl. Acad. Sci. USA* **77**:2876–2880.
40. Van Ness, B. J., Weigert, M., Coleclough, C., Mather, E. L., Kelley, D. E., and Perry, R. P., 1981, Transcription of the unrearranged mouse C_κ locus sequence of the initiation region and comparison of activity with a rearranged V.-C. gene, *Cell* **27**:593–602.
41. Alt, F. W., Rosenberg, N., Enea, V., Siden, E., and Baltimore, D., 1982, Multiple immunoglobulin heavy-chain transcripts in Abelson murine leukemia virus-transformed cell lines, *Mol. Cell. Biol.* **2**:386–400.
42. Alt, F. W., Rosenberg, N., Casanova, R. J., Thomas, E., and Baltimore, D., 1982, Immunoglobulin heavy-chain expression and class switching in a murine leukemia cell line, *Nature* **296**:325–331.
43. Gruss, P., 1984, Magic enhancers, *DNA* **3**:1–5.
44. Gillies, S. C., Morrison, S. L., Oi, V. T., and Tonegawa, S., 1983, A tissue-specific transcription enhancer element is located in the major intron of a rearranged immunoglobulin heavy chain gene, *Cell* **33**:717–728.
45. Banerij, J., Olson, L., and Schaffner, W., 1983, A lymphocyte-specific cellular enhancer is located downstream of the joining region in immunoglobulin heavy chain genes, *Cell* **33**:729–740.
46. Queen, C., and Baltimore, D., 1983, Immunoglobulin gene transcription is activated by downstream sequence elements, *Cell* **33**:741–748.
47. Mercola, M., Wang, X., Olsen, J., and Calame, K., 1983, Transcriptional enhancer elements in the mouse immunoglobulin heavy chain locus, *Science* **221**:663–665.
48. Blattner, F. R., and Tucker, P. W., 1984, The molecular biology of immunoglobulin D, *Nature* **307**:417–422.
49. Mather, E. L., Nelson, K. J., Haimovich, J., and Perry, R. P., 1984, Mode of regulation of immunoglobulin μ- and δ-chain expression varies during B-lymphocyte maturation, *Cell* **36**:329–338.
50. Earley, P., Rogers, J., Davis, M., Calame, K., Bond, M., Wall, R., and Hood, L., 1980, Two mRNAs can be produced from a single immunoglobulin μ gene by alternative RNA processing pathways, *Cell* **20**:313–320.
51. Rogers, J. W., Earley, P., Carter, C., Calame, K., Bond, M., Hood, L., and Wall, R., 1980, Two RNAs with different 3′ ends encode membrane-bound and secreted forms of immunoglobulin μ chain, *Cell* **20**:303–312.

52. Alt, F. W., Bothwell, A. L. M., Knapp, M., Siden, E., Mather, E., Koshland, M., and Baltimore, D., 1980, Synthesis of secreted and membrane-bound immunoglobulin mu heavy chains is directed by mRNAs that differ at their 3′-ends, *Cell* **20:**293–301.
53. Rice, D., and Baltimore, D., 1982, Regulated expression of an immunoglobulin kappa gene introduced into a mouse lymphoid cell line, *Proc. Natl. Acad. Sci. USA* **79:**7862–7865.
54. Oi, V., Morrison, S. L., Herzenberg, L. A., and Berg, P., 1983, Immunoglobulin gene expression in transformed cells, *Proc. Natl. Acad. Sci. USA* **80:**825–829.
55. Stafford, J., and Queen, C., 1983, Cell-type specific expression of a transfected immunoglobulin gene, *Nature* **306:**77–79.
56. Ochi, A., Hawley, R. G., Shulman, M. J., and Hozumi, N., 1983, Transfer of a cloned immunoglobulin light-chain gene to mutant hybridoma cells restores specific antibody production, *Nature* **302:**340–342.
57. Ochi, A., Hawley, R. G., Hawley, T., Schulman, M. J., Traunecker, A., Kohler, G., and Hozumi, N., 1983, Functional immunoglobulin production after transfection of cloned immunoglobulin heavy and light chain genes in lymphoid cells, *Proc. Natl. Acad. Sci. USA* **80:**6351–6355.
58. Sharon, S., Gefter, M. L., Manser, T., Morrison, S. L., Io, V. T., and Ptashne, M., 1984, Expression of a V_HC_K chimaeric protein in mouse myeloma cells, *Nature* **309:**364–367.
59. Picard, D., and Schaffner, W., 1983, Correct transcription of a cloned mouse immunoglobulin gene *in vivo, Proc. Natl. Acad. Sci. USA* **80:**417–421.
60. Graham, F. L., and van der Eb, A. J., 1973, A new technique for the assay of infectivity of human adenovirus 5DNA, *Virology* **52:**456–467.
61. Chu, G., and Sharp, P. A., 1981, SV40 DNA transfection of cells in suspension: Analysis of the efficiency of transcription and translation of T-antigen, *Gene* **13:**197–202.
62. Sandri-Goldin, R. M., Goldin, A. L., Levine, M., and Glorioso, J. C., 1981, High-frequency transfer of cloned herpes simplex virus type 1 sequence to mammalian cells by protoplast fusion, *Mol. Cell. Biol.* **1:**743–752.
63. Morrison, S. L., and Oi, V. T., 1984, Transfer and expression of immunoglobulin genes, *Annu. Rev. Immunol.* **2:**239–256.
64. Gluzman, Y., 1982, *Eukaryotic Viral Vectors,* Cold Spring Harbor Laboratory Press, Cold Spring Harbor, New York.
65. Boss, M. A., Kenten, J. H., Wood, C. R., and Emtage, J. S., 1984, Assembly of functional antibodies from immunoglobulin heavy and light chains synthesized in *E. coli, Nucleic Acids Res.* **12:**3791–3806.
66. Wood, C. L., Boss, M. A., Patel, T. P., and Emtage, J. S., 1984, The influence of mRNA secondary structure on expression of an immunoglobulin heavy chain in *E. coli, Nucleic Acids Res.* **12:**3937–3950.
67. Costantini, F., and Lacy, E., 1981, Introduction of rabbit beta-globin into the mouse germ line, *Nature* **294:**92–94.
68. Brinster, R. L., Chen, H. Y., Trumbauer, M., Senear, A. W., Warren, R., and Palmiter, R. D., 1981, Somatic expression of Herpes thymidine kinase in mice following injection of a fusion gene into eggs, *Cell* **27:**223–231.
69. Brinster, R. L., Ritchie, K. A., Hammer, R. E., O'Brien, R. L., Arp, B., and Storb, U., 1983, Expression of a microinjected immunoglobulin gene in the spleen of transgenic mice, *Nature* **306:**332–336.
70. Storb, U., O'Brien, R. L., McMullen, M. D., Gollahan, K. A., and Brinster, R. L., 1984, High expression of cloned immunoglobulin gene in transgenic mice is restricted to B lymphocytes, *Nature* **310:**238–241.
71. Crosschedl, R., Weaver, D., Baltimore, D., and Costantini, F., 1984, Introduction of a μ Ig gene into the mouse germline: Specific expression in lymphoid cells and synthesis of functional antibody, *Cell* **38:**647–658.
72. Alt, F. W., Enea, V., Bothwell, A. L. M., and Baltimore, D., 1980, Activity of multiple light chain genes in murine myelomas producing a single functional light chain, *Cell* **21:**1–12.

73. Ritchie, K. A., Brinster, R. L., and Starb, U., 1984, Allelic exclusion and control of endogenous immunoglobulin gene rearrangement in κ transgenic mice, *Nature* **312**:517–520.
74. Rusconi, S., and Köhler, G., 1985, Transmission and expression of a specific pair of rearranged immunoglobulin μ and κ genes in a transgenic mouse line, *Nature* **314**:330–334.
75. Manison, S. L., Johnson, M. J., Herzenberg, L. A., and Oi, U. T., 1984, Chimeric human antibody molecules: mouse antigen-binding domains with human constant region domains, *Proc. Natl. Acad. Sci.* **81**:6851–6855.
76. Neuberger, M. S., Williams, G. T., and Fox, R. O., 1984, Recombinant antibodies possessing novel effector functions, *Nature* **312**:604–608.
77. Boulianne, G. L., Hozumi, N., and Schulman, M. J., 1984, Production of functional chimaeric mouse/human antibody, *Nature* **312**:643–646.

Part II

Monoclonal Antibodies in Biomedical Research: Principles and Applications

Chapter 8

The Immunochemistry of Monoclonal Antibodies: Studies on One Immunologic Supergene (HLA) with the Products of Another

PETER PARHAM

1. Introduction

Since the H-2 and HLA systems were defined and have continued to be described by serologic methods, the introduction of monoclonal antibodies into these areas was an obvious and inevitable development.[1] The potential exists for redefining the charts of H-2 public and private specificities and the complex and ever-changing diagrams of HLA cross-reactivities in terms of epitopes defined by panels of monoclonal antibodies. Fundamental questions about the number and arrangement of polymorphic sites could be more rigorously addressed and the involvement of different epitopes in restricting antigen recognition by T cells investigated. At a more practical level it would provide abundant and reliable reagents for assay, localization, and purification of HLA molecules.

Previous reviews have focused on the production, specificity, and applications of monoclonal antibodies against MHC products.[2,3] In this discussion, I will analyze some of these findings from an immunochemical standpoint, considering HLA-A, B molecules as a general model for membrane glycoproteins. One reason for adopting this tack is that many of the novel molecules so far identified and being studied with monoclonal antibodies are membrane glycoproteins. A second is that the following properties make HLA-A, B a good model system:

1. HLA-A, B is present on the surface of cells in amounts that can be easily detected.

PETER PARHAM • Department of Cell Biology, Stanford University School of Medicine, Stanford, California 94305.

2. HLA-A, B can be studied on a wide variety of cell types and with considerable variation in cell surface amount and density.
3. HLA-A, B is representative of a common class of membrane glycoproteins that have most of their mass outside the cell and are anchored into the membrane by a hydrophobic tail.
4. HLA-A, B is biochemically well characterized (for review see Ref. 4).
5. Monoclonal antibodies against many polymorphic and monomorphic epitopes of HLA-A, B are available.[3]
6. HLA-A, B is a large family of polymorphic molecules, which allows for tight genetic control of experiments.
7. The properties of HLA-A, B as an intrinsic cell surface glycoprotein and as a globular water-soluble glycoprotein can be studied. Papain cleaves the molecule close to the membrane to produce a fragment that retains all the antigenic properties of the cell surface form.[4]

2. Fragmentation of IgG to Give F(ab')$_2$ and Fab

The effects of multivalent interactions are of profound consequence for reactions that take place at cell surfaces. In studying the interaction of monoclonal antibodies with cell surface molecules it is therefore important to be able to compare the reactions of bivalent and univalent forms of an antibody. The most controlled comparison is given by F(ab')$_2$ and Fab', which also eliminates possible artifacts due to Fc binding.

Until the introduction of monoclonal antibodies there had been little documentation of methods for the generation of F(ab')$_2$ and Fab from mouse IgG. This was clearly because the mouse was generally not the animal of choice for the production of antisera. Our preliminary experiments showed that direct production of Fab was not a problem,[5] but that cleavage to give F(ab')$_2$ was rather unpredictable. The protocols recommended for human and rabbit IgG by compendia of methods were often not successful. As a consequence of this experience we made a more systematic analysis of the fragmentation patterns of the more common classes of mouse Ig: IgG1, IgG2a, and IgG2b.[6,7] The results for pepsin degradation are combined with those of Lamoyi and Nisonoff[8] and summarized in Fig. 1. There is a trend both in the susceptibility to proteolytic cleavage and in the pattern of cleavage. The susceptibility to cleavage was IgG1 > IgG2a > IgG3 > IgG2b.

For IgG1, cleavage was at heavy chain sites on the carboxy-terminal side of the inter-heavy chain disulfide bonds. This produced an F(ab')$_2$ fragment that was relatively resistant to further proteolysis. It can be effected by pepsin at pH 3.5–4.1 or thiol-free papain at neutral pH. With pepsin the Fc becomes degraded, with papain it is preserved.[3,6]

The initial cleavage of IgG2a was at a similar site to that described for IgG1 and gave an F(ab')$_2$ fragment. A secondary heavy chain site on the amino-terminal side of the inter-heavy chain disulfide bonds was also susceptible to

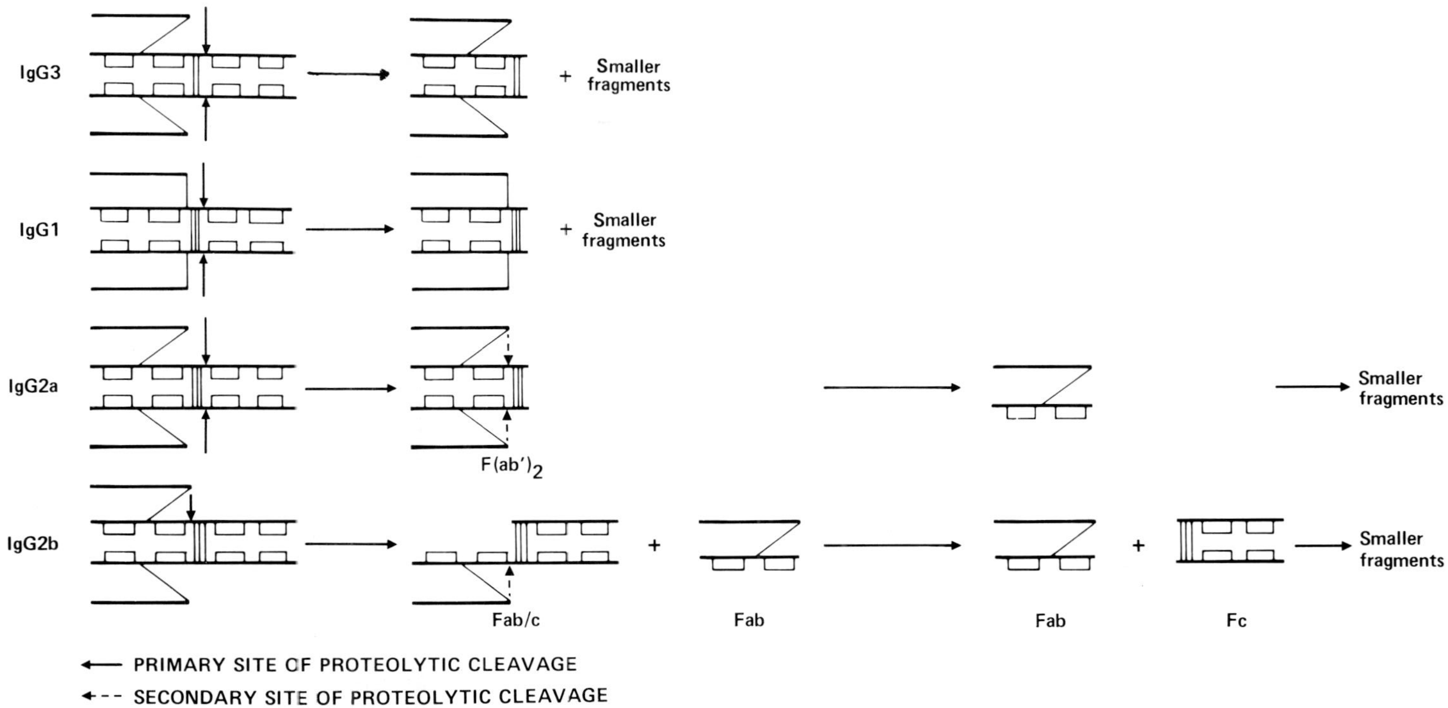

Figure 1. The patterns of fragmentation of different subclasses of mouse IgG obtained with pepsin. (From Ref. 7.)

cleavage. Thus, $F(ab')_2$ is produced, but can then be degraded to Fab. For the three different IgG2a monoclonal antibodies that we have studied digestion can be stopped at a point to yield useful amounts of $F(ab')_2$. However, there are clearly exceptions to all the generalizations one tries to make about monoclonal antibodies. For example, Lamoyi and Nisonoff[8] found one IgG1 that was highly sensitive to proteases, whereas the general experience is that they are resistant.

The trend seen in going from IgG1 to IgG2a is completed with IgG2b. Sites on the amino-terminal side of the inter-heavy-chain disulfides are now the preliminary site of cleavage and Fab fragments are produced directly. We have therefore been unable to prepare $F(ab')_2$ from IgG2b.

From these studies it has emerged that IgG1 is the best class of monoclonal antibody for production of matched preparations of $F(ab')_2$ and Fab'. For our studies this was fortunate, since the majority of the monoclonal anti-HLA-A, B were of the IgG1 class. Limit digests can be done in which $F(ab')_2$ is the only high-molecular-weight product and can then be easily purified. Part of this preparation is then reduced and alkylated to give Fab'. The simplicity of this scheme is such that enzymatic degradations can be carried out on crude ascitic fluid or cell culture supernatant.[6] It is possible that the class-switching methods described in Section 4 may be used to convert monoclonal antibodies from isotypes that do not yield $F(ab')_2$ to ones that do.

3. Fab/c: A Univalent Fragment with Effector Function

Although we were unable to produce $F(ab')_2$ from IgG2b, another fragment called Fab/c can specifically be produced from monoclonal antibodies of this isotype.[6] It consists of the Fc region and one Fab and is the product of a single proteolytic cleavage that removes the other Fab from the intact IgG. The characteristics of Fab/c on sodium dodecyl sulfate polyacrylamide gel electrophoresis (SDS–PAGE) are shown in Fig. 2. In the absence of reducing agents, it migrates as a single band that is a little slower than $F(ab')_2$, with apparent molecular weight of ~115,000. On reduction, it gives three polypeptides: one heavy chain, one light chain, and one heavy chain fragment equivalent to that of the Fc fragment.

When IgG2b is digested with any one of a number of proteases, Fab/c is the first product formed and has a significant lifetime under the conditions of proteolysis. During the course of digestion, a steady state concentration of Fab/c builds up, which in the most favorable cases can be ~25% of the input IgG2b. Continued digestion results in complete degradation of Fab/c to Fab, Fc, and then to small peptides. This pattern of degradation suggests that asymmetric cleavage of IgG2b is occurring. Precedent for this exists with rabbit IgG of the A12 allotype, where glycosylation of one heavy chain in the hinge region renders it more resistant to proteolytic attack.[9] Two additional pieces of evidence suggest that this may also be the case for mouse IgG2b. First, the heavy chain of IgG2b shows heterogeneity on SDS–PAGE, migrating as a doublet. Second,

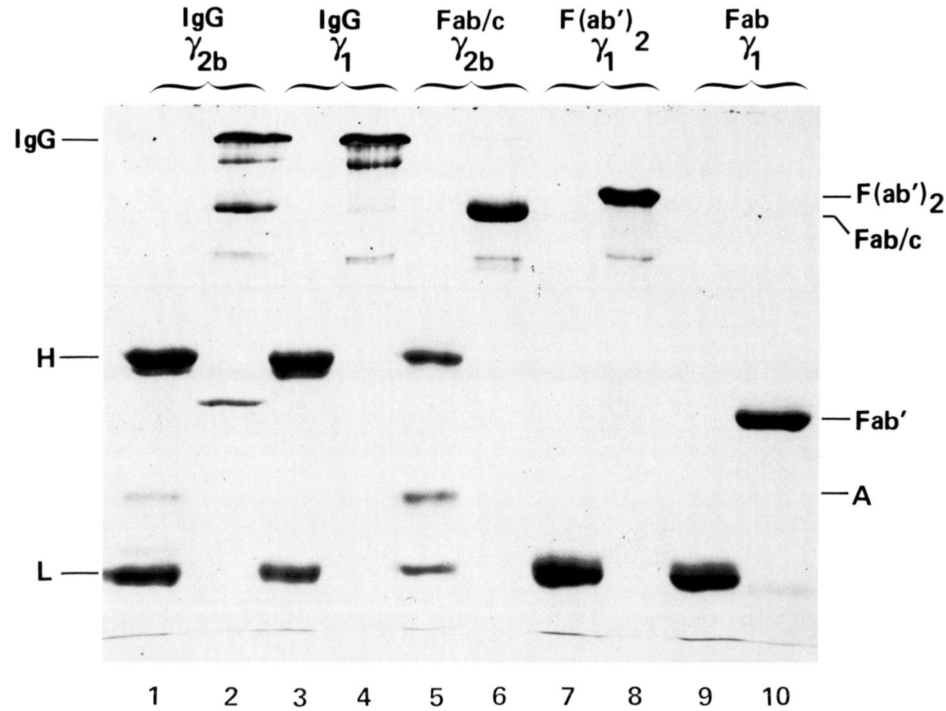

Figure 2. Analysis of Fab/c by sodium dodecyl sulfate–polyacrylamide gel electrophoresis (SDS–PAGE). All samples are derived from the ME1 hybridoma,[13] which is of the IgG1 class, and an IgG2b switch variant derived from ME1. Lanes 2, 4, 6, 8, 10 show samples analyzed without reduction; lanes 1, 3, 5, 7, 9 show samples analyzed with reduction. Samples are (1,2) a preparation of purified IgG2b that has partly degraded to Fab/c and Fab during storage at 4°C (3,4) a purified preparation of IgG1, (5,6) purified Fab/c prepared from IgG2b, (7,8) purified $F(ab')_2$ prepared from IgG1, and (9,10) purified Fab′ prepared form IgG1.

biosynthetic radiolabeling showed that the two bands of the heavy chain doublet had different carbohydrate content.[10]

There is potential for the Fab/c fragment in the use of monoclonal antibodies against cell surface molecules as therapeutic reagents for the elimination of tumor cells.[9] A problem with the use of intact IgG is that antigenic modulation can be induced, rendering the tumor cell resistant. Modulation is only induced by multivalent antibody species and not by Fab fragments. Although the critical mechanisms of antibody-mediated tumor cell elimination have not been defined, they do require the Fc fragment and its associated effector functions. The advantage of Fab/c is that it combines univalency and thus no modulation with effector function. In an animal model using rabbit antibodies of the appropriate allotype, Glennie and Stevenson[9] demonstrated that Fab/c fragments could be superior immunotherapeutic reagents to intact IgG. Similar comparisons could now be carried out with mouse monoclonal antibodies, providing they are of the IgG2b subclass. This requirement need not be restrictive, since monoclonal antibodies of suitable combining site specificity can be switched to the appropriate isotype (see Section 4).

In assessing which antibodies are suitable for use as Fab/c fragments, an important consideration is that since only single-site attachment is possible, the potential strength of the binding to the tumor cell is less for Fab/c than IgG. In practice this would be of little importance for some antibodies and of profound consequence for others. As first shown by Mason and Williams,[11] there are monoclonal IgGs of relatively high affinity that predominantly bind to cells in a univalent mode and do not "need to" make use of their second combining site. For such antibodies Fab/c would bind as strongly as IgG and would give no surprises on that score. In contrast, there are antibodies of relatively low affinity that bind to cells in a bivalent mode and for which the difference in binding strength between univalent and bivalent attachment is large.[12] The Fab/c from such antibodies would not be useful reagents.

For further study of the Fab/c fragment we choose the IgG2b switch variant of the ME1 hybridoma.[13,14] It is of high affinity and we already knew that the Fab′ fragment bound tightly to the target antigens, HLA-B7 or HLA-B27. With elastase digestion a 20% yield of Fab/c was achieved, giving a preparation that was contaminated with Fab, Fc, small peptides, and intact IgG2b. A column of protein A–Sepharose was used to purify Fab/c, IgG2b, and Fc away from Fab, elastase, and other contaminants.[15] Chromatography on Sephadex G200 then removed Fc and gave a partial separation of IgG and Fab/c. Fractions in which Fab/c was the predominant component were pooled and concentrated on a column of protein A–Sepharose with elution at pH 3.5.[15] High-pressure liquid chromatography on a TSK3000SW size exclusion column gave a preparation of highly purified Fab/c as shown in Fig. 2. In collaboration with Dr. H. Coppin (Department of Medical Microbiology, Stanford), we assessed the effector function of the Fab/c fragment in complement-dependent, antibody-mediated cytotoxicity. It specifically killed cells of the appropriate HLA-B specificity with a potency that was about one-tenth that of the intact IgG2b. This is probably a reflection of the different strength of binding of the bivalent IgG compared to univalent Fab/c, since similar differences in titer were observed between the inhibition of ME1 IgG1 binding by $F(ab')_2$ and Fab′.

These results show that at least one major effector function is preserved in the Fab/c fragment, indicating their potential as immunotherapeutic reagents. The immediate problem to be overcome is the development of a more efficient purification scheme.

4. Isotype Switch Variants

Although the physiological role of the different subclasses of IgG is unknown, they individually have distinct advantages and disadvantages as biological tools. Some have been discussed above. IgG1 is the best for making $F(ab')_2$, but rarely fixes complement, and binds protein A from *Staphylococcus aureus* with relatively low affinity. IgG2a is the best reagent for complement fixation or for binding to Fc receptors, but these same properties can be an encumbrance in other systems. IgG2b is most sensitive to degradation, yet is the best source of Fab/c.

A monoclonal antibody against a cell surface molecule becomes a more versatile tool if the isotype can be changed at will while preserving the antigen-combining site. Certain changes of isotype occur spontaneously during normal growth of hybridoma cells and these "switch variants" can then be isolated with the fluorescence activated cell sorter[16] (see Kipps, this volume, Chapter 5). This strategy has been used to develop "families" of monoclonal immunoglobulins with each member having different isotype but identical combining sites. Although the use of this technique to increase the versatility of useful monoclonal antibodies is an obvious one, it has mostly been used for comparative studies of immunoglobulins in which the combining site specificity is a hapten and only of academic importance.[17]

I mentioned in Section 2 that most of our anti-HLAs were IgG1 and how this is an advantage for making $F(ab')_2$. The major and considerable disadvantage is that these antibodies do not fix complement and cannot be used in the standard antibody-dependent, complement-mediated cytotoxicity assay that is used for HLA typing. This has two ramifications; first, the large panels of lymphocytes in HLA-typing laboratories would not be available for further characterization of the specificity of monoclonal anti-HLAs that were IgG1, and second, those monoclonal antibodies would not have potential as HLA typing reagents. A solution to this problem was to isolate variants of the IgG1 hybridomas that had switched isotype to give one of the complement-fixing IgG2 subclasses. Fortunately, this particular switch goes with relatively high frequency, and in collaboration with Drs. T. J. Kipps and L. A. Herzenberg (Genetics Department, Stanford), we have had some success in isolating cytotoxic switch variants of monoclonal anti-HLA.[14,18]

The first switch variants were obtained from the Genox 3.53 hybridoma that secretes a monoclonal antibody specific for DC1, a class II HLA molecule that is homologous to mouse I-A products.[18] The selection is based on staining the surface of cells with fluorescent antibodies that are specific for the isotype required. With a fluorescein-conjugated goat anti-mouse IgG2 preparation, we were able to select for both IgG2a and IgG2b. After expansion of the selected cells the secreted antibodies were simultaneously checked for specificity and isotype in a radioimmune cell binding assay using radioiodinated second-step antibodies that were isotype-specific. IgG2a and IgG2b antibodies that retained the DC1 specificity of the parental IgG1 were tested in the standard HLA typing assay by Dr. Frances Ward of Duke University.

The IgG2 switch variants of Genox 3.53 were found to be cytotoxic and excellent reagents for typing the DC1 specificity.[18] There are considerable advantages in using such monoclonal reagents for HLA typing in preference to the traditionally used human alloantisera:

1. They are stable and homogeneous reagents that can be retrieved from the biological source at any time. The specificity and availability of

given human alloantisera are variable and rather dependent on the "lifestyle" of the donor.

2. They are available in practically unlimited amounts, which can be made available to all HLA-typing laboratories. Therefore, better international standardization becomes possible. Amounts of human alloantisera are limited and their availability is dependent upon an ill-defined system of international barter.
3. The active antibody is quantifiable and present in high concentrations, which means that more controlled and sensitive assays are possible.
4. In practice, the capacity for discrimination of different HLA molecules appears to be greater for monoclonal antibodies made in rodents than the polyclonal antibodies available for humans.

We have since isolated IgG2 switch variants from the ME1 and MA2.1 (anti-HLA-A2 and B17) hybridoma cell lines.[13,19] ME1 provides an example where making the antibody compatible with the HLA typing assay has enabled a more complete definition of its specificity. This IgG1 was first characterized by radioimmune binding assays on a limited panel of cells as being specific for HLA-B7, HLA-B27, and HLA-Bw22.[13] Analysis of the IgG2 switch variants by cytotoxicity assay shows that these are indeed the common and strongest reactions. However, a strong reaction is also found with Bw42, an antigen found in black populations, and specific low-affinity reactions can be picked up with HLA-B14, Bw62, and Bw46. Since the binding assay, in contrast to the cytotoxicity assay, involves considerable washing of the cells, these weaker reactions do not produce very significant levels of binding. These studies are being performed in collaboration with Dr. F. Ward (Duke), Dr. D. Antonelli (Seattle), and Drs. A. Ahern and T. Fuller (Boston).

The switch variants of ME1 have been used by Dr. T. J. Kipps to study the capacity of mouse monoclonal antibodies to mediate antibody-dependent cellular cytotoxicity of human B lymphoblastoid cells by human peripheral blood cells.[14] This is possibly a mechanism by which specific monoclonal antibodies eliminate cells when used as therapeutic reagents. Peripheral blood cells from healthy donors are able to kill cells of an HLA-B7-expressing cell line (JY) when they were coated with ME1 of IgG2 but not IgG1 isotype. There is also a considerable quantitative difference between IgG2a, which is most potent, and IgG2b. A control experiment showed that prebinding of the IgG1 would completely inhibit a subsequent attempt to effect cytotoxicity with the IgG2a. This provides another example of an application of monoclonal antibodies where choice of isotype is important and where isotype switching can be of use. Furthermore, our analysis of antibody-dependent cellular cytotoxicity with a panel of monoclonal anti-HLA reagents indicates that it requires high-affinity antibodies and saturation of all the antigenic sites.

5. Binding of Monoclonal Antibodies to Cell Surface Antigens

From the previous discussion, we have been shown one experimental situation in which the affinity of a monoclonal antibody for a cell surface molecule is critical. This is generalizable to any application of monoclonal antibodies, and in many instances, affinity and specificity will not be independent variables.

Let us first consider the processes by which an IgG molecule binds to an HLA-A, B molecule on the surface of a lymphoblastoid B cell. Assuming a spherical cell with diameter 12 μm and 10^6 HLA molecules randomly distributed per cell, then the average separation of two HLA molecules will be ~400 Å, which is about six times the distance that the two combining sites of an IgG molecule can span. Therefore, antibody will in general diffuse from solution to the cell surface and bind a single HLA molecule to form a univalent complex that can then diffuse in the plane of the membrane. As this complex diffuses, it can either (1) dissociate, (2) encounter a second HLA molecule and either form or not form a bivalent complex, or (3) encounter a second HLA molecule that is already bound to antibody. Which of these reactions predominates depends upon the rate constants of the antibody, the stability of the complexes formed, and other parameters, such as the free antibody concentrations. For illustrative purposes, I shall rationalize the experimentally determined behavior of certain antibodies. Throughout this discussion, affinity will refer to the binding constant of a single antibody-combining site.

1. MA2.1 is of high affinity (1.2×10^9 M^{-1}), due to a high association rate constant and a low dissociation rate constant.[12] Once a complex is formed it will not dissociate during the time course of most experiments (1–6 hr). The rates at which free HLA is bound by the second combining site of an antibody already part of an univalent complex is comparable to the rate at which it will be bound by a free antibody coming from solution. The reaction will for practical purposes stop when all HLA molecules are bound and a mixture of univalent and bivalent complexes will exist at the cell surface. This reaction is thus kinetically and not thermodynamically controlled.

If the initial concentration of free antibody is reduced, this will slow the rate of association from solution and increase the probability of forming bivalent complexes.

If the antigen density at the cell surface is increased, for example, by treating the cells with interferon,[20,21] the univalent complex will have a greater probability of encountering a free HLA molecule and the proportion of bivalent complexes will be increased. Reciprocally, if the HLA antigen density is reduced by using peripheral blood cells or non-B-lymphocyte hematopoietic cell lines, then the proportion of univalent complexes will increase. For example, when the B-cell line JY and the myeloid cell line HL-60 were compared for MA2.1 binding under identical conditions, it was found that JY expressed about four times as much HLA and that the percentage of univalent complexes was 85% for HL-60 and 19% for JY.[12]

The ratio of univalent to bivalent complexes is not very sensitive to changes in the numbers of cells, because the antigenic environment in which an individual antibody finds itself once it reaches a cell surface is not a function of cell density. When antibody is limiting or if cell density becomes very high, such as exists in a lymphoid tissue, this will not necessarily be true.

2. For some combinations of cell surface molecule and epitope specificity of the monoclonal antibody, the formation of a bivalent complex might be thermodynamically unfavorable. In this case, only univalent complexes will be formed. This could be due to the antigen molecules being so large that the IgG could not bridge the gap. Alternatively, the strain induced in either antigen or antibody by bivalent interaction is not compensated by the gain in energy.

3. PA2.1 is an antibody of low affinity (1.9×10^7 M^{-1}), due to a high dissociation rate constant, and an association rate constant comparable to that of the high-affinity antibody MA2.1.[12] A univalent complex formed by PA2.1 and its target HLA molecule (A2 or Aw69) has a 50% chance of dissociating within 4 min. If it encounters a free HLA molecule before dissociating, then a bivalent complex is formed that is considerably more stable, taking 50 min for 50% dissociation. Thus, all univalent complexes will either rapidly dissociate or form stable bivalent complexes. Providing the free antibody concentration is high enough, the HLA will, with time, end up in bivalent complexes. The situation is somewhat analogous to that of a simple enzyme reaction in which there is a reversible reaction between antigen (substrate) and antibody (enzyme) to form univalent complexes (enzyme–substrate) and an effectively irreversible reaction to form bivalent complexes (products) from univalent complexes. The stability of the bivalent complex is the result of two factors. First, dissociation of one of the interactions does not allow the antibody to diffuse away, since it is held to the cell by the second interaction. Second, although dissociation of one of the interactions will allow the relevant HLA molecule to diffuse freely, the diffusion rate in the lipid bilayer is so much slower than in solution that the rate of rebinding of the antibody to reform the bivalent attachment predominates over the rate of escape of the antigen.

If the antigen density is lowered, the rate of formation of bivalent complexes decreases until a point is reached where it is effectively zero. At this point, the probability of a univalent complex finding a second HLA molecule before it dissociates becomes vanishingly small. Unless precautions are taken to avoid wash steps, the univalent complexes of antibodies of this type cannot be detected. The result of these two effects can be that the detection of antigen requires a threshold antigen density that is quite high. For example, the antibody MRC OX3 was made against rat class II histocompatibility molecules and cross-reacts with low affinity on human DC1 molecules, which are expressed on both peripheral B lymphocytes and B-lymphoblastoid cell lines.[22] In conventional radioimmune cell binding assays, MRC OX3 could only be shown to bind to cell lines that have a relatively high density of DC1 and not to peripheral B lymphocytes with a relatively low density. However, the number of DC1 molecules on peripheral B lymphocytes is at least 5000 per cell. From this example, one can see how antibodies of low affinity could give misleading data on the tissue distribution of cell surface molecules.

It is possible to make quantitative comparisons between the strength of univalent vs. bivalent binding. For example, by equilibrium binding and Scatchard analysis we found a 50-fold difference for PA2.1. Although this clearly demonstrates the significance of the effect, it is probably not an accurate assessment of the differences in the binding energies. This is because the Scatchard analysis is based on a simpler bimolecular interaction between antibody and cell surface molecule and the reaction that gives rise to bivalent attachment of antibody is, as described above, more complex. When the results obtained with PA2.1 were analyzed by methods that sought to include these complicating factors, rather higher values ($\sim 10^4$) for the difference between the binding constant of Fab′ and $F(ab')_2$ were obtained.[12]

4. MB40.3 is of low affinity ($9 \times 10^{-7}\ M^{-1}$), due to a low association rate constant, and a dissociation rate constant comparable to that of the high-affinity antibody MA2.1.[23] Antibody thus takes a long time to form a univalent complex, but, once formed, this complex does not dissociate. With free antibody concentrations of up to 1 mg/ml, the rate of association of antibody from solution to the cell surface does not compete with the rate of formation of bivalent from univalent complexes. All antibody reaching the cell surface will end up in bivalent complexes. Unlike the low-affinity antibodies described in the previous section, the mode of binding and the detectibility of binding are not particularly sensitive to antigen density.

From this brief summary, I hope to indicate not only the complexity of the interaction between a cell surface antigen and a monoclonal antibody, but also the range in the affinity and rate constants of antibodies all identified by the same cell-based screening assay. For comparisons of the reactions between different monoclonal antibodies against distinct cell surface molecules or epitopes of the same cell surface molecule to be meaningful, a working knowledge of their binding properties is essential. For example, comparison of the competition for antibody between soluble and cell surface HLA shows that for MB40.3 soluble antigen wins, for PA2.1 cell surface antigen wins, and they compete equally for MA2.1. These properties are readily understood in terms of the relative rate constants.

6. Hybrid Antibodies

The bivalency of IgG molecules can be manipulated to produce molecules that have two distinct combining sites. The hybrid antibody can then be used to cross-link two different molecules in a noncovalent and chemically gentle fashion. Milstein and Cuello[24] produced hybrid antibodies by fusing the cells of two hybridoma cell lines and selecting hybrid cells that biosynthetically assembled mixed molecules including an active hybrid. We have adopted a different approach, which is to use chemical procedures on purified preparation of the two immunoglobulins.[25]

The example I shall describe is a hybrid made from the IgG1 monoclonal antibodies PA2.1, specific for HLA-A2, and BB7.1, specific for HLA-B7.[2] Both of these antibodies are of low affinity and require bivalent attachment to bind strongly to cells. We reasoned that a hybrid antibody would only be able to bind strongly to cells expressing both the HLA-A2 and HLA-B7 molecules. A radioiodinated preparation of PA2.1 was mixed with BB7.1 and mildly reduced

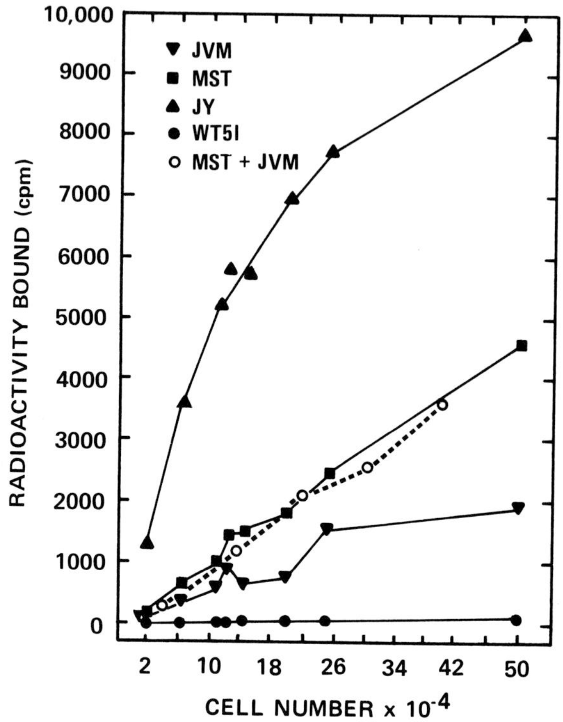

Figure 3. The binding of the ^{125}I-PA2.1–BB7.1 hybrid antibody cells that express (▲) A2 and B7, (■) only B7, (▼) only A2, (●) neither A2 nor B7, and (○) an equimixture of cells having A2 or B7. The names of the B-cell lines are as indicated. In each assay the input radioactivity was 40,000 cpm, the incubation volume was 200 μl, and the incubation time was 1 hr.

with dithiothreitol to break interchain disulfide bonds. The mixture was then desalted into 25 mM NaCl and the pH lowered to 2.5 by addition of 1.0 N HCl. This results in the splitting of the IgG into half molecules consisting of one heavy and one light chain.[25] Raising the pH back to neutrality induces a random reassociation of the half molecules to form hybrid antibodies in addition to the parental forms. At this point, the only radioactive molecules were the hybrid and the reformed PA2.1.

Separation of the three populations of molecules was achieved by exploiting the change in affinity of BB7.1 with temperature. The mixed population of molecules was incubated at 4°C with cells expressing HLA-B7 but not HLA-A2. The nonradioactive BB7.1 molecules bound in a bivalent mode, the radioactive hybrid molecules bound in a univalent mode, and the radioactive PA2.1 molecules did not bind. Washing of the cells at 4°C removed the unbound molecules.

The cells were then resuspended in buffer at 37°C and incubated at that temperature for ½ hr. At the higher temperature, the affinity of BB7.1 decreases and the univalently bound hybrids preferentially dissociate. Centrifugation removes the cells and bound BB7.1 and the supernatant consists of a radiochemically pure preparation of the PA2.1–BB7.1 hybrid.

The binding properties of the hybrid are shown in Fig. 3. It retains specificity of the two parental antibodies and only shows binding to cells expressing either HLA-A2 or HLA-B7. To cells expressing either HLA-A2 or HLA-B7, the binding is weak, whereas binding to cells expressing both HLA-A2 and HLA-B7 is strong. In the control where cells expressing A2 or B7 are mixed, the binding is also weak, showing that, as expected, the two target antigens must be present in the same membrane for the enhancing effect of bivalent interaction to occur.

7. Enhancing Effects of Monoclonal Antibodies in Solution

In the previous two sections I have emphasized how multivalency can increase the strength of the interaction between antibody and membrane-associated antigen. This can also be true in reactions with soluble antigenic molecules.

The simplest situation is where the antigen has repeating epitopes and a closed antigen–antibody complex can be formed by multivalent attachment. This is more stable than the simple bimolecular complex because rebinding is a highly favored reaction when a single interaction dissociates. For experimental purposes repeating epitopes are often made by covalently coupling many identical haptenic groups onto a protein molecule. Natural compounds such as the complex carbohydrates and proteoglycans often have repeating epitopes, and there are examples, such as the malarial sporozoite surface antigen, of single polypeptides with repeating sequences and epitopes. Multisubunit proteins containing more than one copy of a polypeptide will generally have repeating epitopes.

An interesting example of this was an IgG1 antibody made against the creatine kinase of human brain, which consists of two identical subunits.[26] The native antibody bound to the enzyme forming a 1:1 complex with a binding constant that was similar to that of the Fab. This showed that either univalent attachment predominated or that formation of the bivalent complex did not increase the effective strength of interaction. (The latter possibility has been shown to operate in the case of MB40.3 antibody interacting with cell surface HLA-B7 or HLA-B40; see Section 5.) In contrast, when the intra-heavy chain disulfides were broken by mild reduction, a complex of 50-fold higher strength consisting of two molecules of antibody and two molecules of enzyme was formed. Reduction allowed a greater flexibility of the two Fab arms of the IgG molecule and the formation of a cyclic complex into which each component is held by two independent interactions.

Similar high-avidity complexes can be formed with soluble antigenic molecules, such as the papain fragment of HLA-A, B, which do not have repeating epitopes, providing combinations of antibodies against topographically distinct epitopes are used. We have called them tetramolecular complexes (TMC), since they consist of four molecules.[27] As in the case of the antibody against creatine kinase, we have found examples where reduction of inter-heavy chain disulfides is required to form the circular complex. For those antibodies that require bivalent attachment for strong binding to cells we have invariably found that their reactions in solution with solubilized HLA are difficult to detect. For example, they do not immunoprecipitate or form a complex that can be analyzed by high-pressure size exclusion chromatography. When such antibodies are used in pairwise combinations highly stable tetramolecular complexes are often formed. A particularly striking example is shown in Fig. 4 involving the two antibodies BB7.1 and BB7.6 with specificity for two epitopes of HLA-B7.[28] When either antibody alone is incubated with B7 and analyzed by size exclusion HPLC, only peaks corresponding to free antibody and free antigen are observed. This is because the half-times of dissociation of the complexes are short compared to the time for chromatographic analysis. When both antibodies are incubated together with B7 and analyzed, a complex peak corresponding to a tetramolecular complex consisting of one molecule of BB7.1, one molecule of BB7.6, and two molecules of B7 is formed. The role of antibody bivalency in determining the stability of these complexes is simply demonstrated by forming the tetramolecular complex with $F(ab')_2$ fragments. Then addition of 2 mM dithiothreitol reduces the $F(ab')_2$ to Fab′, resulting in complete loss of the complex peak.

Thus, by using combinations of monoclonal antibodies, one can more easily analyze the interactions of lower affinity antibodies. This has proved particularly useful in performing topographic analysis of the epitopes of HLA-A, B, since it has freed us from the constraint of having to use cells or membranes as the antigenic target for low-affinity antibodies. Comparison of different methods for mapping epitopes of HLA-A, B has clearly shown that many artifacts arise in cell-based assays.[28,29]

The formation of cyclic tetramolecular complexes is just the first step one can take in making complexes with enhanced affinity. By enhanced I mean that the resulting strength or avidity of interaction is considerably greater than the arithmetic sum of the individual affinities. It is likely that the tetramolecular complex is a common intermediate in the formation of macromolecular complexes and precipitates with polyclonal antisera. The maximum strength of interaction possible with combinations of antibodies will always be greater than for a single antibody of comparable affinity. It is probably for this reason rather than a qualitative difference in the individual antibodies that polyclonal antisera are generally found to be stronger than available monoclonal antibodies. For applications where the highest avidity possible is preferable, appropriate mixtures of monoclonals should be able to produce an avidity equivalent to the best polyclonal antiserum.

Enhancement in which one antibody facilitates the binding of a second can also result from factors other than antibody bivalency. A second mechanism that has been identified probably involves conformational changes in the antigen induced by antibody binding. In studies on rat class I MHC antigens, Howard and colleagues have analyzed the enhanced binding of the YR1/1 antibody to the $RT1A^a$ molecule in the presence of the R3/47 antibody.[30] The effect was due to a decrease in the dissociation rate constant. It was mediated by Fab fragments and could be detected with both cell surface and solubilized antigen. These two properties rule out the involvement of antibody bivalency

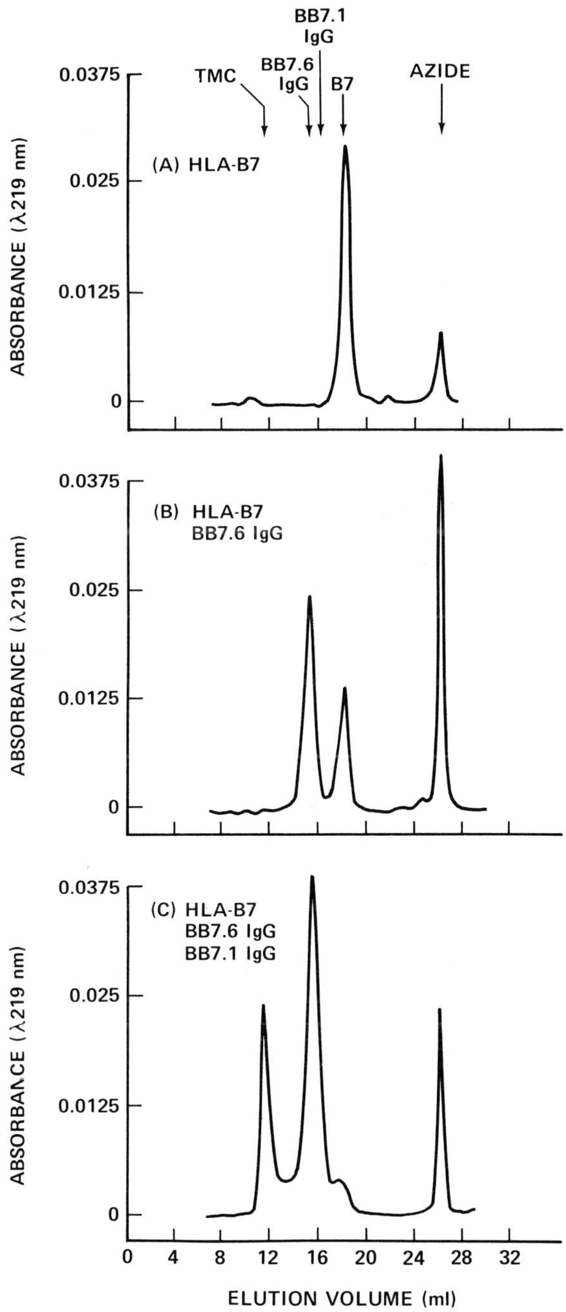

Figure 4. Tetramolecular complexes (TMC) formed by B7, BB7.1, and BB7.6. The three components, papain-solubilized B7, BB7.1, and BB7.6, were incubated in all combinations and the mixtures and the individual components analyzed by size exclusion HPLC. (A) The chromatogram for B7 alone, (B) a mixture of B7 and BB7.6, and (C) a mixture of all three. The elution positions of sodium azide, B7, BB7.1, BB7.6, and the tetramolecular complex are as indicated. That the two IgG1 monoclonal antibodies elute at different positions is not unusual. (From Ref. 28.)

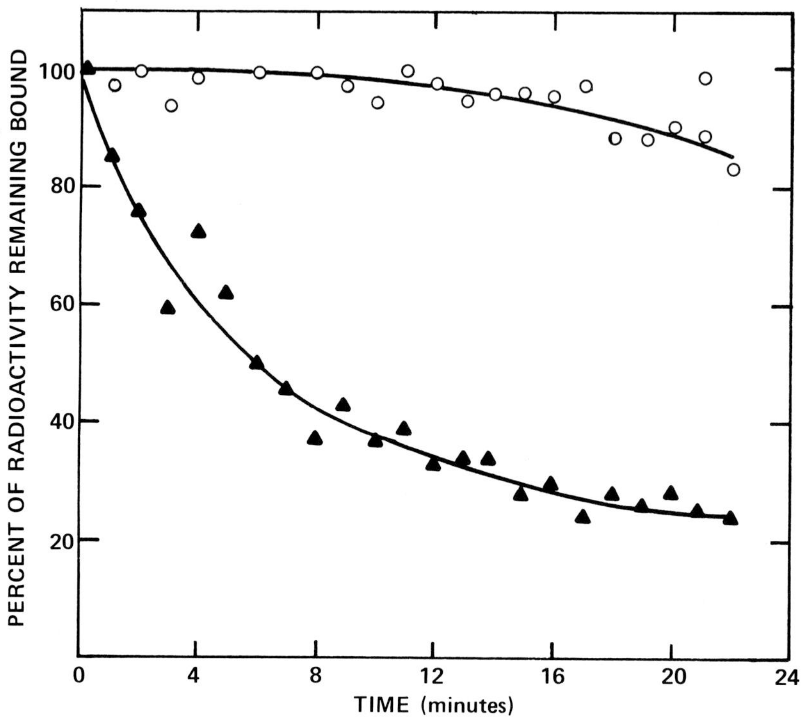

Figure 5. Induction of the release of ME1 from a complex with B7 by MB40.3. The wells of microtiter plates were coated with ME1 and 25 μl of ^{125}I-B7 (200,000 cpm) added. After incubation for 8 hr at 4°C the unbound material was removed and the wells washed; 23,000 cpm were bound to each well; (○) 50-μl aliquots of ME1–Fab′ or (▲) MB40.3–Fab′ at 10 μg/ml were added for different time periods and the residual, bound radioactivity measured. (From Ref. 29.)

and indicate that R3/47 alters the conformation of RTlA^a to a form with higher affinity for YR1/1. A similar phenomenon involving antibodies directed against epitopes of HLA-A, B, C molecules has also been described by Lemonnier *et al.*[31]

I have analyzed[29] a phenomenon complementary to that described by Diamond *et al.*[30] and Lemonnier *et al.*[31] In this case the monoclonal antibodies ME1 and MB40.3 are directed against two separate epitopes of HLA-B7 and binding of one antibody changes the conformation so that affinity for the second antibody is reduced. This is illustrated by the results shown in Fig. 5.

In this experiment the wells of microtiter plates were coated with ME1–IgG and then saturated with radioactive, papain-solubilized HLA-B7, forming a stable complex. After removal of unbound B7, nonradioactive aliquots of saturating amounts of Fab′ fragments of ME1 or MB40.3 were added to the wells. The amount of B7 remaining bound to the wells after various time periods of incubation was measured. In the control wells, to which ME1–Fab′ was added, the intrinsic rate of dissociation of B7 from ME1 was determined. As

B7 dissociated from the solid phase ME1 it would stay in solution due to excess of ME1 in solution. The results show that about 15% dissociation occurred during the 24-min time course of the experiment. In contrast, a faster and more extensive dissociation was observed in the presence of MB40.3–Fab′. This dissociation was clearly not limited by the intrinsic rate of dissociation of B7 from ME1. In fact, the analysis showed that it was determined by the association rate of MB40.3 to the ME1/B7 complexes. Once MB40.3 binds to the ME1/B7 complex it changes the conformation of B7, causing a reduction in affinity for ME1 and a rapid dissociation of the MB40.3/B7 complex from the plate. The conformational changes of B7 are reversible, providing that appropriate concentrations of antibodies are used.

This phenomenon introduces complications into the interpretation of antibody competition experiments that are designed to determine if two monoclonal antibodies are directed against the same or different epitopes. Reciprocal blocking of antibody binding occurs when two antibodies are against the same or closely juxtaposed epitopes, and this is how such data are normally interpreted. However, the antibodies of ME1 and MB40.3, which are against spatially separate epitopes of B7, do reciprocally cross-block.[29] This is because in the presence of excess first "blocking" antibody, all the B7 molecules are in a conformation that binds the radioactive second antibody with considerably lowered affinity.

8. Quantitative Serologic Analysis of HLA-A, B Molecules

Our reason for measuring the strengths and modes of binding of monoclonal antibodies with cell surface antigens was to permit a more quantitative analysis of the cross-reactions of HLA-A, B. The definition of specificity in both the H-2 and HLA serology has been done in a qualitative and somewhat arbitrary fashion, leading to different serologic descriptions of these two homologous systems.[32–34] Each H-2 molecule is described in terms of a collection of private and public specificities, emphasizing complexity in the numbers of epitopes and the sharing of determinants between different H-2 products. In HLA serology each molecule is described in terms of a unique specificity that shows cross-reactivities with various other HLA products. Despite the general appreciation of the existence of the cross-reactivities and, in some cases, the description of shared determinants responsible for these reactions, they have not been systematically incorporated into HLA typing or nomenclature. Thus HLA serology arbitrarily emphasizes the uniqueness of individual HLA molecules. With quantitative analysis one can distinguish different serologic relationships between molecules. For convenience two distinct HLA molecules are defined as sharing an epitope when a monoclonal antibody binds those two molecules with the same affinity. At the other end of the spectrum are what are defined as cross-reactions, i.e., when an antibody binds different HLA molecules with different affinity. From our studies, it appears as though both phenomena are common in the HLA-A, B system. It is also apparent, as described below, that as a consequence of antibody bivalency, large intrinsic serologic differences can become underestimated. For this reason it is preferable to perform analyses with Fab fragments.

Examples of shared epitopes emerged from analysis of antibodies defining epitopes of the HLA-A2 molecule.[35] Determination of the equilibrium binding constant and the rate constants for Fab fragments of the MA2.1 antibody showed that they reacted identically with cells expressing either HLA-A2 or HLA-B17.[12] Thus these two molecules share an epitope, which presumably reflects an underlying structural relationship. It was similarly shown that the PA2.1 antibody defined an epitope shared by HLA-A2 and a novel variant of HLA-A28 that was in fact discovered with this antibody.[12,36] This antigen, which we termed A28*, has now been called HLA-Aw69.

For both MA2.1 and PA2.1, quantitative binding studies with IgG, $F(ab')_2$, and Fab′ led to identical conclusions. This was not true for MB40.3, which was initially found to react with HLA-B7 and HLA-B40 by nonquantitative cell binding assay.[37] Quantitative binding analysis with IgG showed that the interaction with various cells expressing B7 and B40 was similar, indicating that a shared epitope was being recognized. With Fab′ fragments the binding constant for B7 and some B40 molecules was identical, but for other cells expressing B40 the binding was no longer detectable. This showed that B40 could be split into two groups, one reacting more strongly with MB40.3 and sharing an epitope with B7, the other reacting weakly with MB40.3 and thereby showing a cross-reaction with B7 and the other group of B40.

Two other interesting phenomena were encountered with MB40.3. First, $F(ab')_2$ bound more strongly to cells than IgG, and second, neuraminidase treatment of the cells produced an increase in the strength of interaction of either species. These effects were the result of an increased rate of association and were additive, as shown in Fig. 6. The Fc fragment of IgG1 is more negatively charged than the Fab, and neuraminidase removes negatively charged sialic acid from the cell surface. It is therefore possible that removal of negative, electrostatically repulsive charges is responsible for these effects.

We also found that the affinity of MB40.3 for cell surface HLA decreased with the amount of antibody that was already bound to the cell. This negative cooperativity meant that relatively large concentrations of ~0.5 mg/ml antibody are required to achieve saturation.

When cells were treated with neuraminidase and $F(ab')_2$ fragments employed, a weak but significant binding of MB40.3 to cells expressing the B27 antigen could be detected. This represents another weak cross-reaction of this antibody, since no binding was detected with Fab′.

MB40.3 is thus an antibody that binds to at least four distinct HLA molecules. In comparison to antibodies like MA2.1, the reactions are all of low affinity due to a low association rate constant. For B27 and one group of B40 molecules, the dissociation rate is high and bivalent attachment is required for a detectable interaction. For B7 and the other group of B40 molecules, the dissociation rate is low, and in consequence, the measured binding constant for bivalently bound $F(ab')_2$ is not much greater than for Fab′.[23]

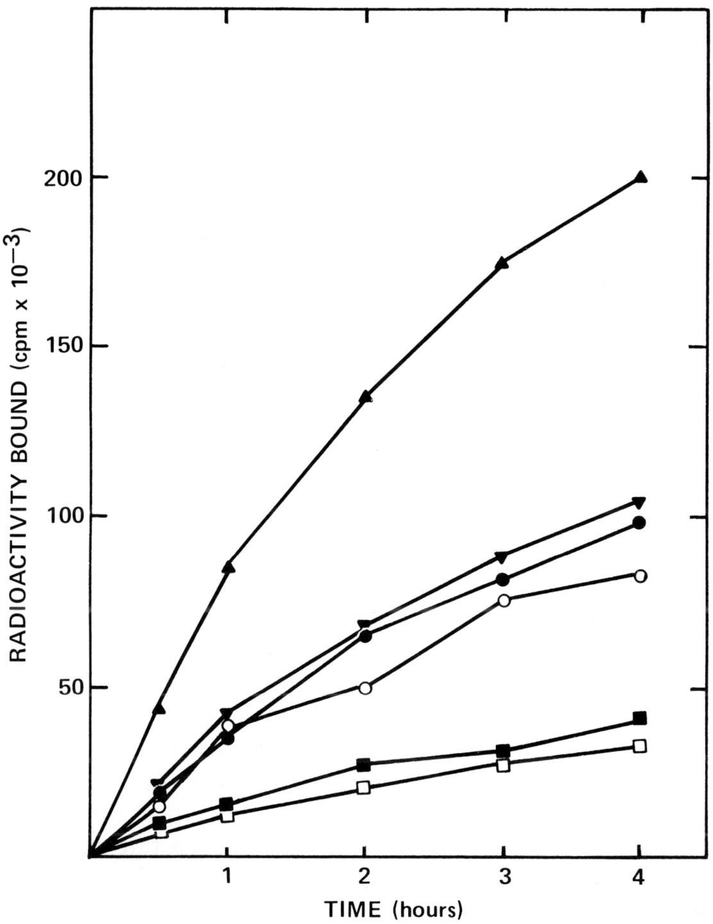

Figure 6. Removal of antibody Fc and cell surface sialic acid increases the rate of association of MB40.3: Association of ^{125}I-MB40.3–IgG and –F(ab′)$_2$ to neuraminidase-treated, mock-treated, and untreated LB cells. Association reactions were with 10^6 cells in 1 ml of PBS/BSA with 10% v/v normal rabbit serum and either 450,000 cpm of ^{125}I-F(ab′)$_2$ or 400,000 cpm of ^{125}I-IgG. Untreated cells with (■) IgG (●) and F(ab′)$_2$ mock-treated cells with (□) IgG and (○) F(ab′)$_2$, and neuraminidase-treated cells with (▼) IgG and (▲) F(ab′)$_2$ (From Ref. 23.)

9. Epitope Mapping

The experiments just described compared the reactions of a single antibody with a panel of HLA-A, B molecules. This provides an assessment of the relatedness between the structures recognized by the antibody on the different antigens. Epitope mapping is a term that is used to describe the opposite process, where the relative interactions of a panel of monoclonal antibodies that all react with a single HLA-A, B molecule are analyzed. In its minimal form this involves a series of experiments that determines whether prebinding of one antibody inhibits subsequent binding of another. The interpretation of blocking when it is observed is not straightforward, because (1) the probes and targets are generally of the same size, (2) antibodies against separate sites can give apparent blocking via conformational changes, and (3) at cell surfaces many blocking reactions are due to membrane effects.

The interpretation of nonblocking is more straightforward, providing one knows that the blocking antibody is saturating its target epitope. For these reasons we have tried to combine the data from the negative blocking assay with additional data derived from positive assays in which we determine if two antibodies can simultaneously bind to the same antigen molecule. This result, when it is obtained, shows conslusively that two antibodies are directed against topographically distinct determinants. Four basic assays have been used.

1. Additive binding assay, in which the maximum numbers of molecules bound by antibody A, antibody B, and a mixture of the two under conditions of saturation are compared.[3,37]
2. Sandwich style of solid phase radioimmunoassay, in which antibody A is bound to the plate and then saturated with antigen. Radioactive antibody B will only bind to the plate if A and B can bind antigen at the same time.[27,29]
3. Enhancing solid phase radioimmunoassay, in which antibody A is bound to the plate and the binding of radioactive antigen in the presence of antibody B assessed. This is primarily used for low-affinity antibodies, for which an enhanced binding over that obtained in the absence of second antibody can be seen when both A and B bind simultaneously.[27,28]
4. Size exclusion HPLC analysis of the immune complexes formed by combinations of antibodies.[27,29]

From studies on a number of different HLA-A, B products it has been shown that each molecule has many topographically distinct polymorphic epitopes.

For B7 we have defined a B7-specific epitope (BB7.1), a B7,B40 epitope (MB40.3), a B7,B27 epitope (ME1), and a Bw6 epitope (BB7.6) that are all topographically distinct. As one pursues this analysis in finer detail with monoclonal antibodies having more complex polymorphic specificities, one can define additional determinants that overlap and join together these four discrete epitopes. This indicates that a considerable part of the molecular surface is involved in forming polymorphic epitopes. An analysis of rat class I MHC antigens came to similar conclusions.[38] From the patterns of sequence variability in the primary structure of HLA-A, B and the results of exon shuffling experiments, we know that most, if not all, of the polymorphic determinants of HLA-B7 are formed by α_1 and α_2, the two amino-terminal domains of the B7 heavy chain (Dr. V. Engelhard, University of Virginia, unpublished data). These findings do not support a model in which the polymorphism of HLA-

A, B molecules is the result of structural alterations within a highly localized area or active site, analogous to the antigen-combining site of immunoglobulins.

One goal of epitope mapping is to define the parts of a molecule that make up an antigenic site. The most direct method of doing this is to identify small peptides that interact with the antibody and then analyze which amino acid residues are important for the activity. This can be done by chemical modification or by synthesis of peptides in which single amino acid substitutions are incorporated. We have successfully applied this approach to show that the arginine at position 45 is important for the epitope of β_2-microglobulin (β_2-m) recognized by the BBM.1 monoclonal antibody.[39]

Another approach is to use monoclonal antibodies to select for mutant cells expressing variant HLA-A, B molecules that have lost single epitopes of the parent molecule.[40] Structural analysis of the mutant molecules will then reveal the amino acid substitution or substitutions responsible for the change in serologic characteristics. Although this will provide information on structural changes that affect epitopes, it will not necessarily identify residues that are actually involved in contacting the antibody combining site. One possibility is that a substitution at one site will produce a conformational change at a distant site. From what we know about the structure of class I antigens and the conformational nature of the antigenic determinants, this is a likely possibility. Once candidate residues have been identified through the immunoselected mutants, additional experiments are required to demonstrate a role in antibody binding.

Figure 7 shows an experiment in which the capacity of HLA, β_2-m, and the peptide SWH.5 corresponding to residues 38–50 of human β_2-m to inhibit monoclonal antibodies against three different monomorphic determinants of HLA molecules is assessed. All three antibodies are inhibited by purified HLA-A2. BBM.1 is also inhibited by free β_2-m, since it is directed against an epitope of the β_2-m subunit. In contrast, W6/32 is against a determinant of the HLA heavy chain and BB7.7 is against a combinatorial determinant formed from both subunits.[41] The SWH.5 peptide also inhibits BBM.1, but on a molar basis is 35,000-fold less effective than β_2-m. This emphasizes a common problem in the use of peptides and fragments of proteins to determine the structural basis of antigenic determinants. For HLA-A, B molecules it is particularly acute, since almost all the determinants are conformational in nature. For example, only one antibody with specificity for the HLA heavy chain reacts in immunoblotting.[3] It is also our experience that monoclonal antibodies made against synthetic peptides with sequences derived from HLA-A, B do not show measurable affinity to the native molecules.

In addition to providing a better definition of the serology of HLA-A, B antigens, it is hoped that by mapping out of the epitopes of HLA-A, B molecules, one will be able to dissect the functional parts of these molecules. These molecules form part of the system by which cytotoxic T lymphocytes (CTLs) specifically recognize cells that are virally infected or expressing foreign membrane antigens. The results of experiments with *in vitro* cellular assays show that the foreign antigen is only recognized by the T lymphocyte when it is in the same

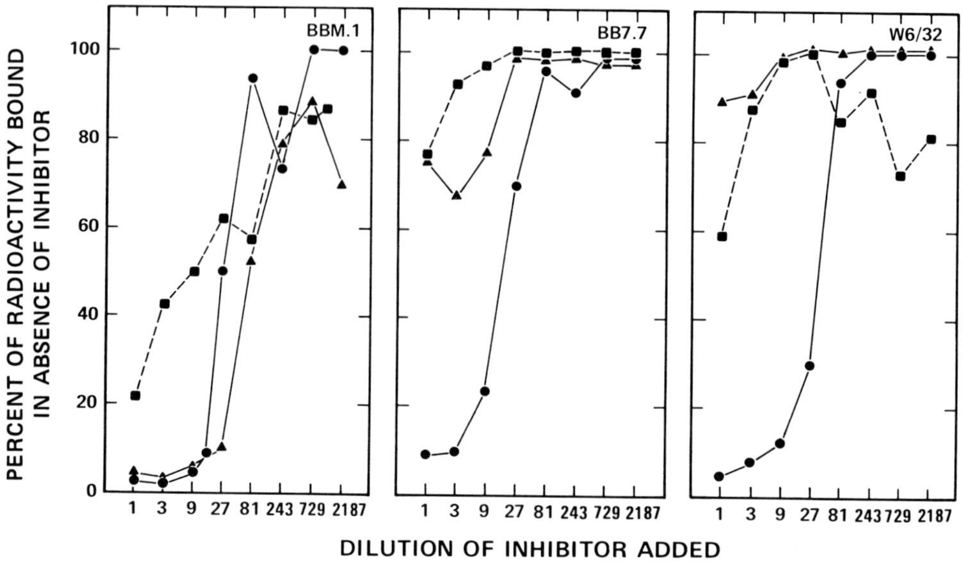

Figure 7. Specific inhibition of the BBM.1 antibody by peptide SWH.5 corresponding to amino acids 38–50 of human β_2-microglobulin (β_2-m). In this assay the effect of the inhibitors; purified β_2-m, purified HLA-A2, and peptide SWH.5, on the binding of monoclonal antibodies BBM.1, BB7.7, and W6/32 against different epitopes of the HLA/β_2-m complex to cell surface antigen is measured. Dilutions of (▲) β_2-m, (●) HLA-A2, and (■) SWH.5 were incubated with limiting amounts of BBM.1, BB7.7, and W6/32 antibodies, which were then tested for binding by indirect trace assay on 10^5 LB cells. Dilutions of 1 corresponded to 2.2 μM for β_2-m, 0.5 μM for HLA-A2, and 6 mM for SWH.5. Hybridoma supernatants at a dilution of 1:50 for BBM.1, 1:16 for W6/32, and 1:4 for BB7.7 were used as sources of antibody and gave specific binding of 29,200, 16,500, and 28,900 cpm in the absence of inhibitors. (From Ref. 39.)

membrane as a histocompatibility antigen of the correct polymorphic type.[42,43] The molecular interactions involved in this process are not known, but it seems likely that a complex involving foreign antigen, HLA-A, B molecule, and receptor molecules of the T lymphocyte is involved. Since the function is essentially one involving the interaction between two cells, and since conjugates of target and effector cells are formed, it is also likely that the complex is formed between components in the opposing plasma membranes. Our initial experiments showed that binding of anti-HLA-A, B monoclonal antibodies to the target cells inhibited killing by cytotoxic lymphocytes.[44] It is not known for certain whether this is the result of covering up epitopes and preventing essential interactions or because modulation, internalization, or shedding of the antigen is induced. Circumstantial evidence favors the covering up hypothesis. For example, in the antibody-dependent cellular cytotoxicity assay described in Section 4, we found that target cells coated with the same monoclonal antibodies were killed. This showed that significant HLA-A, B antigen complexed with antibody remained on the cell surface under conditions that were similar to those used in the CTL assay. Surprisingly, it has been shown that monoclonal antibodies against the supposed foreign antigens such as the influenza hemagglutinin on influenza-infected cells do not inhibit the CTL assay.[45]

It was initially hoped that one could identify the functionally important epitopes of HLA-A, B molecules by using a panel of monoclonal antibodies, whose target epitopes had been mapped by serologic analysis, to inhibit CTL function. The realization from antibody blocking studies showing that artifactual blocking effects were commonplace cast some doubt on the feasibility of this approach. The results so far have reinforced this view. Most of the antibodies that saturate their epitopes under the conditions of the assay cause blocking of CTL function.[44] This suggests that either all of the epitopes are functionally important or that the probes are nonspecifically interfering with the functional interactions. The fact that a monoclonal antibody is three times the size of an HLA-A, B molecules suggests that the latter possibility is likely. However, it is worth attempting a similar anslysis with Fab fragments, since many of the potential artifacts are the consequence of bivalency. However, this necessitates more antibodies of higher affinity than are now generally available.

References

1. Möller, G. (ed), 1979, Hybrid myeloma monoclonal antibodies against MHC products, *Immunol. Rev.* **47**:1–252.
2. Brodsky, F. M., Parham, P., Barnstable, C. J., Crumpton, M. J., and Bodmer, W. F., 1979, Monoclonal antibodies for analysis of the HLA system, *Immunol. Rev.* **47**:3–61.
3. Parham, P., Androlewicz, M. J., Brodsky, F. M., Holmes, N. J., and Ways, J. P., 1982, Monoclonal antibodies: Purification and application to structural and functional studies of class I MHC antigens, *J. Immunol. Meth.* **53**:133–173.
4. Ploegh, H. L., Orr, H. T., and Strominger, J. L., 1981, Major histocompatibility antigens: The human (HLA-A, -B, -C) and murine (H-2K, H-2D) class I molecules, *Cell* **24**:287–299.
5. Mage, M. G., 1980, Preparation of Fab fragments from IgGs of different animal species, *Meth. Enzymol.* **70**:142–150.
6. Parham, P., 1983, On the fragmentation of monoclonal IgG1, IgG2a, IgG2b from BALB/c mice, *J. Immunol.* **131**:2895–2902.
7. Parham, P., 1985, Preparation and purification of active fragments from mouse monoclonal antibodies, in: *Handbook of Experimental Immunology*, 4th ed. (D. M. Weir, C. C. Blackwell, L. A. Herzenberg, L. A. Herzenberg, eds.), Blackwell, Oxford, In press.
8. Lamoyi, E., and Nisonoff, A., 1983, Preparation of $F(ab')_2$ fragments from mouse IgG of various subclasses, *J. Immunol. Meth.* **56**:235–243.
9. Glennie, M. J., and Stevenson, G. T., 1982, Univalent antibodies kill tumour cells *in vitro* and *in vivo*, *Nature* **295**:712–714.
10. Köhler, G., Hengartner, H., and Shulman, M. J., 1978, Immunoglobulin production by lymphocyte hybridomas, *Eur. J. Immunol.* **8**:82–88.
11. Mason, D. W., and Williams, A. F., 1980, The kinetics of antibody binding to membrane antigens in solution and at the cell surface, *Biochem. J.* **187**:1–20.
12. Ways, J. P., and Parham, P., 1983, The binding of monoclonal antibodies to cell surface molecules: A quantitative analysis with IgG against two alloantigenic determinants of HLA-A2, *Biochem. J.* **216**:423–432.
13. Ellis, S. A., Taylor, C., and McMichael, A., 1982, Recognition of HLA, B27 and related antigens by a monoclonal antibody, *Hum. Immunol.* **5**:49–59.

14. Kipps, T. J., Parham, P., and Herzenberg, L. A., 1984, The importance of immunoglobulin isotype in human antibody dependent cell-mediated cytotoxicity directed by murine monoclonal antibodies, *J. Exp. Med.* **161**:1–17.
15. Ey, P. L., Prowse, S. J., and Jenkin, C. R., 1978, Isolation of pure IgG1, IgG2a and IgG2b immunoglobulins from mouse serum using protein-A–sepharose, *Immunochemistry* **15**:429–436.
16. Dangl, J. L., and Herzenberg, L. A., 1982, Selection of hybridomas and hybridoma variants using the fluorescence activated cell sorter, *J. Immunol. Meth.* **52**:1–14.
17. Oi, V. T., Vuong, T. M., Hardy, R., Reidler, J., Dangl, J., Herzenberg, L. A., and Stryer, L., 1984, Correlation between segmental flexibility and effector function of antibodies, *Nature* **307**:136–140.
18. Parham, P., Kipps, T. J., Ward, F. E., and Herzenberg, L. A., 1983, Isolation of heavy chain class switch variants of a monoclonal anti-DC1 hybridoma cell line. Effective conversion of non-cytotoxic IgG_1 antibodies to cytotoxic IgG_2 antibodies, *Hum. Immunol.* **8**:141–151.
19. McMichael, A. J., Parham, P., Rust, N., and Brodsky, F., 1980, A monoclonal antibody that recognizes an antigenic determinant shared by HLA A2 and B17, *Hum. Immunol.* **1**:121–129.
20. Heron, I., Hokland, M., and Berg, K., 1979, Enhanced expression of β_2-microglobulin and HLA antigens on human lymphoid cells by interferon, *Proc. Natl. Acad. Sci. USA* **75**:6215–6219.
21. Fellous, M., Kamoun, M., Gresser, I., and Bono, R., 1979, Enhanced expression of HLA antigens and β_2-microglobulin on interferon-treated human lymphoid cells, *Eur. J. Immunol.* **9**:446–449.
22. McMaster, W. R., Winearls, B. C., and Parham, P., 1979, A monoclonal mouse anti-rat Ia antibody which cross-reacts with a human HLA-DRw determinant, *Tissue Antigens* **14**:543–548.
23. Parham, P., 1984, The binding of monoclonal antibodies to cell surface molecules: Quantitative analysis of the reactions and cross-reactions of an antibody (MB40.3) with four HLA-B molecules, *J. Biol. Chem.* **259**:13077–13083.
24. Milstein, C., and Cuello, A. C., 1983, Hybrid hybridomas and their use in immunohistochemistry, *Nature* **305**:537–540.
25. Nisonoff, A., and Palmer, J. L., 1964, Hybridization of half molecules of rabbit gamma globulin, *Science* **143**:376–379.
26. Thompson, R. J., and Jackson, A. P., 1984, Cyclic complexes and high avidity antibodies, *Trends Biochem. Sci.* **9**:1–3.
27. Holmes, N. J., and Parham, P., 1983, Enhancement of monoclonal antibodies against HLA-A2 is due to antibody bivalency, *J. Biol. Chem.* **258**:1580–1586.
28. Parham, P., 1983, Antigenic determinants of the B7 molecule; Bw6 and B7 specific determinants are spatially separate, *Immunogenetics* **18**:1–16.
29. Parham, P., 1984, Changes in conformation with loss of alloantigenic determinants of a histocompatibility antigen (HLA-B7) induced by monoclonal antibodies, *J. Immunol.* **132**:2975–2983.
30. Diamond, A. G., Butcher, G. W., and Howard, J. C., 1984, Localized conformational changes induced in a class I major histocompatibility antigen by the binding of monoclonal antibodies, *J. Immunol.* **132**:1169–1175.
31. Lemonnier, F. A., Bouteiller, D., Olive, D., Malissen, B., Mishal, Z., Layet, C., Dubreuil, J., Caillol, D. H., Kourilsky, F. M., and Jordan, B. M., 1984, Transformation of $LMTK^-$ cells with purified class I genes V. Antibody-induced structural modification of HLA class I molecules results in potentiation of the fixation of a second monoclonal antibody, *J. Immunol.* **132**:1176–1182.
32. Klein, J., 1975, *Biology of the Mouse Histocompatibility-2 Complex*, Springer-Verlag, Berlin.
33. Festenstein, H., and Demant, P., 1978, HLA and H-2, in: *Current Topics in Immunology*, Volume 9, Edward Arnold, London, pp. 1–212.
34. Bodmer, W. F., 1978, The HLA system, *Br. Med. Bull.* **34**:213–320.
35. Ways, J. P., and Parham, P., 1983, The antigenic structure of HLA-A2: An analysis with competitive binding assays and monoclonal antibodies, *J. Immunol.* **131**:856–863.
36. Holmes, N., and Parham, P., 1984, Molecular characteristics of HLA-A28*, A novel HLA product, and its relationship to HLA-A28 and HLA-A2, *Immunogenetics* **20**:103–115.
37. Parham, P., 1981, Monoclonal antibodies against two separate alloantigenic sites of HLA-B40, *Immunogenetics* **13**:509–527.

38. Diamond, A. G., Larkins, A. P., Wright, B., Ellis, S. T., Butcher, G. W., and Howard, J. C., 1984, The alloantigenic organization of RTIA[a], a class I major histocompatibility complex molecule of the rat, *Eur. J. Immunol.* **14:**405–412.
39. Parham, P., Androlewicz, M. J., Holmes, N. J., and Rothenberg, B. E., 1983, Arginine 45 is a major part of the antigenic determinant of human β_2-microglobulin recognized by mouse monoclonal antibody BBM.1, *J. Biol. Chem.* **258:**6179–6186.
40. Pious, D., Krangel, M. S., Dixon, L. L., Parham, P., and Strominger, J. L., 1982, HLA antigen structural gene mutants selected with an allospecific monoclonal antibody, *Proc. Natl. Acad. Sci. USA* **79:**7832–7836.
41. Brodsky, F. M., and Parham, P., 1982, Monomorphic anti-HLA-A,B,C monoclonal antibodies detecting molecular subunits and combinatorial determinants, *J. Immunol.* **128:**129–135.
42. Zinkernagel, R. M., and Doherty, P. C., 1974, Restriction of *in vitro* T cell-mediated cytotoxicity in lymphocytic choriomeningitis within a syngeneic or semiallogeneic system, *Nature* **248:**701–702.
43. Zinkernagel, R. M., and Doherty, P. C., 1978, MHC-restricted cytotoxic T cells: Studies on the biological role of polymorphic major transplantation antigens determining T-cell restriction-specificity, function, and responsiveness, *Adv. Immunol.* **27:**51–177.
44. McMichael, A. J., Parham, P., Brodsky, F. M., and Pilch, J. R., 1980, Influenza virus-specific cytotoxic T lymphocytes recognize HLA molecules, *J. Exp. Med.* **152:**195s–203s.
45. Askonas, B. A., and Webster, R. G., 1980, Monoclonal antibodies to hemagglutinin and to H-2 inhibit the cross-reactive cytotoxic T cell populations induced by influenza, *Eur. J. Immunol.* **10:**151–156.

Chapter 9

Purification of Membrane Glycoproteins with Monoclonal Antibody Affinity Columns

PAULINE JOHNSON, ALAN F. WILLIAMS, and GILLIAN R. WOOLLETT

1. Introduction

By preparing monoclonal antibodies (MAbs) across species it is possible to identify previously unknown molecules in a complex mixture.[1] In many cases the antibody can then be used to purify the antigen it recognizes and this then opens up a wide range of structural and functional studies (Fig. 1). In particular, MAb affinity chromatography integrates with determination of protein sequence at the nucleic acid level. A limited number of peptides can be prepared from pure antigen and an oligonucleotide probe can then be synthesized from their sequence and used to detect cDNA clones for the antigen.[2] The use of MAbs in affinity chromatography was first applied in studies on cell surface antigens[3,4] (reviewed in Refs. 5–7) and has since been widely applied to purify molecules of all types. The steps from antigen identification with MAb to nucleotide sequence as shown in Fig. 1 have been applied to the EGF receptor,[8] the IL-2 receptor,[9] the MRC OX-2 antigen,[10] and the leukocyte-common antigen (L-CA).[11]

In this chapter we discuss MAb affinity chromatography with reference to lymphocyte membrane glycoproteins. Two recent applications of the technique are described, namely the purification of a denatured glycoprotein chain from the rat T-cytotoxic/suppressor (Tc/s) glycoprotein, and the purification of an antigenically active peptide from rat L-CA.

PAULINE JOHNSON, ALAN F. WILLIAMS, and GILLIAN R. WOOLLETT • MRC Cellular Immunology Unit, Sir William Dunn School of Pathology, University of Oxford, Oxford OX1 3RE, England.

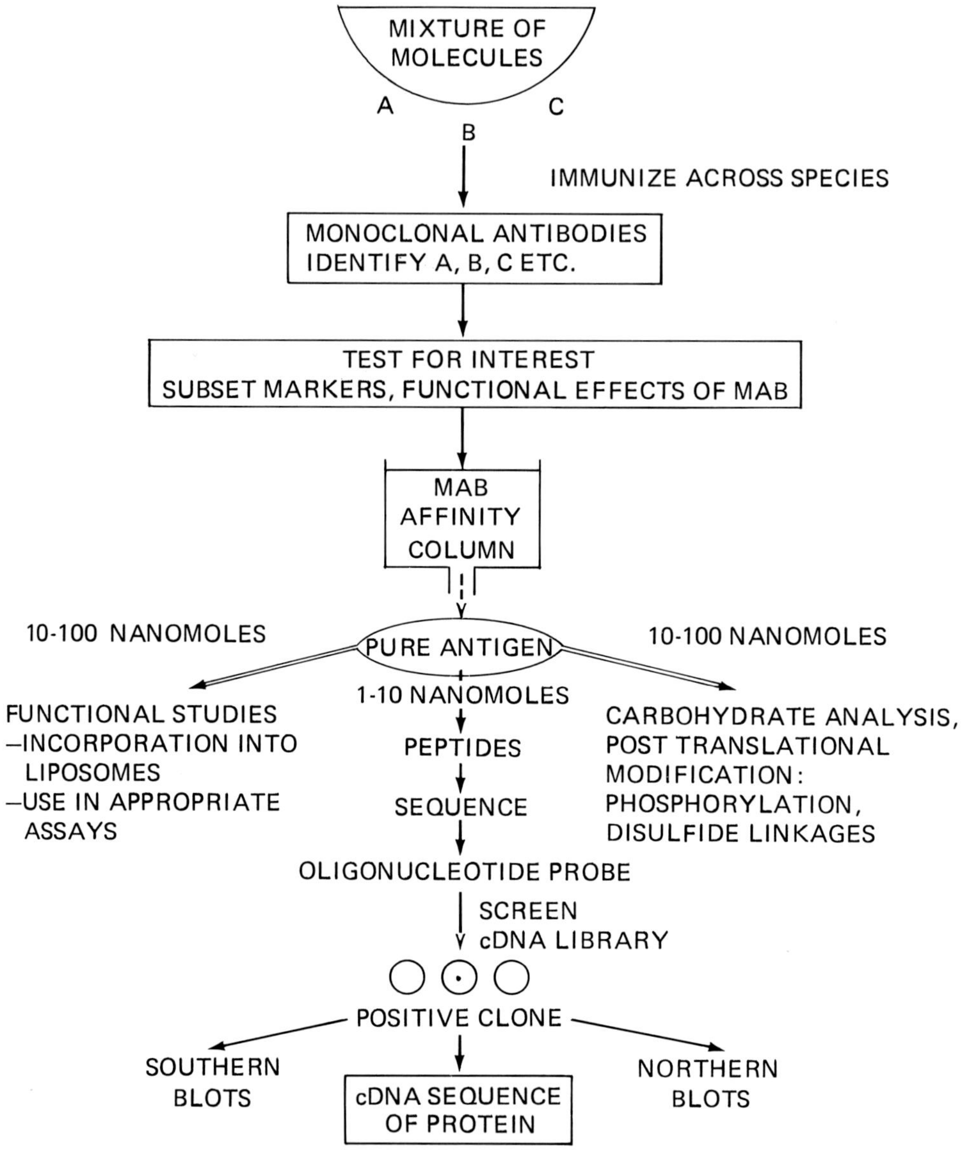

Figure 1. The uses of monoclonal antibodies to purify molecules for structural and functional studies.

2. Key Aspects in Monoclonal Antibody Affinity Chromatography

Here we discuss strategies for antibody affinity chromatography. Detailed protocols for membrane glycoproteins are given elsewhere.[5–7]

2.1. Nature of Antigenic Determinants

Protein antigenic determinants are usually unique to one molecule[12] and antibodies against these should thus allow purification of a single entity. Carbohydrate structures are usually common to a diverse set of polypeptides and thus anticarbohydrate antibodies would not be generally useful in purifying glycoprotein components. However, in the case of the EGF receptor, which is a major glycoprotein of A431 cells, an anticarbohydrate antibody was used to obtain substantially purified material without the need for elution with denaturing agents, since antigen could be eluted with saccharides.[13] In immunizations of mice or rats with mammalian glycoproteins antibodies against protein determinants are commonly obtained.

Irrelevant cross-reactions[14] are a potential source of confusion with antiprotein antibodies. These occur when an antibody reacts with its antigen and also with an unrelated molecule that either shares a small amount of sequence with the relevant antigen or reacts with a different part of the antibody combining site. In our experience such cross-reactions are not an important problem in affinity chromatography, probably because this technique depends upon a monovalent reaction of moderately high affinity. The irrelevant cross-reaction would be likely to have a much lower affinity than the correct reaction and in the systems that have been reported the cross-reactions may only have been seen because techniques that allow multivalent binding were used (for example, Ref. 15).

2.2. Assays of Antigenic Activity

It is important that antigenic activity should be assayed at all stages during a purification procedure and that the amount of purified antigen seen with biochemical techniques should be appropriate to the purification factor (e.g., see purification of the leukocyte sialoglycoprotein[16]). Inhibition of radioactive binding assays is appropriate for measuring antigenic activity and these have been discussed in detail elsewhere.[17,18] In some cases a purification may be performed on the basis that the eluted antigen is the "correct" one in terms of biochemical parameters determined by immunoprecipitation of radiolabeled material or immunoblotting. This can be hazardous because contaminants are always present at some level. With this approach multiple criteria should be used, including determination of apparent molecular weight and isoelectric point.

2.3. Antibody Affinity and Kinetics

Monovalent affinity must be such that an antigen can be almost totally depleted from an extract and retained on the column during washing procedures. If a column contained 10 mg/ml of antibody and 10% of the binding sites were free to react, then the concentration of binding sites would be 12×10^{-6} M. In practice it might be desirable to pass 1 liter of extract through a 20-ml column and deplete antigen to the level of 10% of extract concentration when the column had become 90% saturated. To do this, bound to free antigen would be about 500:1 when the last of the extract was passing through, free antibody would be at 12×10^{-7}M, and an antibody affinity of 4×10^{8} M^{-1} would be needed. In practice the MRC OX-7 monoclonal antibody was effective in purifying mouse Thy-1.1 antigen from large volumes of extract[5] and for this antibody the monovalent affinity is 3×10^{8} M^{-1}.[17] The anti-HLA antibody PA2.1 was effective in an affinity column[6] even though the affinity in this case was only 2×10^{7} M^{-1}. In terms of the above calculation this would be sufficient if the column were used at levels considerably below saturation.

Antibodies suitable for affinity chromatography can be detected empirically by looking for those that are effectively inhibited in binding assays in the presence of detergent[17] or that show good results in immunoprecipitation. Both these techniques theoretically would require higher affinities than needed for affinity chromatography.[18] In contrast, an antibody that works well in immunoblotting[19] may not be effective in affinity chromatography, since in immunoblotting, multivalent binding can occur and low-affinity antibodies can thus give positive results. This might particularly apply to IgM antibodies.

Given that there is a high concentration of antibody on columns, the kinetics of the reaction will usually be sufficient such that binding will be complete at the usual flow rates of 1–2 column volumes per hour. However, the kinetics of antibody–antigen interactions with protein antigens are much slower and more variable than has been commonly accepted,[18] and with some high-affinity antibodies to IL-2, affinity chromatography was ineffective because of slow kinetics (R. Budd and K. Smith, personal communication).

The temperature used for running columns is important with regard to both kinetics and affinity. With an increase in temperature both on-rates and off-rates usually increase, but the off-rate often goes up more than the on-rate, resulting in a drop in affinity.[17] The magnitude of the temperature effects will vary with different antibodies and the use of different temperatures might be exploited to speed the binding reaction or to facilitate antigen elution. In one case HLA antigen that bound to a column at 4°C was eluted by raising the temperature to 37°C.[20] We routinely run antibody columns at 4°C.

2.4. Antibody Coupling, Binding Capacity, Column Size, and Flow Rates

Sepharose 4B and CL-4B (Pharmacia) are the most commonly used column materials, but we have also used Sepharose 2B in the purification of L-CA in an attempt to make more antibody combining sites accessible to a large antigen (the column worked, but the capacity was not quantitated). Standard coupling procedures with cyanogen bromide are used[21] and protocols are outlined in Refs. 5 and 6.

The binding capacities of columns with antibody at 10 mg/ml have been determined to be in the range of 2–20% of theoretical, allowing two binding sites per antibody.[5] The lowest value was for the very large molecule L-CA (150,000 molecular weight), while the highest value was for Thy-1 antigen (18,000 molecular weight). Parham[22] used anti-HLA coupled at 2–3 mg/ml and in this case achieved capacities of about 40% of theoretical.

It might be argued that the coupling of antibodies with spacer groups would improve capacity. One approach along these lines was the use of protein A–Sepharose 4B to bind antibody via its Fc piece and then to cross-link the complex with dimethylpimelimidate.[23] However, no quantitative comparison was made between this column and an equivalent one prepared by conventional methods and it can be calculated from the data in Ref. 23 that the binding capacity of the protein A–antibody column was not proven to be more than 6%. It is not obvious that spacer groups should make a great difference to antibody columns, since one Fab or the Fc should act as a satisfactory spacer group to provide at least one free binding site per molecule. Systematic investigation of the factors that affect column capacities is clearly needed.

Antibody columns routinely leak small amounts of antibody, but in our experience this has not been a major problem if antigen is being purified in amounts >0.2 mg. The antibody is usually a minor contaminant and can often be removed by gel filtration after the affinity column step or by passage through an anti-Ig column. To minimize antibody contamination in eluted material, columns should be preeluted with the dissociating buffer and then reequilibrated with standard buffer prior to application of the extract that contains antigen.

We usually use columns containing at least 5 ml of beads (and up to 60 ml) with antibody at 10 mg/ml. In large-scale preparations it is best to saturate columns with antigen, since this may improve yield, and also will decrease the ratio of leaked antibody to eluted antigen. We have not noticed that yield of antigen decreases if columns are not saturated, but this could happen if some affinity was retained between antigen and antibody under conditions of elution.

Convenient flow rates are 1–2 column volumes per hour. These can be increased or decreased on the basis of whether or not antigen is coming through the column as determined by inhibition of radioactive binding assays.

2.5. Solubilization of Membrane Antigens

Weakly ionic or nonionic detergents[24] are suitable for use in antibody affinity chromatography since these detergents do not usually interfere with antigen–antibody interactions. Deoxycholate is the most commonly used weakly ionic detergent, but its use requires low salt concentrations and $\text{pH} > 8$. Whole cells cannot be solubilized in deoxycholate, since DNA is released. The advantages of deoxycholate are that it is very effective at solubilizing membrane molecules to a monomeric form,[25] that it does not absorb light of 280 nm wavelength, that it has a small micelle size and thus a minor effect on the hydrodynamic properties of a molecule, and that it is easily removed from pure antigen by dialysis or by precipitating antigen with ethanol, in which the detergent remains soluble.

Commonly used nonionic detergents are NP-40, Triton X-100, Brij-96, and Lubrol-PX, the latter two of which give little absorption of light at 280 nm. Nonionic detergents do not release DNA and thus can be used to solubilize antigens from whole cells or membranes and at acid or alkali pH. One major disadvantage of nonionic detergents is that they are virtually nondialyzable because of their low critical micelle concentration and large micelle size. Also, the hydrodynamic properties of a molecule are greatly altered by its binding to a large nonionic detergent micelle.[25]

Detailed protocols for the bulk preparation of membranes and solubilization of glycoproteins are given elsewhere.[5]

2.6. Elution of Antigen

In most cases this requires denaturing conditions and usually high- or low-pH buffers are used. With deoxycholate detergent high pH must be maintained and we have routinely used 0.05 M diethylamine HCl buffer at pH 11.5 to elute antigens.[26] In studies on HLA antigens where high- and low-pH buffers were tried the former conditions were found to give a better yield of antigenic activity.[4] Another alternative is to elute with chaotropic agents,[27] and raised temperature may be exploited, as discussed above. In most cases antigenic activity is recovered when eluted material is neutralized, but this does not necessarily mean that the full biological activity of a molecule has been recovered. However, in the case of the macrophage Fc receptor[28] and the N-CAM adhesion molecule[29] biological activity was retained in material eluted from a column at high pH.

3. Purification Based on Antigenic Determinants Stable to Denaturation

Most of the protein antigenic determinants that have been studied in detail have been found to depend on conformation of the molecule.[12,30] However, this is not always the case and the recently discovered antigens of malaria parasites,[31] which have a repeating sequence of a small number of amino acids, provide a clear example of a protein with immunodominant regions that are independent of conformation. Also, a number of antigenic determinants of cell surface molecules have been found to be resistant to reduction and alkylation in denaturing conditions, for example, the MRC OX-6 determinant, which can be localized to the β chain of the rat Ia-A class II major histocompatibility antigen,[32] and the W3/13 determinant found on the leukocyte sialoglycoprotein.[16] Below we discuss the MRC OX-8 and MRC OX-22 antibodies, which also recognize determinants not dependent on conformation, and illustrate the exploitation of this in chain separation and peptide purification by antibody chromatography.

3.1. Separation of the Denatured Chains of the T-Cytotoxic/ Suppressor Glycoprotein

MRC OX-8 antibody is a mouse monoclonal IgG1 antibody which binds to thymocytes, cytotoxic and suppressor T cells, and the majority of natural killer cells. Immunoprecipitation studies with radiolabeled antigen show the OX-8 antigen to consist of two glycoprotein chains of 39,000 and 34,000 molecular weight that were found in disulfide-linked dimers and higher multimers.[33] This antigen appears to be the homologue of the mouse Lyt-2/3 and human T8 antigens, which show similar but not identical chain compositions. Lyt-2/3 has three bands, two of which seem to constitute different polypeptides,[34] while with T8 there may only be one main glycoprotein chain.[35] cDNA coding for human T8 has now been cloned[36] and this has led to the cloning of one chain of the Lyt-2/3 complex. If the dissimilar glycoprotein chains were purified in mouse or rat, the approach shown in Fig. 1 could be taken to obtain cDNA clones for the second chain of the rodent antigens.

Using an MRC OX-8 affinity column, OX-8 antigen was obtained substantially pure by two cycles of affinity chromatography carried out exactly as in Ref. 5. The antigen was then reduced and alkylated in 2% sodium dodecyl sulfate (SDS) and was found to retain its antigenic, activity as shown in Fig. 2. To remove minor contaminants the reduced and alkylated material was subjected to gel filtration in 0.2% SDS, and this gave a fraction as shown in Fig. 3, track 1. This material was made to 0.5% with deoxycholate and the affinity chromatography step was repeated with the result shown in Fig. 3, track 2 (unretarded) and track 3 (eluted). Both bands were obtained pure and have been used to prepare peptides for sequencing. The yield of antigenic activity from starting cells through to the substantially purified oligomer prior to reduction and alkylation was about 25% and the final yield of the low-molecular-weight band was 6% of starting activity.

3.2. Purification of an Antigenically Active Peptide of the Leukocyte-Common Antigen

The MRC OX-22 antibody labels all rat B cells and T-cytotoxic/suppressor cells, but splits T helper cells into two sets with different functional activities.[37] The OX-22 antigenic determinant is found on a subfraction of L-CA glycoproteins and it is unusual in that it was stable after reduction and alkylation and also was not destroyed by trypsin digestion.[38] These results are shown in Fig. 4 in comparison with similar assays for the OX-1 antigenic determinant, which is found on all the L-CA glycoproteins and is destroyed by denaturation. The OX-22 antigenic determinant appears to be protein in nature, since, when

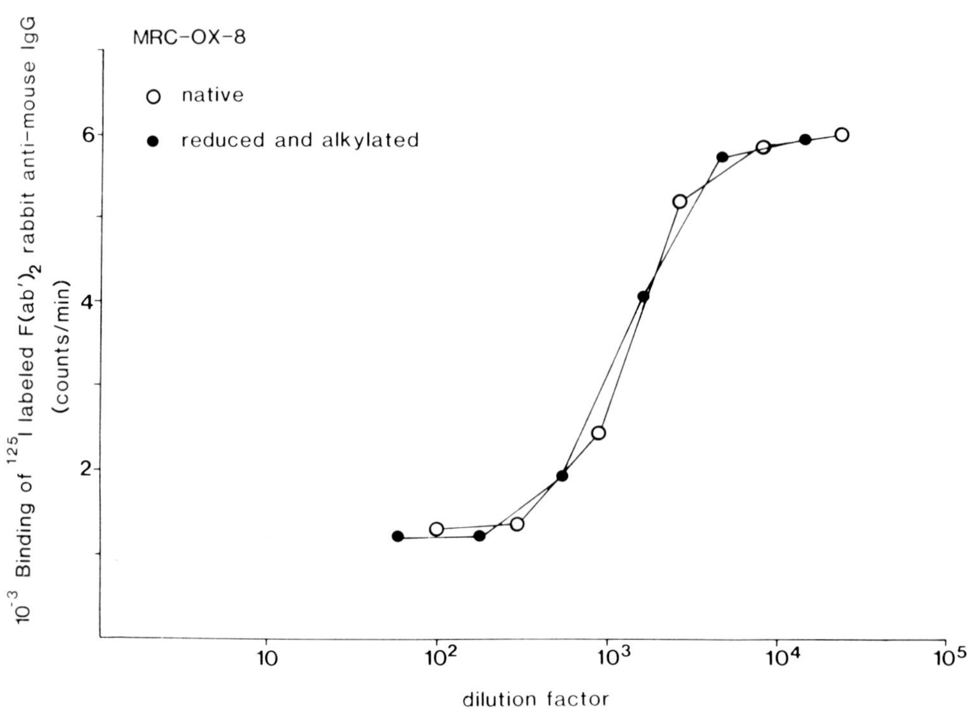

Figure 2. The effect of reduction and alkylation on the activity of OX-8 antigen assessed by the inhibition of a radioactive binding assay. OX-8 antigen obtained after two cycles of antibody affinity chromatography (Fig. 3) was reduced in 2% w/v SDS, 0.4 M Tris-HCl pH 8, 50 mM EDTA, 2.5 mM, dithiothreitol (DTT) at 37°C for 1 hr. ^{14}C-labeled iodoacetic acid at 5 mM was added and the mixture was incubated in the dark at room temperature for 15 min. A second aliquot of DTT at 8 mM was added, followed by incubation at 37°C for 4 hr, and then unlabeled iodoacetic acid was added in threefold excess over DTT and incubated as before. Dilutions of the antigen were made into 0.5% BSA, 150 mM NaCl, and 10 mM Tris-HCl, pH 8, and they were incubated with tissue culture supernatant containing MRC OX-8 antibody at 1/25. Antibody activity was assayed[1] by incubating 50-μl aliquots of the mixture with 2.5×10^6 glutaraldehyde-fixed rat thymocytes, washing, and then incubating with ^{125}I-rabbit F(ab')$_2$ anti-mouse IgG antibody.

tryptic peptides were further digested with pronase, the activity was lost (Fig. 4B).

The tryptic peptide with OX-22 antigenic activity was purified in the scheme shown in Fig. 5 and two antigenically active peptides were obtained after the HPLC step. Peptide A contained about 2 nmoles of peptide and this was sequenced by Dr J. Gagnon, MRC Immunochemistry Unit, Oxford to give the unambiguous partial sequence:

Gly Ala Asp Thr Gly (—) Leu Ser Ser Gln Ala Asp Leu

↑ possible glycosylation site

RAT THYMOCYTES

↓

MEMBRANE (TWEEN-40 METHOD)

↓

DEOXYCHOLATE EXTRACT

↓

OX-8 AFFINITY COLUMN (x2) → SUBSTANTIALLY PURE ANTIGEN

↓

REDUCTION AND ALKYLATION AND GEL FILTRATION IN SDS → MINOR CONTAMINANTS REMOVED

↓

OX-8 AFFINITY COLUMN → CHAINS SEPARATED

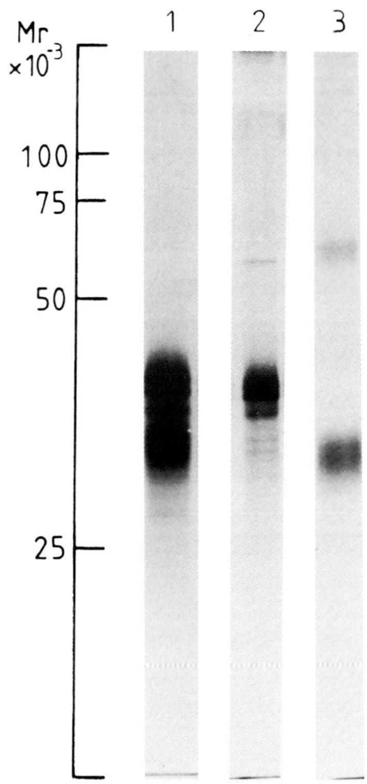

Figure 3. Flow diagram for the purification of MRC OX-8 antigen. Typically 4×10^{11} thymocytes were used in one preparation. The Tween 40 method for membrane preparation is described in Ref. 5. The results of the last affinity column step showing chain separation is illustrated on a 12% SDS–polyacrylamide gel with protein identified by the silver stain method. Track 1 is the purified antigen after gel filtration in 0.2% SDS. Track 2 is the protein not bound to the OX-8 column. Track 3 is protein specifically bound and eluted from a 1-ml OX-8 antibody column.

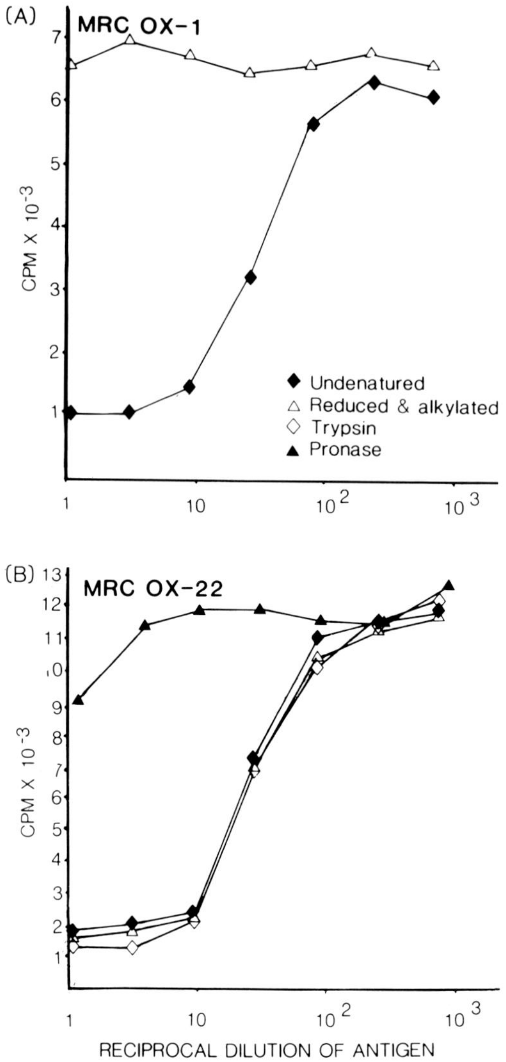

Figure 4. A comparison of the effects of chemical and enzymatic treatments on two different antigenic determinants of the L-CA assessed by the inhibition of radioactive binding assays. Tween 40 membrane was prepared from rat spleens, solubilized in deoxycholate, and subjected to affinity chromatography on an OX-22 antibody column. The eluted material was used in the assays. Some of this was precipitated with ethanol and the pellet resuspended in 7 M guanidine-HCl, 0.5 M Tris-HCl, 2 mM EDTA, and 5 mM DTT, pH 8.2, and incubated at 37°C for 1 hr. Iodoacetamide was added to 11 mM and the mixture left for 30 min on ice before dialysis back into 0.5% deoxycholate and 10 mM Tris-HCl, pH 8. An aliquot of this reduced and alkylated material was then digested with trypsin for 24 hr (1% w/w of trypsin was added to the protein at 0 and 4 hr). An aliquot of this material was then treated with pronase as for trypsin. The dilutions of the antigens used in the assay were adjusted so as to represent equal concentrations of the original eluted antigen.

The same sequence was given by peptide B and the difference in the position of elution of peptides from HPLC could be due to differences in glycosylation.

The rat L-CA molecule is currently being sequenced at the cDNA level[11] and the location of the above peptide in the sequence of the B-cell L-CA form will help in understanding the antigenic heterogeneity in the L-CA molecules.

ACKNOWLEDGMENT P. Johnson is a Beit Memorial Research Fellow.

	RECOVERY OF ANTIGENIC ACTIVITY
400 RAT SPLEENS	100%
↓	
MEMBRANE FRACTION (TWEEN 40 METHOD)	43%
↓	
DEOXYCHOLATE EXTRACT	26%
↓	
OX-22 AFFINITY COLUMN	21%
↓	
REDUCED AND ALKYLATED	17%
↓	
TRYPSINIZED	21%
↓	
OX-22 AFFINITY COLUMN	14.4%
↓	
HPLC A	4.0%
B	0.8%

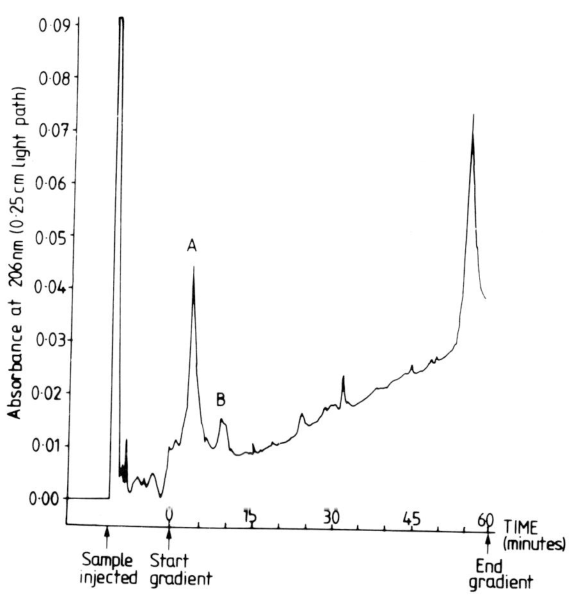

Figure 5. Flow diagram for the purification of a tryptic peptide with OX-22 antigenic activity. The percentage of recovery of antigenic activity after each step is given on the right. OX-22 antigen was prepared as described in Ref. 4 and reduced and alkylated and trypsinised as described in the legend to Fig. 4. This was then applied to the same 40-ml OX-22 antibody column and the tryptic peptide eluted at high pH. After neutralization it was then extensively dialyzed in dialysis tubing with a 1000-molecular-weight cutoff into 0.1 M ammonium bicarbonate and applied to a Waters μ Bondapak C_{18} HPLC common equilibriated in 10 mM ammonium acetate, pH 6.8, and eluted using a gradient of 0–60% v/v acetonitrile. The absorbance was monitored at 206 nm and peaks A and B were assayed for antigenic activity.

References

1. Williams, A. F., Galfre, G., and Milstein, C., 1977, Analysis of cell surfaces by xenogeneic myeloma-hybrid antibodies: Differentiation antigens of rat lymphocytes, *Cell* **12:**663–673.
2. Suggs, S. V., Wallace, R. B., Hirose, T., Kawashima, E. H., and Itakura, K., 1981, Use of synthetic oligonucleotides as hybridization probes: Isolation of cloned cDNA sequences for human β2-microglobulin, *Proc. Natl. Acad. Sci. USA* **78:**6613–6617.
3. Sunderland, C. A., McMaster, W. R., and Williams, A. F., 1979, Purification with monoclonal antibody of a predominant leukocyte-common antigen and glycoprotein from rat thymocytes, *Eur. J. Immunol.* **9:**155–159.
4. Parham, P., Barnstable, C. J., and Bodmer, W. F., 1979, Use of a monoclonal antibody (W6/32) in structural studies of HLA-A, B, C antigens, *J. Immunol.* **123:**342–349.
5. Williams, A. F., and Barclay, A. N., 1985, Glycoprotein antigens of the lymphocyte surface and their purification by antibody affinity chromatography, in: *Handbook of Experimental Immunology*, 4th ed. (D. M. Weir, and L. A. Herzenberg, eds.), Blackwell, Oxford, In press.
6. Parham, P., 1983, Monoclonal antibodies against HLA products and their use in immunoaffinity chromatography, *Meth. Enzymol.* **92:**110–138.
7. Mescher, M. F., Stallcup, K. C., Sullivan, C. P., Turkewitz, A. P., and Herrman, S. H., 1983, Purification of murine MHC antigens by monoclonal antibody affinity chromatography, *Meth. Enzymol.* **92:**86–109.
8. Ullrich, A., Coussens, L., Hayflick, J. S., Dull, T. J., Gray, A., Tam, A. W., Lee, J., Yarden, Y., Libermann, T. A., Schlessinger, J., Downward, J., Mayes, E. L. V., Whittle, N., Waterfield, M. D., and Seeburg, P. H., 1984, Human epidermal growth factor receptor cDNA sequence and aberrant expression of the amplified gene in A431 epidermoid carcinoma cells, *Nature* **309:**418–425.
9. Leonard, W. J., Depper, J. M., Crabtree, G. R., Rudikoff, S., Pumphrey, J., Robb, R. J., Kronke, M., Svetlik, P. B., Peffer, N. J., Waldmann, T. A., and Greene, W. C., 1984, Cloning and expression of cDNAs for human I-L2 receptor, *Nature* **311:**626–631.
10. Clark, M. J., Gagnon, J., Williams, A. F., and Barclay, A. N., 1985, MRC OX-2 antigen: A lymphoid/neuronal membrane glycoprotein with a structure like a single Ig light chain, *EMBO J.* **4:**113–118.
11. Thomas, M., Barclay, A. N., Gagnon, J., and Williams, A. F., 1985, Evidence from cDNA clones that the rat leucocyte-common antigen (T200) spans the lipid bilayer and contains a cytoplasmic domain of 80,000 Mr, *Cell*, In press.
12. Benjamin, D. C., Berzofsky, J. A., East, I. J., Gurd, F. R. N., Hannum, C., Leach, S. J., Margoliash, E., Michael, J. G., Miller, A., Prager, E. M., Reichlin, M., Sercarz, E. E., Smith-Gill, S. J., Todd, P. E., and Wilson, A. C., 1984, The antigenic structure of proteins: A reappraisal, *Annu. Rev. Immunol.* **2:**67–101.
13. Parker, P. J., Young, S., Gullick, W. J., Mayes, E. L. V., Bennett, P., and Waterfield, M. D., 1984, Monoclonal antibodies against the human epidermal growth factor receptor from A431 cells. Isolation, characterization, and use in the purification of active epidermal growth factor receptor, *J. Biol. Chem.* **259:**9906–9912.
14. Lane, D., and Koprowski, H., 1982, Molecular recognition and the future of monoclonal antibodies, *Nature* **296:**200–202.
15. Dulbecco, R., Unger, M., Bologna, M., Battifora, H., Syka, P., and Okada, S., 1981, Cross-reactivity between Thy-1 and a component of intermediate filaments demonstrated using a monoclonal antibody, *Nature* **292:**772–774.
16. Brown, W. R. A., Barclay, A. N., Sunderland, C. A., and Williams, A. F., 1981, Identification of a glycophorin-like molecule at the cell surface of rat thymocytes, *Nature* **289:**456–460.
17. Mason, D. W., and Williams, A. F., 1980, The kinetics of antibody binding to membrane antigens in solution and at the cell surface, *Biochem. J.* **187:**1–20.
18. Mason, D. W., and Williams, A. F., 1985, Kinetics of antibody reaction and the analysis of cell surface antigens, in: *Handbook of Experimental Immunology*, 4th ed (D. M. Weir and L. A. Herzenberg, eds.) Blackwell, Oxford, In press.

19. Towbin, H., Staehelin, T., and Gordon, J., 1979, Electrophoretic transfer of proteins from polyacrylamide gels to nitrocellulose sheets: Procedure and some applications, *Proc. Natl. Acad. Sci. USA* **76:**4350–4354.
20. Garotta, G., and Trucco, M., 1980, HLA antigens, temperature dependent elution from specific monoclonal antibody columns, in: *Protides Biol. Fluids, Colloquium 28* (H. Peeters, ed.), Pergamon Press, Oxford, pp. 463–466.
21. Porath, J., 1974, Coupling reactions and general methodology. General methods and coupling procedures, *Meth. Enzymol.* **34:**13–29.
22. Parham, P., 1979, Purification of immunologically active HLA-A and -B antigens by a series of monoclonal antibody columns, *J. Biol. Chem.* **254:**8709–8712.
23. Schneider, C., Newman, R. A., Sutherland, D. R., Asser, U., and Greaves, M. F., 1982, A one-step purification of membrane proteins using a high efficiency immunomatrix, *J. Biol. Chem.* **257:**10766–10769.
24. Helenius, A., and Simons, K., 1975, Solubilization of membranes by detergents, *Biochim. Biophys. Acta* **415:**29–79.
25. Letarte-Muirhead, M., Acton, R. T., and Williams, A. F., 1974, Preliminary characterization of Thy-1.1 and Ag-B antigens from rat tissues solubilized in detergents, *Biochem. J.* **143:**51–61.
26. Letarte-Muirhead, M., Barclay, A. N., and Williams, A. F., 1975, Purification of the Thy-1 molecule, a major cell-surface glycoprotein of rat thymocytes, *Biochem. J.* **151:**685–697.
27. Edgington, T. S., 1971, Dissociation of antibody from erythrocyte surfaces by chaotropic ions, *J. Immunol.* **106:**673–680.
28. Mellman, I. S., and Unkeless, J. C., 1980, Purification of a functional mouse Fc receptor through use of a monoclonal antibody, *J. Exp. Med.* **152:**1048–1069.
29. Rutishauser, U., Hoffman, S., and Edelman, G. M., 1982, Binding properties of a cell adhesion molecule from neural tissue, *Proc. Natl. Acad. Sci. USA* **79:**685–689.
30. Crumpton, M. J., 1974, Protein antigens: The molecular bases of antigenicity and immunogenicity, in: *The Antigens*, Volume II (M. Sela, ed.), Academic Press, New York, pp. 1–78.
31. Dame, J. B., Williams, J. L., McCutchan, T. F., Weber, J. L., Wirtz, R. A., Hockmeyer, W. T., Maloy, W. L., Haynes, J. D., Schneider, I., Roberts, D., Sanders, G. S., Reddy, E. P., Diggs, C. L., and Miller, L. H., 1984, Structure of the gene encoding the immunodominant surface antigen on the sporozoite of the human malaria parasite *Plasmodium falciparum*, *Science* **225:**593–599.
32. McMaster, W. R., 1981, A monoclonal antibody which detects a polymorphic Ia antigenic determinant reacts with purified β polypeptide chain, *Immunogenetics* **13:**347–350.
33. Thomas, M. L., and Green, J. R., 1983, Molecular nature of the W3/25 and MRC OX-8 marker antigens for rat T lymphocytes: Comparisons with mouse and human antigens, *Eur. J. Immunol.* **13:**855–858.
34. Naim, H. Y., Luescher, B., Corradin, G., and Bron, C., 1984, The mouse Lyt-2/3 antigen complex—II. Structural analysis of the subunits, *Mol. Immunol.* **21:**337–341.
35. Snow, P. M., and Terhorst, C., 1983, The T8 antigen is a multimeric complex of two distinct subunits on human thymocytes but consists of homomultimeric forms on peripheral blood T lymphocytes, *J. Biol. Chem.* **258:**14675–14681.
36. Kavathas, P., Sukhatme, V., Parnes, J., and Herzenberg, L. A., 1984, cDNA clones for the human T cell differentiation antigen Leu-2 isolated from transfectants, *Fed. Proc.* **43:**1593.
37. Spickett, G. P., Brandon, M. R., Mason, D. W., Williams, A. F., and Woollett, G. R., 1983, MRC OX-22, a monoclonal antibody that labels a new subset of T lymphocytes and reacts with the high molecular weight form of the leukocyte-common antigen, *J. Exp. Med.* **158:**795–810.
38. Woollett, G. R., Barclay, A. N., Puklavec, M., and Williams, A. F., 1985, Molecular and antigenic heterogeneity of the rat leucocyte-common antigen from thymocytes and T and B lymphocytes. *Eur. J. Immunol.* **15:**168–173.

Chapter 10

Transferrin Receptor

IAN S. TROWBRIDGE

1. Introduction

In 1963, Jandl and Katz[1] showed that the binding of serum transferrin to immature red cells was a specific and saturable process and postulated that the iron required for heme synthesis was delivered from transferrin to these cells via specific cell surface receptors. In the next two decades, as the requirements for the growth of mammalian cells in tissue culture were defined, it was found that transferrin was an essential growth factor for virtually all cells.[2] This latter observation stimulated interest in the role of transferrin in cell growth, and transferrin binding studies carried out in the late 1970s showed that transferrin receptors could be detected on a wide variety of cultured cell lines and that their expression on the cell surface was coordinately regulated with cell growth.[3–6] At about this time, in studies aimed at defining changes in the cell surface of human hematopoietic cells during differentiation and malignant transformation, an immunodominant proliferation-associated cell surface antigen was detected on cultured human tumor cells by means of a murine monoclonal antibody (MAb).[7] Further characterization of this molecule showed that it was the human transferrin receptor.[8–10] Subsequently MAbs against the transferrin receptor of human and mouse cells have provided the tools not only to establish the general structural features of the receptor, but also to investigate various functional aspects of the receptor and to isolate successfully the human transferrin receptor gene by an approach based on gene transfer and selection by fluorescence activated cell sorting. This body of work provides an indication of some of the varied and productive uses to which MAbs can be applied in the analysis of cell surface receptors.

IAN S. TROWBRIDGE • Department of Cancer Biology, Salk Institute for Biological Studies, San Diego, California 92138.

2. Structure of the Transferrin Receptor

2.1. Identification of Monoclonal Antibodies against Transferrin Receptor

One of the major advantages of MAbs in the study of cell surfaces is that specific cell membrane molecules can be identified on the basis of their antigenicity and isolated from a complex mixture of components without prior knowledge of their properties. They can then be readily characterized in terms of cellular distribution and structure and, under favorable circumstances, insight into their function may be acquired. In the case of the transferrin receptor, MAbs specific for the human receptor were selected for study from a collection of MAbs against previously undefined cell surface antigens because they were found to recognize a major cell surface glycoprotein of cultured human hematopoietic tumor cell lines whose expression appeared to be linked to cell proliferation.[7] The relationship to cell proliferation was shown most clearly by the fact that the glycoprotein was induced on the surface of peripheral blood lymphocytes after mitogenic stimulation and conversely was lost from the surface of inducible human promyelocytic cell line HL-60, since, after treatment with chemical inducers, the cells stopped growing and differentiated along the myeloid pathway. The distribution of the antigen on normal and leukemic hematopoietic cells also suggested that the molecule was selectively expressed on rapidly dividing cells.[7–9] Different lines of evidence led ourselves[8] and others[9,10] to suspect that this immunologically defined glycoprotein was the transferrin receptor. This idea was tested by asking whether MAbs against the glycoprotein could immunoprecipitate cell surface-associated transferrin from detergent solubilized cell lysates (Fig. 1). Since these MAbs did not interact directly with transferrin, and MAbs against other cell surface glycoproteins did not nonspecifically precipitate transferrin from cell lysates, the ability of MAbs B3/25[8] and OKT9[9,10] to coprecipitate transferrin firmly established that they recognized the human transferrin receptor. This exemplifies a general point: that the coprecipitation of a receptor–ligand complex by a MAb is probably the most rigorous single criterion to define an antireceptor antibody.

2.2. Structure of the Transferrin Receptor

MAbs against the transferrin receptor have played an important role in defining the general structural features of the molecule (Fig. 2). The data summarized schematically in Fig. 2 are derived from both biochemical studies of the mature surface-iodinated receptor and biosynthetic radiolabeling experiments of the receptor with a variety of precursors.[7,11–13] In each kind of experiment, the radiolabeled transferrin receptor was isolated from cell lysates by immunoprecipitation and analyzed by SDS–polyacrylamide gel electrophoresis. Analysis of the mature receptor under reducing and nonreducing conditions showed that it is a disulfide-bonded dimer consisting of two ap-

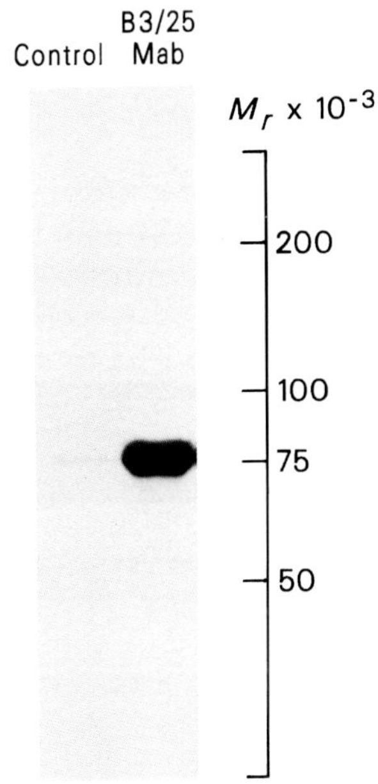

Figure 1. Coprecipitation of ^{125}I-labeled transferrin with the human transferrin receptor by MAb B3/25. RPMI 8402 cells, a human leukemic T cell line, were incubated with ^{125}I-labeled human transferrin. The cells were washed to remove unbound ligand and then detergent lysates were prepared. The figure shows the specific immunoprecipitation of transferrin complexed to its receptor by MAb B3/25. MAb T29/33 specific for human T200 (control lane) does not precipitate transferrin. For further experimental details see Ref. 8.

parently identical subunits of M_r 95,000. Treatment of intact ^{125}I-labeled human cells with as little as 2 μg/ml of trypsin results in the quantitative release from the cell surface of a soluble 70,000-M_r fragment of the transferrin receptor that is resistant to further proteolysis. This fragment contains essentially all the radioactivity associated with the surface-iodinated intact receptor and can be immunoprecipitated by MAbs that react with the extracellular portion of the receptor. This establishes that the bulk of the transferrin receptor must be exposed on the external side of the cell surface.[11,13] Furthermore, the tryptic fragment of the receptor has an apparent M_r of 70,000 under both reducing and nonreducing conditions. Although proteolysis might take place at more than

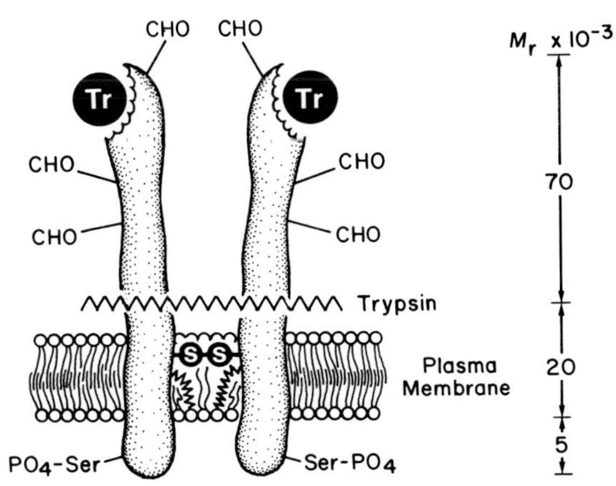

Figure 2. Schematic representation of the transferrin receptor based upon the structural data described in the text.

one site, the simplest interpretation of this result is that the disulfide bond(s) that covalently link the two receptor subunits are located in the portion of the transferrin receptor that presumably remains embedded in the membrane after proteolysis.

The stoichiometry of the binding of transferrin to the receptor has been studied by Schneider *et al.*[13] using the cross-linking reagents disuccinimidyl suberate and dithiobis (succinimidyl proprionate). If cells labeled with ^{125}I- or [^{35}S]methionine were cross-linked to ^{125}I-labeled transferrin with either reagent and the transferrin receptor isolated by immunoprecipitation, a band of M_r 340,000 was seen on SDS–polyacrylamide gel electrophoresis under nonreducing conditions. Under reducing conditions, dithiobis (succinimidyl proprionate) was cleaved and the 340,000-M_r cross-linked product could be shown to contain both transferrin receptor and transferrin. However, if the nonreducible cross-linker disuccinimidyl suberate was used, after reduction, the cross-linked product was partially reduced to a molecular species which ran as a diffuse band of approximately 180,000–200,000 M_r, which by differential labeling could be shown to contain both transferrin and transferrin receptor. This has been interpreted as showing that the dimeric receptor binds two molecules of transferrin and that each subunit probably has a single independent binding site for the ligand (Fig. 2).

The clearest evidence that the transferrin receptor is a transmembrane molecule, as depicted in Fig. 2, comes from proteolysis experiments in which microsomes from cells briefly labeled with [^{35}S]methionine were digested with protease K.[13] Insertion of a transmembrane protein into the endoplasmic reticulum membrane is a cotranslational event and, as previously shown for the HLA-A, B, C glycoprotein,[14] the extracellular domain of a transmembrane molecule is consequently protected from proteolysis in intact microsomes, whereas the cytoplasmic portion of the molecule is completely digested. In the case of the transferrin receptor, the molecule isolated by immunoprecipitation from protease K-treated microsomes was found to be approximately 5000 daltons smaller than the receptor isolated from untreated microsomes. It is inferred from this result that the receptor has a cytoplasmic tail of 5000 daltons.

Studies of the biosynthesis of the transferrin receptor in cultured human cells have also been informative.[11–13] As shown in Fig. 3 pulse-chase experiments of the transferrin receptor isolated by immunoprecipitation from cells labeled with [^{35}S]methionine show that the newly synthesized receptor has an apparent M_r of 88,000 and that within 4 hr this precursor is converted into the mature cell surface form of the receptor with an apparent molecular weight of 95,000. Digestion of the immature form of the receptor with endoglycosidase H converts the 88,000-M_r species to one of M_r 80,000 (Figs. 3a and 3b), whereas the apparent M_r of the mature receptor was reduced from 95,000 to 89,000 (Figs. 3i and 3j). In other experiments, the apparent M_r of the transferrin receptor isolated from cells treated with the antibiotic tunicamycin was 79,000.[12] The interpretation of these results, supplemented by additional data from similar experiments with receptors metabolically labeled with 2[^{3}H]mannose, is that the protein moiety of the transferrin receptor is of M_r about 80,000 and that,

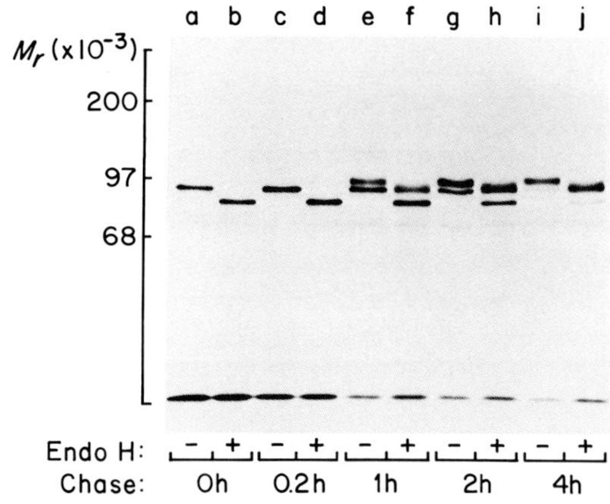

Figure 3. Pulse-chase experiment showing the glycosylation of the human transferrin receptor. Cells were labeled for 10 min with [^{35}S]methionine, then chased for the indicated periods of time. Immunoprecipitates were prepared using a MAb against the human transferrin receptor and analyzed by SDS–PAGE with or without prior treatment with endoglycosidase H. The data are taken from Ref. 12, where further experimental details can be found.

during its synthesis, the protein is modified by the addition of probably three *N*-asparagine-linked oligosaccharides. The mature cell surface form of the receptor contains both complex and high-mannose *N*-asparagine-linked oligosaccharides that are derived from a lipid-linked oligosaccharide precursor via a high-mannose intermediate present on the immature intracellular form of the glycoprotein as described for other secreted and membrane-bound glycoproteins. There is no indication that the transferrin receptor is extensively modified by the addition of *O*-linked sugars as described for the low-density lipoprotein (LDL) receptor.[15]

In addition to glycosylation, the transferrin receptor is modified by the covalent addition of fatty acid as shown by metabolic labeling with [^{3}H]palmitate.[11] The acylation of the transferrin receptor is a posttranslational event, since only the mature form of the receptor can be labeled with [^{3}H]palmitate.[12] There is evidence that acylation can occur more than 1–2 days after the synthesis of the receptor and, as shown in Fig. 4, the fatty acid moiety turns over more rapidly than the receptor itself, which has a half-life of 2–3 days in CCRF-CEM cells. Tryptic cleavage of the palmitate-labeled receptor localizes the acylation site(s) to the 20,000-M_r portion of the molecule associated with the cell membrane.[11] It is not presently known which amino acid residue is modified by the addition of fatty acid. However, by analogy with the vesicular stomatitis virus (VSV) G protein[16] and an HLA-B heavy chain,[17] the most likely candidate would seem to be a cysteine residue located either in or proximal to the lipid bilayer. Although there have been a number of suggestions as to the function of the fatty acids covalently bound to membrane proteins (reviewed in Ref. 18), their role remains to be established. One obvious possibility is that the lipid moiety is involved in the interaction of membrane glycoproteins with the lipid bilayer. In the case of VSV G protein, acylation does not appear to be required for transport of the glycoprotein to the cell surface.[16]

The transferrin receptor is also phosphorylated,[13,19] although in some cell lines detectable metabolic labeling of the receptor with [^{32}P]phosphate is not

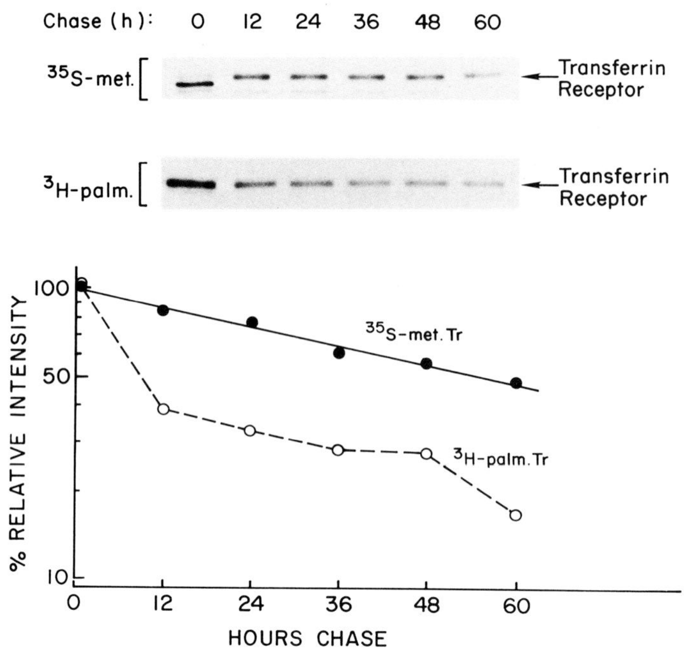

Figure 4. Turnover rate of [^{35}S]methionine- or [^{3}H]palmitate-labeled transferrin receptors. Transferrin receptor was isolated from pulse-labeled cells at various times by immunoprecipitation, and autoradiograms of the labeled receptor were scanned to derive the graph shown. The data are taken from Ref. 12, where further experimental details can be found.

observed under the usual labeling conditions employed. Serine is the principal site of phosphorylation, and in HL-60 cells[19] and some human T leukemic cell lines (D. Shackelford, unpublished results), it has been shown that phosphorylation is enhanced in the presence of phorbol esters.

Most of the information about the structure of the transferrin receptor is derived from studies of the receptor of cultured human cell lines. However, MAbs have also been obtained against the mouse transferrin receptor[20,21] and it appears that the mouse homologue is similar to the human receptor in most respects, with the exception that it is less sensitive to tryptic cleavage at the cell surface.[21]

3. Functional Aspects of the Transferrin Receptor

3.1. Monoclonal Antibodies That Block Receptor Function

An important use of MAbs against the transferrin receptor has been to study the relationship of transferrin receptor function and cell growth. The MAbs against the human transferrin receptor that were originally described did not interfere with receptor function.[7–10,22] The first question that arose, therefore, was whether such antibodies could be obtained. We took the approach to this question of preparing a second generation of MAbs against the receptor by immunizing mice with purified human transferrin receptor glycoprotein isolated by affinity chromatography on an immunoabsorbant column prepared with an existing MAb against the receptor. MAbs against the transferrin receptor were first identified in immunoprecipitation studies and then tested for their capacity to block the binding of ^{125}I-labeled human transferrin to the human leukemic cell line CCRF-CEM. This led to the detection of a single MAb, designated 42/6, that could inhibit the binding of transferrin to its receptor on human cells.[23] It should be apparent that this strategy of using a MAb against a specific component of a complex mixture such as cell membrane molecules for affinity purification in order to facilitate the preparation of additional MAbs with more desirable properties is of general applicability.

MAb 42/6 has been shown to specifically inhibit transferrin-mediated iron uptake by a variety of cultured human cell lines.[23,24] The degree of inhibition varies from cell line to cell line, but in the case of the human T leukemic cell lines CCRF-CEM and RPMI 8402 transferrin-mediated iron uptake is virtually completely inhibited by saturating amounts of the MAb. This result firmly establishes the functional importance of the cell surface transferrin receptor defined by 42/6 and other MAbs in cellular iron uptake. The importance of transferrin receptor function during cell growth was shown by the fact that MAb 42/6 also profoundly inhibits the growth of CCRF-CEM cells in tissue culture.[23,24]

Shortly after MAb 42/6 was obtained, a rat antibody, designated RI7 208, that was specific for the murine transferrin receptor was identified.[20] This antibody is similar to MAb 42/6 in that it inhibits transferrin-mediated iron uptake into cultured mouse cell lines and also inhibits cell growth. In contrast to MAb 42/6, however, MAb RI7 208 does not inhibit binding of transferrin to mouse cells.[25] Studies of the physiological effects of these two antibodies on iron uptake and cell growth provide insight into several aspects of this problem. First, the question arises as to what properties of the MAbs are important for their effects on transferrin receptor function. In reciprocal competitive binding studies, both MAb 42/6 and RI7 208 partially or completely block the binding of other antibodies against the receptor that do not interfere with function.[23,25] This indicates that the antigenic sites recognized by both classes of antibody are juxtaposed on the transferrin receptor molecule, suggesting that the fine specificity of the antibodies is not a major factor in determining whether they interfere with receptor function. However, the class of antibody may be important; MAb 42/6 is an IgA, whereas MAb RI7 208 and another rat antibody, REM 17, that blocks murine transferrin receptor function (J. Lesley and R. Schulte, unpublished results) are both IgMs. In contrast, all the MAbs against the human and murine transferrin receptors that do not interfere with receptor function are IgG antibodies. This strongly suggests that either the size of the polymeric IgA and IgM antibodies or their ability to extensively cross-link receptors is a crucial factor in their ability to block growth. However, at present we have very little idea of the precise mechanism by which these antibodies inhibit iron uptake and block growth. Even MAb 42/6 may not only inhibit transferrin binding but also interfere with other steps in transferrin-mediated iron uptake.

Another question is whether the effects of MAbs that block transferrin receptor function inhibit the growth of all cells equally effectively. Transferrin receptors are expressed on actively growing normal cell types in tissue culture and these cells require transferrin for growth. For this reason it was not unexpected that MAbs that block transferrin receptor function inhibit the growth of some normal cells in primary culture as well as established malignant cell lines. MAb 42/6 inhibits phytohemagglutinin-induced mitogenesis of human peripheral blood lymphocytes[26] and the *in vitro* growth of normal human granulocyte/macrophage progenitor (CFU-GM) cells.[27] Similarly, continuous exposure to MAb RI7 208 inhibits the growth of both myeloid (CFU-C) and early and late erythroid progenitors (BFU-E and CFU-E) (J. Lesley and R. Schulte, unpublished results). An unanticipated finding, however, was that the MAbs do not inhibit the growth of all cell types *in vitro*. For example, the growth of many human carcinoma cell lines and melanoma cell lines are not inhibited by MAb 42/6.[24] These cells express similar numbers of transferrin receptors as hematopoietic cell lines that are sensitive to the growth inhibitory effects of the antibody and there is no significant difference in the affinity of antibody binding to sensitive and resistant cells. Similarly, inhibition by MAb RI7 208 of transferrin-mediated iron uptake is as great for mouse L cells as for hematopoietic cell lines that are exquisitely sensitive to the growth inhibitory effects of the antibody. Nevertheless, L cells can be grown for several weeks in saturating amounts of the antibody without affecting their growth rate.[20,24] The differential effects of the antibodies on the growth of different cell types is paradoxical, but may reflect either differences in their total capacity to transport iron or to differences in their metabolic adaptation to iron deprivation.[24]

One interesting use of the MAb RI7 208 has been to select mutant cells from sensitive murine lymphoma cell lines that are resistant to growth inhibition by this antibody.[25] Inhibition of transferrin-mediated iron uptake by the antibody in the resistant mutants is much less than with the parental cell lines, suggesting that iron deprivation is indeed the cause of the growth inhibition. Resistance to the antibody is codominantly expressed in somatic hybrids between parental and mutant cell lines and there is evidence that there is a subtle difference in antibody binding to the transferrin receptor of the mutant cell lines.[25] Overall, the evidence suggests that the mutants arise by a mutation in one of the two transferrin receptor structural genes and that both the aberrant and normal receptor polypeptides are expressed on the cell surface. These mutants should be amenable to rigorous analysis now that the appropriate molecular probes are available for the transferrin receptor gene (see below). These and other classes of mutants that can be selected with MAbs that block transferrin receptor function might be expected to contribute to an understanding of the relationship between transferrin-mediated iron uptake and cell growth.

3.2. Receptor-Mediated Endocytosis

In the last few years, some aspects of transferrin-mediated iron uptake have been worked out.[28–35] On the basis of both biochemical and morphological studies it has been established that after transferrin binds to its receptor, the receptor–ligand complex is rapidly taken up into the cell via coated pits.[28–30] The receptor–ligand complex becomes localized predominantly in endocytic vesicles, which become acidified as the result of the action of a proton pump.[33,34] Under these acidic conditions, iron dissociates from transferrin but apotransferrin remains bound to the receptor and is recycled back to the cell surface. At pH 7 apotransferrin rapidly dissociates from the receptor,[31,32] leaving it to undergo another round of endocytosis. MAbs against the transferrin receptor have been useful in following the fate of the receptor independently from transferrin itself. By using a MAb against the human transferrin receptor complexed to colloidal gold, Hopkins and Trowbridge[30] carried out a series of electron microscopic studies of transferrin receptor distribution during transferrin-mediated iron uptake into A431 cells, a human carcinoma cell line. After endocytosis via coated pits, antibody–receptor complexes can be seen localized in the peripheral cytoplasm within the immediate vicinity of the plasma membrane. In this region of the cell the antibody–receptor complexes are found primarily in narrow tubular cisternae and small vesicles (20–50 nm in diameter). Later, the complexes become concentrated in larger vesicles in the perinuclear region of the cell on the *trans* side of the Golgi complex. In these structures, the majority of gold particles could be seen to lie close to the limiting membrane. By using transferrin–peroxidase complexes in combination with gold-labeled antibodies against the transferrin receptor, it was shown that both ligand and the receptor remained associated during their passage through these various cell compartments.[35]

The use of MAbs to study transferrin receptor endocytosis and recycling is a relatively recent development and it is likely that antibodies, especially MAbs against defined regions of the receptor, will play an important role in the future in understanding various aspects of the process. Furthermore, studies with antibody–toxin conjugates against the transferrin receptor[36,37] are likely to contribute to a more complete understanding of the limiting factors in the entry of antibody-targeted ligands into cells.

4. Gene Transfer and Molecular Cloning of the Human Transferrin Receptor

A recent application of monoclonal antibodies has been their use in the molecular cloning of cell surface antigens by means of gene transfer followed by cell sorting (see Refs. 38–41 and this volume, Chapter 22 and 23). The approach is based upon the stable transformation of cultured recipient cells by total genomic donor DNA using the technique of DNA-mediated gene transfer.[42] If an appropriate selection technique is available, then rare transformed recipient cells can be isolated that express the acquired gene of interest. Strategies can then be designed to retrieve this gene from the transformed cell. MAbs provide the tools for selecting transformants expressing particular cell surface antigens by fluorescence activated cell sorting. Since MAbs against the human transferrin receptor do not react with the murine receptor, the expression of the human receptor on transformed mouse cells can be detected even though the cells express their own endogenous receptor.

Mouse L-cell transformants expressing the human transferrin receptor on their cell surface have been obtained by a two-step selection procedure.[40,41] Mouse L (thymidine kinase negative) cells were cotransformed with the Herpes simplex virus thymidine kinase (*tk*) gene and total human DNA using the calcium phosphate method. Cells expressing the *tk* gene were then selected in hypoxanthine/aminopterin/thymidine (HAT) medium. Pools of several thousand HAT-resistant colonies were stained by indirect immunofluorescence for the human transferrin receptor and then sorted by flow cytometry. By selecting the brightest viable fluorescent cell population and repeated cycles of cell sorting, mouse transformants expressing the human transferrin receptor were obtained. In two independent studies, one by ourselves[40] and the other by Kuhn *et al.*,[41] two or three rounds of sorting were found to be necessary before significant populations of fluorescent cells were observed, and the frequency with which stable transformants expressing the human receptor were obtained was in the range of one in 10^4 HAT-resistant colonies. In our hands, there was considerable variability in the stability with which independent transformants expressed their human transferrin receptor despite being continuously cultured in selective HAT medium. Analysis of stable transformants showed that the human transferrin receptor is expressed in amounts similar to the murine receptor itself and antibody blocking experiments showed that the human receptor was functional in mediating iron uptake into the cells.[40] Subsequently, Kuhn *et al.*[41] derived a series of secondary transformants expressing the human transferrin receptor that contained only small amounts of human DNA. From a phage library prepared from one of the secondary transformants, they were able to select recombinant phage containing human transferrin receptor DNA by screening the library for human repetitive sequences with nick-translated total human DNA. This approach offers a general method for the isolation of structural genes of cell surface molecules that can be detected on the basis of their antigenicity.[38,39]

5. Concluding Remarks

MAbs have made a major contribution to our understanding of the structure and function of the transferrin receptor. The primary structure of the transferrin receptor will probably be known in the next few months as sequencing of human transferrin receptor cDNA is carried out. It should then be possible to prepare MAbs against defined regions of the molecule by immunization with synthetic polypeptides. Such reagents should provide further insight into various aspects of transferrin receptor structure and function.

ACKNOWLEDGMENTS I would like to acknowledge the contributions of my colleagues in the Department of Cancer Biology at the Salk Institute to the work discussed in this chapter. Bishr Omary, Derrick Domingo, Jayne Lesley, Roberta Schulte, Robert Hyman, Roland Newman, and Frederick Lopez have all been involved in various aspects of the studies described. I also thank Ami Koide for her help in preparation of the manuscript. The work cited from my laboratory was supported by grant CA 34787 from the National Cancer Institute.

References

1. Jandl, J. H., and Katz, J. H., 1963, The plasma to cell cycle of transferrin, *J. Clin. Invest.* **43**:314–326.
2. Barnes, D., and Sato, G., 1980, Serum-free cell culture: A unifying approach, *Cell* **22**:649–655.
3. Larrick, J. W., and Cresswell, P., 1979, Modulation of cell-surface iron transferrin receptors by cellular density and state of activation, *J. Supramol. Struct.* **11**:421–428.
4. Galbraith, G. M. P., Galbraith, R. M., and Faulk, W. P., 1980, Transferrin binding by human lymphoblastoid cell lines and other transformed cells, *Cell Immunol.* **49**:215–222.
5. Hamilton, T. A., Wada, H. G., and Sussman, H. H., 1979, Identification of transferrin receptors on the surface of human cultured cells, *Proc. Natl. Acad. Sci. USA* **75**:6406–6410.
6. Galbraith, R. M., and Galbraith, G. M. P., 1981, Expression of transferrin receptors on mitogen-stimulated human peripheral blood lymphocytes: Relation to cellular activation and related metabolic events, *Immunology* **44**:703–710.
7. Omary, M. B., Trowbridge, I. S., and Minowada, J., 1980, Human cell-surface glycoprotein with unusual properties, *Nature* **286**:888–891.
8. Trowbridge, I. S., and Omary, M. B., 1981, Human cell surface glycoprotein related to cell proliferation is the receptor for transferrin, *Proc. Natl. Acad. Sci. USA* **78**:3039–3043.
9. Sutherland, R., Delia, D., Schneider, C., Newman, R., Kemshead, J., and Greaves, M., 1981, Ubiquitous cell surface glycoprotein on tumor cells is proliferation associated receptor for transferrin, *Proc. Natl. Acad. Sci. USA* **78**:4515–4519.
10. Goding, J. W., and Burns, G. F., 1981, Monoclonal antibody OKT9 recognizes the receptor for transferrin on human acute lymphocytic leukemia cells, *J. Immunol.* **127**:1256–1258.
11. Omary, M. B., and Trowbridge, I. S., 1981, Covalent binding of fatty acid to the transferrin receptor in cultured human cells. *J. Biol. Chem.* **256**:4715–4718.
12. Omary, M. B., and Trowbridge, I. S., 1981, Biosynthesis of the human transferrin receptor in cultured cells, *J. Biol. Chem.* **256**:12888–12892.
13. Schneider, C., Sutherland, R., Newman, R. A., and Greaves, M. F., 1982, Structural features of the cell surface receptor for transferrin that is recognized by the monoclonal antibody OKT9, *J. Biol. Chem.* **257**:8516–8522.
14. Owen, M. J., Kissonerghis, A.-M., and Lodish, H. F., 1980, Biosynthesis of HLA-A and HLA-B antigens *in vivo*, *J. Biol. Chem.* **255**:9678–9684.
15. Cummings, R. D., Kornfeld, S., Schneider, W. J., Hobgood, K. K., Tolleshang, H., Brown, M. S., and Goldstein, J. L., 1983, Biosynthesis of the N- and O-linked oligosaccharides of the low density lipoprotein receptor, *J. Biol. Chem.* **258**:15261–15273.
16. Rose, J. K., Adams, G. A., and Gallione, C. J., 1984, The presence of cysteine in the cytoplasmic domain of the vesicular stomatitis virus glycoprotein is required for palmitate addition, *Proc. Natl. Acad. Sci. USA* **81**:2050–2054.
17. Kaufman, J. F., Krangel, M. S., and Strominger, J. L., 1984, Cysteines in the transmembrane region of the major histocompatibility complex antigens are fatty acylated via thioester bonds, *J. Biol. Chem.* **259**:7230–7238.

18. Schmidt, M. F. G., 1983, Fatty acid binding: A new kind of posttranslational modification of membrane proteins, *Curr. Top. Microbiol. Immunol.* **102**:101–129.
19. May, W. S., Jacobs, S., and Cuatrecasas, P., 1984, Association of phorbol ester-induced hyperphosphorylation and reversible regulation of transferrin membrane receptors in HL60 cells, *Proc. Natl. Acad. Sci. USA* **81**:2016–2020.
20. Trowbridge, I. S., Lesley, J., and Schulte, R., 1982, Murine cell surface transferrin receptor: Studies with an anti-receptor monoclonal antibody, *J. Cell. Physiol.* **112**:403–410.
21. van Agthoven, A., Goridis, C., Naquet, P., Pierres, A., and Pierres, M., 1984, Structural characteristics of the mouse transferrin receptor, *Eur. J. Biochem.* **140**:433–440.
22. Haynes, B. F., Hemler, M., Cotner, T., Mann, D., Eisenbarth, G. S., Strominger, J. L., and Fauci, A. S., 1981, Characterization of a monoclonal antibody (5E9) that defines a human cell surface antigen of cell activation, *J. Immunol.* **127**:347–351.
23. Trowbridge, I. S., and Lopez, F., 1982, Monoclonal antibody to transferrin receptor blocks transferrin binding and inhibits human tumor cell growth *in vitro*, *Proc. Natl. Acad. Sci. USA* **79**:1175–1179.
24. Trowbridge, I. S., and Newman, R. A., 1984, Monoclonal antibodies to transferrin receptors, in: *Antibodies to Receptors: Probes for Receptor Structure and Function* (M. F. Greaves, ed.), Academic Press, London, pp. 235–261.
25. Lesley, J. F., and Schulte, R. J., 1984, Selection of cell lines resistant to anti-transferrin receptor antibody: Evidence for a mutation in transferrin receptor, *Mol. Cell. Biol.* **4**:1675–1681.
26. Mendelsohn, J., Trowbridge, I., and Castagnola, J., 1983, Inhibition of human lymphocyte proliferation by monoclonal antibody to transferrin receptor, *Blood* **62**:821–826.
27. Taetle, R., Honeysett, J. M., and Trowbridge, I., 1983, Effects of anti-transferrin receptor antibodies on growth of normal and malignant myeloid cells, *Int. J. Cancer* **32**:343–349.
28. Bleil, J. D., and Bretscher, M. S., 1982, Transferrin receptor and its recycling in HeLa cells, *EMBO J.* **1**:351–355.
29. Harding, C., Heuser, J., and Stahl, P., 1983, Receptor-mediated endocytosis of transferrin and recycling of the transferrin receptor in rat reticulocytes, *J. Cell. Biol.* **97**:329–339.
30. Hopkins, C. R., and Trowbridge, I. S., 1983, Internalization and processing of transferrin and the transferrin receptor in human carcinoma A431 cells, *J. Cell Biol.* **97**:508–521.
31. Dautry-Varsat, A., Ciechanover, A., and Lodish, H. F., 1983, pH and the recycling of transferrin during receptor-mediated endocytosis, *Proc. Natl. Acad. Sci. USA* **80**:2258–2262.
32. Klausner, R. D., Ashwell, G., van Renswoude, J., Harford, J. B., and Bridges, K. R., 1983, Binding of apotransferrin to K562 cells: Explanation of the transferrin cycle, *Proc. Natl. Acad. Sci. USA* **80**:2263–2266.
33. van Renswoude, J., Bridges, K. R., Hartford, J. B., and Klausner, R. D., 1982, Receptor-mediated endocytosis of transferrin and the uptake of Fe in K562 cells: Identification of a nonlysosomal acidic compartment. *Proc. Natl. Acad. Sci. USA* **79**:6186–6190.
34. Yamashiro, D. J., Tycko, B., Fluss, S. R., and Maxfield, F. R., 1984, Segregation of transferrin to a mildly acidic (pH 6.5) para-Golgi compartment in the recycling pathway, *Cell* **37**:789–800.
35. Hopkins, C. R., 1983, Intracellular routing of transferrin and transferrin receptors in epidermoid carcinoma A431 cells, *Cell* **35**:321–330.
36. Trowbridge, I. S., and Domingo, D., 1981, Anti-transferrin receptor monoclonal antibody and toxin–antibody conjugates affect growth of human tumor cells. *Nature* **294**:171–173.
37. Lesley, J., Domingo, D. L., Schulte, R., and Trowbridge, I. S., 1984, Effect of an anti-murine transferrin receptor–ricin A conjugate on bone marrow stem and progenitor cells treated *in vitro*, *Exp. Cell. Res.* **150**:400–407.
38. Kavathas, P., and Herzenberg, L. A., 1983, Stable transformation of mouse L cells for human membrane T-cell differentiation antigens, HLA and β-microglobulin: Selection by fluorescence-activated cell sorting, *Proc. Natl. Acad. Sci. USA* **80**:524–528.
39. Kuhn, L. C., Barbosa, J. A., Kamarck, M. E., and Ruddle, F. H., 1983, An approach to the cloning of cell surface protein genes, *Mol. Biol. Med.* **1**:335–352.
40. Newman, R., Domingo, D. L., Trotter, J., and Trowbridge, I. S., 1983, Selection and properties of a mouse L-cell transformant expressing human transferrin receptor, *Nature* **304**:643–645.

41. Kuhn, L. C., McClelland, A., and Ruddle, F. H., 1984, Gene transfer, expression and molecular cloning of the human transferrin receptor gene, *Cell* **37:**95–103.
42. Pellicer, A., Robins, D., Wold, B., Sweet, R., Jackson, J., Lowy, I., Roberts, J. M., Sim, G. K., Silverstein, S., and Axel, R., 1980, Altering genotype and phenotype by DNA-mediated gene transfer, *Science* **209:**1414–1422.

Chapter 11

Functional and Structural Interrelationships among the Mac-1, LFA-1 Family of Leukocyte Adhesion Glycoproteins, and their Deficiency in a Novel Heritable Disease

TIMOTHY A. SPRINGER and DONALD C. ANDERSON

1. Introduction

Cell surface adherence reactions are of central importance in the immune functions of lymphocytes, monocytes, and granulocytes. Lymphocytes adhere to antigen-presenting macrophages or dendritic cells in the induction of T-lymphocyte immune responses, and to target cells in cell-mediated killing. Adhesive interactions are fundamental to a wide sprectrum of functions of granulocytes, monocytes, and macrophages. Specific recognition of opsonized microorganisms is facilitated by membrane receptors for IgG and for the third component of complement (C3), which mediate microbe–cell adhesion prior to the triggering of cytoskeletal events leading to endocytosis. Adhesion mediated by IgG (Fc) receptors can also trigger antibody-dependent killing of target cells, independently of endocytosis. In the absence of opsonins, some microorganisms/particles may adhere to granulocytes/monocytes without undergoing ingestion or may be phagocytized inefficiently, depending on the physical properties of the microorganisms.[1]

Cell translocation *in vitro* and *in vivo* has also been shown to be influenced by the precise nature of cell–substrate adherence interactions.[1–3] Studies employing time-lapse photography or photomicrography have shown that granulocytes adhere preferentially to vascular endothelium adjacent to a site of inflammation.[4] Evidence exists that physical properties of endothelial cells or

TIMOTHY A. SPRINGER • Laboratory of Membrane Immunochemistry, Dana-Farber Cancer Institute and Department of Pathology, Harvard Medical School, Boston, Massachusetts 02115. DONALD C. ANDERSON • Baylor College of Medicine, Department of Pediatrics, Houston, Texas 77050.

experimental substrates (glass, plastic, albumin, fibrinogen, fibronectin) influence adherence, and secondarily the extent and direction of cell migration.[3,5] Substrates that promote irreversible adhesion or those that significantly diminish or prevent adherence effectively impair cell translocation. Directed migration (chemotaxis) appears to require intermittent adhesion that is sufficiently strong to allow attachment to a substrate but sufficiently localized temporally to allow selective detachment.[6]

A family of high-molecular-weight glycoproteins with identical β subunits has recently been characterized on leukocyte surfaces that is important in many of the above adhesion reactions. Monoclonal antibodies have been instrumental in elucidating the structural interrelationships and functions of these three glycoproteins, macrophage antigen 1 (Mac-1), lymphocyte function-associated antigen 1 (LFA-1), and p150,95. Furthermore, this research has led to the definition, with monoclonal antibodies, of a novel heritable disease that manifests itself in defects in leukocyte adherence and motility.

Using this glycoprotein family as an example, this chapter emphasizes advances in research on the structure and function of cell surface proteins and their abnormalities in disease that have uniquely been made possible by the monoclonal antibody technique of Köhler and Milstein.

2. Probing Cell Surface Functions with Monoclonal Antibodies

The lymphoid immune system has been extensively studied as a model of cell adhesion, both because its cells circulate and can be readily obtained in suspension, and because adhesive interactions between T cells and other cells are extremely important in the development, regulation, and expression of specific immunity. The interaction between cytolytic T lymphocytes (CTL) and target cells has proved particularly amenable to study. CTLs are readily elicited to virus-infected cells or to histoincompatible foreign cells. CTLs adhere to and lyse target cells bearing specific antigen. Prior to the introduction of monoclonal technology, CTL-mediated killing had been shown to consist of a Mg^{2+}-dependent adhesion step and a Ca^{2+}-dependent lethal hit delivery step[8]; however, at the molecular level, CTL-mediated killing was essentially a "black box." With monoclonal antibody probes, the structure and function of a number of molecules participating in the cytolytic T lymphocyte–target cell interaction have now been elucidated (reviewed by Krensky *et al.*, this volume, Chapter 35). These include the T-lymphocyte receptor for specific antigen and a molecule with a more general role in leukocyte adhesion reactions, lymphocyte function-associated antigen (LFA-1).

The use of highly specific "functional screening" strategies has allowed MAbs to cell interaction molecules on CTLs to be readily identified, despite the use of whole cells to elicit the antibodies[9] (Fig. 1). In studies on mouse CTL-mediated killing, rats were immunized to mouse CTLs and 1000 rat × mouse hybridoma cultures were established per spleen. Culture supernatants containing secreted antibodies were harvested from the hybridomas 2 weeks

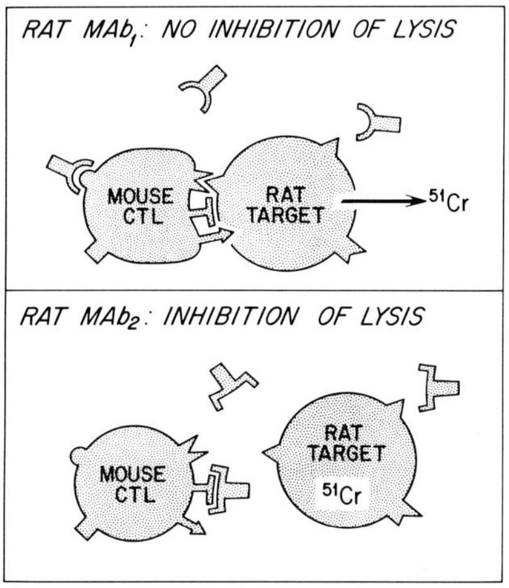

Figure 1. Screening for monoclonal antibodies blocking CTL effector cell function. Rat anti-mouse CTL MAbs are tested for blocking of mouse CTLs with specificity for rat lymphoma target cells. Antibodies that might block by binding to the target are avoided, since the target cell is syngeneic with the rat antibody donor in the system shown.[9] Screening for mouse MAbs to human anti-human histocompatibility antigen CTLs has also led to the identification of function-associated antigens on the CTL effector, and additionally, to the identification of antigens on the target cell important in CTL recognition.[49]

after fusion and incubated with CTLs. Then ^{51}Cr-labeled target cells were added and lysis of target cells was assessed by ^{51}Cr release (Fig. 1). This assay has allowed rapid screening of MAbs that inhibited CTL-mediated killing, and the identification of LFA-1 in mouse[9,10] and human.[11]

The paradigm of inhibiting (or stimulating; see Kaye, this volume, Chapter 32) specific cellular functions with MAbs appears to be generally applicable to the identification and study of cell surface receptors. The concentrations of MAbs secreted into tissue culture medium (20–200 μg/ml)[12] are high enough to give saturation binding to cells for most MAbs. The antibodies we have selected inhibit cellular function at concentrations of 1–5 μg/ml (Refs. 11 and 13 and T. A. Springer and D. C. Anderson, unpublished results). Most effective blocking is obtained when excess antibody is present throughout the functional assay. This is particularly important for receptors for which increased surface expression can be functionally triggered (see below). Possible artifactual effects on function due to binding to antigens with a high number of sites/cell or due to cell agglutination, toxicity, or binding to Fc receptors must always be considered. Such artifacts have been ruled out for anti-LFA-1,[13] but one example of an apparently artifactual inhibition of CTL-mediated killing has been found. An IgM anti-Thy-1 MAb was obtained that agglutinated CTLs and gave variable but sometimes strong inhibition of killing.[10]

3. Functional Properties of LFA-1

LFA-1 is expressed on the surface of T and B lymphocytes, monocytes, and granulocytes, but is absent from nonhematopoietic cells. Functional studies in the mouse and human have given concordant results. Anti-LFA-1 MAbs inhibit the first step in T-cell-mediated killing, i.e., the adherence of the killer cell to the target cell.[13,14] Non-antigen-specific "natural" killing[11,15] and polymorphonuclear leukocyte antibody-dependent cellular cytotoxicity[16] are also inhibited.

The broad distribution of LFA-1 on leukocytes, and the inhibition of granulocyte-mediated, antibody-dependent cellular cytotoxicity as well as T-cell functions by anti-LFA-1 MAb, suggested that LFA-1 might be of general importance in leukocyte cell interactions. Further support for this idea has come from experiments showing that LFA-1 can mediate adhesion between lymphocytes in the apparent absence of any other ligand–receptor interactions. LFA-1 MAbs inhibit spontaneous and phorbol ester-induced self-aggregation of B-cell lymphoblastoid lines.[17] In common with the adhesion step in CTL-mediated killing, this self-aggregation is divalent cation-dependent. Overall, the findings suggest that LFA-1 acts as a cell adhesion molecule, which can synergize with antigen-specific receptors, Fc receptors, or other receptors to increase the efficiency of cell–cell interactions.

4. Functional Properties of Mac-1, a Molecule Related to LFA-1

The macrophage 1 (Mac-1) molecule of mouse and human has a β subunit identical to that of LFA-1, but contains a different α subunit.[18,19] In contrast to LFA-1, Mac-1 is absent from B and T lymphocytes. It is present on monocytes, granulocytes, and large granular lymphocytes.[20]

A MAb to Mac-1 was found to inhibit the complement receptor type 3 (CR3) on mouse and human cells.[21] The CR3 mediates adherence and phagocytosis of particles opsonized with iC3b, a cleaved, hemolytically inactive form of the third component of complement. MAbs to the Mac-1, OKM10, and in some cases the OKM1 determinants on the human Mac-1 molecule also inhibit CR3 function.[19,22,23] MAbs that bind to other determinants on Mac-1 but do not inhibit CR3 activity have also been obtained.[23,24] Such MAb–Mac-1 antigen complexes bound to *Staphylococcus aureus* bacteria specifically agglutinate iC3b opsonized erythrocytes,[23] positively demonstrating that the Mac-1 molecule has CR3 activity. In common with the adherence reactions in which LFA-1 is implicated, CR3-mediated adherence is dependent on divalent cations.[23]

5. Glycoprotein Family Interrelationships

Serology has for many years been a sensitive method for detecting similarities and differences between molecules. However, pure antigen preparations were required either for immunization or absorption. This was because it was important to distinguish between (1) a true cross-reaction between a subpopulation of antibodies to antigen 1 with related antigen 2, or (2) immunization with an antigen 1 preparation contaminated with a small amount of antigen 2, resulting in an antiserum with independent populations of antibodies to unrelated antigens 1 and 2. Since at the forefront of research on newly discovered molecules pure antigen preparations are almost never at hand, it is a tremendous advantage to be able to obtain monospecific, cloned hybridoma lines after immunization with impure antigen. Using this technique, highly specific MAbs, as well as those recognizing potential cross-reactions, may be obtained.

Both types of MAb were obtained to the Mac-1, LFA-1 glycoprotein family, allowing the interrelationships of its glycoprotein subunits to be elucidated by immunochemical techniques. The cross-reaction of monoclonal and conventional antibodies between LFA-1 and Mac-1 was one of the first clues that these surface molecules were related.[18,25] Three types of MAb were obtained: those specific for Mac-1 (Fig. 2A, lane 2), those specific for LFA-1 (Fig. 2A, lane 4), and those cross-reacting between Mac-1 and LFA-1 (Fig. 2A, lane 3).[19,24] Both molecules contain α and β subunits noncovalently associated in $\alpha_1\beta_1$ complexes, as shown by cross-linking experiments.[24,26] The α subunits of Mac-1 and LFA-1 are M_r 170,000 and 180,000, respectively; the β subunits are each M_r 95,000. Western blotting of murine Mac-1 and LFA-1 showed that the cross-reactive MAb reacted with the β subunits of both antigens.[24] None of five MAbs specific for LFA-1 or four MAbs specific for Mac-1 reacted in Western blotting. The subunit reactivity of two of the MAbs specific for LFA-1 was elucidated during elution of LFA-1 from MAb–Sepharose columns with increasing pH. The β subunit was eluted in early fractions, followed by the α subunit in later fractions. Thus, disruption of the noncovalent association between the α and the β subunits preceded dissociation of the α subunit from the MAb. These results showed that two determinants specific to LFA-1 are present on its α subunit. Polyclonal rat antisera, but none of seven rat anti-mouse MAbs tested, were reactive with the Mac-1 or LFA-1 α subunits after pH-induced dissociation.

Since polyclonal antisera sample a wide variety of antigen epitopes, they are useful for obtaining more general conclusions about the immunochemical relationships between proteins. Mac-1 and LFA-1 were purified on MAb affinity columns. Antisera were then prepared to Mac-1 and to the LFA-1 α subunit, which was separated from the β subunit by an SDS–PAGE purification step. Antisera were tested with preparations of subunits dissociated at high pH. No cross-reactions between the α subunits were found at antibody concentrations 100- to 500-fold higher than required for reaction with the homologous α subunits. Thus, the α subunits are completely immunologically distinct. In contrast, cell lysates containing LFA-1 were as effective as those containing Mac-1 in absorbing antibodies to the Mac-1 β subunit present in anti-Mac-1 serum. Thus, the LFA-1 and Mac-1 β subunits are immunologically identical.[24]

Most mouse anti-human Mac-1 and LFA-1 MAbs were found to be immunoreactive with subunits dissociated by high pH. As in the mouse, MAbs specific for an individual member of the family were found to be α subunit-specific, while MAbs reacting with all types of αβ complex were found to react with the common β subunit.[19]

These results are in agreement with chemical characterization. The β subunits are identical by isoelectric focusing and peptide mapping; the α subunits

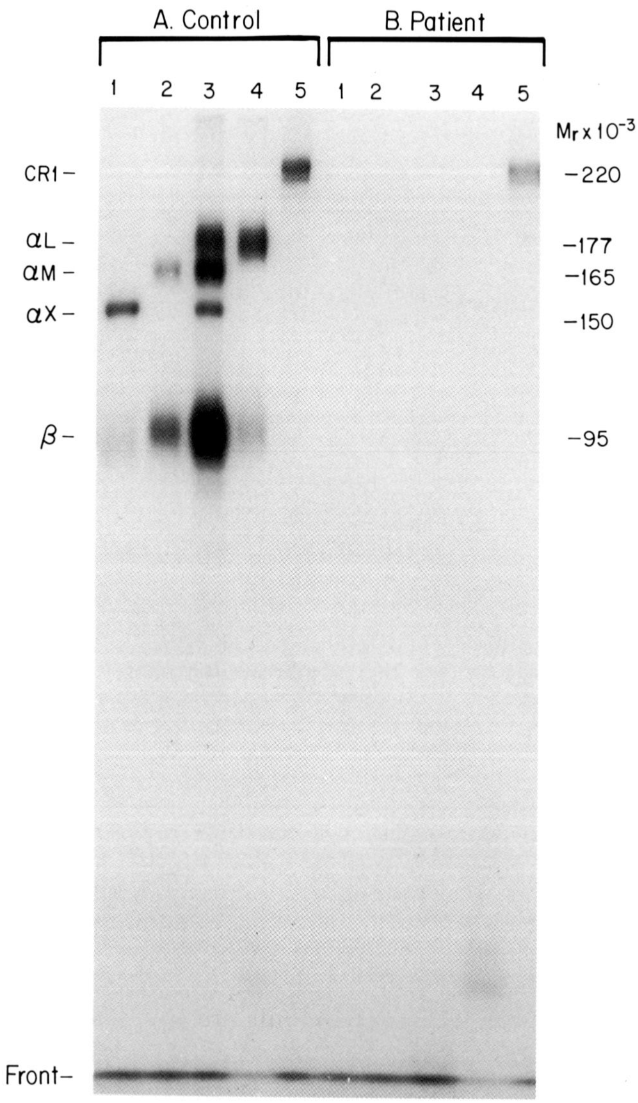

Figure 2. Immunoprecipitation of Mac-1, LFA-1, and p150,95 from healthy adults and deficient patient granulocytes. Granulocytes were surface-labeled with ^{125}I using lactoperoxidase. Triton X-100 lysates of (A) healthy control or (B) patient granulocytes were immunoprecipitated with anti-p150,95 MAb SHCL3 (lane 1), anti-Mac-1 α MAb OKM10 (lane 2), anti-β MAb TS1/18 (lane 3), anti-LFA-1 α MAb TS1/22 (lane 4), or anti-CR1 MAb 44D (lane 5). Precipitates were subjected to SDS 7% PAGE and autoradiography.

focus at distinct pI values and share at most one out of 17 tyrosyl tryptic peptides.[18,25,26] The NH_2-terminal amino acid sequences of the LFA-1 and Mac-1 α subunits show 33% homology (T. A. Springer, D. B. Teplow, and W. J. Dreyer, *Nature*, in press). This is highly significant homology, suggesting that the genes arose by a duplication event, but this degree of homology is generally too low to be immunochemically detected. As a rule, for globular proteins, 60% sequence homology is required for cross-reaction to occur.[27,28]

Polyclonal antiserum to Mac-1 has been useful in molecular biology experiments.[29,30] Polyclonal rabbit antiserum prepared to Mac-1 purified on MAb immunoaffinity columns[26] was found to immunoprecipitate Mac-1 translated in an *in vitro* reticulocyte lysate system, while none of several MAbs tested were effective. With polyclonal anti-Mac-1 IgG, Mac-1 mRNA preparations were purified approximately 1000-fold using the polysome purification procedure described by Kraus (this volume, Chapter 25). cDNA prepared to immunopurified mRNA, and oligonucleotide probes specified by the NH_2-terminal sequence, have been used to clone the Mac-1 α subunit gene (L. Sastre, T. Springer, T. Roberts, J. Roman, and W. Dreyer, unpublished results).

A third type of $\alpha\beta$ complex has been identified in humans by precipitation with anti-β MAb.[19] (Fig. 2). This $\alpha\beta$ complex has been termed p150,95 after its subunits of M_r 150,000 and 95,000. Recently, two MAbs specific for the p150,95 molecule were identified among MAbs in the myeloid panel of the second international workshop on human leukocyte differentiation[31] (see Fig. 2A, lane 1). Additionally, an IgM MAb to p150,95 has been obtained by immunizing mice with a mixture of human p150,95, Mac-1, and LFA-1. This antigen preparation was purified from granulocyte lysates using an anti-β subunit MAb coupled to Sepharose (L. Miller and T. A. Springer, unpublished). The p150,95 molecule is expressed on human monocytes and granulocytes but not on B or T lymphocytes.[31,32]

Surface expression of p150,95 and Mac-1 can be dramatically "upregulated" by physiological stimuli. The stimulatory agents include *f*-Met-Leu-Phe, an analogue of bacterial proteins, and C5a, an anaphylactic fragment of the complement component C5. These agents bind to specific receptors on myeloid cells and stimulate a broad spectrum of physiological responses, including increased adherence, chemotaxis, and granule secretion. *In vivo*, these agents stimulate circulating granulocytes and monocytes to aggregate, adhere to endothelial cells, and migrate into inflammatory sites.[4,6] When granulocytes[33] or monocytes (Fig. 3) are stimulated *in vitro* with *f*-Met-Leu-Phe (10^{-8} M), the amount of Mac-1 and p150,95 expressed on the cell surface is increased four- to sevenfold. In contrast, surface expression of LFA-1 is unaffected. These large increases in surface expression occur within $\frac{1}{2}$ hr, suggesting a latent store of Mac-1 and p150,95 in granulocytes and monocytes. Secretion of components stored in secondary granules and perhaps in other secretory vesicles is stimulated under these conditions.[34] This suggests an intracellular location, perhaps in the membrane bilayer surrounding secretory organelles, for the latent store of Mac-1 and p150,95. The lack of such a store of LFA-1 suggests that

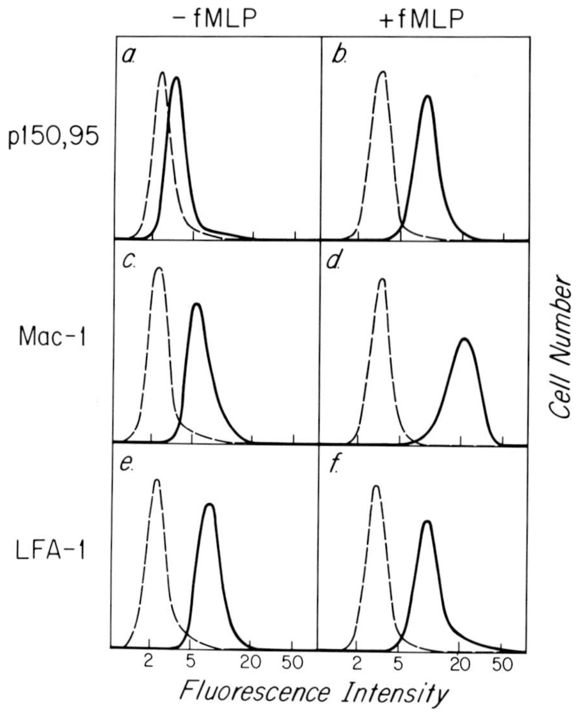

Figure 3. *f*-Met-Leu-Phe selectively stimulates increased Mac-1 and p150,95 expression on monocytes. Mononuclear cells were incubated with 10^{-8} M *f*-Met-Leu-Phe for 30 min at 37°C or were held at 4° to prevent upregulation stimulated by cell preparation,[43] labeled with MAb and FITC anti-mouse IgG at 4°C, and subjected to immunofluorescent flow cytometry on an Epics V.[19] Cells were stained with specific MAbs (solid curves) or P3X63 control IgG1 (dashed curves).

after biosynthesis, targetting of these molecules to the plasma membrane or secretory organelles is influenced by their α subunits.

6. Mac-1, LFA-1 Deficiency Disease

With the use of MAbs, a novel disease has been recognized in which the Mac-1, LFA-1 and p150,95 glycoproteins are deficient. Recurrent bacterial infection, progressive periodontitis, persistent leukocytosis, and/or delayed umbilical cord separation has been described in patients whose neutrophils demonstrated depressed phagocytic function and deficient adherence and chemotaxis.[35–39] When total, surface-labeled granulocyte proteins from these patients were subjected to SDS–PAGE, (a) glycoprotein(s) variously estimated to be M_r 110,000,[35] 180,000,[36] 150,000,[37] or 138,000[38] was found to be lacking. Deficiency of a specific surface molecule in one of these patients was pinpointed using MAbs to the α and β subunits of Mac-1.[38,40,41]

Deficiency on the cell surface of both the α and β subunits of Mac-1 might be secondary to a lack of the α or β subunit. If the primary deficiency were of the β subunit, a lack of LFA-1 and p150,95 would also be predicted. This hypothesis has been tested with MAbs specific for the LFA-1 αL and Mac-1 αM subunits and the common β subunit,[33] and more recently with p150,95-specific MAbs[31,39] which presumably react with the p150,95 αX subunit.

Expression on the surface of patient cells was quantitated by immunofluorescent flow cytometry. Patient granulocytes and mononuclear cells were markedly deficient in the entire glycoprotein family, as shown with MAbs specific for each α subunit and the common β subunit. An interesting quantitative difference was seen between patients. Patients 1 and 2 expressed between 0.2 and 0.5% of the normal amounts of Mac-1, LFA-1, and p150,95, values that are marginally distinguishable from complete absence. In contrast, patients 4–8 expressed clearly higher but subnormal amounts of 3–9% of these molecules. These levels of expression have been termed severe and moderate deficiency, respectively.[39] Incubation of patient granulocytes with 10^{-8} M *f*-Met-Leu-Phe resulted in a small absolute increase in the amount of surface-accessible Mac-1, p150,95, or the common β subunit in moderately deficient patients, but the percent of normal expression remained unchanged in comparison to similarly treated healthy cells.

To examine the deficiency at a molecular level, patients' granulocytes were labeled with ^{125}I and subjected to immunoprecipitation. A representative experiment with patient 1 is shown in Fig. 2. From control cells, the anti-αL MAb, anti-αM MAb, and anti-p150,95 precipitated the respective individual α subunits noncovalently associated with the common β subunit (Fig. 2A, lanes 1, 2, and 4). The anti-β MAb precipitated the β subunit and the three types of α subunits noncovalently associated with it: αL, αM, and the αX subunit of the p150,95 molecule (Fig. 2A, lane 3). In contrast, cells from patients were strikingly deficient in all these molecules (Fig. 2B, lanes 1–4). The normal parents and siblings of the patients were positive for immunoprecipitation.[33] The CR1 was present in similar amounts in normal and patient cells (Figs. 2A and 2B, lane 5).

To test for low levels of expression in patient cells, autoradiograms were subjected to prolonged exposure.[33,39] Precipitation of small amounts of LFA-1, Mac-1, and p150,95 was detected in moderately deficient but not in severely deficient patients. Notably, anti-αL and anti-β MAbs each precipitated both α and β subunits. This shows that when surface expression can be detected on patient cells, it is due to the presence of the normal αβ complex, rather than to the presence of free α or β subunits.

The deficiency appears to be limited to the Mac-1, LFA-1 glycoprotein family. The CR1, the neutrophil Fc receptor, and HLA antigen glycoproteins were present in normal amounts and were of normal mobility in SDS–PAGE. Furthermore, out of 118 antimyeloid MAbs screened in the second international leukocyte workshop, the only negative MAbs were 16 directed to the LFA-1, Mac-1 family or its members.[31] Normal numbers of *f*-Met-Leu-Phe receptors and normal granule secretion triggered by receptors for *f*-Met-Leu-Phe and C5a have previously been described on these patients' cells.[38,42] Furthermore, latent CR1[43] but not Mac-1 or p150,95 was present in patients' granulocytes, which could be expressed on the surface in response to *f*-Met-Leu-Phe or C5a.

A number of lines of evidence show that Mac-1, LFA-1, p150,95 deficiency is a heritable autosomal recessive disease[33,39]: (1) Mothers and fathers were found to express approximately half the normal amount of αL, αM, and β sub-

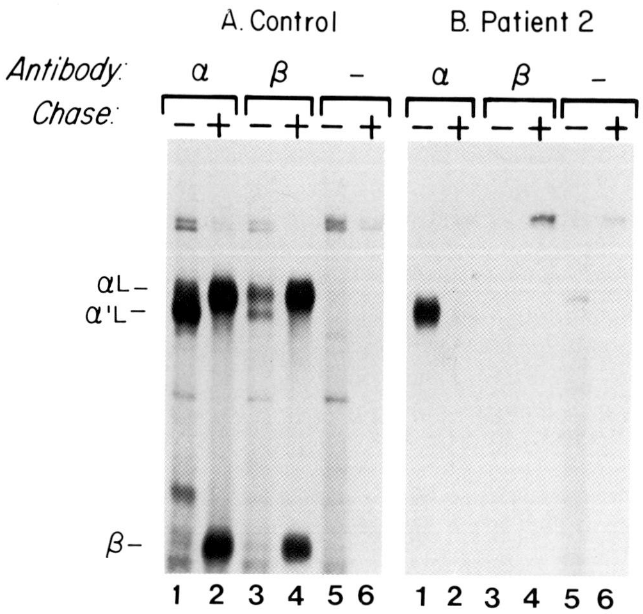

Figure 4. LFA-1 biosynthesis in patient and normal lymphocytes. Lymphocytes of patient 2 were blast-transformed with phytohemagglutinin (identical results were obtained with lymphocytes of patients 1 and 4).[33] Cultured blasts were then labeled with [^{35}S]methionine for 2 hr, and either harvested immediately or chased for 22 hr with unlabeled methionine as indicated. Triton X-100 and sodium deoxycholate-solubilized cell lysates were immunoprecipitated with Sepharose-coupled TS1/22 anti-LFA-1 α MAb, TS1/18 anti-β MAb, or activated, quenched Sepharose as a negative control. Precipitates were subjected to SDS–PAGE and fluorography.

units, both on unstimulated and on *f*-Met-Leu-Phe-stimulated granulocytes. (2) In the case of X-linked inheritance, two populations (normal and defective) of maternal granulocytes would be expected as a result of X-chromosome inactivation, as is observed in the X-linked form of chronic granulomatous disease. However, all four mothers had a single population of granulocytes expressing intermediate levels of each glycoprotein subunit. (3) One recently identified family contains a cluster of an affected father, son, and daughter.[39] (4) Equivalent numbers of male and female patients have been identified. (5) One patient (#3) was the product of a consanguinous marriage.

The molecular pathogenesis of this deficiency was investigated in biosynthesis experiments. Biosynthesis experiments with normal cells have shown that the α and β subunits are derived from separate precursors denoted as α′ and β′, and that association into an α′β′ complex precedes processing to the mature αβ form and expression on the cell surface.[19,44] In patients' cells, the α′L precursor was synthesized in normal amounts and had normal stability; however, α′L never matured to αL (Fig. 4B, lanes 1 and 2), and lack of precipitation of α′L by anti-β MAbs showed that it did not become β-associated (Fig. 4B, lanes 3 and 4). Two lines of evidence strongly suggest that the primary

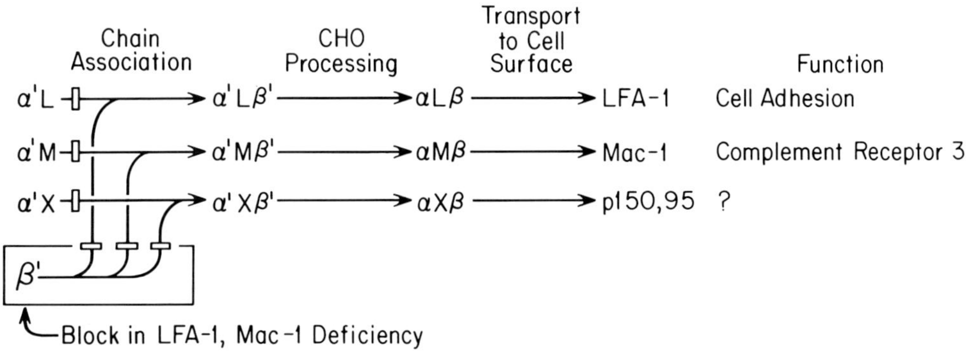

Figure 5. Biosynthesis of the Mac-1, LFA-1 glycoprotein family. The biosynthetic pathway in normal cells is as described in Ref. 19. The evidence for a primary block in β-subunit synthesis, a secondary block in α'L biosynthesis due to lack of β-subunit association, and hypothetically similar blocks in α'M and α'X biosynthesis is discussed in Ref. 33 and the text. Lack of α-subunit processing and transport to the cell surface or to latent pools appears to be due to a requirement for association with the β subunit.

defect is in the β subunit: (1) the presence of normal α'L but absence of any form of αLβ complex either at the cell surface or as an intracellular precursor that would have been detectable by precipitation of αL or α'L by anti-β MAbs, and (2) the lack of three different surface proteins, which have as their only common structural entity the β subunit.

The effect of β deficiency on biosynthesis of the Mac-1, LFA-1 family is summarized in Fig. 5. The presence of α'L precursor but no αL inside patients' cells and the absence of cell surface αL show that association with the β subunit is required for processing and transport to the surface. Biosynthesis experiments have been done thus far with cells that express only LFA-1, but since the biosynthetic pathways of Mac-1, p150,95, and LFA-1 are similar in normal cells,[19] it is proposed that α'M and α'X intracellular precursors are blocked at the same point in their biosynthetic pathway in patient myeloid cells, as shown in Fig. 5.

The lack of three α subunits on the cell surface as the result of β-subunit deficiency represents an interesting example of the effects of gene complementation on the phenotypic expression of an inherited defect. The lack of a latent pool of Mac-1 and p150,95 in patients' cell suggests that subunit association is also required for entry into this pool, which is presumably intracellular. Studies with endoglycosidase H digestion of Mac-1 have shown that the maturation of α'M to αM is due to the conversion of high-mannose to complex-type carbohydrates (T. Kishimoto, L. Sastre, and T. A. Springer, unpublished results). This type of carbohydrate processing is known to occur in the Golgi, suggesting that lack of association with β in patients' cells blocks transport to the Golgi. To further understanding of the nature of the mutation at the mRNA and DNA level, DNA probes specific for the α subunits (see above) and β subunits are being prepared.

Other patients appear to resemble the eight we have studied in lacking multiple members of the Mac-1, LFA-1 glycoprotein family. Two patients in the eastern U.S.,[40,41,45] one in the western U.S.,[46] three in England,[47] and one in France[48] have a similar deficiency of β and of multiple α subunits. Although none of these patients have been characterized by biosynthetic labeling of precursors, the findings in each case are suggestive of a similar β-subunit defect.

Heterogeneity among these patients in their symptoms heretofore hindered their classification into a single clinical entity. A common molecular basis for their disease has now been demonstrated: inherited Mac-1, LFA-1 deficiency. Severe and moderate deficiency variants of the disease have been recognized; heterogeneity with respect to the severity of clinical illness and/or abnormalities of leukocyte functions observed among recognized examples of this disease appears causally related to quantitative differences among the patients in surface expression of this critical glycoprotein family.[39] Granulocytes of patients 4–8 have about 5% of normal amounts on the cell surfaces, whereas patients 1–3 have a clearly more severe, almost complete deficiency. Patients 2 and 3 died before the age of 2; patient 1 is 5 years old. Among our patient population, patients 4–8 appear to have a relatively less severe clinical disease as compared to patients 1–3 and have survived longer (mean age 19 years). The presence of identical molecular deficiencies among these patients has confirmed that they represent examples of the same genetic disease. However, the possibility exists that disease among different recognized kindreds results from independent mutations within or affecting the same gene. This is suggested by the quantitative variations in Mac-1, LFA-1, p150,95 surface expression and the different ethnic backgrounds among the patients, including Anglo-Saxon, Iranian, and Hispanic.

Since a deficiency of the Mac-1, LFA-1 family has been clearly documented on multiple types of leukocytes, including granulocytes, monocytes, and T and B lymphocytes, the observed functional abnormalities of both phagocytic and lymphoid cells of these patients[39,42] are not unexpected. Recurrent soft tissue infections secondary to bacterial microorganisms is unquestionably related to granulocyte dysfunction in this disorder. Patient granulocytes are deficient in multiple adhesion-dependent functions, including attachment and spreading, aggregation, chemotaxis, antibody-dependent cytotoxicity, and CR3-mediated adherence and phagocytosis.[35,38,42,46] Deficiency of CR3 function as measured with iC3b-opsonized particles is in good agreement with the previous identification of Mac-1 as the CR3[21,23] of human myeloid cells. The wide spectrum of adhesion-dependent abnormalities may be related to all three members of this glycoprotein family, since all are expressed on normal granulocytes and monocytes. Treatment with combinations of anti-αL, -αM, and -β MAbs reproduces abnormalities in adhesion-related functions in normal granulocytes,[16,38,42,46] while no blockade of adherence-independent functions, including shape change and specific binding of chemotactic factors, is observed. Interestingly, granulocyte adhesion, in common with other functions in which Mac-1 and LFA-1 are implicated, is divalent-cation dependent.[3]

The failure of patients' granulocytes to hyperadhere in response to chemoattractants *in vitro* may be related to deficient upregulation of Mac-1 and p150,95.[38] Since granulocyte adherence to endothelial cells *in vivo* and to a variety of substrates *in vitro* represents the prerequisite for mobilization to inflammatory sites and for chemotaxis, respectively, the adherence abnormalities in this disorder provide a plausible explanation for clinical features of impaired pus formation, occurrence of necrotic infections of skin and mucous membranes, and impaired wound healing. Lack in patients of granulocyte or monocyte accumulation at abraded skin sites (Rebuck skin window test) is also notable in this respect.[39]

Although lymphocytes express only one member of the family, LFA-1, some evidence supports the clinical pathological importance of lymphoid cell dysfunction in this disorder. Of importance, the death of patient 3 was related to a fulminant and progressive viral (pico RNA virus) respiratory infection. Impaired proliferative responses of patient cells to PHA (10–25% of normal values) and diminished cytolytic T-lymphocyte and natural killing activity have been documented in studies on some of our patients[16,17] as well as in a patient reported elsewhere.[46] Interestingly, the PHA responses and cytotoxic killing by lymphocytes of patients 1, 2, and 4 are even further decreased by anti-LFA-1 MAb, suggesting that even the small amounts of LFA-1 present on patient cells can contribute to their functional responsiveness.[17] The functional defects of LFA-1-deficient lymphocytes appear identical to the defects observed in normal lymphocytes treated with anti-LFA-1 MAb. The excellent agreement between studies on MAb-treated normal cells and on genetically deficient cells, both for LFA-1 and Mac-1, is an important confirmation of the validity of using MAb probes for the study of cell surface function.

Previously, immunodeficiency diseases have been described in which specific cell lineages are absent or abnormally developed, as in severe combined immunodeficiency; secreted components are lacking, as in complement deficiencies; or intracellular enzymes are lacking, as in chronic granulomatous disease. To the best of our knowledge, Mac-1, LFA-1 deficiency is the first reported instance of an immunodeficiency disease related to the lack of specific cell surface proteins. The combined tools of monoclonal antibodies and an inherited deficiency syndrome should allow rapid progress in understanding the important functions of the Mac-1, LFA-1 glycoprotein family in leukocyte adhesion reactions.

ACKNOWLEDGMENTS. We would like to thank the many colleagues who collaborated in studies cited here for their important contributions. This work was supported by NIH grants AI 19031, CA 31798, and CA 31799, and Council for Tobacco Research grant 1307.

References

1. Dawson, P., and Mandell, O., 1980, Phagocyte strategy vs. microbial tactics, *Rev. Inf. Dis.* **2**:817–836.

2. Carter, S. B., 1967, Haptotaxis and the mechanism of cell motility, *Nature* **213**:256–260.
3. Smith, C. W., Hollers, J. C., Patrick, R. A., and Hassett, C., 1979, Motility and adhesiveness in human neutrophils: Effects of chemotactic factors, *J. Clin. Invest.* **63**:221–229.
4. Atherton, A., and Born, G. V. R., 1972, Quantitative investigations of the adhesiveness of circulating polymorphonuclear leucocytes to blood vessel walls, *J. Physiol.* **222**:447–474.
5. Keller, H. U., Barandum, S., Kistler, P., and Ploem, J., 1979, Locomotion and adhesion of neutrophil granulocytes: Effects of albumin, fibrinogen and gammaglobulins studied by reflexion contrast microscopy, *Exp. Cell Res.* **122**:351–362.
6. Wilkinson, P. C., and Lackie, J. M., 1979, The adhesion, migration and chemotaxis of leukocytes in inflammation, *Curr. Top. Path.* **68**:47–88.
7. Köhler, G., and Milstein, C., 1975, Continuous cultures of fused cells secreting antibody of predefined specificity, *Nature* **256**:495–497.
8. Martz, E., 1977, Mechanism of specific tumor cell lysis by alloimmune T-lymphocytes: Resolution and characterization of discrete steps in the cellular interaction, *Contemp. Top. Immunobiol.* **7**:301–361.
9. Davignon, D., Martz, E., Reynolds, T., Kürzinger, K., and Springer, T., A., 1981, Lymphocyte function-associated antigen 1 (LFA-1): A surface antigen distinct from Lyt-2,3 that participates in T lymphocyte–mediated killing, *Proc. Natl. Acad. Sci. USA* **78**:4535–4539.
10. Sanchez-Madrid, F., Davignon, D., Martz, E., and Springer, T. A., 1982, Antigens involved in mouse cytolytic T-lymphocyte (CTL)-mediated killing: Functional screening and topographic relationship, *Cell. Immunol.* **73**:1–11.
11. Krensky, A. M., Sanchez-Madrid, F., Robbins, E., Nagy, J., Springer, T. A., and Burakoff, S. J., 1983, The functional significance, distribution, and structure of LFA-1, LFA-2, and LFA-3: Cell surface antigens associated with CTL-target interactions, *J. Immunol.* **131**:611–616.
12. Springer, T. A., 1982, Quantitation of hybridoma immunoglobulins and selection of myeloma or specific light chain loss variants, *Meth. Enzymol.* **92**:147–160.
13. Davignon, D., Martz, E., Reynolds, T., Kürzinger, K., and Springer, T. A., 1981, Monoclonal antibody to a novel lymphocyte function-associated antigen (LFA-1): Mechanism of blocking of T lymphocyte-mediated killing and effects on other T and B lymphocyte functions, *J. Immunol.* **127**:590–595.
14. Krensky, A. M., Robbins, E., Springer, T. A., and Burakoff, S. J., 1984, LFA-1, LFA-2 and LFA-3 antigens are involved in CTL-target conjugation, *J. Immunol.* **132**:2180–2182.
15. Hildreth, J. E. K., Gotch, M. F., Hildreth, P. D. K., and McMichael, A. J., 1983, A human lymphocyte-associated antigen involved in cell-mediated lympholysis, *Eur. J. Immunol.* **13**:202–208.
16. Kohl, S., Springer, T. A., Schmalstieg, F. C., Loo, L. S., and Anderson, D. C., 1984, Defective natural killer cytotoxicity and polymorphonuclear leukocyte antibody-dependent cellular cytotoxicity in patients with LFA-1/OKM-1 deficiency, *J. Immunol.* **133**:2972–2978.
17. Springer, T. A., Rothlein, R., Anderson, D. C., Burakoff, S. J., and Krensky, A. M., 1985, The function of LFA-1 in cell-mediated killing and adhesion: Studies on heritable LFA-1, Mac-1 deficiency and on lymphoid cell self-aggregation, in: *Mechanisms of Cell-Mediated Cytotoxicity II*, Plenum Press, New York, In press.
18. Kürzinger, K., Ho, M. K., and Springer, T. A., 1982, Structural homology of a macrophage differentiation antigen and an antigen involved in T-cell-mediated killing, *Nature* **296**:668–670.
19. Sanchez-Madrid, F., Nagy, J., Robbins, E., Simon, P., and Springer, T. A., 1983, A human leukocyte differentiation antigen family with distinct alpha subunits and a common beta subunit: The lymphocyte-function associated antigen (LFA-1), the C3bi complement receptor (OKM1-Mac-1), and the p150,95 molecule, *J. Exp. Med.* **158**:1785–1803.
20. Unkeless, J. C., and Springer, T. A., 1984, Macrophages, in: *Handbook of Experimental Immunology*, 4th ed., Volume IV: *Applications of Immunological Methods in Biomedical Sciences* (D. M. Weir, C. C. Blackwell, L. A. Herzenberg, and L. A. Herzenberg, eds.), Blackwell, Oxford, In press.
21. Beller, D. I., Springer, T. A., and Schreiber, R. D., 1982, Anti-Mac-1 selectively inhibits the mouse and human type three complement receptor, *J. Exp. Med.* **156**:1000–1009.

22. Arnaout, M. A., Todd, R. F., III, Dana, N., Melamed, J., Schlossman, S. F., and Colten, H. R., 1983, Inhibition of phagocytosis of complement C3- or immunoglobulin G-coated particles and of C3bi binding by monoclonal antibodies to a monocyte-granulocyte membrane glycoprotein (Mol), *J. Clin. Invest.* **72**:171–179.
23. Wright, S. D., Rao, P. E., Van Voorhis, W. C., Craigmyle, L. S., Iida, K., Talle, M. A., Westberg, E. F., Goldstein, G., and Silverstein, S. C., 1983, Identification of the C3bi receptor of human monocytes and macrophages with monoclonal antibodies, *Proc. Natl. Acad. Sci. USA* **80**:5699–5703.
24. Sanchez-Madrid, F., Simon, P., Thompson, S., and Springer, T. A., 1983, Mapping of antigenic and functional epitopes on the alpha and beta subunits of two related glycoproteins involved in cell interactions, LFA-1 and Mac-1, *J. Exp. Med.* **158**:586–602.
25. Trowbridge, I. S., and Omary, M. B., 1981, Molecular complexity of leukocyte surface glycoproteins related to the macrophage differentiation antigen Mac-1, *J. Exp. Med.* **154**:1517–1524.
26. Kürzinger, K., and Springer, T. A., 1982, Purification and structural characterization of LFA-1, a lymphocyte function-associated antigen, and Mac-1, a related macrophage differentiation antigen, *J. Biol. Chem.* **257**:12412–12418.
27. Ibrahimi, I. M., Prager, E. M., White, T. J., and Wilson, A. C., 1979, Amino acid sequence of California quail lysozyme. Effect of evolutionary substitutions on the antigenic structure of lysozyme, *Biochemistry* **13**:2736–2744.
28. Prager, E. M., Wilson, A. C., Perin, J. P., and Jolles, P., 1978, Further studies of an anomalous cross-reaction involving worm and vertebrate lysozymes, *Immunochemistry* **15**:577–583.
29. Springer, T. A., Sastre, L., Schmalstieg, F. C., and Anderson, D. C., 1985, Inherited LFA-1, Mac-1 deficiency and its molecular biology, in: *Mononuclear Phagocytes and Inflammation* (R. van Furth and Z. A. Cohn, eds.), Martinus Nijhoff, in press.
30. Springer, T. A., Sastre, L., and Anderson, D. C., 1985, The LFA-1, Mac-1 Leukocyte adhesion glycoprotein family and its deficiency in a heritable human disease, *Biochem. Soc. Trans.* **13**:3–6.
31. Springer, T. A., and Anderson, D. C., 1985, Antibodies specific for the Mac-1, LFA-1, p150,95 glycoproteins or their family, or for other granulocyte proteins, in: *Leukocyte* Typing II (E. Reinherz, ed.), Springer-Verlag, Berlin, (in press).
32. Schwarting, R., Stein, H., and Wang, C. Y., 1984, The monoclonal antibodies anti S-HCL 1 (anti Leu 14) and anti S-HCL 3 (anti Leu M5) allow the diagnosis of hairy cell leukemia, *Blood* (in press).
33. Springer, T. A., Thompson, W. S., Miller, L. J., Schmalstieg, F. C., and Anderson, D. C., 1984, Inherited deficiency of the Mac-1, LFA-1, p150,95 glycoprotein family and its molecular basis, *J. Exp. Med.* **160**:1901–1918.
34. Gallin, J. I., Fletcher, M. P., Seligman, B. E., Hoffstein, S., Cehes, K., and Mounessa, N., 1982, Human neutrophil-specific granule deficiency: A model to assess the role of neutrophil-specific granules in the evolution of the inflammatory response, *Blood* **59**:1317–1329.
35. Crowley, C. A., Curnutte, J. T., Rosin, R. E., Andre-Schwartz, J., Gallin, J. I., Klempner, M., Snyderman, R., Southwick, F. S., Stossel, T. P., and Babior, B. M., 1980, An inherited abnormality of neutrophil adhesion: Its genetic transmission and its association with a missing protein, *N. Engl. J. Med.* **302**:1163–1168.
36. Buchanan, M. R., Crowley, C. A., Rosin, R. E., Gimbrone, M.A., and Babior, B. M., 1982, Studies on the interaction between GP-180-deficient neutrophils and vascular endothelium, *Blood* **60**:160–165.
37. Arnaout, M. A., Pitt, J., Cohen, H. J., Melamed, J., Rosen, F. S., and Colten, H. R., 1982, Deficiency of a granulocyte-membrane glycoprotein (gp150) in a boy with recurrent bacterial infections, *N. Engl. J. Med.* **306**:693–699.
38. Anderson, D. C., Schmalstieg, F. C., Kohl, S., Arnaout, M. A., Hughes, B. J., Tosi, M. F., Buffone, G. J., Brinkley, B. R., Dickey, W. D., Abramson, J. S., Springer, T. A., Boxer, L. A., Hollers, J. M., and Smith, C. W., 1984, Abnormalities of polymorphonuclear leukocyte function associated with a heritable deficiency of high molecular weight surface glycoproteins (GP138): Common relationship to diminished cell adherence, *J. Clin. Invest.* **74**:536–551.

39. Anderson, D. C., Schmalstieg, F. C., Finegold, M. J., Hughes, B. J., Rothlein, R., Miller, L. J., Kohl, S., Tosi, M. F., Jacobs, R. L., Waldrop, T. C., Goldman, A., Shearer, W. T., and Springer, T. A., 1985, The severe and moderate phenotypes of heritable Mac-1, LFA-1 deficiency: their quantitative definition and relation to leukocyte dysfunction and clinical features, *J. Inf. Dis.* (in press).

40. Springer, T. A., 1985, The LFA-1, Mac-1 glycoprotein family and its deficiency in an inherited disease: Introduction, *Fed. Proc.* (in press).

41. Dana, N., Todd, R. F., III, Pitt, J., Springer, T. A., and Arnaout, M. A., 1984, Deficiency of a surface membrane glycoprotein (Mol) in man, *J. Clin. Invest.* **73:**153–159.

42. Anderson, D. C., Schmalstieg, F. C., Shearer, W., Freeman, K., Kohl, S., Smith, C. W., and Springer, T., 1985, Abnormalities of PMN monocyte function and recurrent infection associated with a heritable deficiency of adhesive surface glycoproteins, *Fed. Proc.* (in press).

43. Fearon, D. T., and Collins, L. A., 1983, Increased expression of C3b receptors on polymorphonuclear leukocytes induced by chemotactic factors and by purification procedures, *J. Immunol.* **130:**370–375.

44. Ho, M. K., and Springer, T. A., 1982, Mac-1 antigen: Quantitative expression in macrophage populations and tissues, and immunofluorescent localization in spleen, *J. Immunol.* **128:**2281–2286.

45. Arnaout, M. A., Dana, N., Pitt, J., and Todd, R. F., III, 1985, Deficiency of two human leukocyte surface membrane glycoproteins (Mol and LFA-1), *Fed. Proc.* (in press).

46. Beatty, P. G., Harlan, J. M., Rosen, H., Hansen, J. A., Ochs, H. D., Price, T. D., Taylor, R. F., and Klebanoff, S. J., 1984, Absence of monoclonal-antibody-defined protein complex in boy with abnormal leucocyte function, *Lancet* **I:**535–537.

47. Ross, G. D., Thompson, R. A., Walport, M. J., Springer, T. A., Watson, J. V., Ward, R. H. R., Lida, J., Newman, S. L., Harrison, R. A., and Lachmann, P. J., 1984, Characterization of patients with an increased susceptibility to bacterial infections and a genetic deficiency of leukocyte membrane complement receptor type three (CR3) and the related membrane antigen LFA-1, *Blood*, manuscript submitted.

48. Fischer, A., Seger, R., Durandy, A., Grospierre, B., Virelizier, J. L., Griscelli, C., Fischer, E., Kazatchkine, M., Bohler, M. C., Descamps-Latscha, B., Trung, P. H., Springer, T. A., Olive, D., and Mawas, C., 1984, Deficiency of the adhesive protein complex LFA-1, C3bi complement receptor, p150,95 in a girl with recurrent bacterial infections, *Blood* (in press).

49. Sanchez-Madrid, F., Krensky, A. M., Ware, C. F., Robbins, E., Strominger, J. L., Burakoff, S. J., and Springer, T. A., 1982, Three distinct antigens associated with human T lymphocyte-mediated cytolysis: LFA-1, LFA-2, and LFA-3, *Proc. Natl. Acad. Sci. USA* **79:**7489–7493.

Chapter 12

Demonstration of Receptor Function of Membrane Proteins by Selection and Immobilization with Monoclonal Antibodies

JANIS JACKS WEIS and DOUGLAS T. FEARON

1. Background

Monoclonal antibodies (MAbs) that are specific for certain types of cells and for stages of ontogenetic development can be produced without prior knowledge of antigenic differences between the cell types. Once identified, however, the elucidation of the function of these interesting antigens may represent a formidable task. In this chapter, we discuss the technique of selection and immobilization of membrane proteins by MAbs bound to *Staphylococcus aureus* bacteria. This technique allows visualization of receptor interactions with ligands on cells or in solution. Since multivalent interactions between *S. aureus* bacteria–MAb-receptor complexes and ligand-coated particles can be established, the method is particularly useful for studies on receptors where univalent reactions are of low affinity. The use of this method to identify two different membrane proteins as receptors for fragments of the third component of complement (C3) and one of these additionally as an Epstein–Barr virus (EBV) receptor, is described. To introduce these studies, the biology of C3, C3 receptors, and EBV is first briefly reviewed.

1.1. C3 Ligands

C3 consists of two polypeptide chains, an α chain of 120,000 M_r and a β chain of 75,000 M_r, which are covalently linked by disulfide bonds (Fig. 1). C3 is activated when the α chain is cleaved by the C3 convertases of either the

JANIS JACKS WEIS and DOUGLAS T. FEARON • Department of Medicine, Harvard Medical School, and Department of Rheumatology and Immunology, Brigham and Women's Hospital, Boston, Massachusetts 02115.

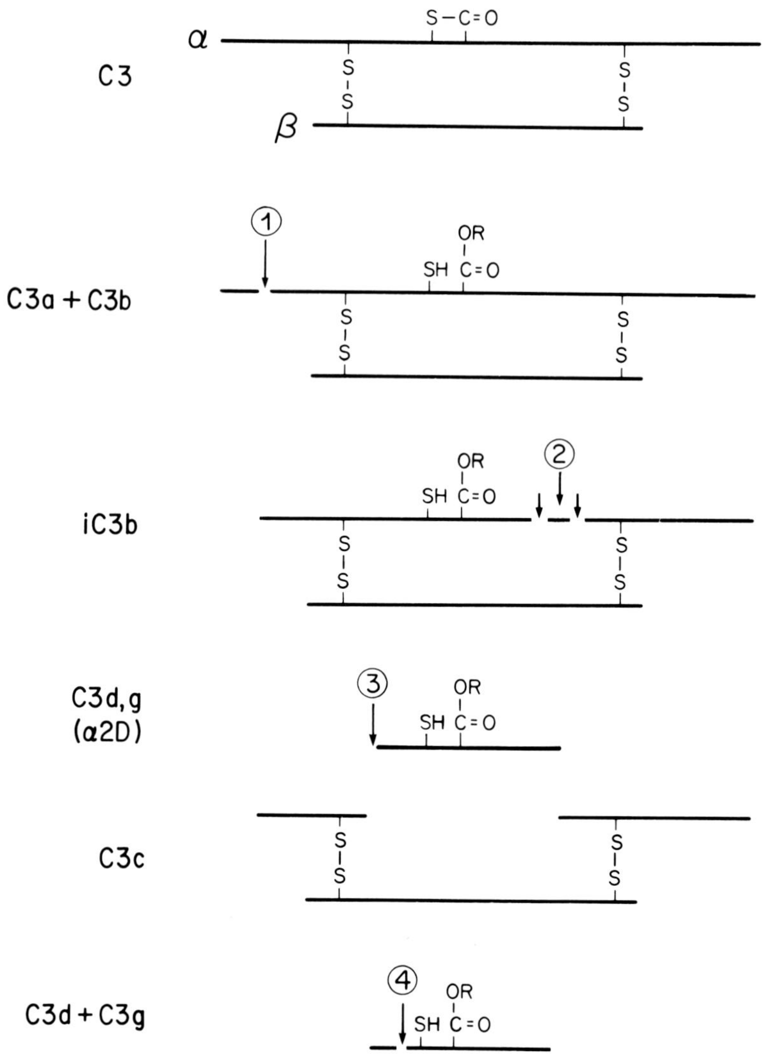

Figure 1. Sequential generation of the C3b, iC3b, C3dg, and C3d fragments from C3. In reaction 1 the α chain is cleaved by a C3 convertase to generate C3a and C3b. The thiolester in the latter fragment undergoes a transacylation reaction to mediate relatively nonspecific covalent binding to the activator of complement (R). In reaction 2 the C3b is hydrolyzed by factor I at two sites, releasing a 3000-M_r peptide and forming iC3b. In reaction 3 the iC3b is cleaved at third site by factor I to release C3c and leave the C3dg fragment bound to the activator of complement. Reactions 2 and 3 require either factor H or CR1 as cofactors. In reaction 4 the C3g fragment is hydrolyzed from the C3d fragment by noncomplement enzymes. The C3e fragment, not shown in the figure, is derived from the COOH terminus of the lower molecular weight α-polypeptide chain fragment of C3c.

Table I. Characteristics of Receptors for C3 Fragments Bound to Complement Activators

Receptor	Molecular weight	Ligands	Cells
CR1	160,000–260,000	C3b, iC3b, C4b	Erythrocytes, neutrophils, monocytes/macrophages, B lymphocytes, some T lymphocytes, glomerular podocytes
CR2	145,000	C3dg, C3d, iC3b, C3b (weak), EBV	B Lymphocytes
CR3	165,000 α, 95,000 β	iC3b, C3dg (?)	Neutrophils, monocytes, macrophages, large granular lymphocytes

classical or alternative pathways, resulting in release of the 9000-M_r C3a peptide. Within the α chain of the remaining C3b fragment a thiolester is transiently exposed, which mediates attachment to the target of complement activation by formation of an ester or amide bond between its glutamyl component and a hydroxyl or amino group of the target.[1–3] The bound C3b is then converted to iC3b by cleavage of the α chain at two sites by factor I, in the presence of cofactors H or the C3b receptor, resulting in α-chain fragments of 68,000 and 40,000 M_r and the release of a 3000-M_r fragment.[4] The covalent binding site is retained within the 68,000-M_r fragment and the β chain remains disulfide-linked to the α-chain fragments. The 68,000 M_r fragment of the α chain is susceptible to further cleavage by I in the presence of these cofactors to generate the C3dg fragment of 43,000 M_r which remains covalently attached to the target of complement activation.[5,6] The β chain is not attached to C3dg and is released with the 40,000- and 25,000-M_r α-chain fragments as C3c. The C3dg is susceptible to further degradation by non-complement-derived enzymes such as trypsin, neutrophil elastase, and bacterial enzymes to generate the 30,000-M_r C3d fragment,[5] which also remains covalently bound to the target of activation.

1.2. Complement Receptor Type 1 (CR1)

The bound fragments of C3, C3b, iC3b, C3dg, and C3d mediate the binding of complement-coated particles and immune complexes to various cell types involved in immune and inflammatory reactions by interacting with at least three types of receptors (Table I). Complement receptor type 1 (CR1), or the C3b receptor, has primary specificity for the C3c region of C3b, but also binds iC3b and C4b,[7–10] the major cleavage fragment of C4. This receptor is present on erythrocytes, neutrophils, monocytes/macrophages, B cells,[7,8,11] some T cells,[12] mast cells,[13] and glomerular podocytes.[14–16] CR1 has endocytic functions on myelomonocytic cells, a role in clearance of circulating immune complexes on erythrocytes, and possible immunoregulatory effects on B lymphocytes.[17] CR1 is comprised of a single polypeptide chain and has several allotypic forms of 160,000–260,000 M_r, which are expressed in a codominant fashion.[18–21] The number of CR1 expressed by erythrocytes is under genetic control by another autosomal locus with two codominant alleles. Low CR1 expression on erythrocytes has been found with high frequency in patients with systemic lupus erythematosus and in their unaffected family members.[22,23] Loss or degradation of receptor due to the pathological process of the disease also may contribute to the observed low receptor number on patients' cells.[24,25]

1.3. Complement Receptor Type 2 (CR2)

Complement receptor type 2, CR2, is a B-cell-specific receptor with specificity for the d region of C3, which is most exposed in the C3dg and iC3b fragments, but also to a limited extent in C3b.[26–31] CR2 has recently been identified as a 140,000- to 145,000-M_r glycoprotein recognized by the monoclonal antibodies HB-5 and anti-B-2 based, in part, on the capacity of these antibodies to inhibit rosette formation between transformed B-lymphoblastoid cells and sheep erythrocytes coated with C3b, iC3b, and C3d[28–31] (EC3b, EiC3b, and EC3d, respectively). Efficient inhibition of rosette formation by these Mabs required a second, goat anti-mouse antibody.[30,31] The requirement for second antibody, indicating that neither antibody was directed against the ligand binding site of the CR2, probably represented capping of the receptor–MAb complex or greater steric hindrance of the ligand binding region by the polyclonal antibody than was conferred by the monoclonal. In order to prove definitively that the antigen recognized by the HB-5 antibody was CR2 and not simply spatially associated with it, the MAb was used to select the antigen from lysates of receptor-bearing cells and to immobilize it on protein A-bearing *S. aureus* particles.[31] This conferred on these particles the ability to bind C3b, iC3b, and C3d, demonstrating that the antigen recognized by the HB-5 MAb had CR2 function, as will be discussed in Section 2.1.

1.4. Complement Receptor Type 3 (CR3)

Complement receptor type 3, CR3, binds iC3b[9] in a cation-dependent manner, and is expressed by neutrophils, monocytes/macrophages, and large granular lymphocytes having natural killing and antibody-dependent, cell-mediated cytotoxic activity[32] (Table I). Like the binding of C3b-coated complexes by CR1 on myelomonocytic cells, CR3 promotes the phagocytosis of complement-activating complexes by binding iC3b. CR3 is a glycoprotein having two polypeptide chains of 165,000 and 95,000 M_r and has been identified as the membrane antigen termed Mac-1,[33] OKM1,[34] or Mo1.[35] Anti-Mac-1 and anti-Mo1 MAbs were shown to inhibit rosette formation between human monocytes and sheep erythrocytes coated with iC3b.[33,35] In addition, cells from patients genetically deficient in surface expression of Mac-1 and two related antigens had several adherence and phagocyte defects, including the inability to form rosettes with EiC3b (see Springer and Anderson, this volume, Chapter 11). Several MAbs directed against CR3 have been used to immobilize CR3 on protein A-bearing *S. aureus* particles, which conferred on these particles the ability to bind to EiC3b,[34] as will be reviewed in Section 2.2.

1.5. Epstein–Barr Virus Receptor and Its Relationship to CR2

The Epstein–Barr virus is a human herpesvirus that is endemic in all human populations. Of the hematopoietic cells, EBV infects only B lymphocytes, which it immortalizes, and which are the only cells with a receptor for this virus.[36] However, the virus can infect oropharyngeal epithelial cells and, in fact, it is suggested that these cells produce and shed infectious virus, while infected B cells rarely produce virus but do become transformed.[37,38] It has been hypothesized that epithelial cells become infected after fusion with infected B lymphocytes or that they are directly infected *in vivo*,[38] although a virus receptor has not been identified. In 1976, Jondal *et al.*[39] suggested that the B-lymphocyte receptor for EBV (EBVR) was associated with the B-lymphocyte receptor for mouse complement-coated erythrocytes, which was presumed to be the C3d receptor. The evidence was based on coexpression of EBV receptor and the C3d receptor as detected by indirect immunofluorescence for EBV binding and rosette formation with mouse complement-coated erythrocytes for C3d receptors.[39–41] Additionally, EBV was able to block rosette formation between B-lymphoblastoid cell lines and mouse complement-coated erythrocytes, and treatment of lymphoblastoid cells with human C3 plus rabbit anti-C3 and goat anti-rabbit IgG blocked binding of EBV. By indirect fluorescence for EBV and deposited C3 the receptors were also found to cocap[42] and to be removed together in receptor stripping experiments.[43] A linear correlation between complement receptor activity and the ability to absorb EBV by human cell lines was found.[44] Additionally, the expression of both EBVR and complement receptors was induced by theophylline treatment of human undifferentiated lymphomas.[45] However, due to the ambiguities in rosetting assays for complement receptors and the indirect nature of assays used for virus receptors, this has remained a controversial issue. Furthermore, within the literature there are conflicting data, since B lymphocytes from patients with common variable agammaglobulinemia are not transformed with EBV, yet their lymphocytes do contain cells capable of forming rosettes with C3b-coated and mouse complement-coated erythrocytes.[46] Furthermore, mouse–human hybrids of B-lymphoblastoid cell lines have been analyzed that appear to express EBVR, but do not form rosettes with C3d-coated erythrocytes.[47]

The identification of CR2 and the availability of specific antibody probes for the two complement receptors expressed on B lymphocytes, CR1 and CR2, allowed reassessment of the relationship among CR1, CR2, and EBVR.[48] The relative expression of EBVR, CR1, and CR2 on human lymphoblastoid cell lines was determined by cytofluorographic analysis of cells stained with directly fluoresceinated EBV or with polyclonal anti-CR1 or monoclonal anti-CR2 (HB-5) followed by fluoresceinated second antibody. The rank order of expression of EBVR and CR2 by the cell lines was identical, while two lines positive for EBVR did not express CR1. A cell line that expresses CR1, CR2, and EBVR was treated with polyclonal anti-CR1 or monoclonal anti-CR2 plus the appropriate second antibody to determine if uptake of virus could be inhibited. Treatment with anti-CR2 plus second antibody, but not anti-CR1 plus second antibody, completely blocked binding of fluoresceinated EBV, suggesting that the virus was binding to CR2. The requirement for second antibody for blocking of virus uptake suggested that the monoclonal was not directed against the virus binding site. Thus, the same technique used to identify the HB-5 antigen as CR2 could be used to isolate and immobilize the receptor and demonstrate its EBV binding properties.

2. Demonstration of Specificity of Monoclonal Antibody-Immobilized Antigen for Particulate Ligand

2.1. Identification of CR2: Methodology and Results

The ability of E coated with fragments of C3 to adhere to *S. aureus* particles to which the HB-5 antigen had been specifically immunoabsorbed was used to assay for CR2 function of this B-cell protein[31] (Fig. 2). *Staphylococcus aureus* cell wall particles, 3.2×10^7 (Bethesda Research Laboratories), were incubated for 30 min at 0°C with 40 μg of either HB-5 or UPC10 (Bionetics), an irrelevant MAb directed to levan, and were washed three times with phosphate-buffered saline containing 0.5% Nonidet P-40 (BDH), 0.5 mM phenylmethylsulfonyl fluoride, 5 mM diisopropyl fluorophosphate, 0.02% sodium azide, and 0.1% soybean trypsin inhibitor (lysis buffer). Each of the two types of monoclonal antibody bearing *S. aureus* particles was incubated for 90 min at 4°C with lysates of 2×10^7 Raji cells in 0.8 ml of lysis buffer. The *S. aureus* particles were then washed once with lysis buffer, washed three times with Veronal-buffered saline containing 0.1% gelatin (GVB), and assessed for their capacity to form rosettes during incubation of 8×10^6 particles with 5×10^5 E, EC3b, EiC3b, and EC3d, respectively, in 0.05 ml of GVB for 2 hr at 37°C. The adherence of the particles to the cells was assessed by phase contrast microscopy utilizing a Leitz Orthoplan microscope (Fig. 3). Ninety-eight to ninety-nine percent of EC3d and EiC3b were coated with *S. aureus* particles, while 25–40% of EC3b were coated with the particles. There was no adherence of particles to control E, nor did particles primed with control antibody of irrelevant specificity, UPC10, bind to E coated with C3 fragments. Similar results were obtained when the source of CR2 was lysate of B-lymphocyte-enriched peripheral blood mononuclear cells. Because the conditions used for the immunoabsorption of the HB-5 antigen led to the absorption of only one cell surface protein, as determined by immunoprecipitation from ^{125}I-surface-labeled Raji cells,[31] this experiment demonstrated that the HB-5 antigen was CR2.

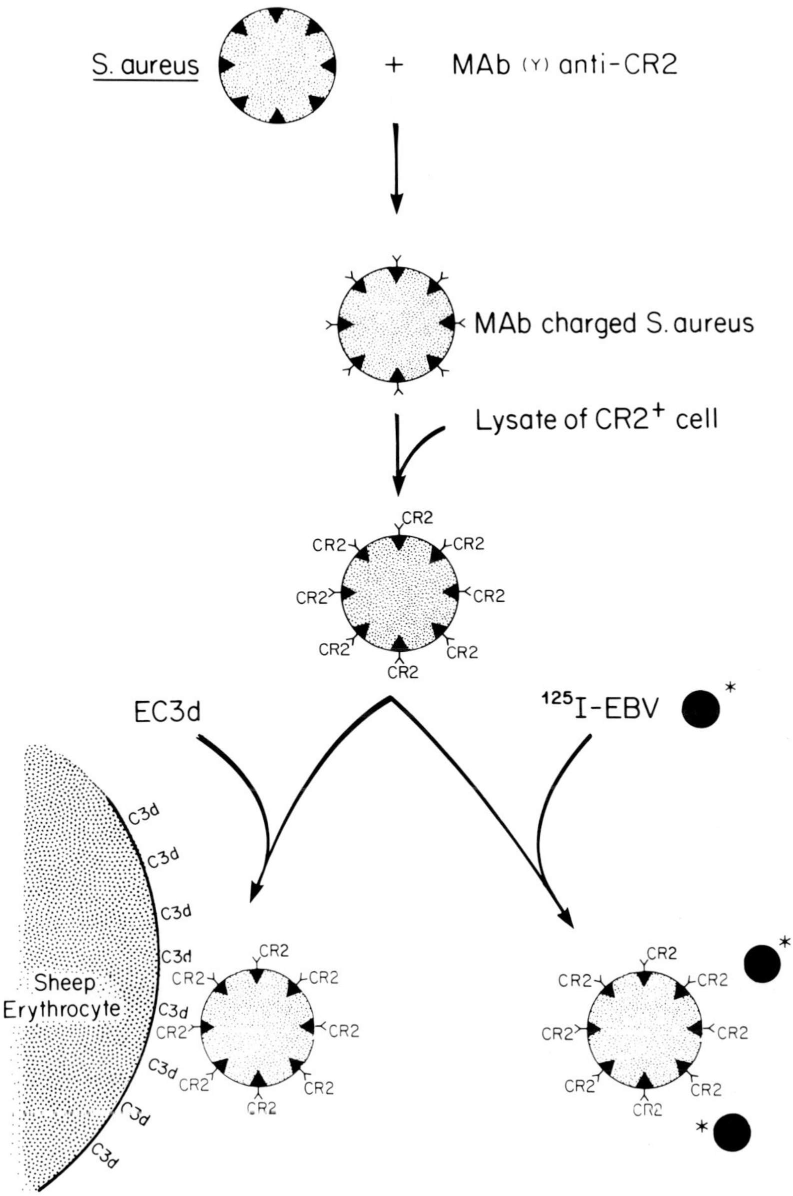

Figure 2. Demonstration of receptor function of immobilized HB-5 antigen. *Staphylococcus aureus* particles were primed with the HB-5 MAb and incubated in a detergent lysate of CR2/EBVR-positive cells. The CR2 function of the HB-5 antigen-bearing particles was assayed by adherence to EC3d (Fig. 3). The EBVR function of the HB-5 antigen-bearing particles was assayed by uptake of ^{125}I-labeled EBV (Fig. 4).

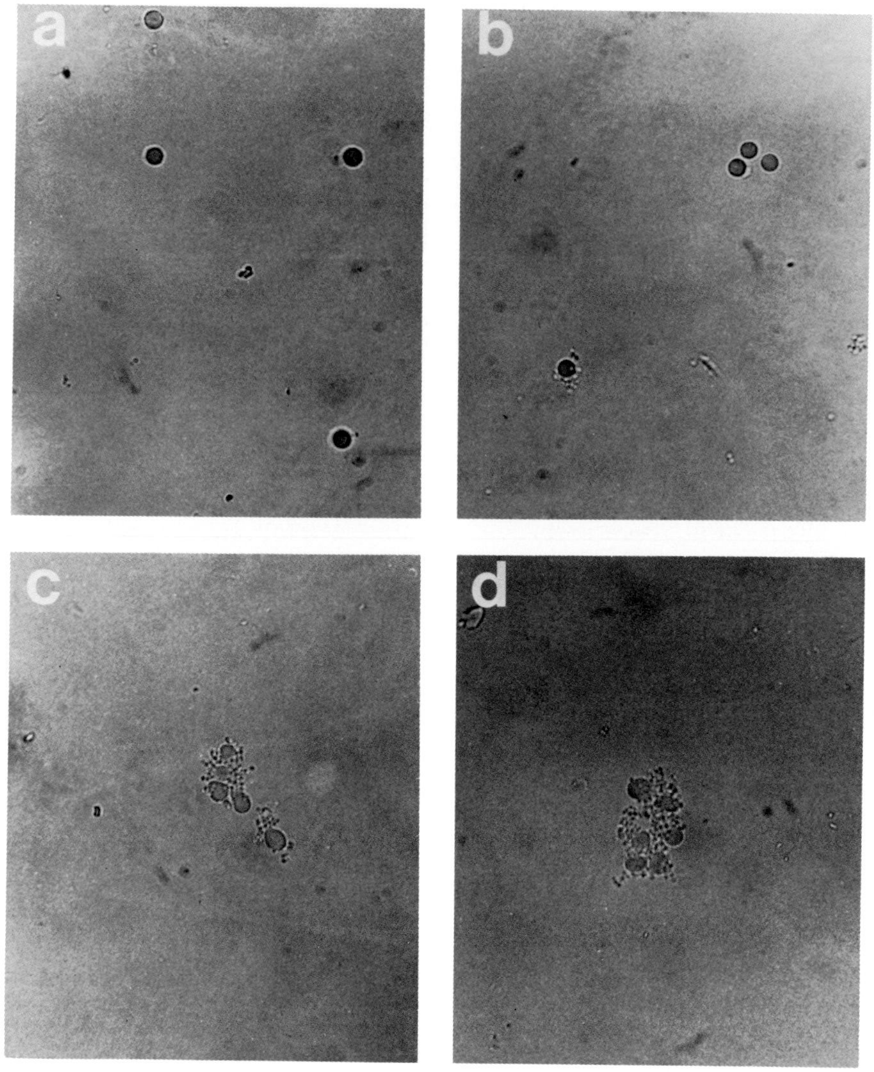

Figure 3. Phase-contrast micrographs of adherence of *S. aureus* particles bearing the HB-5 antigen to (a) E, (b) EC3b, (c) EiC3b, and (d) EC3d. (From Ref. 31.)

2.2. Identification of CR3

The identity of the antigen recognized by the monoclonal antibodies anti-Mac 1, anti-Mo1, and OKM1 as CR3 was confirmed in the same manner as for CR2. The first use of this receptor immobilization assay was to establish that the antibodies OKM1 and IB4, both directed against this antigen, could be used to immobilize the protein on *S. aureus* particles by incubating Mab primed particles with lysate of human macrophages.[34] These particles acquired the ability to adhere weakly to EiC3b, a reaction that reflected CR3 function of the intact cell, since it required divalent cations. Unrelated MAb did not allow immunoabsorption of this function from the macrophage lysate. Furthermore, when a MAb that was very efficient in blocking CR3 function of the intact cell and was suspected to be directed against the ligand binding site was used to prime the S. *aureus* particles under conditions in which immunoprecipitation of the antigen by the MAb could be demonstrated, the particles did not acquire CR3 function. This was further evidence that the MAb was indeed directed against the ligand binding site.

2.3. Properties of the Antibody and the Antigen

For this technique to be applicable in other systems several properties of the monoclonal antibody must be established. There should be some functional data suggesting that the antibody is indeed directed against the relevant receptor. For example, inhibition or stimulation of a receptor-dependent function by the monoclonal antibody in the presence or absence of a second antibody would constitute suggestive evidence for the specificity of the MAb. It is also essential that the MAb not block the ligand binding site, which would preclude its use in the immobilization assay, except as a confirmatory reagent. However, the limited experience with anti-C3 receptor MAbs suggests that most bind to epitopes sufficiently distant from the ligand binding site so that the receptor function of the antigen is preserved.[33–35] An additional requirement for the MAb is that its affinity for the antigen be great enough to immunoprecipitate the protein from a detergent lysate. For example, the anti-Mac 1 MAb, which was raised against a mouse macrophage antigen and cross-reacts with a homologous antigen in humans, blocks rosette formation between human macrophages and EiC3b, but is unable to immunoprecipitate the human protein, and therefore would not be useful in the assay.[32,33] Presumably detergent solubilization of the membrane prevented divalent binding by the antibody that was necessary for low-affinity cross-reactivity. It is not necessary that the MAb bind protein A, since second antibodies are commercially available and the S. *aureus* particles can be primed with an anti-mouse antibody prior to incubation with the MAb. Certain properties of the antigen are also required for a positive result. For example, the membrane protein must retain receptor function after extraction from the membrane. Also, if two polypeptide chains are required for ligand binding, they must be firmly associated such that both are immobilized with the monoclonal.

2.4. Application to Determining Receptor Function When the Purified Ligand Is Available

Whenever there is presumptive evidence identifying an antigen as the receptor for a defined ligand this technique employing monoclonal antibody immobilization of the receptor may be used to confirm the finding. Particularly useful will be situations when a MAb has inhibitory or stimulatory effect on a specific function or ligand binding that is greatly enhanced by or requires the presence of second antibody. This will indicate that the MAb is probably not directed against the ligand binding site of the receptor and can be used to immobilize the protein without blocking its activity. When the ligand is available in purified form it can be conjugated to an insoluble particle to take advantage of the increased avidity of receptor for particles bearing many copies of the ligand. Methods for conjugating the ligand to a sheep erythrocyte include glutaraldehyde[49] and chromic chloride[50] coupling. Results could then be obtained from phase contrast microscopy of adherence by the *S. aureus*–MAb-receptor complexes to the ligand bearing E, much as was done for CR2 and CR3. This approach is applicable when the ligand can readily be purified in large amounts, such as a complement protein, or when the molecule has been generated by recombinant DNA technology and is therefore available in large quantities.

3. Demonstration of Specificity of Monoclonal Antibody-Immobilized Antigen for Soluble Ligand

When the ligand is labile and must be used in soluble form, or when purified ligand is not available, the receptor activity of the antigen immobilized by monoclonal antibody can be assayed by binding of the soluble ligand to the receptor-bearing *S. aureus* particle. The ability of CR2 to bind EBV was confirmed by the binding of purified, ^{125}I-labeled EBV to *S. aureus* to which CR2 had been immobilized by the HB-5 MAb.

3.1. Identification of CR2 as the Epstein–Barr Virus Receptor: Methodology and Results

The binding of purified virus and the HB-5 MAb indicated that the EBV receptor and CR2 were found to be expressed in the same rank order by all human cell lines tested, whereas expression of CR1 and HLA were not correlated with EBV receptor expression.[48] The anti-CR2 MAb HB-5 was also found to block uptake by the human B-lymphoblastoid cell line SB of directly fluoresceinated EBV. This inhibition required the presence of a second, goat anti-mouse antibody indicating that the HB-5 did not interact with the EBV binding site of CR2. To assess directly the ability of CR2 to bind EBV, CR2 was immobilized on protein A-bearing *S. aureus* particles with the HB-5 monoclonal, and the binding of soluble ^{125}I-labeled EBV was quantitated[48] (Fig. 2). *Staphylococcus aureus* particles bearing immobilized HB-5 antigen were prepared exactly as described for demonstration of its CR2 function except the cell lysates were of the CR2/EBVR-positive cell line SB or of the CR2/EBVR-negative cell line HSB-2 which is derived from the same individual as SB. The particles

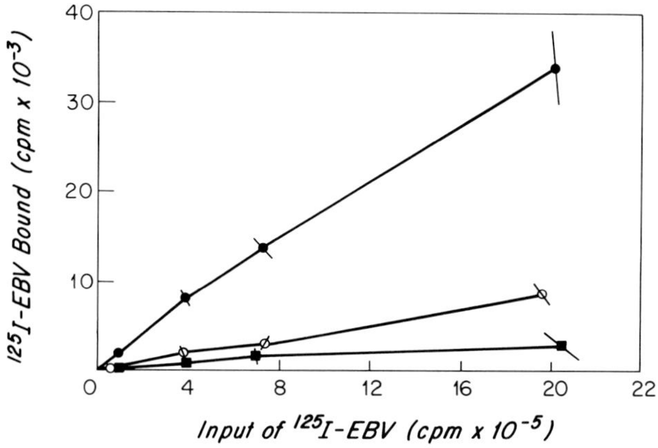

Figure 4. ^{125}I-labeled EBV binding to *S. aureus* particles coated with monoclonal antibody and cell lysate; (●) HB-5, SB lysate; (○) UPC10, SB lysate; (■) HB-5, HSB-2 lysate. Background values determined from binding of ^{125}I-labeled EBV to *S. aureus* particles coated with UPC10 and HSB-2 lysate were subtracted from each sample. (Modified from Ref. 48.)

were washed once with lysis buffer and three times with Hank's balanced salt solution containing 0.1% bovine serum albumin (HBSS-BSA). These conditions led to uptake of only one protein as determined by immunoprecipitation from surface-labeled cells.[48] Binding of EBV was assessed by incubating 3.2×10^7 *S. aureus* particles with increasing increments of ^{125}I-labeled EBV, ranging from 0.2×10^6 to 5×10^6 cpm, in 0.08 ml of HBSS-BSA with 12.5% heat-inactivated human serum for 60 min at 37°C. Duplicate 0.025-ml samples were removed, layered on 0.2 ml of a 3:1 mixture of dibutylphthalate (Eastman) and dinonylphthalate (ICN) in 0.4-ml polypropylene Microfuge tubes, and particles were pelleted by centrifugation at $8000 \times g$ for 90 sec. The tubes were cut and the cell pellets and supernatants were assessed for radioactivity. The technique of centrifugation through oil rapidly separates bound from free ligand and permits detection of low-affinity interactions. Background binding of ^{125}I-EBV was determined by the uptake of virus by particles primed with the irrelevant antibody UPC10 and exposed to lysate from the CR2/EBVR-negative cell line HSB-2. The *S. aureus* particles that were incubated with HB-5 prior to exposure to lysate of the CR2/EBVR-positive SB cells bound 5- to 13-fold more ^{125}I-EBV than did particles primed with irrelevant MAb prior to incubation with receptor containing lysate or particles primed with HB-5 but subsequently incubated with lysate from the receptor-negative HSB-2 cells (Fig. 4). Therefore, the specifically immobilized CR2 bound EBV.

3.2. Application to Determining Receptor Function of Membrane Proteins When Purified Ligand Is Not Available

This technique will be applicable to confirming receptor function in situations previously outlined when the ligand is either too labile to be immobilized, such as an enveloped virus, or when purified ligand is not available. For example, it would be possible to determine if a particular MAb were directed against a receptor for a growth factor by using the MAb to immobilize the putative receptor on *S. aureus* particles and determining if these particles could deplete a crude source of the growth factor. In this way a single membrane protein could be assayed for the ability to bind a given factor. This type of demonstration requires a sensitive assay for the ligand, but does not require that the ligand be purified, radiolabeled, or coupled to a particulate substrate.

4. Summary

A novel technique involving the immobilization of antigens recognized by monoclonal antibodies on protein A-bearing *S. aureus* particles has been used to demonstrate receptor function of two complement receptors, CR2[31] and CR3.[34] This technique has also been used to demonstrate that one of these receptors, CR2, is the B-lymphocyte receptor for Epstein–Barr virus.[48] There is general applicability of this technique for the confirmation of receptor activity of an antigen for which there are preliminary data suggesting this function. Receptor function of the antigen immobilized by monoclonal antibody can be demonstrated using either particulate ligand, as for CR2 and CR3, or soluble ligand, as for EBVR. The general methodology employed is outlined in the following flow chart:

Insolubilized MAb
+
Source of receptor
+
Source of ligand
↓
Demonstration of ligand binding
or Depletion of biological activity

ACKNOWLEDGMENT. This work was supported by Grants AI-07722, AI-10356, AI-17917, AI-06838, AM-05577, and RR-05669 from the National Institutes of Health.

References

1. Law, S. K., and Levine, R. P., 1977, Interaction between the third complement protein and cell surface macromolecules, *Proc. Natl. Acad. Sci. USA* **74**:2701–2705.
2. Tack, B. F., Harrison, R. A., Janatova, J., Thomas, M. L., and Prahl, J. W., 1980, Evidence for presence of an internal thiolester bond in third component of human complement, *Proc. Natl. Acad. Sci. USA* **77**:5764–5768.
3. Pangburn, M. K., and Müller-Eberhard, H. J., 1980, Relation of a putative thiolester bond in C3 to activation of the alternative pathway and the binding of C3b to biological targets of complement, *J. Exp. Med.* **152**:1102–1114.
4. Harrison, R. A., and Lachman, P. J., 1980, Novel cleavage products of the third component of human complement, *Mol. Immunol.* **17**:9–20.

5. Lachmann, P. J., Pangburn, M. K., and Oldroyd, R. G., 1982, Breakdown of C3 after complement activation: Identification of a new fragment, C3g, using monoclonal antibodies, *J. Exp. Med.* **156:**205–216.
6. Ross, G. D., Lambris, J. D., Cain, J. A., and Newman, S., 1982, Generation of three different fragments of bound C3 with purified Factor I or serum. I. Requirements for Factor H vs. CR1 cofactor activity, *J. Immunol.* **129:**2051–2060.
7. Fearon, D. T., 1980, Identification of the membrane glycoprotein that is the C3b receptor of the human erythrocyte, polymorphonuclear leukocyte, B lymphocyte, and monocyte, *J. Exp. Med.* **152:**20–30.
8. Dobson, N. J., Lambris, J. D., and Ross, G. D., 1981, Characteristics of isolated erythrocyte complement receptor type one (CR1, C4b–C3b receptor) and CR1-specific antibodies, *J. Immunol.* **126:**693–698.
9. Ross, G. D., Newman, S. L., Lambris, J. D., Devery-Pocius, J. E., Cain, J. A., and Lachmann, P. J., 1983, Generation of three different fragments of bound C3 with purified Factor I or serum. II. Location of binding sites in the C3 fragments for factors B and H, complement receptors, and bovine conglutinin, *J. Exp. Med.* **158:**334–352.
10. Cooper, N. R., 1969, Immune adherence by the fourth component of complement, *Science* **165:**396–398.
11. Tedder, T. F., Fearon, D. T., Gartland, G. L., and Cooper, M. D., 1983, Expression of C3b receptors on human B cells and myelomonocytic cells but not on natural killer cells, *J. Immunol.* **120:**1668–1673.
12. Wilson, J. G., Tedder, T. F., and Fearon, D. T., 1983, Characterization of human T lymphocytes that express the C3b receptor, *J. Immunol.* **131:**684–689.
13. Vranian, G., Jr., Conrad, D. H., and Ruddy, S., 1981, Specificity of C3 receptors that mediate phagocytosis by rat peritoneal mast cells, *J. Immunol.* **126:**2302–2306.
14. Gelfand, M. C., Frank, M. M., and Green, I., 1975, A receptor for the third component of complement in the human renal glomerulus, *J. Exp. Med.* **142:**1029–1034.
15. Kazatchkine, M. D., Fearon, D. T., Appay, M. D., Mandet, C., and Bariety, J., 1982, Immunohistochemical study of the human glomerular C3b receptor in normal kidney and in seventy-five cases of renal diseases, *J. Clin. Invest.* **69:**900–912.
16. Emancipator, S. N., Iida, K., Nussenzweig, V., and Gallo, G. R., 1983, Monoclonal antibodies to human complement receptor (CR1) detect defects in glomerular diseases, *Clin. Immunol. Immunopathol.* **27:**170–175.
17. Daha, M. R., Bloem, A. C., and Ballieux, R. E., 1984, Immunoglobulin production by human peripheral lymphocytes induced by anti-C3 receptor antibodies, *J. Immunol.* **132:**1197–1201.
18. Wong, W. W., Wilson, J. G., and Fearon, D. T., 1983, Genetic regulation of a structural polymorphism of human C3b receptor, *J. Clin. Invest.* **72:**685–693.
19. Dykman, T. R., Cole, J. L., Iida, K., and Atkinson, J. P., 1983, Polymorphism of human erythrocyte C3b/C4b receptor, *Proc. Natl. Acad. Sci. USA* **80:**1698–1702.
20. Dykman, T. R., Hatch, J. A., and Atkinson, J. P., 1984, Polymorphism of the human C3b/C4b receptor. Identification of a third allele and analysis of receptor phenotypes in families and patients with systemic lupus erythematosus, *J. Exp. Med.* **159:**691–703.
21. Dykman, T., Hatch, J., Aqua, M., and Atkinson, J., 1984, Identification of novel C3b/C4b receptor (C3bR) phenotypes in normal individuals and SLE, *Fed. Proc.* **43:**1454 (abstract).
22. Miyakawa, Y., Yamada, A., Kosaka, K., Tsuda, F., Kosuga, E., and Mayumi, M., 1981, Defective immune adherence (C3b) receptor on erythrocytes of patients with systemic lupus erythematosus, *Lancet* **2:**493–497.
23. Wilson, J. G., Wong, W. W., Schur, P. H., and Fearon, D. T., 1982, Mode of inheritance of decreased C3b receptors on erythrocytes of patients with systemic lupus erythematosus, *N. Engl. J. Med.* **307:**981–986.
24. Iida, K., Mornaghi, R., and Nussenzweig, V., 1982, Complement receptor (CR1) deficiency in erythrocytes from patients with systemic lupus erythematosus, *J. Exp. Med.* **155:**1427–1438.
25. Ross, G. D., Walport, M. J., Parker, C. J., Lentine, A. F., Fuller, C. R., Yount, W. J., Myones, B. L., Winfield, J. B., and Lachmann, P. J., 1984, Acquired loss of erythrocyte (E) CR1 (C3b-receptor)

in systemic lupus erythematosus and other diseases with autoantibodies and/or complement activation, *Arthritis Rheum.* **27:**S28.

26. Eden, A., Miller, G. W., and Nussenzweig, V., 1973, Human lymphocytes bear membrane receptors for C3b and C3d, *J. Clin. Invest.* **52:**3239–3242.
27. Ross, G. D., Polley, M. J., Rabellino, E. M., and Grey, H. M., 1973, Two different complement receptors on human lymphocytes; one specific for C3b and one specific for C3b inactivator-cleaved C3b, *J. Exp. Med.* **138:**798–811.
28. Nadler, L. M., Stashenko, P., Hardy, R., van Agthoven, A., Terhorst, C., and Schlossman, S. F., 1981, Characterization of a human B cell-specific antigen (B2) distinct from B1, *J. Immunol.* **126:**1941–1947.
29. Tedder, T. F., Clement, L. T., and Cooper, M. D., 1984, Expression of C3d receptors during human B cell differentiation: Immunofluorescence analysis with the HB-5 monoclonal antibody, *J. Immunol.* **133:**678–683.
30. Iida, K., Nadler, L., and Nussenzweig, V., 1983, Identification of the membrane receptor for the complement fragment C3d by means of a monoclonal antibody, *J. Exp. Med.* **158:**1021–1033.
31. Weis, J. J., Tedder, T. F., and Fearon, D. T., 1984, Identification of a 145,000 M_r membrane protein as the C3d receptor (CR2) of human B lymphocytes, *Proc. Natl. Acad. Sci. USA* **81:**881–885.
32. Ault, K. A., and Springer, T. A., 1981, Cross-reaction of a rat anti-mouse phagocyte-specific monoclonal antibody (anti-Mac-1) with human monocytes and natural killer cells, *J. Immunol.* **126:**359–364.
33. Beller, D. I., Springer, T. A., and Schreiber, R. D., 1982, Anti-Mac-1 selectively inhibits the mouse and human type three complement receptor, *J. Exp. Med.* **156:**1000–1009.
34. Wright, S. D., Rao, P. E., Van Voorhis, W. C., Craigmyle, L. S., Iida, K., Talle, M. A., Westberg, E. F., Goldstein, G., and Silverstein, S. C., 1983, Identification of the C3bi receptor of human monocytes and macrophages by using monoclonal antibodies, *Proc. Natl. Acad. Sci. USA* **80:**5699–5703.
35. Arnaout, M. A., Todd, R. F., III, Dana, N., Melamed, J., Schlossman, S. F., and Colten, H. R., 1983, Inhibition of phagocytosis of complement C3- or immunoglobulin G-coated particles and of C3bi binding by monoclonal antibodies to a monocyte-granulocyte membrane glycoprotein (Mo1), *J. Clin. Invest.* **72:**171–179.
36. Jondal, M., and Klein, G., 1973, Surface markers on human B and T lymphocytes. II. Presence of Epstein–Barr virus receptors on B lymphocytes, *J. Exp. Med.* **138:**1365–1378.
37. Sixbey, J. W., Vesterinen, E. H., Nedrud, J. G., Raab-Traub, N., Walton, L. A., and Pagano, J. S., 1983, Replication of Epstein–Barr virus in human epithelial cells infected *in vitro, Nature* **306:**480–483.
38. Sixbey, J. W., Nedrud, J. G., Raab-Traub, N., Hanes, R. A., and Pagano, J. S., 1984, Epstein–Barr virus replication in oropharyngeal epithelial cells, *N. Engl. J. Med.* **310:**1225–1230.
39. Jondal, M., Klein, G., Oldstone, M. B. A., Bokish, V., and Yefenof, E., 1976, Surface markers on human B and T lymphocytes. VIII. Association between complement and Epstein–Barr virus receptors on human lymphoid cells, *Scand. J. Immunol.* **5:**401–410.
40. Einhorn, L., Steinitz, M., Yefenof, E., Ernberg, I., Bakacs, T., and Klein, G., 1978, Epstein–Barr virus (EBV) receptors, complement receptors and EBV infectibility of different lymphocyte fractions of human peripheral blood. II. Epstein–Barr virus studies, *Cell Immunol.* **35:**43–58.
41. Yefenof, E., Klein, G., and Kvarnung, K., 1977, Relationships between complement activation, complement binding, and EBV absorption by human hematopoietic cell lines, *Cell. Immunol.* **31:**225–233.
42. Yefenof, E., Klein, G., Jondal, M., and Oldstone, M. B. A., 1976, Surface markers on human B- and T-lymphocytes. IX. Two-color immunofluorescence studies on the association between EBV receptors and complement receptors on the surface of lymphoid cell lines, *Int. J. Cancer* **17:**693–700.
43. Yefenof, E., and Klein, G., 1977, Membrane receptor stripping confirms the association between EBV receptors and complement receptors on the surface of human B lymphoma lines, *Int. J. Cancer* **20:**347–352.

44. Jonsson, V., Wells, A., and Klein, G., 1982, Receptors for the complement C3d component and the Epstein–Barr virus are quantitatively coexpressed on a series of B-cell lines and their derived somatic cell hybrids, *Cell Immunol.* **72**:263–276.

45. Magrath, I., Freeman, C., Santaella, M., Gadek, J., Frank, M., Spiegel, R., and Novikovs, L., 1981, Induction of complement receptor expression in cell lines derived from human undifferentiated lymphomas. II. Characterization of the induced complement receptors and demonstration of simultaneous induction of EBV receptor, *J. Immunol.* **127**:1039–1043.

46. Schwaber, J. F., Klein, G., Ernberg, I., Rosen, A., Lazarus, H., and Rosen, F. S., 1980, Deficiency of Epstein–Barr virus (EBV) receptors on B lymphocytes from certain patients with common varied agammaglobulinemia, *J. Immunol.* **124**:2191–2196.

47. Hutt-Fletcher, L. M., Fowler, E., Lambris, J. D., Feighny, J., Simmons, J. G., and Ross, G. D., 1983, Studies of the Epstein–Barr virus receptor found on Raji cells. II. A comparison of lymphocyte binding sites for Epstein–Barr virus and C3d, *J. Immunol.* **130**:1309–1312.

48. Fingeroth, J. D., Weis, J. J., Tedder, T. F., Strominger, J. L., Biro, P. A., and Fearon, D. T., 1984, Epstein–Barr virus receptor of human B lymphocytes is the C3d receptor CR2, *Proc. Natl. Acad. Sci. USA* **81**:4510–4514.

49. Lemieux, S., Avrameas, S., and Bussard, A. E., 1974, Local haemolysis plaque assay using a new method of coupling antigens on sheep erythrocytes by glutaraldehyde, *Immunochemistry* **11**:261–269.

50. Poston, R. N., 1974, A buffered chromic chloride method of attaching antigens to red cells: Use in haemagglutination, *J. Immunol. Meth.* **5**:91–102.

Chapter 13

Production of Rat × Mouse Hybridomas for the Study of the Nicotinic Acetylcholine Receptor

SUSAN M. HOCHSCHWENDER, LORENE K. LANGEBERG, DOUGLAS W. SCHNEIDER, and JON M. LINDSTROM

1. Introduction

In this chapter we will discuss methods used in our laboratory for the production of monoclonal antibodies (MAbs) to acetylcholine receptors (AChRs) and their use in obtaining information on AChR structure, function, and synthesis, the autoimmune response to AChR, and the identification of putative AChRs in neurons. Space limitations preclude extensive discussion and referencing of work done in other laboratories in this field.

The AChR is an integral membrane protein found in fish electric organs and in the postsynaptic membrane of mammalian skeletal muscle consisting of five subunits with an $\alpha_2\beta\gamma\delta$ stoichiometry (reviewed in Ref. 1). The amino acid sequences of all the subunits of (Torpedo) (see Refs. 2–4 and references therein), the α subunit of calf muscle, and the α subunit of human muscle[5] AChRs have been deduced from the cDNA sequences and are all quite homologous. Calculated molecular weights are α 50,116, β 53,681, γ 56,601, and δ 57,565.[2–4] The α subunits each contain an ACh binding site.[6] Certain snake venom toxins, such as α-bungarotoxin (αBgt), bind specifically to the ACh binding sites with high affinity.

Myasthenia gravis (MG) is characterized by impaired neuromuscular transmission due to antibody-mediated loss of AChR. Autoantibodies appear to act primarily by two mechanisms that increase the rate of AChR destruction. One is antigenic modulation, which is an increase in the normal rate of endocytosis due to antibody cross-linking of AChRs. The other is complement-mediated destruction of the postsynaptic membrane. MG and its animal model induced by immunization with AChR, experimental autoimmune myasthenia gravis (EAMG), have been recently reviewed.[7]

SUSAN M. HOCHSCHWENDER, LORENE K. LANGEBERG, DOUGLAS W. SCHNEIDER, and JON M. LINDSTROM • Receptor Biology Laboratory, Salk Institute, San Diego, California 92138.

A number of laboratories have produced MAbs to fish electric organ AChRs[8–15] and mammalian muscle AChRs.[16–18] We have produced a library of more than 200 MAbs to AChR from *Torpedo*[13] and *Electrophorus* organ,[14] human muscle,[18] fetal bovine muscle,[19] purified *Torpedo* AChR subunits,[20] AChR-rich membrane vesicles (unpublished results), and synthetic peptides.[21]

2. Production of Rat Monoclonal Antibodies

2.1. Immunization

AChR from electric organs or muscle can be purified by affinity chromatography.[22] Denatured subunits of *Torpedo californica* AChR are purified by electrophoresis.[23] To produce MAbs against the denatured subunits of muscle AChR, we immunize with AChR that has been denatured by boiling for 2 min in 2% sodium dodecyl sulfate (SDS). Complete denaturation is crucial, since a large fraction of MAbs against native AChR are directed against a single region,[13,14] which we call the main immunogenic region (MIR). Synthetic peptides to be used as immunogen are coupled to a carrier protein such as serum albumin or keyhole limpet hemocyanin.[21,24]

We have varied many parameters of immunization, but not systematically. The majority of rats used to produce MAbs are Lewis rats, but Sprague-Dawley and Lou rats have also been immunized successfully. Generally, several rats are immunized. The rats with the highest titers are used for the fusion; the rest are bled out for antisera. Our most productive fusions have occurred with spleen cells from rats without clinical signs of EAMG, with titers greater than 1×10^{-7} M, after three immunizations over the course of 1 month, and with the final boost given 3 days prior to the fusion. We have had many successful fusions that did not meet all of these criteria. For example, we obtained several antipeptide MAbs using rats with titers of 1×10^{-9} M or less (unpublished results). Immunogen doses range from 5 to 100 μg in 200–600 μl of complete Freund's adjuvant[22] and have been delivered by a variety of methods: subcutaneous, intradermal, intraperitoneal, and in foot pads. For a discussion of immunization schedules, see Refs. 19 and 22 and references therein.

2.2. Fusion and Direct Cloning in Soft Agarose

Most of our hybridoma lines are from fusions of rat spleen cells with the mouse myeloma S194/5.XXO.BU.1 (S194).[25] This cell line has several advantages. It does not secrete IgG, and it grows both in suspension and in soft agarose. The major disadvantage is that we cannot inexpensively grow up antibodies in ascites. We have also fused rat spleen cells to P3-NS1/1-Ag4-1,[26] a mouse myeloma, and 210.RCY3.Ag1.2.3 (Y3),[27] a Lou rat myeloma. The Y3 myeloma has the advantage that the hybridomas from Lou rat spleen cells fused with it could be grown in ascites. There are several disadvantages: the myeloma secretes κ chains, hybridomas cannot be cloned in soft agar, and feeder cells are necessary.

Since S194 is used in most of our fusions, only methods applicable to S194 will be discussed. Methods for the other two myelomas have been described.[19,22] S194 myeloma cells are thawed about 2 weeks prior to the fusion and are maintained in logarithmic growth in either Dulbecco's modified Eagle's medium (DMEM) or Iscove's modified DMEM supplemented with 10% horse serum, 2×10^{-3} M glutamine, and 1×10^{-4} M 2-mercaptoethanol. Five days before the fusion they are cultured in the presence of 1×10^{-4} M bromodeoxyuridine, a thymidine analogue. Bromodeoxyuridine is light-sensitive, so all manipulations are done in minimal light. Stock solutions of 100× bromodeoxyuridine are prepared in 0.15 M sodium chloride, sterile filtered, and stored in foil-wrapped aliquots at −20°C.

The fusion procedure[19,22] follows the basic principles of Köhler and Milstein.[28] All instruments and reagents are prepared before the day of the fusion. The following reagents are required: 20× hypoxanthine (H), 50× thymidine and aminopterin (TA), and 20× hypoxanthine and thymidine (HT). These are prepared, sterile filtered, aliquoted, and stored frozen at −20°C. Media are prepared: 1× Iscove's HAT,* 2× Iscove's HAT, 3% Sea Prep 15/45 agarose,[29] Iscove's DMEM with 2% horse serum, and Iscove's DMEM. Twenty Costar (cat. no. 3524) 24-well plates per fusion are numbered, filled with Iscove's 2% horse serum, and stored overnight in a 37°C, 10% CO_2 incubator. Preincubation of the plates reduces cytotoxicity.

The following are prepared the day of the fusion. Polyethylene glycol (PEG) is autoclaved for 15 min, then cooled to 37°C, and Iscove's DMEM and dimethylsulfoxide are added at the following ratio, PEG:Iscove's:dimethylsulfoxide 1:0.9:0.1 (w/v/v). In the past we have used BDH 1500 PEG, but recently changed to Merck 4000 GK,[30] since in our system it seems to give a slightly higher fusion efficiency. Prepare HAT-agarose† and maintain at 37°C. In the past we used Difco Bacto agar, which is difficult to use because it gels at about 35°C. The one disadvantage to the Sea Prep agarose, which gels at 15°C, is that cell colonies are very compact and more difficult to see than colonies in Difco Bacto agar. Completely aspirate the medium from the 24-well plates and dispense approximately 200 μl HAT-agarose per well (two drops from a 10-ml shortie glass pipette). Place the plates on trays of ice to solidify the agarose. Store the plates in a 37°C, 10% CO_2 incubator.

Rats are sacrificed and the spleens collected under sterile conditions. We have used lymphocyte-to-myeloma ratios varying from 2:1 to 10:1 successfully. Generally, 1×10^8 lymphocytes (half a rat spleen) and 5×10^7 S194 myeloma cells are mixed in a 50-ml centrifuge tube and centrifuged 7 min at

* 1× Iscove's HAT: Iscove's DMEM, 1×10^{-4} M hypoxanthine, 8×10^{-7} M aminopterin, 1.6×10^{-5} M thymidine, 10% serum, 2×10^{-3} M glutamine, 1×10^{-4} M 2-mercaptoethanol.

† HAT-agarose: 50% 2× Iscove's HAT, 50% 3% Sea Prep 15/45 agarose, Iscove's 1% (Iscove's DMEM, 2×10^{-3} M glutamine, 1×10^{-4} M 2-mercaptoethanol, 1% fetal bovine serum, 10 μg/ml insulin, 10 μg/ml transferrin).

2000 rpm in a clinical centrifuge. The supernatant is aspirated and the tube tapped to loosen the pellet. The following procedure is done in a 37°C water bath and timing is critical. Add 1 ml of 37°C PEG solution dropwise over 1 min with shaking, shake 1 min, and then add 1 ml of 37°C Iscove's DMEM over 1 min with gentle shaking. Twenty milliliters of Iscove's DMEM is added over 8 min with shaking. Allow the fusion mix to stand 5 min, then centrifuge for 7 min at 2000 rpm. Aspirate the supernatant and resuspend the pellet in 1 ml of 1× Iscove's HAT, and clone in soft agarose.

Mix 500 μl of cell suspension per 100-ml bottle of HAT-agarose, then dispense approximately 300 μl (three drops from a glass 10-ml shortie pipette) per well of a 24-well plate with agarose base prepared earlier. Two 100-ml bottles of HAT-agarose cell suspension will cover 24–25 24-well plates. Place the plates on trays of ice until the agarose solidifies, then overlay with 0.5 ml 1× Iscove's HAT. The cells are maintained in a humidified 37°C, 10% CO_2 incubator.

Four to five days after the fusion add 0.5–1 ml of 1× Iscove's HAT. Starting with the following week, change the medium two times per week. The medium has to be aspirated carefully. The best approach we have found is to use a Pasteur pipette with a 90° bend in the tip and aspirate under reduced vacuum, then carefully replace with fresh medium. A successful fusion will produce 20–40 colonies per well.

Screening assays are done 2–3 weeks postfusion. The time of the screening depends on the size of the colonies, but is performed 3 days after a medium change. Screening assays will be discussed in Section 2.3. At this stage, start replacing medium with 1× Iscove's HT.

Colonies from wells containing antibody of interest are individually picked with sterile, plugged Pasteur pipettes and transferred to 0.2-ml wells of 96-well plates containing 50–100 μl of medium. The colonies are disrupted by gentle pipetting and a medium control well is created prior to picking the colonies. Continue maintenance of the 24-well plates. The medium in the 96-well plates, both the control and cell containing wells, is changed two times the next day. Generally, 3 days later the supernatants are assayed for specific antibody. If no wells are positive, go back to the original well in the 24-well plate and repeat the procedure. Cells in wells containing antibody of interest are cultured and expanded to 48-, then 24-, then 6-well plates. As soon as possible, freeze at least three 1-ml vials of 1×10^7 cells/ml and reclone.

Recloning is done in soft agarose. Three percent Sea Prep 15/45 agarose is mixed with an equal volume of 2× Iscove's DMEM containing 2× concentrations of serum, glutamine, and 2-mercaptoethanol. Dispense 1.4 ml Iscove's agarose into the first well of a 24-well tissue culture plate, dispense 0.4 ml into the next nine wells, and leave wells 11 and 12 empty. Repeat the procedure for the next 12 wells. Add approximately 300 cells to the first well, pipette up and down to mix, transfer 1 ml to the next well, mix, and continue to serially dilute the rest of the wells; split the last milliliter of suspension between wells 11 and 12. Aspirate any air bubbles. Agarose is solidifed on trays of ice. Overlay with medium and change medium as described for direct cloning. After about

2 weeks, colonies should be visible to the eye. If there are no colonies, repeat the procedure starting with 1000 cells. Screen supernatants for antibody. Transfer colonies from one or two positive wells containing the least number of colonies to a 96-well plate. At this point, cells are weaned into our mass culturing medium as discussed in Section 2.4. The cell culture supernatants are assayed and a clone is selected for mass culture.

2.3. Screening Assays

Because making MAbs is very labor-intensive, we try to refine our screening assays so that desirable hybridomas are identified at an early stage. The initial screening assays should be simple. After the number of wells of potential interest is reduced, a number of assays can be performed. Appropriate selection of reagent concentrations can select for affinity. Many of the assays discussed in Section 3 are applicable screening assays at this stage. Before a specific property is assigned to MAb, it is usually confirmed by several different assays, because every type of assay has its biases and limitations.

Radioimmunoassays have been described in detail.[19,22] AChR labeled with ^{125}I-αBgt is incubated with cell culture supernatant in 96-well polyvinylchloride plates (Cat. no. 1-220-25B, Dynatech Laboratories), normal rat serum is added, then goat anti-rat immunoglobulin G (IgG). The plates are centrifuged and the pellets washed. Radioactivity in the pellets is measured either by cutting and counting individual wells in a gamma counter or by autoradiography. The AChR contains two αBgt binding sites. If AChR is half-labeled with ^{125}IαBgt, MAbs directed against its binding site can be detected.

Whenever possible, we use some type of enzyme-linked immunosorbant assay (ELISA) as our method of screening. The advantages are not having to deal with radioactivity or radioactive waste, long-term stability of the enzyme-labeled protein, and speed. There are, however, limitations. The assay requires fairly pure antigen ($>25\%$). AChR does not bind randomly to the surface of Immulon I plates (Dynatech, flat bottom). Ninety percent of the AChRs may have the same determinants obscured. Binding of an antigen to the plate can cause localized denaturation, which can obscure some determinants,[31] but reveal other determinants.[32] We have several MAbs that appear to fit that description. Some bind to AChR immobilized on plastic, but do not bind to soluble AChR, and some bind to soluble AChR but not immobilized AChR.

Glucose oxidase (Type II, Sigma) is the enzyme label used for ELISA assays. Antiserum is affinity-purified on antigen, which is immobilized on agarose. MAbs are purified as described in Section 2.5. Glucose oxidase is conjugated to antibody by periodate oxidation of the enzyme carbohydrate, followed by Schiff's base formation with the IgG essentially by the method of Harper and Orengo.[33] Glucose oxidase (9–10 mg/ml) and IgG (9–10 mg/ml) are dialyzed against 0.1 M sodium bicarbonate, pH 9.5. Add 0.1 M sodium metaperiodate in distilled water to the glucose oxidase so that the final concentration is 0.029 M and stir in a foil-wrapped tube at room temperature for 3 hr. Add an amount of IgG equal (by weight) to the glucose oxidase and 24% PEG 6000 to a final concentration of 5.7%. Stir for 3 hr at room temperature. Add 5 mg/ml sodium borohydride in 0.01 M sodium hydroxide so that the final concentration is 8.7 mM. Stir 30 min and add threefold more sodium borohydride. Stir for 1 hr. The conjugate is dialyzed against 0.01 M sodium phosphate, 0.1 M sodium chloride, 0.01 M sodium azide, pH 7.4 (PBS + azide). Then unconjugated enzyme is removed by gel filtration on an Ultragel ACA 34 column. Fractions are monitored for absorbance at 280 nm and for enzyme activity. The conjugate is concentrated to 10 mg/ml and stored at −20°C in 50% glycerol (v/v). Enzyme activity is detected by measuring the 414-nm absorbance at 1.5 min after mixing 600 μl of substrate with 400 μl of a 1/200 dilution of fraction. The reaction is stopped with 150 μl of 1 N sulfuric acid. No change in 414-nm absorbance is detected for up to 15 min post-sulfuric acid addition. The substrate is the same used in our ELISA and for one plate consists of 18 ml PBS, 3 mg 2,2′-azino-di-[3-ethylbenzthiazoline sulfonate] (Boehringer Mannheim), 2.25 ml 18% glucose, and 150 μl of 1 mg/ml horseradish peroxidase (SIGMA, Type VI.)[34] The glucose must be allowed to stand at room temperature to allow for mutarotation to the β-d isomer. If the horseradish peroxidase is greater than 300 U/mg, we decrease the concentration to about 275 U/ml.

The screening assay is as follows. Antigen is diluted to 2×10^{-8} M (for intact AChR, units are moles of αBgt binding sites per liter) in 0.01 M sodium bicarbonate, pH 9.5, 50 μl is added per well to Immulon 1 flat-bottom plates (Dynatech), and the plate is shaken overnight at 4°C. The plate is warmed to room temperature and washed three times with 200 μl/well PBS-Tween-BSA.* One of the washes is allowed to stand in the wells for 20 min to block any protein binding sites on the plastic. Fifty microliters of cell culture supernatant is incubated with shaking for 4 hr at room temperature or overnight at 4°C. After washing the wells three times with PBS-Tween-BSA, 50 μl of the appropriate dilution of a 1:1 mix of glucose oxidase–goat anti-rat immunoglobulin and glucose oxidase–MAR 18.5 is added per well and shaken at room temperature for 2 hr. MAR 18.5 is a mouse anti-rat κ chain MAb[35] and was a gift from Drs. L. Lanier and G. Gutman. The wells are washed four times with PBS-Tween-BSA and 200 μl of substrate is added per well. Absorbance at 410 nm is read with a Dynatech Minireader II microtiter plate reader.

2.4. *In Vitro* Large-Scale Monoclonal Antibody Production

After a hybridoma has been selected and recloned, it is grown in large amounts for stock. Since these MAbs are from rat × mouse hybridomas, production in ascites is not economically practical. A number of laboratories have developed serum-free media,[36–39] which are generally less expensive than serum-containing medium and the MAb purification is easier. We tried three

* PBS-Tween-BSA: 0.01 M sodium phosphate, 0.1 M sodium chloride, 0.01 M sodium azide, pH 7.4, 5% Tween 20, 5 mg/ml bovine serum albumin.

or four serum-free media, but none worked for all of our hybridoma lines. We use Iscove's DMEM (powder mix, Irvine Scientific), 2×10^{-3} M glutamine, 1×10^{-4} M 2-mercaptoethanol, 1% fetal bovine serum, 10 μg/ml insulin (bovine, Sigma), 10 μg/ml transferrin (human, Sigma), and antibiotics and antimycotics (Iscove's 1%).* Although this is not serum-free, the low serum content has many of the same advantages. Both rat × S194 hybridomas and rat × Y3 hybridomas are productive in the medium with tissue culture supernatant titers ranging from 1×10^{-8} to 2×10^{-6} M.

Many times we need relatively large amounts of MAb, 100–1000 mg. The approach taken by Cleveland *et al.*[39] is quite useful. The rat × S194 hybridomas grow in suspension, but will lightly adhere to plastic. Density enhances binding to a point, and then limits binding. Cells are grown in Iscove's 1% in Falcon T175 flasks. Every few days the cell culture supernatant is decanted and fresh medium added. We have cultured some hybridoma lines for 2 months without loss of MAb production, but MAb production should be monitored, since this system has the potential for selecting nonproducing hybridomas. The cells are centrifuged out of the supernatant and the supernatant is concentrated under positive nitrogen pressure in an Amicon stirred cell. MAb is partially purified and concentrated by 18% sodium sulfate fractionation, producing 10–15 mg/ml antibody that is 50–90% of the total protein. The major contaminants are serum albumin and a protein with a molecular weight of about 60,000.

2.5. Monoclonal Antibody Purification

For many appliations, MAbs are needed at purities in excess of 95%. Each MAb has unique biochemical properties, which influence its purification. A good first step is gel filtration on Sephacryl S-300. Ultragel ACA 34 and 44 also work well. A second step is chromatography on DEAE affigel Blue.[40] Generally, the MAb will elute from the column in less than 100 mM sodium chloride. One complicating factor is that some of the MAbs have very reactive sulfhydryls and form covalent complexes with the serum albumin. This has also been observed with human immunoglobulins.[41]

Another approach to purifying MAbs is affinity purification on anti-rat IgG columns. The major disadvantage is that the denaturing conditions required to break the MAb–anti-MAb interaction can denature a large fraction of MAb.

2.6. Preparation and Purification of Monoclonal Antibody Fragments

At times it is useful to have univalent MAb or MAb activity without the interactions that occur with the Fc region. There are papain cleavage sites in the hinge region of the heavy chain of IgG that when split produce Fab and Fc

* Composition given in footnote specifying HAT-agarose.

fragments. The procedure discussed by Mage[42] for the production and purification of Fab fragments has worked consistently with our MAbs of IgG class.

Production of Fab_2 fragments can be accomplished using pepsin[43] or *Staphylococcus aureus* V8 proteinase.[44] We use pepsin and, unlike the Fab production, have found no one set of reaction conditions for all of our MAbs. Usually a series of small-scale digestions varying pH, enzyme concentration, and reaction time is used to determine optimal conditions. If the MAb binds to protein A, protein A–Sepharose can be used to separate intact MAb from Fab_2. Gel filtration on an Ultragel ACA 44 column is used to purify Fab_2.

3. Characterization of Monoclonal Antibodies and Specificity Determination

Bazin *et al.*[45] identified and described the following rat immunoglobulin classes and subclasses: IgM, IgA, IgE, IgG_1, IgG_{2a}, IgG_{2b}, IgG_{2c}. Our collection of MAbs are mostly IgM, IgG1, IgG_{2a}, IgG_{2b}, and one IgG_{2c}. The IgM subclass is easily recognized by its molecular weight. The rest are identified by either radial immunodiffusion or radioimmunoassay using subclass typing sera purchased from Miles. Antisubclass MAbs are available through Boehringer Mannheim, and we are currently looking at their use as enzyme-labeled reagents to determine MAb subclass by ELISA.

A large percentage of rat immunoglobulins do not bind to staphylococcal protein A.[46] Of the 135 MAbs we have tested, 28 bind well to protein A. (Refs. 14 and 18; S. Tzartos and J. Lindstrom, unpublished results; S. Hochschwender and J. Lindstrom, unpublished results). These are mostly IgG_1, but a few are IgM, IgG_{2a}, and IgG_{2b}, which is in agreement with Medgyesi *et al.*[46] Another 59 show limited binding, that is, between 10 and 90% of the MAbs bind to protein A. Of these, IgG_1 is the predominant subclass. Forty-eight of our MAbs do not bind protein A (Pansorbin, Calbiochem-Behring) at all.

An ELISA assay has been used for determining subunit specificity of our MAbs. Electrophoretically purified subunits are bound to the wells. Figure 1 illustrates the data and describes the method.

Subunit determination by radioimmunoassay has been discussed in detail,[19,22] so will be described only briefly here. Test MAb is incubated with either ^{125}I-labeled SDS denatured AChR or purified subunits.[22] Then MAbs bound to ^{125}I subunits are precipitated with goat anti-rat IgG agarose. After washing, MAb and ^{125}I subunit are eluted, electrophoresed, and the ^{125}I subunit identified by autoradiography. This assay is limited to MAbs that bind to denatured subunits.

Competitive binding assays are used to determine subunit specificity of MAbs that do not bind to denatured AChR.[14,19,22] These assays also are used to determine if two mAbs bind to the same region. AChR is immobilized on either agarose or toxin–agarose, then saturated with protecting MAb of known specificity. Unbound MAb is washed off, and test MAb is incubated with an

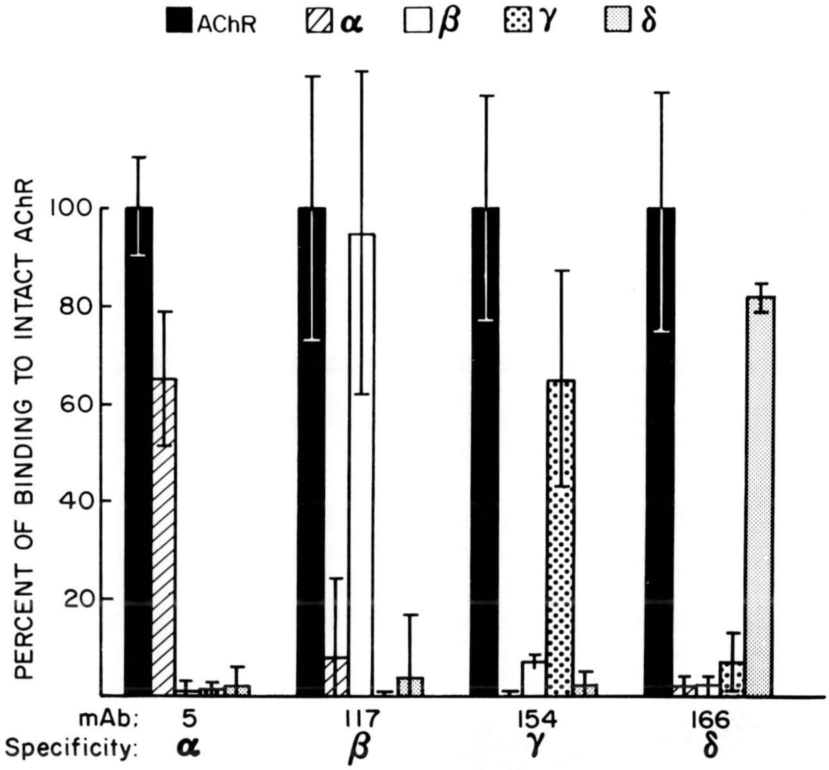

Figure 1. Subunits of *Torpedo* AChR were diluted into 0.01 M sodium bicarbonate, pH 9.5, at concentrations such that 50 μl would bind 0.2×10^{-12} mole per well on Immulon Substrate polystyrene ELISA plates (Dynatech, no longer available): $\alpha = 9.98 \times 10^{-9}$ M, $\beta = 9.91 \times 10^{-9}$ M, $\gamma = 9.92 \times 10^{-9}$ M, $\delta = 1.98 \times 10^{-8}$ M, *Torpedo* acetylcholine receptor $= 4.04 \times 10^{-8}$ M. Subunits, 50 μl, were dried on the microtiter plate wells by vacuum over Drierite. The plates were washed three times with 200 μl PBS-Tween-BSA, with the last wash left in the wells for 15 min to block any protein binding sites. Fifty microliters of 4.0×10^{-9} M MAb was incubated per well for 2 hr at room temperature. After three washes with 200 μl PBS-Tween-BSA, 50μl glucose oxidase goat anti-rat immunoglobulin was added per well and incubated 1 hr at room temperature. Enzyme substrate (see Section 2.3) was added and absorbance at 414 nm read using a Titertek Multiskan (Flow Laboratories).

equimolar amount of AChR in the conjugate. The suspension is centrifuged and the anti-AChR titer of the supernatant is determined.

The most convenient method for measuring MAb cross-reactivity with AChR of different species is determination of the relative titers by radioimmunoassay. Several dilutions of test MAb are incubated with an excess of ^{125}I-αBgt-labeled AChR. Normal rat serum is added and the MAb–^{125}-I-αBgt AChR complexes are precipitated with goat anti-rat IgG. The majority of our species cross-reactive MAbs are directed against the main immunogenic region (Refs.

13, 14, and 18; S. Tzartos, S. Hochschwender, L. Langeberg, P. Vasquez, and J. Lindstrom, unpublished results).

The majority of MAbs obtained from fusions where the rat was immunized with native AChR are directed against a region on the extracellular surface of α subunits that we call the main immunogenic region (MIR).[13,14,18] Since we have quite a few MAbs to this region, screening assays are done as soon as possible to determine if a MAb is against the MIR. If it is, the cells are frozen and no further work is done with them. All of these assays can be applied to epitopes other than the MIR.

Anti-MIR specificity is determined by some type of competition assay with MAb 35, an anti-MIR MAb.[14] If the MAb is cross-reactive with *Torpedo* AChR, its ability to block glucose oxidase–MAb 35 binding to *Torpedo* AChR adsorbed on polystyrene Immulon 1 plates is measured to determine if it is directed at the MIR. Another approach is the competition radioimmunoassay used to determine subunit specificity of conformationally sensitive determinants described earlier. A third approach takes advantage of protein A binding activity. MAb 35 binds to protein A. If the test MAb does not, its ability to block MAb 35 binding to ^{125}I-αBgt AChR is measured by precipitation of MAb 35–^{125}I-αBgt-AChR complexes with Pansorbin. If test MAb does bind protein A, then Fab 35 is used to block test MAb binding to ^{125}I-αBgt-AChR.

An ELISA assay for determining whether two MAbs against *E. coli* tryptophan synthase bind to the same epitope[32] has been applied to the AChR.[21] The basic principle of this assay is that if two MAbs bind simultaneously to antigen in the assay, the absorbances from enzyme label activity will be equal to the sum of the absorbances of each MAb binding alone. AChR is bound to polystyrene assay plates as described in Section 2.3. After the plate is washed, the MAbs at saturating concentrations are added singly and in pairs to the plate and incubated with the AChR overnight at 4°C. Unbound MAb is washed off and glucose oxidase-labeled MAR 18.5 is used to determine MAb binding.

Stoichiometry of MAb–AChR complexes can be measured by sucrose gradient centrifugation.[47] For example, in the case of the α subunit there are two types of MAbs, intramolecular cross-linkers and intermolecular cross-linkers. Intramolecular cross-linkers link the two α subunits in an AChR. Intermolecular cross-linkers, like MAbs to the MIR, cross-link the α subunits in adjacent AChRs, and can form complexes of different sizes depending on the ratio of MAb to AChR. The ability of MAbs to the MIR to cross-link AChRs enables them to cause antigenic modulation.

4. Use of Monoclonal Antibodies to Study Acetylcholine Receptors

MAbs have been used extensively in studies of Torpedo AChRs (reviewed in Refs. 48–50). Specificity determination of MAbs revealed structural homologies between subunits[13,14] and between species (Refs. 13, 14, and 51; S.

Tzartos, L. Langeberg, S. Hochschwender, and J. Lindstrom, unpublished results), which are being confirmed by cDNA sequencing.[2–4] The MIR was identified[13,14] and shown to have pathological significance in MG.[52] MAbs have been used as probes of AChR topology. Fairclough *et al.*[53] have used electron microscopy to show that the two α subunits are not adjacent. Several methods of determining transmembrane orientation of determinants showed that MAbs to native AChR were directed mainly to the extracellular surface, whereas MAbs to denatured subunits were directed at its cytoplasmic surface (Refs. 51 and 54; D. Schneider and J. Lindstrom, unpublished results). Once the amino acid sequence of the *Torpedo* AChR α subunit was known, methods of predicting antigenic determinants were employed[55] to predict the location of the MIR.[2] MAbs from a fusion with spleen cells from a rat immunized with the synthetic peptide α 152–167 showed that the predicted MIR determinant was wrong.[21] Similar conclusions were drawn by Juillerat *et al.*[56] From cDNA sequences three groups predicted that the COOH terminus was on the extracellular surface.[2–4] On the contrary, two predicted that it was on the cytoplasmic surface.[57,58] MAbs and serum antibodies to the COOH terminus showed that it is on the cytoplasmic surface.[21,24] This illustrates the importance of immunochemical techniques for testing structural models.

With the exception of three MAbs, 10,[50,59] 148, and 168,[72] most MAbs bind to AChR without affecting function.[50,59]

Subunit-specific MAbs have been used to study regulation, synthesis, conformational maturation, and assembly of AChRs in the mouse muscle cell line BC3H-1. The MAb 61 recognizes nascent α chains, where MAb 35 does not bind until α subunits undergo a conformation change.[60,61] The time course of AChR assembly was studied by immune precipitation at intervals after pulse labeling with MAb 61 or the β-specific MAb 73. Initially, each MAb bound only its specific subunit, but as the subunits associated to form mature AChRs each MAb precipitated all of the associated subunits. MAb 61 has also been used to detect synthesis of α subunits *in vitro*,[62] and this approach was used to select for a cDNA clone for the α subunit of BC3H-1 AChR.[63]

Proteolytic digests of AChRs from *Electrophorus* electric organ and muscle were electrophoresed and then electrophoretically transferred to covalently reactive paper. This Western blot was exposed to subunit-specific MAbs and antisera and ^{125}I-labeled anti-IgG to produce peptide maps.[64] The blot was erased with SDS and successively exposed to MAbs specific for each subunit. In this way the subunit peptide maps of AChRs from the two tissues were compared. It was found that the two AChRs differed only by minor posttranslational modifications, if at all.

Although αBgt is a very specific probe for AChRs in fish electric organs and mammalian muscle,[6] it has shown mixed specificity in neurons. For example, at some neuronal synapses αBgt blocks AChR function,[65] whereas on other neurons it binds to non-AChR components.[66–68] In the case of chick ciliary ganglion neurons, αBgt binds to high-affinity sites, but these sites are not AChRs and are not located at synapses.[68] MAbs specific for the MIR bind to these neurons, predominantly on the synaptic membrane.[69] Anti-MIR MAbs also bind to neurons in chick brain at sites different from where αBgt binds.[70] Hopefully, MAbs will be useful probes for neuronal AChRs as they have been for muscle and electric organ AChRs.

5. Use of Monoclonal Antibodies to Study Myasthenia Gravis and Experimental Autoimmune Myasthenia Gravis

A number of laboratories have used MAbs as model autoantibodies.[8–14,52,71] We have tested a number of MAbs of different specificities and subclasses. Thus far, only MAbs against the MIR passively transfer the complement-dependent acute form of EAMG (Ref. 14; S. Tzartos, P. Vasquez, and J. Lindstrom, unpublished results; Hochschwender, S., Vasquez, P., and Lindstrom, J., unpublished results), and only anti-MIR MAbs cause antigenic modulation of AChR in fetal bovine muscle cell[47] and BC3H-1 cells (S. Tzartos and J. Lindstrom, unpublished results; S. Hochschwender, D. Schneider, and J. Lindstrom, unpublished results). The properties of MIR antibodies that are different from the MAbs that have no pathological effect are that anti-MIR MAbs cross-link AChRs and are directed against an extracellular determinant.

MAbs were used to determine the spectrum of anti-AChR specificities in MG patient sera in a competitive binding assay using subunit-specific MAbs.[52] On the average, more than half of the autoantibodies were directed at the MIR. The spectrum of specificity does not change in an individual, even though autoantibody concentration or clinical symptoms may change. Also, there is no apparent correlation between specificity spectrum and clinical state.

Acknowledgments. This work was supported by grants to J. L. from the National Institutes of Health (NS11323), the Muscular Dystrophy Association, the McKnight Foundation, the Alexander S. Onassis Charitable Foundation, and the Los Angeles and California Chapters of the Myasthenia Gravis Foundation. S. H. was a postdoctoral fellow of the Muscular Dystrophy Association. We thank Drs. Lewis Lanier and George Gutman for the gift of MAR 18.5.

References

1. *Cold Spring Harbor Symposia on Quantitative Biology*, 1983, Volume XLVIII, Cold Spring Harbor, New York.
2. Noda, M., Takahashi, H., Tanabe, T., Toyosato, M., Kikyotani, S., Furutani, Y., Hirose, T., Takashima, H., Inayama, S., Miyata, T., and Numa, S., 1983, Structural homology of *Torpedo californica* acetylcholine receptor subunits, *Nature* **302**:528–532.
3. Claudio, T., Ballivet, M., Patrick, J., and Heinemann, S., 1983, Nucleotide and deduced amino acid sequences of *Torpedo californica* acetylcholine receptor γ subunit, *Proc. Natl. Acad. Sci. USA* **80**:1111–1115.
4. Devillers-Thiery, A., Giraudat, J., Bentaboulet, M., and Changeux, J.-P., 1983, Complete mRNA coding sequence of the acetylcholine binding α-subunit of *Torpedo marmorata* acetylcholine receptor: A model for the transmembrane organization of the polypeptide chain, *Proc. Natl. Acad. Sci. USA* **80**:2067–2071.

5. Noda, M., Furutani, Y., Takahashi, H., Toyosato, M., Tanabe, T., Shimizu, S., Kikyotani, S., Kayano, T., Hirose, T., Inayama, S., and Numa, S., 1983, Cloning and sequence analysis of calf cDNA and human genomic DNA encoding α-subunit precursor of muscle acetylcholine receptor, *Nature* **305:**818–823.
6. Karlin, A., 1980, Molecular properties of nicotinic acetylcholine receptors, in: *The Cell Surface and Neuronal Function* (G. Poste, G. Nicolson, and C. Cotman, eds.), Elsevier/North-Holland Biomedical Press, New York, pp. 191–260.
7. Lindstrom, J., 1984, Immunobiology of Myasthenia gravis, experimental autoimmune myasthenia gravis and Lambert–Eaton syndrome, *Annu. Rev. Immunol.* **3:**111–133.
8. Dwyer, D. S., Kearney, J. F., Bradley, R. J., Kemp, G. E., and Oh, S. J., 1981, Interaction of human antibody and murine monoclonal antibody with muscle acetylcholine receptor, *Ann. N.Y. Acad. Sci.* **377:**143–157.
9. Gomez, C., Richman, D., Berman, P., Burres, S., Arnason, B., and Fitch, F., 1979. Monoclonal antibodies against purified nicotinic acetylcholine receptors, *Biochem. Biophys. Res. Commun.* **88:**575–582.
10. Lennon, V. A., and Lambert, E. H., 1980, Myasthenia gravis induced by monoclonal antibodies to acetylcholine receptors, *Nature* **285:**238–240.
11. Mochly-Rosen, D., Fuchs, S., and Eshhar, Z., 1979, Monoclonal antibodies against defined determinants of acetylcholine receptors, *FEBS Lett.* **106:**389–392.
12. Froehner, S. C., Douville, K., Klink, S., and Culp, W. J., 1983, Monoclonal antibodies to cytoplasmic domains of the acetylcholine receptor, *J. Biol. Chem.* **258:**7112–7120.
13. Tzartos, S. J., and Lindstrom, J. M., 1980, Monoclonal antibodies used to probe acetylcholine receptor structure: Localization of the main immunogenic region and detection of similarities between subunits, *Proc. Natl. Acad. Sci. USA* **77:**755–759.
14. Tzartos, S. J., Rand, D. E. Einarson, B. L., and Lindstrom, J. M., 1981, Mapping of surface structures of *Electrophorus* acetylcholine receptor using monoclonal antibodies, *J. Biol. Chem.* **256:**8635–8645.
15. Walters, D., and Maelicke, A., 1983, Organization of ligand binding sites at the acetylcholine receptor: A study with monoclonal antibodies, *Biochemistry* **22:**1811–1819.
16. Kamo, I., Furakawa, S., Tada, A., Mano, Y., Iwasaki, Y., Furuse, T., Ito, N., Hayashi, K., and Satoyoshi, E., 1982, Monoclonal antibody to acetylcholine receptor: Cell line established from thymus of patient with myasthenia gravis, *Science* **215:**995–997.
17. Vernet Der Garabedian, B., and Morel, E., 1983, Monoclonal antibodies against the human acetylcholine receptor, *Biochem. Biophys. Res. Commun.* **113:**1–9.
18. Tzartos, S., Langeberg, L., Hochschwender, S., and Lindstrom, J., 1983, Demonstration of a main immunogenic region on acetylcholine receptors from human muscle using monoclonal antibodies to human receptor, *FEBS Lett.* **158:**116–118.
19. Tzartos, S., and Lindstrom, J., 1981, Production and characterization of monoclonal antibodies for use as probes of acetylcholine receptors, in: *Monoclonal Antibodies in Endocrine Research* (R. Fellows and G. Eisenbarth, eds.), Raven Press, New York, pp. 69–86.
20. Gullick, W. J., and Lindstrom, J., 1983, Mapping the binding of monoclonal antibodies to the acetylcholine receptor from *Torpedo californica*, *Biochemistry* **22:**3312–3320.
21. Lindstrom, J., Criado, M., Hochschwender, S., Fox, J. L., and Sarin, V., 1984, Immunochemical tests of acetylcholine receptor subunit models, *Nature* **311:**573–575.
22. Lindstrom, J., Einarson, B., and Tzartos, S., 1981, Production and assay of antibodies to acetylcholine receptors, *Meth. Enzymol.* **74:**432–460.
23. Lindstrom, J., Merlie, J., and Yogeeswaran, G., 1979, Biochemical properties of acetylcholine receptor subunits from *Torpedo californica*, *Biochemistry* **18:**4465–4470.
24. Ratnam, M., and Lindstrom, J,. 1984, Structural features of the nicotinic acetylcholine receptor revealed by antibodies to synthetic peptides, *Biochem. Biophys. Res. Commun.* **122:**1225–1233.
25. Hyman, R., Ralph, P., and Sarkar, S., 1972, Cell-specific antigens and immunoglobulin synthesis of murine myeloma cells and their variants, *J. Natl. Cancer Inst.* **48:**173–184.
26. Köhler, G., Howe, S. C., and Milstein, C., 1976, Fusion between immunoglobulin-secreting and nonsecreting myeloma cell lines, *Eur. J. Immunol.* **6:**292–295.

27. Galfrè, G., Milstein, C., and Wright, B., 1979, Rat × rat hybrid myelomas and a monoclonal anti-Fd portion of mouse IgG, *Nature* **277**:131–133.
28. Köhler, G., and Milstein, C., 1975, Continuous cultures of fused cells secreting antibody of predefined specificity, *Nature* **256**:495–497.
29. Civin, C. I., and Banquerigo, M. L., 1983, Rapid, efficient cloning of murine hybridoma cells in low gelation temperature agarose, *J. Immunol. Meth.* **61**:1–8.
30. Fazekas de St. Groth, S., and Scheidegger, D., 1980, Production of monoclonal antibodies: Strategy and tactics, *J. Immunol. Meth.* **35**:1–21.
31. Mendelson, E., and Bustin, M., 1984, Monoclonal antibodies against distinct determinants of histone HS bind to chromatin, *Biochemistry* **23**:3459–3466.
32. Djavadi-Ohaniance, L., Friguet, B., and Goldberg, M. E., 1984, Structural and functional influence of enzyme–antibody interactions: Effects of eight different monoclonal antibodies on the enzymatic activity of *Escherichia coli* tryptophan synthase, *Biochemistry* **23**:97–104.
33. Harper, J. R., and Orengo, A., 1981, The preparation of an immunoglobulin–amylglucosidase conjugate and its quantitation by an enzyme-cycling assay, *J. Immunol. Meth.* **113**:51–57.
34. Johnson, R. B., and Nakamura, R. M., 1980, Improved techniques in ELISA for viruses and IgG and IgM-type viral antibodies, in: *Immunoassays: Clinical Laboratory Techniques for the 1980s* (R. M. Nakamura, W. R. Dito, and E. S. Tucker III, eds.), Alan Liss, New York, pp. 141–156.
35. Lanier, L. L., Gutman, G. A., Lewis, D. E., Griswold, S. T., and Warner, N. L., 1982, Monoclonal antibodies against rat immunoglobulin kappa chains, *Hybridoma* **1**:125–131.
36. Chang, T. H., Steplewski, Z., and Koprowski, H., 1980, Production of monoclonal antibodies in serum free medium, *J. Immunol. Meth.* **39**:369–375.
37. Kawamoto, T., Sato, J. D., Le, A., McClure, D. B., and Sato, G. H., 1983, Development of a serum-free medium for growth of NS-1 mouse myeloma cells and its application to the isolation of NS-1 hybridomas, *Anal. Biochem.* **130**:445–453.
38. Fazekas de St. Groth, S., 1983, Automated production of monoclonal antibodies in a cytostat, *J. Immunol. Meth.* **57**:121–136.
39. Cleveland, W. L., Wood, I., and Erlanger, B. F., 1983, Routine large-scale production of monoclonal antibodies in a protein-free culture medium, *J. Immunol. Meth.* **56**:221–234.
40. Bruck, C., Portetelle, D., Glineur, C., and Bollen, A., 1982, One-step purification of mouse monoclonal antibodies from ascitic fluid by DEAE Affi-gel blue chromatography, *J. Immunol. Meth.* **53**:313–319.
41. Mohammad, S. F., Sharma, N., and Woodward, S. C., 1983, Disulfide linking of albumin to the hinge region of immunoglobin G in normal human serum, *Biochim. Biophys. Acta* **749**:47–51.
42. Mage, M., 1980, Preparation of Fab fragments from IgGs of different animal species, *Meth. Enzymol.* **70**:142–150.
43. Rousseaux, J., Biserte, G., and Bazin, H., 1980, The differential enzyme sensitivity of rat immunoglobulin G subclasses to papain and pepsin, *Mol. Immunol.* **17**:469–482.
44. Rousseaux, J., Rousseaux-Prevost, R., Bazin, H., and Biserte, G., 1983, Proteolysis of rat IgG subclasses by *Staphylococcus aureus* V8 proteinase, *Biochim. Biophys. Acta* **748**:205–212.
45. Bazin, H., Beckers, A,. and Querinjean, P., 1974, Three classes and four (sub)classes of rat immunoglobulins: IgM, IgA, IgE, and IgG1, IgG2a, IgG2b, IgG2c, *Eur. J. Immunol.* **4**:44–48.
46. Medgyesi, G. A., Fust, C., Gergely, J., and Bazin, H., 1978, Classes and subclasses of rat immunoglobulins: Interaction with the complement system and with staphylococcal protein A, *Immunochemistry* **15**:125–129.
47. Conti-Tronconi, B., Tzartos, S., and Lindstrom, J., 1981, Monoclonal antibodies as probes of acetylcholine receptor structure. 2. Binding to native receptor, *Biochemistry* **20**:2181–2191.
48. Lindstrom, J., 1984, Nicotinic acetylcholine receptors: Use of monoclonal antibodies to study synthesis, structure, function, and autoimmune response in: *Receptor Biochemistry and Methodology*, Volume IV (J. C. Venter, C. M. Frazer, and J. M. Lindstrom, eds.), Alan R. Liss, New York, pp. 21–57.
49. Lindstrom, J., 1983, Using monoclonal antibodies to study acetylcholine receptors and myasthenia gravis, *Neurosci. Commentary* **1**:139–156.

50. Lindstrom J., Tzartos, S., Gullick, W., Hochschwender, S., Swanson, L., Sargent, P., Jacob, M., and Montal, M., 1983, Use of monoclonal antibodies to study acetylcholine receptors from electric organs, muscle, and brain and the autoimmune response to receptor in myasthenia gravis, *Cold Spring Harbor Symp. Quant. Biol.* **XLVIII:**89–99.
51. Sargent, P. B., Hedges, B. E., Tsaveler, L., Clemmons, L., Tzartos, S., and Lindstrom, J. M,. 1984, Structure and transmembrane nature of the acetylcholine receptor in amphibian skeletal muscle as revealed by cross-reacting monoclonal antibodies, *J. Cell Biol.* **98:**609–618.
52. Tzartos, S. J., Seybold, M. E., and Lindstrom, J. M., 1982, Specificities of antibodies to acetylcholine receptors in sera from myasthenia gravis patients measured by monoclonal antibodies, *Proc. Natl. Acad. Sci. USA* **79:**188–192.
53. Fairclough, R. H., Finer-Moore, J., Love, R. A., Kristofferson, D., Desmeules, P. J., and Stroud, R. M., 1983, Subunit organization and structure of an acetylcholine receptor, *Cold Spring Harbor Symp. Quant. Biol.* **XLVIII:**9–20.
54. Anderson, D., Blobel, G., Tzartos, S., Gullick, W., and Lindstrom, J., 1983, Transmembrane orientation of an early biosynthetic form of acetylcholine receptor δ subunit determined by proteolytic dissection in conjunction with monoclonal antibodies, *J. Neurosci.* **3:**1773–1784.
55. Hopp, T. P., and Woods, K. R., 1981, Prediction of protein antigenic determinants from amino acid sequences, *Proc. Natl. Acad. Sci. USA* **78:**3824–3828.
56. Juillerat, M. A., Barkas, T., and Tzartos, S. J., 1984, Antigenic sites of the nicotinic acetylcholine receptor cannot be predicted from the hydrophilicity profile, *FEBS Lett.* **168:**143–148
57. Guy, R., 1983, A structural model of the acetylcholine receptor channel based on partition energy and helix packing calculations, *Biophys. J.* **45:**249–261.
58. Finer-Moore, J., and Stroud, R., 1984, Amphipathic analysis and possible formation of the ion channel in an acetylcholine receptor, *Proc. Natl. Acad. Sci. USA* **81:**155–159.
59. Lindstrom, J., Tzartos, S., and Gullick, B., 1982, Structure and function of acetylcholine receptors studied using monoclonal antibodies, *Ann. N.Y. Acad. Sci.* **377:**1–19
60. Merlie, J. P., and Lindstrom, J., 1983, Assembly *in vivo* of mouse muscle acetylcholine receptor: Identification of an α subunit species that may be an assembly intermediate, *Cell* **34:**747–757.
61. Merlie, J, P., Sebbane, R., Gardner, S., Olson, E., and Lindstrom, J., 1983, The regulation of acetylcholine receptor expression in mammalian muscle, *Cold Spring Harbor Symp. Quant. Biol.* **XLVIII:**135–146.
62. Sebbane, R., Clokey, G., Merlie, J. P., Tzartos, S., and Lindstrom, J., 1983, Characterization of the mRNA for mouse muscle acetylcholine receptor α subunit by quantitative translation *in vitro*, *J. Biol. Chem.* **258:**3294–3303.
63. Merlie, J. P., Sebbane, R., Gardner, S., and Lindstrom, J., 1983, cDNA clone for the α subunit of the acetylcholine receptor from the mouse muscle cell line BC3H-1, *Proc. Natl. Acad. Sci. USA* **80:**3845–3849.
64. Gullick, W. J., and Lindstrom, J. M., 1983, Comparison of the subunit structure of acetylcholine receptors from muscle and electric organ of *Electrophorus electricus*, *Biochemistry* **22:**3801–3807.
65. Marshall, L., 1981, Synaptic localization of α bungarotoxin binding which blocks nicotinic transmission at frog sympathetic neurons, *Proc. Natl. Acad. Sci. USA* **78:**1948–1952.
66. Patrick, J., and Stallcup, B., 1977, α Bungarotoxin binding and cholinergic receptor function on a rat sympathetic nerve line, *J. Biol. Chem.* **252:**8629–8633.
67. Carbonetto, S. T., Fambrough, D. M., and Muller, K. F., 1978, Nonequivalence of α bungarotoxin receptors and acetylcholine receptors in chick sympathetic neurons, *Proc. Natl. Acad. Sci. USA* **75:**1016–1020.
68. Jacob, M., and Berg, D., 1983, The ultrastructural localization of α bungarotoxin binding sites in relation to synapsis on chick ciliary ganglion neurons, *J. Neurosci.* **3:**260–271.
69. Jacob, M. H., Berg, D. K., and Lindstrom, J. M., 1984, Shared antigenic determinant between the *Electrophorus* acetylcholine receptor and a synaptic component on chicken ciliary ganglion neurons, *Proc. Natl. Acad. Sci. USA* **81:**3223–3227.

70. Swanson, L., Lindstrom, J., Tzartos, S., Schmued, L., O'Leary, D., and Cowan, W., 1983, Immunohistochemical localization of monoclonal antibodies to the nicotinic acetylcholine receptor in the midbrain of the chick, *Proc. Natl. Acad. Sci.* **80**:4532–4536.
71. Fuchs, S., Bartfeld, D., Mochly-Rosen, D., Souroujon, M., and Feingold, C., 1981, Acetylcholine receptor: Molecular dissection and monoclonal antibodies in the study of experimental myasthenia, *Ann. N. Y. Acad. Sci.* **377**:110–124.
72. Wan, K., and Lindstrom, J., 1985, Effects of monoclonal antibodies on the functions of purified acetylcholine receptor from *Torpedo californica* reconstituted into liposomes, *Biochemistry*, In press.

Chapter 14

Sperm Surface Domains

DIANA G. MYLES and PAUL PRIMAKOFF

1. Introduction

Pattern formation during differentiation is a fundamental process in biology. Cell differentiation, which results in dramatic changes in cell surface composition, can also result in the localization of cell surface molecules into ordered domains. Formation of cell surface domains has been demonstrated in a wide variety of cell types. Monoclonal antibodies (MAbs) are making a major impact on the ability to localize and identify surface proteins. Some examples of recent investigations of localized surface molecules using monoclonal antibodies are studies on sperm,[1] epithelial cells,[2] hepatocytes,[3] neurons,[4] and muscle cells (Ref. 5; Hochschwender *et al.*, this volume, Chapter 13). In most instances it has not yet been established how these surface domains are created and stabilized. In some cases the biological significance of membrane order is known (e.g., the polarity of certain epithelial cell enzymes), but in other cases the function of localization of cell surface molecules into domains remains a mystery (e.g., sperm). Monoclonal antibodies have great potential as probes for the biological functions and structural basis of membrane order.

In this review we will consider several aspects of sperm cell surface topography. The sperm cell plasma membrane demonstrates remarkable long-range order, so much so that early studies with relatively nonspecific probes such as lectins, heterogeneous antibodies, and cationic ferritin were able to recognize the regional heterogeneity of the sperm surface.[6] The advent of monoclonal antibodies has provided a wider range of probes directed against specific antigenic sites on surface proteins and potentially on glycolipids. Monoclonal antibodies have been utilized by many labortories to define antigen domains on the surface of mammalian sperm (e.g,. Refs. 7–19). They also provide a method for studying sperm cell surface functions, including the exocytotic fusion of the acrosomal membrane with the plasma membrane, ion fluxes into and out of sperm, and interaction with the egg during the various steps of fertilization.

DIANA G. MYLES and PAUL PRIMAKOFF • Department of Physiology, University of Connecticut School of Medicine, Farmington, Connecticut 06032.

2. Production and Characterization of the Monoclonal Antibodies

2.1. Hybridoma Production and Screening

Three separate fusions have generated the 56 hybridoma lines in our collection. C57/Bl/6 female mice were immunized by intraperitoneal injection with 150 μg of a membrane protein (enriched in anterior head membrane) in complete Freund's adjuvant. Two of the mice received the same injection a second time in incomplete Freund's adjuvant, and all three mice received a final intravenous injection of 100 μg of membrane protein in phosphate-buffered saline 3 days prior to the fusion. The myeloma line P3-NS1/1-Ag4-1 was used as a fusion partner.[1,8]

Supernatants from 832 separate hybridoma cultures were screened in a solid phase radioactive binding assay using a sperm sonicate containing membranes as the antigen and a ^{125}I-labeled rabbit F(ab′)$_2$ anti-mouse IgG as the second antibody. By this assay, 38% of the supernatants were scored as positive. Binding to formaldehyde-fixed sperm was tested by indirect immunofluorescence on 176 of the 318 positive supernatants. By indirect immunofluorescence, 60 supernatants were negative, one bound to the entire sperm surface, and 115 bound to localized domains of the sperm surface. The hybridoma line producing antibody that bound to whole sperm was cloned and retested by indirect immunofluorescence. It split into two lines; one line produced antibody directed against the whole head and the other produced antibody to the whole tail. Thus, all the hybridoma antibodies that we have tested by indirect immunofluorescence bind to a localized region of the sperm. Antibodies are given letter designations according to the region to which they localize (Fig. 1A), as follows: anterior head (AH), posterior head (PH), whole head (WH), posterior tail (PT), and whole tail (WT).[1] Number designations from 1 to 100 are assigned to antibodies from cloned lines, and from 1001 to 1100 to antibodies from uncloned lines. Antibodies that bind to surface antigens were selected by demonstrating fluorescent staining of live, swimming sperm in which the plasma membrane was impermeant to calcium ions.[1,8]

Many of the antibody-producing lines have been cloned by limiting dilution, and antibody subclass has been determined by Ouchterlony. Among those antibodies where subclass has been determined, the majority belong to the IgG1 subclass.

2.2. Tissue and Species Specificity of the Antigens

Tissue distribution of antibody binding has been studied for several different antibodies. Four of the antibodies (AH-1, PH-1, WH-1, and PT-1) were tested for their ability to be absorbed by homogenates of kidney, RBC, liver, brain, and spleen.[8] Three additional antibodies (PH-20, PH-30, WH-30) were tested for binding to kidney, RBC, liver, brain, spleen, lung, intestine, skeletal

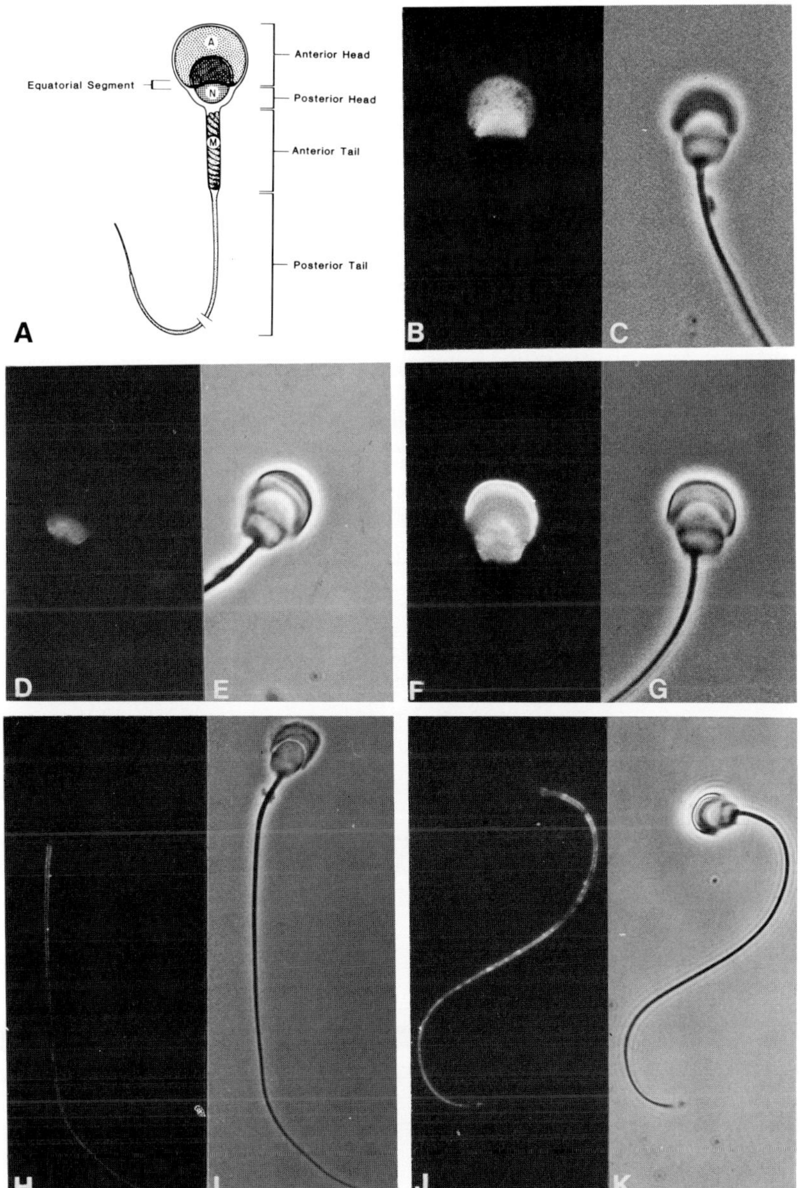

Figure 1. Surface domains of the guinea pig sperm. (A) Diagram showing sperm cell morphology and terminology for surface regions. A, Acrosome; N, nucleus; M, mitochondria. (B–K) MAb binding to sperm freshly removed from the cauda epididymis observed by indirect immunofluorescence. Corresponding phase contrast micrographs are of the same cells. (B, C) AH-1 binding pattern; (D, E) PH-20 binding pattern; (F, G) WH-1 binding pattern; (H, I) PT-1 binding pattern; (J, K) WT-1 binding pattern. (Parts A, J, and K are reproduced from Ref. 1; parts B, C, F, and G from Ref. 8; and parts D and E from Ref. 23; and parts H and I from Ref. 35; by permission of the respective publishers.)

muscle, and cardiac muscle (A. E. Cowan, P. Primakoff, and D. G. Myles, unpublished results). With one exception, there was no detectable antibody binding to any of these tissues. The one exception was a slight absorbtion of AH-1 with the highest concentrations of liver, brain, and spleen homogenates.[8] Thus, as far as they have been tested, six of the seven MAbs with different antigenic specificities (see below) appear to be sperm specific.

The recognized antigens were also not detected for the most part on the surface of other species of sperm that were tested, including sperm from humans, mice, rats, or hamsters.[20] Only three of the antibodies (AH-30, AH-31, and AH-1032) cross-react with hamster sperm. All three antibodies demonstrate a different topographic localization on hamster sperm than was observed on guinea pig sperm. From detergent extracts of guinea pig sperm, all three antibodies immunoprecipitate three ^{125}I-surface-labeled polypeptides, detectable after SDS–polyacrylamide gel electrophoresis, with relative molecular weights of 62,000, 52,000, and 38,000. No immunoprecipitates were obtained from detergent extracts of ^{125}I-surface-labeled hamster sperm.[20] These results suggest the possibility that the antibodies are recognizing the same determinant on unrelated surface molecules from the two species.

3. Topographic Localization of Surface Antigens: A Map of the Guinea Pig Sperm Cell Surface

The surface of any cell where the existence of membrane domains is suspected can be studied strictly from the point of view of overall surface topography. A map of the surface can be constructed using MAbs that will answer the basic questions, "How many domains exist, do the domains overlap, and are there multiple antigens in each domain?" The initial map obtained will of course reflect the relative immunogenicity of the various surface molecules and this may bias it toward antigens of particular topographic distributions. Virtually all the MAbs thus far isolated to mammalian sperm surfaces show localized patterns of binding.[7–19] This may mean that standard hybridoma procedures selectively "see" topographically restricted antigens. Topographically restricted membrane molecules could have specific structural features that on the one hand would allow them to become or remain localized and on the other hand might also be highly immunogenic. Alternatively, the sperm cell may have few surface molecules that are distributed throughout the plasma membrane.

On the surface of guinea pig sperm from the cauda epididymis we have found five distinct localization patterns of surface antigens (Fig. 1). These are extensive membrane domains, each involving a large proportion of the total plasma membrane of the cell. The five regions of antigen localization are: anterior head, posterior head, whole head, posterior tail, and whole tail (Fig. 1). These large surface domains correspond in some degree to internal features of the sperm cell (Fig. 1A): the anterior head region lies over the secretory granule, the acrosome; the posterior head plasma membrane is over the proximal half

Table I. Identification of Sperm Cell Surface Antigens

	Molecular weight of precipitated polypeptides × 10^{-3}	Number of antibodies
Anterior head		
Group 1	52	6
2	70, 62, 46, 25, 18	3
3	62, 52, 38	10
3A[a]	62, 52, 38	5
4	38, 16	1
5	No bands on gel	2
Posterior head		
Group 1	60	1
2	66, 48, 41	3
3	58, 48	2
4	No bands on gel	1
Whole head		
Group 1	42	4
2	89, 45	1
3	No bands on gel	12
Posterior tail		
Group 1	No bands on gel[b]	1
Whole tail		
Group 1	No bands on gel	4

[a] This group gives a surface-labeled immunoprecipitate, but only stains permeabilized cells by indirect immunofluorescence.
[b] The antigen recognized by PT-1 has been identified as a protein and characterized as having a sedimentation coefficient (when complexed with *n*-octyl-β-D-glucopyranoside) of 6.8 S on a sucrose gradient.

of the nucleus, and the posterior surface tail region is the region of the tail posterior to the cell's mitochondria, all of which are confined to the midpiece (or anterior tail region). The whole-head and whole-tail surface antigen localizations correspond to these two obvious morphological divisions of the cell, but do not overlie any single organelle or internal structure. Antibodies binding in these five surface patterns could be further subclassified into groups with unique antigenic specificities according to the analysis of their immunoprecipitates (Table I). The antibody collection detects at least 14 distinct antigens in the five surface regions (Refs. 1 and 21; R. Marrion Halenda, P. Primakoff, and D. G. Myles, unpublished results). Eleven of these are proteins that can be surface-labeled with ^{125}I and identified by immunoprecipitation.[1] Thus, the basic features of the guinea pig sperm surface map are: (1) there exist a minimum of five domains, (2) the domains are overlapping (e.g., the whole-head localization overlaps the anterior and posterior heads), and (3) there can be multiple antigens in each domain. The finding of overlapping domains and several antigens per domain leads to an appreciation of the complexity of the surface mosaic. It also suggests obvious questions concerning the creation,

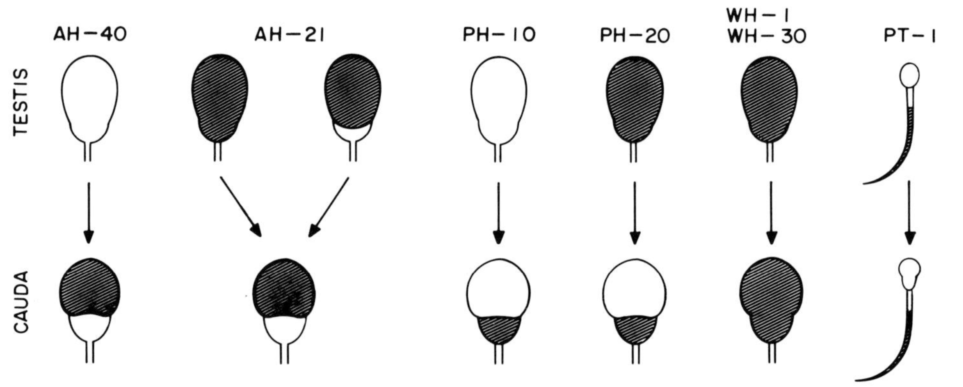

Figure 2. Changes in antibody binding patterns during final stages of sperm differentiation. Diagram shows immunofluorescence (hatched areas) observed on sperm from the testis and sperm from the cauda epididymis. (Reproduced from Ref. 23 by permission.)

maintenance, and function of each domain. The guinea pig sperm surface antigen domains defined with monoclonal antibodies correspond roughly to the guinea pig sperm surface specializations described for freeze-fracture images of the plasma membrane and also to the segregation of lipid probes, indicating heterogeneity of lipid domains.[22]

4. How Do Surface Antigens Become Localized during Differentiation of the Sperm Cell?

The establishment of sperm surface topography might occur at different times in development. Some antigens may become localized during the transformation of a round spermatid into the asymmetric sperm cell, whereas other antigens may only become localized after the sperm, with its basic morphology formed, leaves the testis and passes through the epididymis during the process of epididymal maturation. An example of the first situation is the antigen recognized by the MAb PT-1. The PT-1 antigen is found dispersed on the surface of round spermatids, but is already restricted to the posterior tail region of testicular sperm (Fig. 2) and then shows no further change in position on cauda epididymal sperm.[23] An example of the second situation is the PH-20 antigen, which is distributed on the whole head of testicular sperm, but becomes restricted to the posterior head of cauda epididymal sperm (Fig. 2).[23] Other antigens, for example, those recognized by the MAbs AH-40 and PH-10, only appear during epididymal passage, since they are not detected on testicular sperm, but are present on the anterior head (AH-40) and posterior head (PH-10) of cauda epididymal sperm (Fig. 2).[23]

Our results at this phenomenological level indicate that the recruitment of antigens into domains is an ongoing process during sperm development and that various mechanisms may be involved. Antigens such as PH-20 that initially appear in one pattern and then show an altered distribution may actually be moving in the plane of the membrane to their final location. Alternatively, they may be modified or covered up in a particular region. Whatever the process by which PH-20 changes its localization pattern from whole head of testicular sperm to posterior head of epididymal sperm, it must be a selective process; other whole-head antigens (e.g., WH-1 and WH-30) that are on the whole head of testicular sperm do not alter their position on epididymal sperm (Fig. 2).[23]

The appearance of new antigens (AH-40, PH-10) on the sperm surface during the transformation of testicular sperm into epididymal sperm could result from the addition of new molecules either from inside the cell or from epididymal fluid.[24,25] If the AH-40 and PH-10 antigens are added during epididymal passage, they either become tightly bound to the membrane or are integrally incorporated into it, since they are not washed off easily as is true for some sperm surface antigens.[10] The appearance of new antibody binding sites could alternatively result from the uncovering or modification of existing molecules.

5. What Keeps Antigens in Their Domains? The Maintenance of Surface Topography

The question of how surface domains are created is closely linked to the question of what maintains these suface patterns. However, entirely different mechanisms could act in these phenomena. Theories of antigen domain maintenance can be divided into three main categories: (1) models involving the restricted mobility of surface antigens in their final domain, (2) the existence of a membrane barrier to antigen movement at the domain boundary, and (3) molecular domains resulting from thermodynamic partitioning of molecules into a specific region.

Restricted mobility may occur via interactions with an extracellular matrix, an internal cytoskeleton, or by the formation of aggregates in the membrane. Restricted mobility has been suggested to be involved in domain maintenance of acetylcholine receptors[26] and could play a role in the maintenance of other molecules in localized domains.[27]

We have addressed the question of whether cells use mechanisms other than immobilization to localize surface molecules. With the technique of fluorescence redistribution after photobleaching (FRAP), we have shown that the antigen PT-1, localized on the posterior tail region of the guinea pig sperm cell surface, is freely diffusing in the membrane. In studies of this protein antigen we have measured a diffusion coefficient of 2.5×10^{-9} cm^2/sec involving >90% of the molecules binding PT-1.[21] This diffusion coefficient approaches the theoretical limit for a freely diffusing protein in a lipid bilayer.[28] This result means that any mechanism involving immobilization or a significant reduction in lateral mobility can be ruled out. At this point we cannot distinguish between mechanisms based on thermodynamic partitioning or a membrane barrier.

However, any thermodynamic partitioning would have to result from favored associations with other mobile molecules, such as lipids in a fluid lipid domain.

PT-1 could be constrained to its domain by a barrier in the membrane that prevents its diffusion out of the posterior tail region. Freeze-fracture images of the plasma membrane of the guinea pig sperm reveal a membrane specialization, the annulus, at the anterior–posterior tail junction.[29,30] This annulus is a potential candidate for such a barrier. Membrane barriers have been suggested to maintain molecules in surface domains of other cell types. In particular, it has been suggested that tight junctions may be responsible for maintaining the membrane polarity of epithelial cells by restricting molecules to either the apical or basolateral membrane.[31,32]

6. Dynamics of Surface Localization: The Migration of Surface Molecules from Their Original Domain to a New Domain

In response to external signals or an internal developmental program the distribution of surface molecules can be altered. Clusters of acetylcholine receptors form on the surface of muscle cells from preexisting disperse receptors when exposed to brain extracts.[33] Binding of ligand to dispersed surface receptors can trigger the accumulation of receptors into coated pits.[34] Other examples of altered surface domains exist.

We have described two topographic rearrangements of localized surface molecules that occur prior to fertilization during steps that alter the functional state of the sperm.[35] When sperm are removed from the cauda epididymis and incubated under *in vitro* conditions that will allow them to acquire the capacity to fertilize eggs ("capacitation"), the surface pattern of the PT-1 antigen is altered. The antigen, which is initially localized to the posterior tail (Figs. 1H and 1I), is now detected predominantly on the anterior tail (Figs. 3A and 3B). A second alteration in the pattern of antigen localization occurs immediately following the exocytotic fusion of the outer acrosomal membrane with the plasma membrane (acrosome reaction). This fusion results in the loss of the fused membrane vesicles from the anterior head and the joining of the inner acrosomal membrane to the plasma membrane. The PH-20 antigen is originally detected exclusively on the posterior head plasma membrane (Figs. 1D and 1E) and after exocytosis is found only on the inner acrosomal membrane (Figs. 3C and 3D).

Both cases of antigen redistribution (PT-1 and PH-20) apparently result from a migration of surface antigen, since redistribution is observed on cells with monoclonal antibody bound prior to incubation. Furthermore, redistribution is observed with both antigens when cells stained with monoclonal antibody and a FITC-labeled second antibody are incubated in the presence of a 50 to 100-fold excess of monoclonal antibody in the medium to prevent dissociation and reassociation of the bound antibodies to any newly exposed sites. FITC label is seen in the new region after capacitation or exocytosis in these

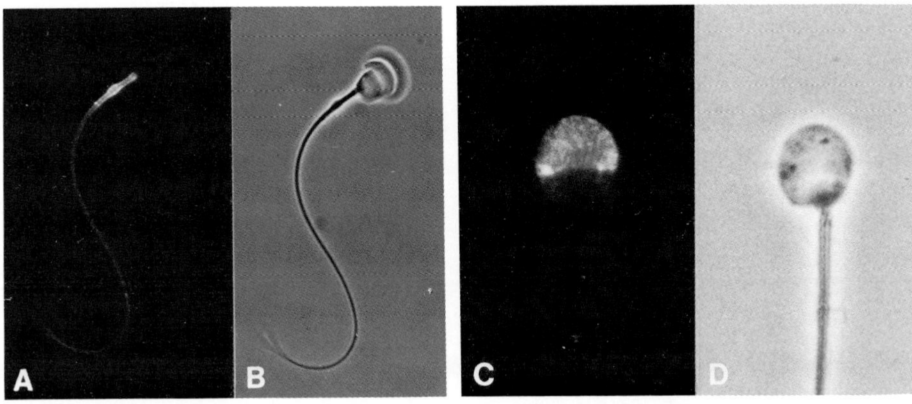

Figure 3. Migration of surface antigens PT-1 and PH-20 to new domains. (A) PT-1 MAb binding after 90 min incubation at 37°C in a capacitating medium. The PT-1 antigen has accumulated on the anterior tail region, but the posterior tail is still stained. (B) Phase contrast micrograph of the same cell. (C) PH-20 MAb binding on a sperm that has undergone exocytosis (acrosome reaction), live staining. No detectable fluorescence remains on the posterior head. (D) Phase contrast micrograph of the same cell. (Micrographs are reproduced from Ref. 35 by permission.)

conditions, indicating that the apparent redistribution of surface molecules results from a migration of existing molecules and not exposure of new antibody binding sites in the new surface domains.

The two migrations occur at different rates. A typical time course for PT-1 migration in a population of cells is shown in Fig. 4A. After 30 min at 37°C, 50% of the sperm show PT-1 antibody binding to the anterior tail, and by 60 min, 95% of the sperm show antigen migration. In contrast, the migration of the PH-20 antigen is much more rapid (Fig. 4B). One minute after induction of exocytosis, the PH-20 antigen has begun migration on all cells in the population. After 10 min, migration is complete: 100% of the sperm show binding of the PH-20 antibody exclusively to the inner acrosomal membrane.[35]

Besides a difference in the kinetics of the two migrations, there also exists a difference in their requirement for ATP synthesis. When incubated in the presence of the metabolic poisons carbonyl cyanide *m*-chlorophenylhydrazone (CCCP) or 2,4-dinitrophenol (DNP), the PT-1 antigen shows little or no migration onto the anterior tail domain. However, the PH-20 antigen migrates even in the presence of CCCP and 2-deoxyglucose.[35]

Several different functions for the migration of surface molecules can be imagined. Migrations could potentially bring molecules into a new environment, thereby regulating their activity. Also, the disappearance of proteins from a particular region, as is seen during PH-20 migration, could alter the composition of the region losing the molecule, leading to an activation or deactivation of a surface function in that region. An alternative function of surface migration would be simply the concentration of a membrane protein in a new surface region where its activity would have a different effect on cellular func-

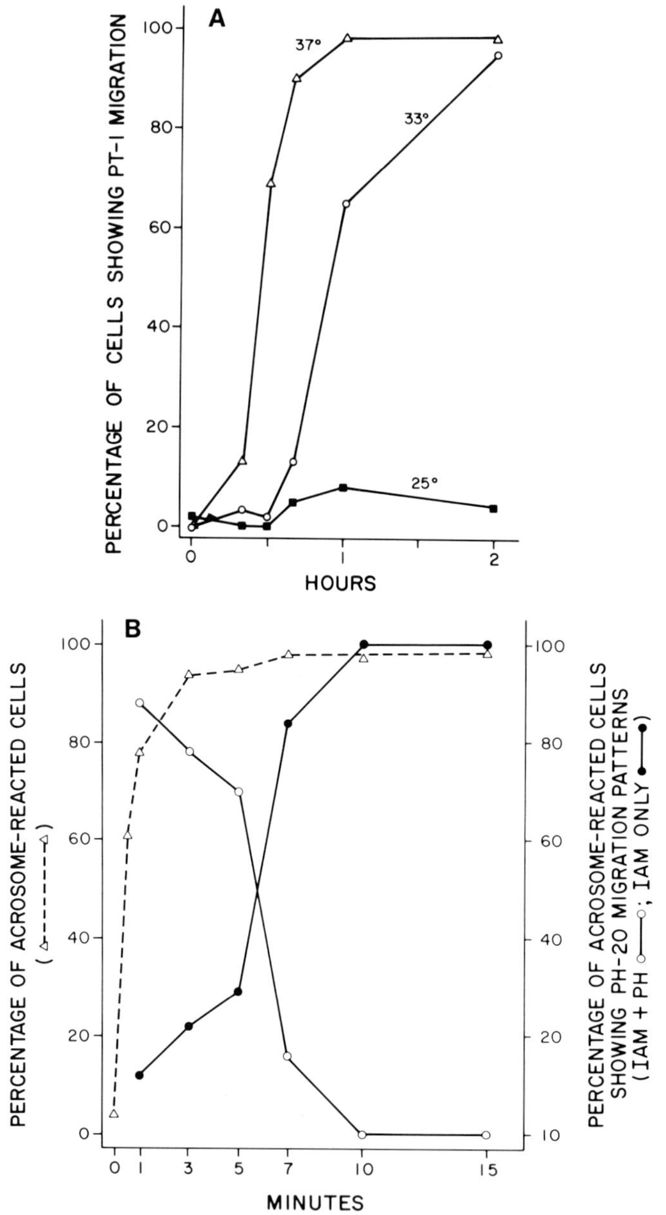

Figure 4. Kinetics of antigen migrations. (A) Kinetics of PT-1 antigen migration onto the anterior tail surface at (△) 37°C, (○) 33°C, or (■) 25°C. Sperm are incubated in capacitating medium, fixed at various times, and scored for the presence or absence of fluorescence on the anterior tail at each time point. (B) Kinetics of PH-20 antigen migration on cells undergoing exocytosis (acrosome reaction) after addition of the Ca^{2+} ionophore A23187. (△) Percentage of acrosome-reacted cells; (●) percentage of acrosome-reacted cells showing PH-20 antibody binding to both the inner acrosomal membrane and the posterior head; (○) percentage of acrosome-reacted cells showing PH-20 antibody binding exclusively to the inner acrosomal membrane. (Reproduced from Ref. 35 by permission.)

tion. The sperm surface migrations provide a favorable experimental system to study both the regulation of surface activity by localization of molecules and the mechanisms involved in establishing and maintaining localizations.

7. Conclusions

Cell surface topography is an area of great importance in the understanding of plasma membrane function. It also provides a view into the general topic of membrane organization. The study of cell surface topography requires appropriate probes; for example, labeled α-bungarotoxin initially contributed much to the investigation of acetylcholine receptor distribution. The advent of monoclonal antibodies has provided the capability of making libraries of specific membrane probes without initially purifying membrane molecules, allowing for the initiation of many new studies on cell surface topography.

ACKNOWLEDGMENTS. The preparation of this manuscript was supported by NIH grant HD 16580 to D. G. M. This work was done during the tenure of an Established Investigatorship of the American Heart Association and was partly supported by a Grant-in-Aid from the American Heart Association, with funds contributed in part by the Connecticut Affiliate, to P. P.

References

1. Primakoff, P., and Myles, D. G., 1983, A map of the guinea pig sperm surface constructed with monoclonal antibodies, *Dev. Biol.* **98:**417–428.
2. Ojakian, G. K., and Herzlinger, D. A., 1984, Analysis of epithelial cell surface polarity with monoclonal antibodies, *Fed. Proc.* **43:**2208–2216.
3. Hixson, D. C., DeLourdes-Ponce, M., Allison, J. P., and Walbors, E. F., Jr., 1984, Cell surface expression by adult rat hepatocytes of a non-collagen glycoprotein present in rat liver biomatrix, *Exp. Cell Res.* **152:**402–414.
4. Buckley, K. M. Schweitzer, E. S., Miljanich, G. P., Clift-O'Grady, L., Kushner, P. D., Reichardt, L. F., and Kelly, R. B., 1983, A synaptic vesicle antigen is restricted to the junctional region of the presynaptic plasma membrane, *Proc. Natl. Acad. Sci. USA* **80:**7342–7346.
5. Tzartos, S. J., 1984, Monoclonal antibodies as probes of the acetylcholine receptor and myasthenia gravis, *Trends Biochem. Sci.* **9:**63–67.
6. Koehler, J. K., 1978, The mammalian sperm surface: Studies with specific labeling techniques, *Int. Rev. Cytol.* **54:**73–108.
7. Bechtol, K. B., Brown, S. C., and Kennett, R. H., 1979, Recognition of differentiation antigens of spermatogenesis in the mouse by using antibodies from spleen-cell–myeloma hybrids after syngeneic immunization, *Proc. Natl. Acad. Sci. USA* **76:**363–367.
8. Myles, D. G., Primakoff, P., and Bellve, A. R., 1981, Surface domains of the guinea pig sperm defined with monoclonal antibodies, *Cell* **23:**433–439.
9. Feuchter, F. A., Vernon, R. B., and Eddy, E. M., 1981, Analysis of the sperm surface with monoclonal antibodies: topographically restricted antigens appearing in the epididymis, *Biol. Reprod.* **24:**1099–1110.
10. Schmell, E. D., Yuan, L. C., Gulyas, B. J., and August, J. T., 1982, Identification of mammalian sperm surface antigens. I. Production of monoclonal anti-mouse sperm antibodies, *Fertil. Steril.* **37:**249–257.

11. Gaunt, S. J., 1982, A 28K-dalton cell surface autoantigen of spermatogenesis: Characterization using a monoclonal antibody, *Dev. Biol.* **89**:92–100.
12. Naz, R. K., Saxe, J. M., and Menge, A. C., 1983, Inhibition of fertility in rabbits by monoclonal antibodies against sperm, *Biol. Reprod.* **28**:249–254.
13. Wolf, D. P., Sokoloski, J. E., Dandekar, P., and Bechtol, K. B., 1983, Characterization of human sperm surface antigens with monoclonal antibodies, *Biol. Reprod.* **29**:713–723.
14. Jones, R., Brown, C. R., Cran, D. G., and Gaunt, S. J., 1983, Surface and internal antigens of rat spermatozoa distinguished using monoclonal antibodies, *Gamete Res.* **8**:255–265.
15. Saling, P. M., Raines, L. M., and O'Rand, M. G., 1983, Monoclonal antibody against mouse sperm blocks a specific event in the fertilization process, *J. Exp. Zool.* **227**:481–486
16. Moore, H. D., and Hartman, T. D., 1984, Localization by monoclonal antibodies of various surface antigens of hamster spermatozoa and the effect of antibody on fertilization *in vitro*, *J. Reprod. Fertil.* **70**:175–183.
17. O'Rand, M. G., Irons, G. P., and Porter, J. P., 1984, Monoclonal antibodies to rabbit sperm autoantigens. I. Inhibition of *in vitro* fertilization and localization on the egg, *Biol. Reprod.* **30**:721–729.
18. Isahakia, M., and Alexander, N. J., 1984, Interspecies cross-reactivity of monoclonal antibodies directed against human sperm antigens, *Biol. Reprod.* **30**:1015–1026.
19. Koyama, Y. I., Shinomiya, T., Sakai, Y., Shiba, T., and Yanagisawa, K. O., 1984, Identification of sperm antigenic determinants with phylogenetically diverse and limited distribution using monoclonal antibodies, *J. Reprod. Immunol.* **6**:141–150.
20. Primakoff, P., Heaton, M. R., and Myles, D. G., 1983, Species specificity of hybridoma antibodies to surface antigens of guinea pig sperm, *Gamete Res.* **8**:385–394.
21. Myles, D. G., Primakoff, P., and Koppel, D. E., 1984, A localized surface protein of guinea pig sperm exhibits free diffusion in its domain, *J. Cell Biol.* **98**:1905–1909.
22. Friend, D. S., 1982, Plasma membrane diversity in a highly polarized cell, *J. Cell Biol.* **93**:243–249.
23. Myles, D. G., and Primakoff, P., 1983, Establishment of sperm surface topography analyzed with monoclonal antibodies, in: *The Sperm Cell* (J. Andre, ed.), Martins Nijhoff, The Hague, pp. 127–130.
24. Vernon, R. B., Muller, C. H., Herr, J. C., Feuchter, F. A., and Eddy, E. M, 1982, Epididymal secretion of a mouse sperm surface component recognized by a monoclonal antibody, *Biol. Reprod.* **26**:523–535.
25. Brown, C. R., vonGlos, K. I. and Jones, R., 1983, Changes in plasma membrane glycoproteins of rat spermatozoa during maturation in the epididymis, *J Cell Biol.* **96**:256–264.
26. Stya, M., and Axelrod, D., 1983, Mobility and detergent extractability of acetylcholine receptors on cultured rat myotubes: A correlation, *J. Cell Biol.* **97**:48–51.
27. McCloskey, M., and Poo, M.-M., 1984, Protein diffusion in cell membranes: some biological implications, *Int. Rev. Cytol.* **87**:19–81.
28. Peters, R., and Cherry, R. J., 1982, Lateral and rotational diffusion of bacteriorhodopsin in lipid bilayers: Experimental test of Saffman–Delbruck equation, *Proc. Natl. Acad. Sci. USA* **79**:4317–4321.
29. Friend, D. S., and Fawcett, D. W., 1974, Membrane differentiation in freeze-fractured mammalian sperm, *J. Cell Biol.* **63**:641–664.
30. Elias, P. M., Friend, D. S., and Goerke, J., 1979, Membrane sterol heterogeneity. Freeze fracture detection with saponins and filipin, *J. Histochem. Cytochem.* **27**:1247–1260.
31. Rodriguez-Boulan, E., 1983, Membrane biogenesis, enveloped RNA viruses, and epithelial polarity, *Modern Cell Biol.* **1**:119–170.
32. Herzlinger, D. A., and Ojakian, G. K., 1984, Studies on the development and maintenance of epithelial cell surface polarity with monoclonal antibodies, *J. Cell Biol.* **98**:1777–1787.
33. Buc-Caron, M.-H., Nystrom, P., and Fishbach, G. D., 1983, Induction of acetylcholine receptor synthesis and aggregation: Partial purification of low-molecular-weight activity, *Dev. Biol.* **95**:378–386.
34. Anderson, R. G. W., and Kaplan, J., 1983, Receptor-mediated endocytosis, *Modern Cell Biol.* **1**:1–52.
35. Myles, D. G., and Primakoff, P., 1984, Localized surface antigens of guinea pig sperm migrate to new regions prior to fertilization, *J. Cell Biol.* **99**:1634–1641.

Chapter 15

The Cytoskeleton

LAN BO CHEN, SHARON ROSENBERG, KAREN K. NADAKAVUKAREN, ELIZABETH S. WALKER, ELIZABETH L. SHEPHERD, and GLENN D. STEELE, JR.

1. Introduction

One of the active areas in cell biology involves the attempt to identify, characterize, and localize cytoskeletal components in nonmuscle cells. The standard approaches in this field have been the detection of a protein by gel electrophoresis or chromatography, the purification to homogeneity, the preparation of specific antibodies, and the localization by immunocytochemistry. The number of cytoskeleton-associated proteins is on the order of 1000. The rate-limiting step has been the isolation of individual components to a sufficient purity for raising highly specific antibodies.

The advent of hybridoma–monoclonal antibody technology has dramatically changed the outlook of this field. Protein purification is no longer a prerequisite. For immunization, 10% purity is more than sufficient to raise useful antibodies. Most significantly, hybridomas allow the generation of antibodies recognizing different antigenic determinants of a protein and different monoclonal antibodies for the same determinant with varying affinities. Since each of these antibody populations is separated, unlike the polyclonal antiserum in which they are all mixed, monoclonal antibodies become useful for probing biological activities of cytoskeletal components as well. In the absence of useful mutants defective in cytoskeletal components in mammalian cells, the availability of homogeneous antibodies able to bind and perturb the activity of cytoskeletal components is an alternative to studying the eventual question in this field: the function of these proteins in living cells. To date, even the functions of actin, tubulin, and intermediate filament proteins in interphase nonmuscle cells are still at the exploratory stage.

Over the last few years, we have explored the possibility of using total cytoskeleton without purifying the individual components to raise monoclonal

---

LAN BO CHEN, SHARON ROSENBERG, KAREN K. NADAKAVUKAREN, ELIZABETH S. WALKER, ELIZABETH L. SHEPHERD, and GLENN D. STEELE, Jr. • Division of Cell Growth and Regulation, Dana-Farber Cancer Institute Harvard Medical School, Boston, Massachusetts 02115.

antibodies. Almost all cytoskeletal components can be isolated in one fraction by nonionic detergent. We have used such a fraction to immunize mice and successfully raised monoclonal antibodies specific for actin, tubulin, vimentin, keratin, tropomysin, and several new components.

2. Experimental Procedures

2.1. Generation of Monoclonal Antibodies against Cytoskeleton

The procedure for producing the hybridoma lines was essentially that of Köhler and Milstein.[1] BALB/c mice were immunized intraperitoneally with the detergent-insoluble cytoskeletal fraction of any human carcinoma line prepared by extraction with a buffer containing 1% Triton X-100, 10 mM 1,4-piperazinediethanesulfonic acid, 100 mM KCl, 300 mM sucrose, 2.5 mM $MgCl_2$, and 1 mM PMSF ("CSK buffer") as described previously.[2–4] Two 100-mm dishes of confluent cells were used as starting material for the antigen for each injection. All injections were intraperitoneal, with a suspension of antigen in 0.4 ml complete (for the first injection) or incomplete (days 18 and 30) Freund's adjuvant. Two days later, the immunized mice were sacrificed and the spleen cells isolated. NS-1 mouse myeloma cells (2×10^8) were fused with spleen cells (8×10^8) in the presence of 1 ml of 50% polyethylene glycol (PEG 1000, Koch-Light Laboratories, Berks, England) in RPMI 1640 medium (GIBCO, Grand Island, New York) and 1.5% dimethylsulfoxide for 2 min at 37°C. The cells were washed in medium RPMI 1640, resuspended in 200 ml of complete medium (RPMI 1640 plus 15% fetal calf serum, 2 mM glutamine, 100 μg/ml garamycin), and plated in 10 96-well plates (Flow Laboratories, McClean, Virginia). The cultures were fed with HAT selection medium (13.6 μg/ml hypoxanthine, 0.18 μg/ml aminopterin, 3.9 μg/ml thymidine) for 2 weeks and then changed to the same medium without aminopterin. After screening, selected wells were weaned to complete medium without hypoxanthine and thymidine. Cloning was carried out in medium made semisolid by the addition of Methocel (1.4%) (Sigma, St. Louis, Missouri), using a serum lot (M. A. Bioproducts, Walkersville, Maryland) selected to give a cloning efficiency equivalent to that obtained with the use of a 3T3 cell feeder layer.

Antibody-containing ascites fluid was obtained by injecting cloned hybridoma cells [(1–10) $\times 10^7$ per mouse] intraperitoneally into BALB/c mice primed with pristane (2,6,10,14-tetramethylpentadecane; Aldrich Chemical Co., Milwaukee, Wisconsin). The ascites fluid was stored at 4°C, either under sterile conditions or in the presence of 0.01% sodium azide. Both conditioned culture medium and ascites fluid stored this way were stable for at least 1 year. Each batch of ascites fluid was checked by immunofluorescence to ascertain that at dilutions greater than 1:50 the staining pattern was the same as that of conditioned medium.

Table I. Fixation Procedures for Immunofluorescence

1.	3.5% Formaldehyde in PBS for 20 min; acetone at −20°C for 2 min
2.	3.5% Formaldehyde in PBS for 20 min; methanol at −20°C for 2 min
3.	3.5% Formaldehyde in PBS for 20 min; 1% Triton X-100 in PBS for 10 min
4.	Acetone at −20°C for 5 min
5.	Methanol at −20°C for 5 min
6.	Penman's CSK buffer (see text) for 3 min at 4°C; 3.5% formaldehyde in PBS for 3 min at 4°C
7.	Penman's CSK buffer for 3 min at 4°C; methanol at −20°C for 2 min
8.	0.025% Glutaraldehyde in PBS for 3 min; 3.5% formaldehyde in PBS for 10 min; acetone at −20°C for 2 min
9.	0.025% Glutaraldehyde in PBS for 3 min; dithiobis (succinimidyl propionate) (0.2 mg/ml in PBS) at 37°C for 5 min; methanol at −20°C for 2 min
10.	Dithiobis (succinimidyl propionate) (0.2 mg/ml) at 37°C for 5 min; acetone at −20°C for 2 min

2.2 Antibody Screening

Cells were grown to confluence in UV-sterilized polyvinylchloride 96-well plates (Dynatech Laboratories, Alexandria, Virginia), fixed in −20°C methanol for 5 min, and washed in PBS. Hybridoma-conditioned medium was incubated with fixed cells overnight at 4°C. After washing in PBS, each well was tested for the presence of bound antibody with either an alkaline phosphatase-conjugated second antibody or I^{125}-labeled goat anti-mouse mixed Igs (New England Nuclear, Billerica, Massachusetts). Conditioned media positive by this initial screening were tested further by immunofluorescence. Selected cultures were then cloned immediately.

2.3 Fixation Procedures for Immunofluorescent Stainings of Cytoskeleton

One of the most important considerations in using monoclonal antibodies to study cytoskeleton is how to preserve the native location of each of the antigens. This problem has not been easy to solve. To date, we know very little about the location of cytoskeleton components in living cells, except in the well-known cases of tubulin in mitotic spindles, actin in stress fibers. In the absence of "living cell standard," any fixation procedure should be considered as tentative. Better fixation may always be forthcoming to replace the old one. When a new monoclonal antibody is generated, there is no rule one can follow as to what fixation procedure should be used. Our experience suggests that the safest approach is to choose a cell type and fix it with ten different procedures as outlined in Table I. If only one fixation procedure is followed, sometimes one can miss very useful antibodies. One of our actin monoclonal antibodies is the best example. Had we only used the standard formaldehyde–acetone fixation, we would have completely missed this very useful actin monoclonal antibody during the initial screenings. It turns out that the antigenic site(s) for this antibody is exquisitely sensitive to acetone. Once methanol or detergent is used instead of acetone, excellent actin localization is revealed with this antibody.

Once all ten different fixations have been tried, how can one decide which one comes closest to the living cell condition? If the antibody is recognizing a well-established component such as actin, tubulin, or an intermediate filament component, it is easier to choose because there are numerous published photographs to compare. If it is a new component, there is almost no logic to follow. In most cases one needs additional biochemical evidence to guide the guessing. If a component clearly has a high affinity for other known components, the good fixation should show at least the association of the new component with the established component. The best examples are the localizations of microtubule-associated protein(s) and vimentin-associated protein(s). However, one should bear in mind that this new component may interact with more than one component, and one fixation procedure may preserve one of the associations but not the other. There is no easy answer for such a situation. It remains one of the challenges in this field.

Perhaps it should be admitted that the decision on fixation is often made by intuition, which is strongly influenced by how pretty the image is. Myosin localization is the best example. When all ten fixation protocols were tried, only acetone at $-20°C$ gave a clean and "believable" image. This fixation was adopted 10 years ago and to date no one knows whether myosin in living cells is similar to the image revealed by acetone fixation; however, no one dares to change this fixation because no other fixation gives rise to a prettier picture. The lack of a scientific basis for fixation reflects the infant stage of this field and the need for further research. Monoclonal antibodies provide an excellent opportunity to move this field forward. Microinjection of fluorescently labeled monoclonal antibody into living cells is becoming a routine procedure, allowing one to choose a fixation that leads to an image identical to that in living cells.

It should be emphasized that the protocols shown in Table I are the procedures used in this laboratory. Other laboratories have different variations. Moreover, better procedures and fixatives are being sought. The fact that most of these fixations for immunofluorescence are not suitable for electron microscopy suggests that there is a long way to go in fixation science. Glutaraldehyde is widely used in electron microscopy, but it readily leads to high levels of background fluorescence. Perhaps better cross-linking reagents should be synthesized and screened.

2.4 Immunofluorescence Staining of Cytoskeleton

Cells grown on glass coverslips were fixed by one of the procedures listed in Table I, washed in water and PBS, and incubated with antibodies. Either undiluted conditioned medium or ascites fluid (diluted >1:100) was used as the source of the monoclonal antibody. The rabbit polyclonal antiserum raised against cytoskeletal component was used at a dilution of >1:40. For double immunofluorescence labeling, mouse monoclonal and rabbit polyclonal antibodies were mixed. The second antibody was a mixture of fluorescein-conjugated goat anti-rabbit IgG and rhodamine-conjugated goat anti-mouse mixed Igs (Cappel Laboratories, West Chester, Pennsylvania). All incubations with antibodies were for 30 min at 37°C in a humidified chamber, and each incubation was followed by a 1 min wash in PBS. Coverslips were mounted on glycerol-gelatin (Sigma Chemical Co., St. Louis, Missouri) containing 0.1 M *n*-propyl gallate[5] to retard photobleaching.

Frozen sections of mouse, human, and rabbit tissues were prepared as described.[6] Unmasking experiments were performed by incubating methanol-fixed sections for 1 hr at 37°C in 0.13% trypsin, 0.1% $CaCl_2$, followed by washing in PBS and application of antibodies. Immunofluorescence was performed as described above, except that the second antibody was usually a mixture of fluorescein-conjugated goat anti-mouse Igs and rhodamine-conjugated goat anti-rabbit IgG (Cappel).

Fluorescence microscopy was carried out with a Zeiss Photomicroscope III equipped with epifluorescence optics and Planapo 63× and 40× objective lenses. For the double immunofluorescence experiments, exposures on Kodak Tri-X films were first made for fluorescein and second for rhodamine at EI 3600 and 6300, respectively. The film was developed in Kodak HC110 (dilution B) for 12 min.

3. Examples of Monoclonal Antibodies Specific for Cytoskeletal Components

3.1. Actin Localization with Monoclonal Antibodies

Polyclonal antibodies specific for actin have traditionally been difficult to prepare. Not until the last decade was actin antiserum generated in rabbits and used for localization of actin in cultured cells.[7] One of the important factors for this success was the use of SDS to denature actin to expose antigenic site(s). In the subsequent 10 years, there was a worldwide effort to raise actin antiserum in rabbits, with very little success. There were fewer than five out of 1000 rabbits producing high-titer actin antisera in the course of this worldwide effort. The advent of hybridoma-monoclonal antibodies encouraged a new hope initially. However, during the last 8 years, there has not been a great deal of success in making actin monoclonal antibodies. Fewer than ten hybridoma lines producing useful actin antibodies have been generated.[8,9] In contrast, almost every laboratory engaging in this area of research has easily raised monoclonal antibodies specific for tubulin, vimentin, keratin, tropomyosin, etc. The likely explanation is that actin is indeed a poor antigen.

The first widely used actin monoclonal antibody was developed by Lin at Cold Spring Harbor Laboratory.[8] This antibody, JLA20, has remarkable avidity and specificity, as evidenced by a number of publications using it. The only reason that it has not become the standard in this field, as was the case for

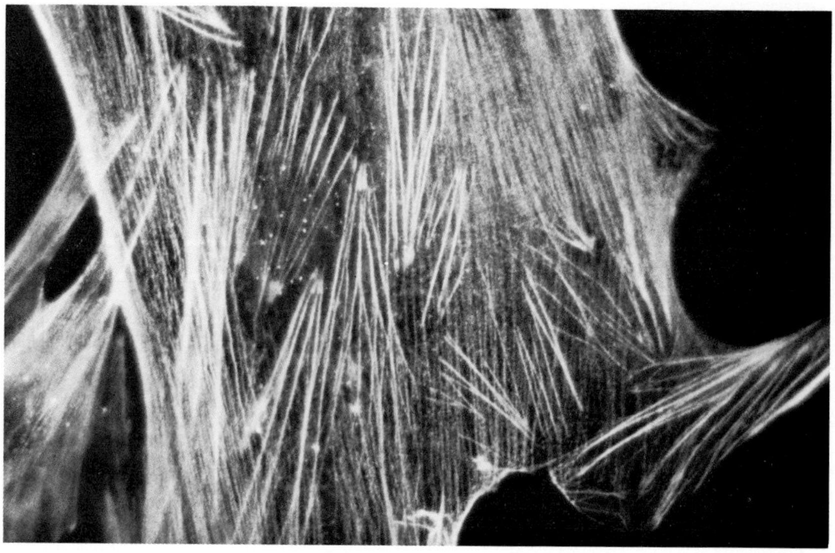

Figure 1. Immunofluorescent staining with actin monoclonal antibody (SR-C) of human fibroblast FS-2.

Lazarides and Weber's rabbit antiactin antibodies for many years, is that this antibody is an IgM. Although in some cases it is advantageous to have large antibodies, the less stable nature of this IgM against actin discourages the attempt to make it a standard. The titer of this antibody in less experienced hands can drop 1000-fold in a few weeks. Nonetheless, this actin antibody has remained the best thus far in the field. Two of Parham's actin monoclonal antibodies have been deposited at the American Type Culture Collection (ATCC). Rarely do these two hybridoma lines produce useful actin antibodies in laboratories purchasing the cell lines from ATCC.

Using total platelet cytoskeleton as antigen, one of us (S. R.) has generated an actin monoclonal antibody that is mouse IgG. Immunoblottings of total cell proteins and purified actin with this antibody show that it recognizes only actin, not the microfilament-associated protein(s). Immunofluorescent staining of cultured cells demonstrates that this antibody is useful for localizing actin-containing stress fibers (Fig. 1). This antibody is unusual in that the antigenic site(s) is sensitive to acetone even at −20°C. Our fixation procedure for this antibody has been formaldehyde followed by methanol. Cells extracted with Penman's CSK buffer, then fixed in formaldehyde, can also be stained for actin with this antibody. All stainings can be blocked by the presence of highly purified skeletal muscle actin.

The distribution of actin filaments in tumorigenic cells has been studied by Pollack with Lazaride and Weber's rabbit antiactin antisera.[7,10] In general, there are far fewer actin cables in transformed cells than in normal cells, although exceptions exist. We have used our actin monoclonal antibodies to

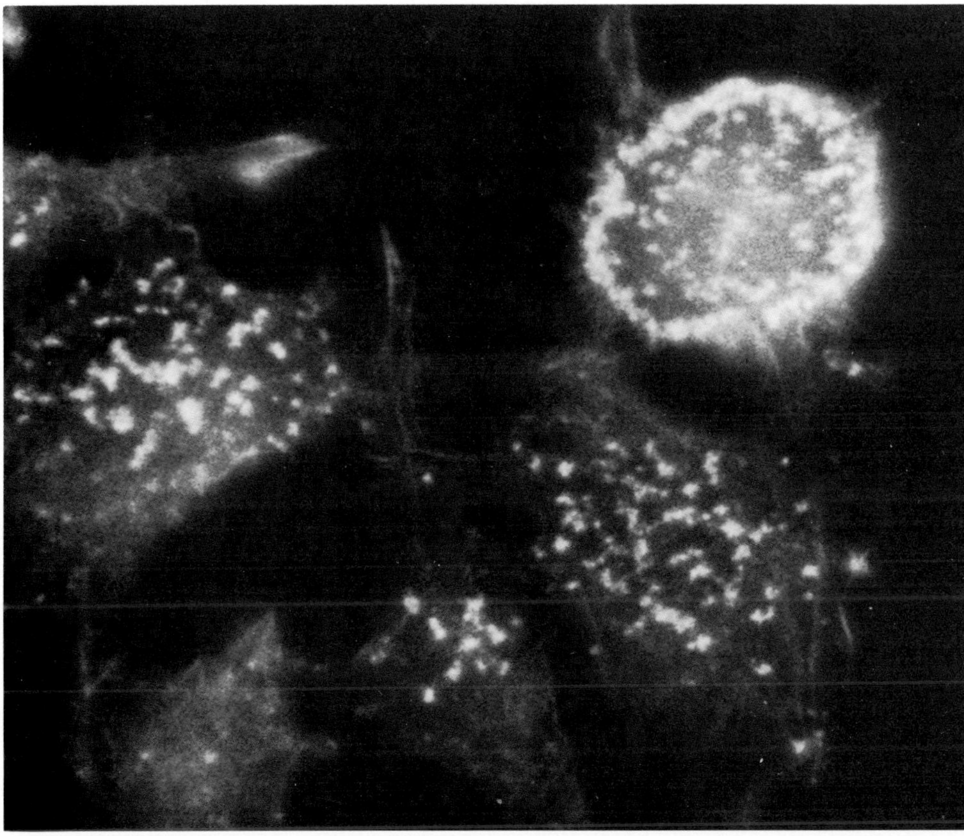

Figure 2. Immunofluorescent staining with actin monoclonal antibody (SR-C) of Rous sarcoma virus-transformed rat cells AnAn.

screen a variety of tumor-derived and transformed cell lines. The most striking example of alteration in actin distribution is found in rat cells transformed by Rous sarcoma virus. Only actin aggregates are detected in these cells (Fig. 2). Electron microscopy also revealed the unusual aggregates of microfilaments in RSV–rat cells. In human carcinoma-derived cells, using our actin monoclonal antibody, we find in numerous cases that actin cables can readily be detected, in contrast to sarcoma or transformed fibroblasts, where actin cables appear to be far fewer. The significance of alterations in actin distribution in some tumor cells is still unknown.

3.2. Tubulin Monoclonal Antibodies

A large number of hybridomas producing tubulin antibodies have been generated by numerous laboratories. In the course of our screenings of hybri-

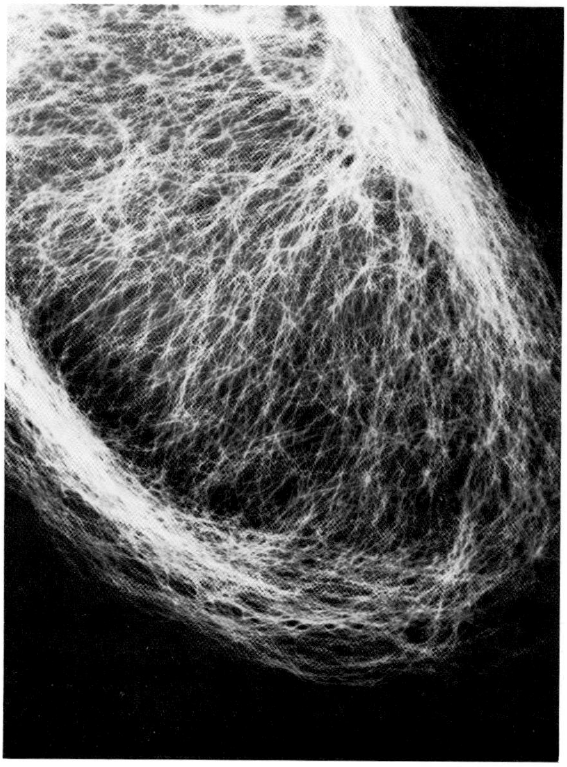

Figure 3. Immunofluorescent staining with tubulin monoclonal antibody (H2-1B2) of a primary human kidney epithelial cell.

domas raised against total cytoskeleton, clones producing tubulin antibodies are often detected. These antibodies are in general useful for microtubule localization (Fig. 3). Mitotic spindles and microtubules in normal interphase cells are easily stained with such monoclonal antibodies.

Tubulin antibody is useful for microinjection because the unpolymerized tubulin pool represents a significant portion of total tubulin and the constant treadmilling of microtubule–tubulin allows perturbation by tubulin monoclonal antibody.[11] Unfortunately, cell shape is not changed, suggesting that microtubules may not be absolutely essential for shape maintenance of interphase cells. However, intracellular motility of mitochondria is severely curtailed by the injection of tubulin monoclonal antibodies. Double stainings of mitochondria with rhodamine 123 and microtubules with tubulin monoclonal antibody show a good correlation in distributions of these two cellular components. It is likely that microtubules play a role in mitochondrial movement and distribution.[12–14]

Microtubules initially were reported to be disorganized in tumor cells.[15] Now there appears to be a consensus that microtubules in tumor cells are very difficult to preserve.[16] Many fixation protocols that work for normal cells are simply unable to maintain microtubules for immunofluorescence staining in tumor cells. One of us (K. K. N.) found that with fixation by the cross-linker dithiosuccinimidyl propionate, microtubules in a variety of tumor cells, in particular, the human carcinoma-derived cells, are not disorganized. No gross difference between normal and tumor cells can be detected except that the tumor cells tend to be thicker and therefore have a thicker layer of microtubules.

3.3. Vimentin Monoclonal Antibodies

Once it became known that the expression of intermediate filament proteins is linked to differentiation, monoclonal antibodies became a powerful tool for distinguishing cell types based on intermediate filaments.[17–19] Vimentin is expressed in mesenchymal cells but not in adult muscle cells, neuronal cells, epithelial cells, or glial cells. On the other hand, among other intermediate filament proteins, keratin is expressed only in epithelial cells, desmin in muscle cells, neurofilaments in neuronal cells, and glial acidic protein in glial cells but not in any other types of normal cells. However, in culture most cell types express vimentin, in particular, the epithelial cells. Therefore, for those studying intermediate filaments in cultured cells, vimentin is a subject of great interest.

Polyclonal antivimentin antibodies raised in rabbits sometimes contain antibody species recognizing the common antigenic determinants of all intermediate filament proteins. Although these undesirable antibody species can be removed by absorption with keratin, it is highly desirable to prepare monoclonal antibodies specific for determinants unique to vimentin. Many laboratories have engaged in this work and numerous clones of vimentin antibodies are now available. As expected, in addition to vimentin-specific monoclonal antibodies, those recognizing the common determinants of all intermediate filament proteins have also been identified.[20]

Figure 4 shows the immunofluorescence staining of vimentin in cultured fibroblasts with a monoclonal antibody specific for vimentin, not cross-reacting with keratin, desmin, glial acidic protein, or neurofilament proteins. The distribution of vimentin in tumor cells is generally unchanged. Even in a fully rounded cell, vimentin filaments can still be discerned.

3.4. Keratin Monoclonal Antibodies

Of the intermediate filament proteins found in vertebrate cells, the keratin class, specifically expressed in epithelial cells, is the most complex.[17–19] Distinctive subsets of 2–10 of the 15–20 different keratin polypeptides are expressed by different types of epithelial cells and tissues. Keratin expression also changes as a function of differentiation within the same tissue, as illustrated by the epidermal keratinocyte.[21] The biological reason for these diverse patterns of keratin expression is unknown. By use of monoclonal antibody technology, it is possible to generate antibodies that recognize all the keratins, a specific subset, or even a single keratin.[21–26] Figure 5 shows immunofluo-

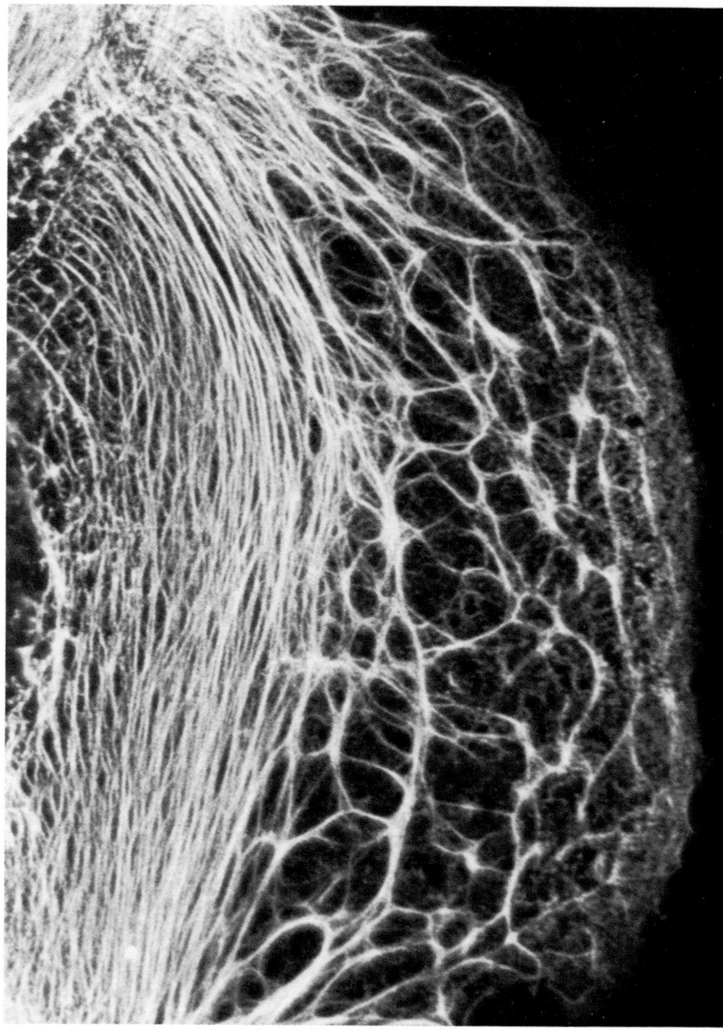

Figure 4. Immunofluorescent staining with vimentin monoclonal antibody of a human fibroblast FS-2.

rescence staining of human breast carcinoma cells with a keratin monoclonal antibody recognizing most keratin species, raised by immunizing mouse with total cytoskeleton of human colon carcinoma cell line CCL187.

When we screened the hybridomas raised against total cytoskeleton of human bladder transitional cell carcinoma line EJ, one clone (H10-1) producing antibody recognizing a minor, keratin filament-associated antigen appeared to be unusually specific, limited to a subset of simple glandular epithelia and part of the transitional epithelia of bladder, but not found in nonglandular simple epithelia or stratified squamous epithelia. Frozen sections of mouse,

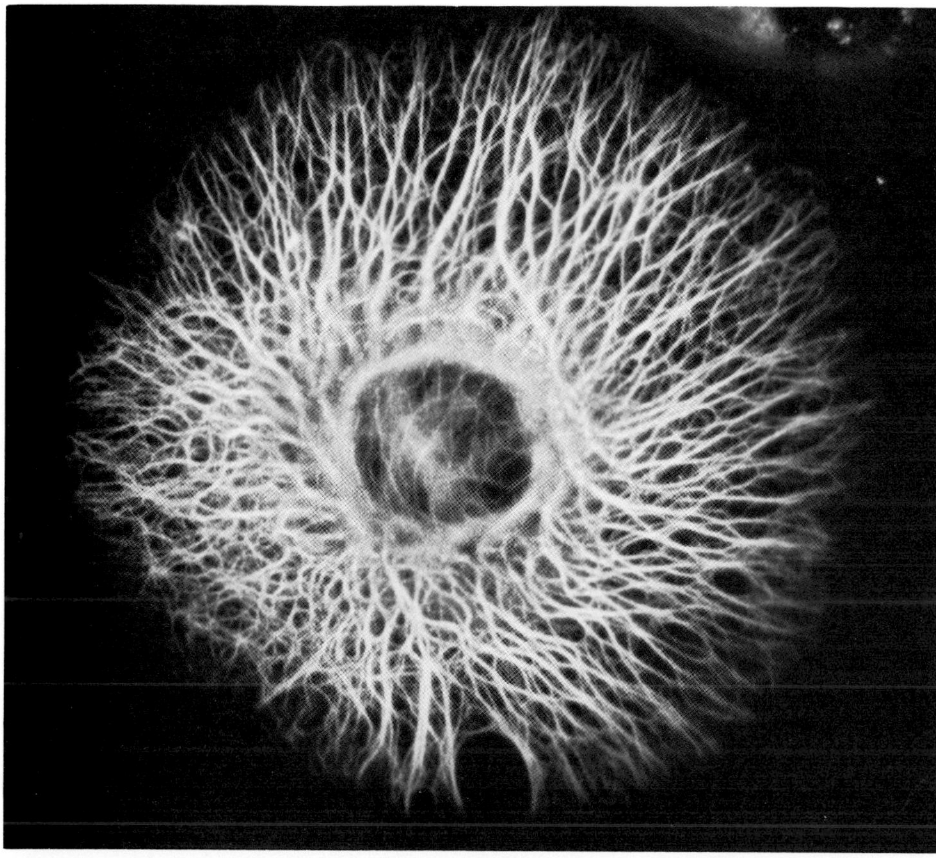

Figure 5. Immunofluorescent staining with keratin monoclonal antibody (J1B3) of a human breast carcinoma cell MCF-7.

human, and rabbit tissues were examined by double immunofluorescence using H10-1 monoclonal antibody and a rabbit anti-(total epidermal stratum corneum keratins) to provide an internal comparison of total keratin levels. Figures 6A–6C show a cross section of mouse epidermis, which was strongly stained by the rabbit anti-(total keratins) (Fig. 6A), but not by H10-1 (Fig. 6B). Identical results were seen with examples of human stratified squamous epithelia: epidermis, esophagus, and rectal epithelium. Figures 6D–6F show a cross section through the ridge dividing the glandular and nonglandular regions of the mouse stomach. Anti-(total keratins) stained both the keratinized stratified squamous epithelium of the nonglandular region and the simple columnar epithelium of the stomach glands (Fig. 6D), whereas H10-1 stained only the epithelium of the glands. In a section through the glandular portion of the stomach, the anti-(total keratins) labeled all the epithelia in the field (Fig. 6G), whereas H10-1 labeled the epithelium lining the stomach glands but not the simple

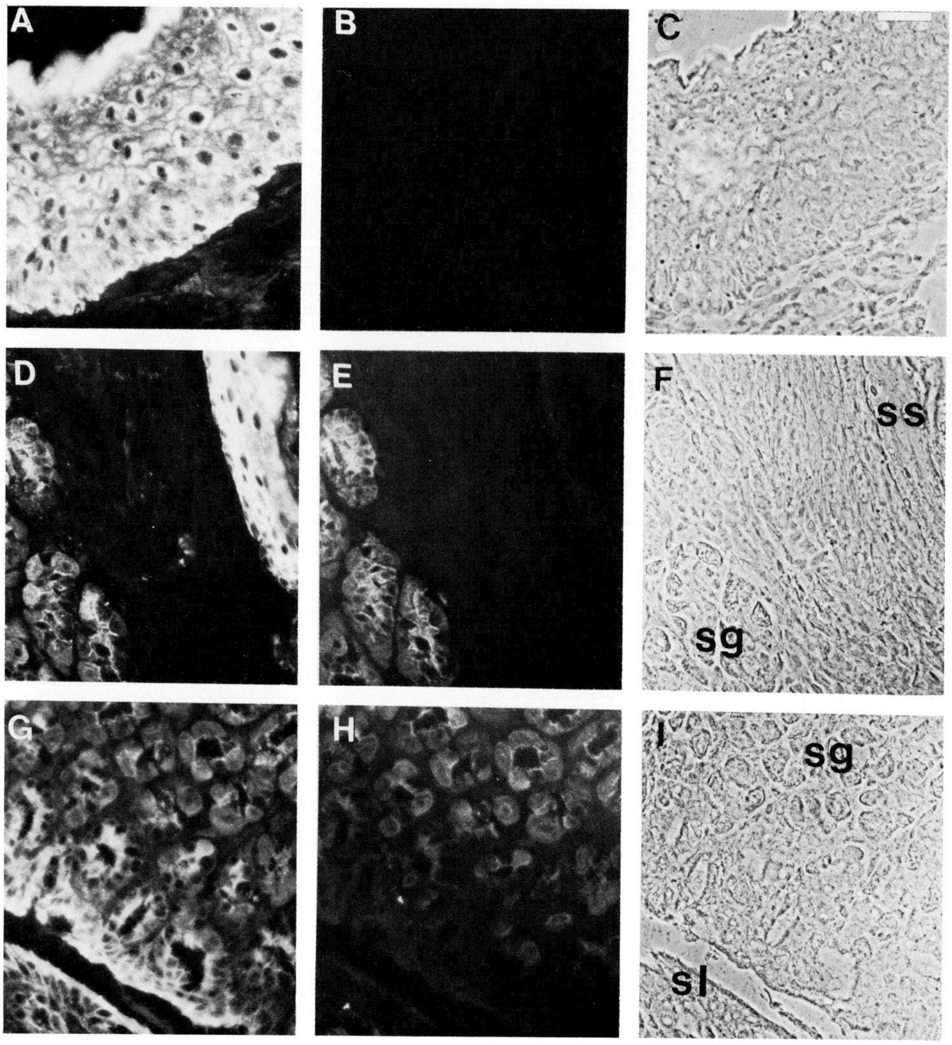

Figure 6. Double immunofluorescence on frozen sections of mouse tissues, using (A, D, G) rabbit anti-(total callus keratins) and (B, G, H) the H10-1 monoclonal antibody; (C, F, I) phase. (A–C) Epidermis; (D–F) junctional region of stomach showing nonglandular keratinized stratified squamous epithelium (ss) and glandular epithelium containing stomach glands (gastric pits; sg); (G–I) glandular region of stomach showing simple epithelial stomach lining (sl) and stomach glands (sg). Bar = 34 μm.

glandular epithelium (Fig. 6H). It was possible to see H10-1-positive mucosal glands in sections of both human (Figs. 7A and 7B) and mouse colon, but negative mucosal glands were also observed. Human breast was heterogeneous for H10-1-positive and -negative epithelia. The H10-1 monoclonal antibody also recognized nine of 14 human colon (Figs. 7C and 7D) and four of six human

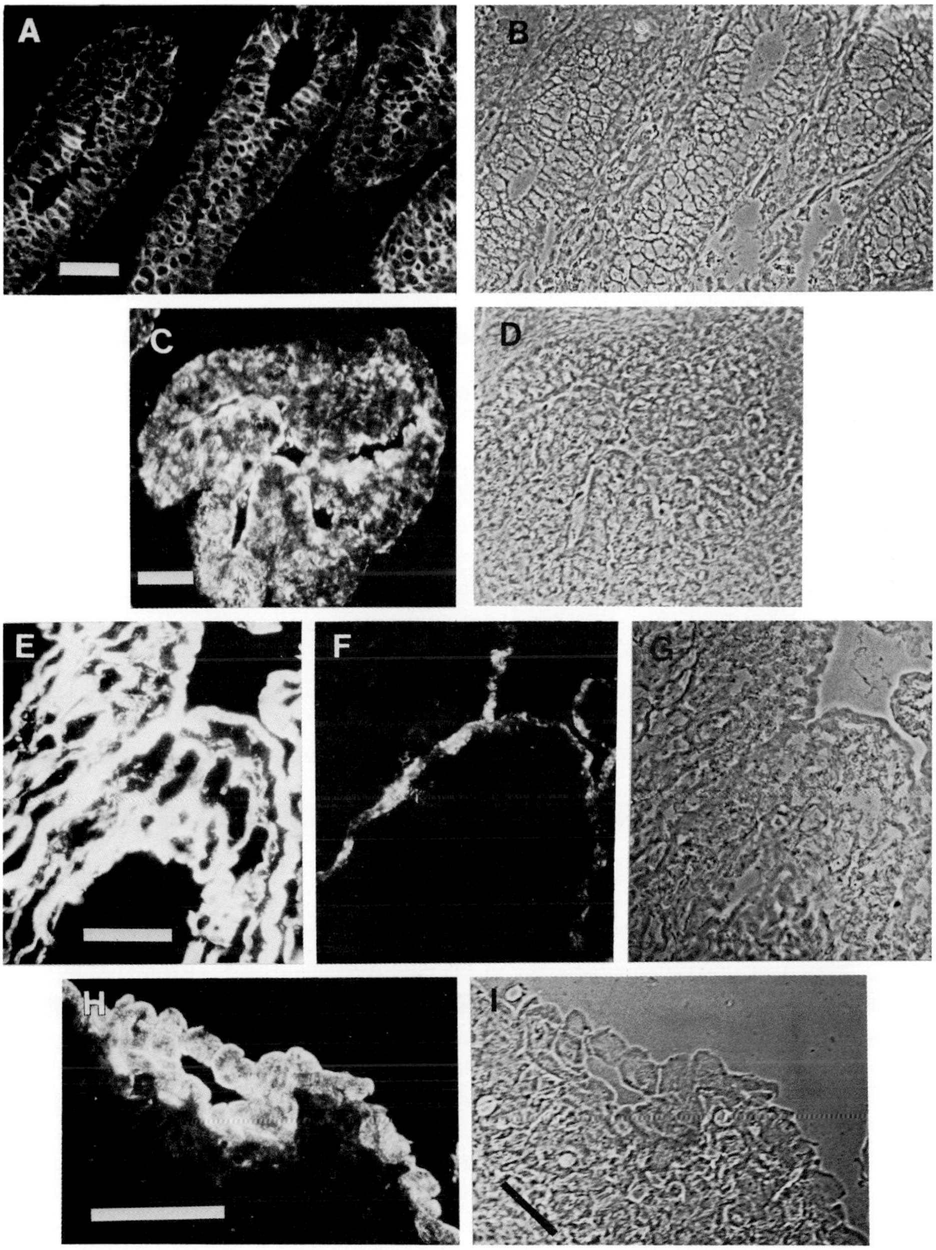

Figure 7. Immunofluorescence with the H10-1 monoclonal antibody on sections of (A, B) normal human colon mucosal glands and (C, D) colon carcinoma. Double immunofluorescence on a frozen section of mouse bladder using (E) rabbit anti-(total callus keratins) and (F) the H10-1 monoclonal antibody; (G) phase; (H) H10-1 staining on rabbit bladder; the depth of the transitional epithelium is indicated in the phase (I). Bar for part A and C, 50 μm; for part E, 25 μm; for part H, 100 μm.

breast carcinomas and did not stain nonepithelial tumors (two sarcomas and a melanoma). Human liver was heterogeneously stained, while mouse small intestinal and kidney tubule, and mouse and human endometrial epithelium, were not stained. Trypsin treatment of sections to expose "masked" antigens did not alter these results. Sections through mouse bladder were strongly stained by the H10-1 monoclonal antibody in the upper but not the basal layers of the transitional epithelium, whereas the rabbit antibody stained the entire transitional epithelium (Figs. 7E–7G). A similar observation was made on rabbit bladder (Figs. 7H and 7I). It appears that the antigen recognized by the H10-1 monoclonal antibody distinguishes a subpopulation of cells within transitional cell epithelia, and certain glandular simple epithelia.

4. Examples of Utility of Monoclonal Antibodies against Cytoskeleton

4.1. Unusual Cells without Intermediate Filaments

The nearly ubiquitous nature of intermediate filaments suggests their involvement in essential cellular functions. However, here we describe the first example of a human cell line that does not appear to express intermediate filaments. Cell line SW13 (obtainable from the American Type Culture Collection as CCL 105) was derived from a carcinoma of the adrenal cortex. These cells grow well in culture, and have an epithelial "cobblestone" morphology. Cells of epithelial origin usually express keratin characteristic of the originating cell type. However, immunofluorescence with three monoclonal and two polyclonal antibodies recognizing human keratins did not reveal keratin-containing intermediate filaments in SW13 cells. A small percentage (less than 5%) of SW13 cells as obtained from the ATCC expressed vimentin filaments, but subcloning yielded several clones in which immunofluorescence for vimentin was negative. Triton-insoluble cytoskeletal fractions of metabolically labeled SW13 subclones were also analyzed by two-dimensional gel electrophoresis, in parallel with cell types that express vimentin. No polypeptide spots corresponding to the position of vimentin were seen.

In contrast to the single polypeptide coded by the vimentin gene, keratins have molecular weights from 40 to 70 kD and a wide range of pI.[15] In addition, it has been reported that some cell types express keratinlike polypeptides that are not detectible by immunofluorescence, but can be identified in cytoskeletal fractions by the technique of immunoblotting. Therefore, cytoskeletal protein fractions of SW13 were also analyzed by one-dimensional gel electrophoresis followed by immunoblotting. A mixture of keratin monoclonal antibodies AE1 and AE3,[27] as well as a rabbit anti-human-keratins antiserum, both recognized keratin bands in the cytoskeletal fraction of the human breast carcinoma line MCF-7, but did not recognize SW13.

SW13 cells were further screened by immunofluorescence for expression of intermediate filament proteins other than vimentin or keratins. Monoclonal antibodies recognizing the neurofilament 200-kD protein, and an antigenic determinant common to all classes of intermediate filament proteins ("Pruss" antibody)[20] all failed to reveal intermediate filaments within these cells. In addition, monoclonal antibody JLB7, recognizing a 95-kD, IF-associated protein,[8] did not stain SW13, suggesting that there may be coordinate regulation of intermediate filaments and intermediate filament-associated-protein gene expression. Immunoblotting of SW13 cytoskeletal fractions with the neurofilament and the Pruss antibodies also revealed no intermediate filament protein bands. Immunofluorescence staining of SW13 with rabbit polyclonal antibodies against human glial filaments also failed to detect any antigen. Transmission electron microscopy of thin sections of SW13 cells revealed no intermediate filaments.

Intermediate filaments have been proposed to play roles in a variety of cellular functions, including cell division and maintenance of cell shape. The absence of any intermediate filaments in SW13 cells suggests that a new perspective is required to understand the function of this cytoskeletal system, since maintenance of an epitheloid morphology and mitosis in SW13 cells evidently does not require intermediate filaments.

4.2 Microinjection of Monoclonal Antibodies into Living Cells

One of the distinct advantages of monoclonal over polyclonal antibodies is that their homogeneity makes them suitable for microinjection into living cells. The most striking example is injection of the JLB7 monoclonal antibody specific for the vimentin-associated 95-kD protein, which causes the distribution of vimentin to retract toward the nuclear region.[28,29] Using this monoclonal antibody, we have confirmed Lin and Feramisco's finding and to our surprise it did not alter the distribution of mitochondria (Fig. 8). As a result of such experiments, we realize that the interactions between cellular organelles and the cytoskeleton are likely to be complex, not as simple as previously suggested, and that monoclonal antibodies are probably an excellent tool for elucidating the role of cytoskeleton in intracellular motility.

5. Concluding Remarks

Monoclonal antibodies are clearly useful for the study of the cytoskeleton. The field is still at the infant stage. More new monoclonal antibodies need to be made—in particular, those that may be useful for the functional studies of cytoskeleton. The most important application of hybridoma technology in cytoskeletal research might be the identification of new components without the need for first purifying the component, since mice can be immunized with unfractionated total cytoskeleton. All monoclonal antibodies described in this chapter were raised by this method. Several monoclonal antibodies that we have not described here because of space limitations appear to recognize new

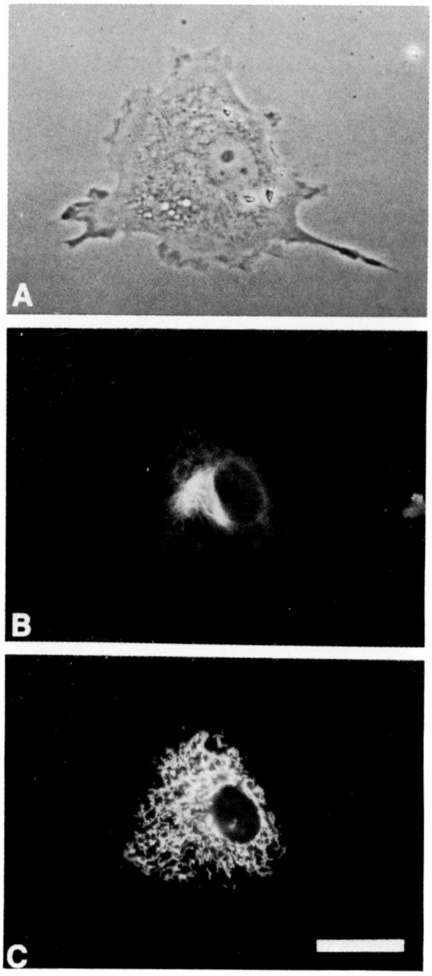

Figure 8. Microinjection of monoclonal antibody (JBL7; generously provided by J. Lin, Cold Spring Harbor Laboratory) into gerbil fibroma cells (CCL146). (A) Phase-contrast photograph; (B) vimentin staining in a fixed cell; (C) mitochondrial staining with rhodamine 123 in a living cell. Bar represents 100 μm.

components, since these antibodies do not react with any known cytoskeletal components. Most of the potential new components are likely to be minor proteins, in contrast to the abundant proteins such as actin, tubulin, vimentin, or keratin. Without hybridoma technology, it would be difficult to identify, characterize, and raise specific antibodies to these minor components.

ACKNOWLEDGMENTS. This work has been supported by grants from the National Cancer Institute (NCI) and Council for Tobacco Research to L. B. C.; K. K. N. was supported by a training grant from the National Cancer Institute to A. B. Pardee and a postdoctoral fellowship from NCI. S. R. was supported by a postdoctoral fellowship from NCI. L. B. C. is the recipient of an American Cancer Society Faculty Research Award.

References

1. Köhler, G., and Milstein, C., 1975, Continuous cultures of fused cells secreting antibody of predefined specificity, *Nature* **256**:495–497.
2. Bernal, S. D., and Chen, L. B., 1982, Induction of cytoskeleton-associated proteins during differentiation of human myeloid leukemic cell lines, *Cancer Res.***42**:5106–5116.
3. Cervera, M., Dreyfuss, G., and Penman, S., 1981, Messenger RNA is translated when associated with the cytoskeletal framework in normal and VSV infected HeLa cells, *Cell* **23**:113–120.
4. Cheng, Y.-S. and Chen, L. B., 1981, Detection of phosphotyrosine-containing 34,000-dalton protein in the framework of cells transformed with Rous sarcoma virus, *Proc. Natl. Acad. Sci.* **78**:2388–2392.
5. Giloh, H., and Sedat, J. W., 1982, Fluorescence microscopy: Reduced photobleaching of rhodamine and fluorescein protein conjugates by *n*-propyl gallate, *Science* **217**:1252–1255.
6. Shi, S.-R., Bhan, A. K., Pilch, B. Z., Chen, L. B., and Goodman, M. L., 1984, Immunohistochemical localization of keratin in head and neck neoplasms and normal tissues, *Am. J. Pathol.* **117**:53–63.
7. Lazarides, E., and Weber, K., 1974, Actin antibody: The specific visualization of actin filaments in non-muscle cells, *Proc. Natl. Acad. Sci. USA* **71**:2268–2272.
8. Lin, J. J. C., 1981, Monoclonal antibodies against myofibrillar components of rat skeletal muscle decorate the intermediate filaments of cultured cells, *Proc. Natl. Acad. Sci. USA* **78**:2335–2339.
9. Simpson, P. A., Spudich, J. A., and Parham, P., 1984, Monoclonal antibodies prepared against *Dictyostelium* actin: Characterization and interactions with actin, *J. Cell Biol.* **99**:287–295.
10. Pollack, R., Osborn, M., and Weber, K., 1976, Patterns of organization of actin and myosin in normal and transformed cultured cells, *Proc. Natl. Acad. Sci. USA* **73**:994–998.
11. Cleveland, D. W., Pittenger, M. F., and Feramisco, J. R., 1983, Elevation of tubulin levels by microinjection suppresses new tubulin synthesis, *Nature* **305**:738–740.
12. Wang, E., and Goldman, R. D., 1978, Functions of cytoplasmic fibers in intracellular movements in BHK-21 cells, *J. Cell Biol.* **79**:708–726.
13. Heggeness, M. J., Simon, M., and Singer, S. J., 1978, Association of mitochondria with microtubules in cultured cells, *Proc. Natl. Acad. Sci. USA* **75**:3863–3866.
14. Summerhayes, I. C., Wong, D.,, and Chen, L. B., 1983, Effect of microtubules and intermediate filaments on mitochondrial distribution, *J. Cell Sci.* **61**:87–105.
15. Brinkley, B. R., Fuller, G. M., and Highfield, D. P., 1975, Cytoplasmic microtubules in normal and transformed cells in culture: Analysis by tubulin antibody immunofluorescence, *Proc. Natl. Acad. Sci. USA* **73**:4981–4985.
16. Osborn, M., and Weber, K., 1977, The display of microtubules in transformed cells, *Cell* **12**:561–571.
17. Osborn, M., Altmannsberger, M., Shaw, G., Schauer, A., and Weber, K., 1982, Various sympathetic derived human tumors differ in neurofilament expression: Use in diagnosis of neuroblastoma, ganglioneuroblastoma and pheochroblastoma, *Virchows Arch. B Cell Pathol. Mol. Pathol.* **40**:141–152.
18. Moll, R., Franke, W. W., Schiller, D. L., Geiger, B., and Krepler, R., 1982, The catalogue of human cytokeratins: Patterns of expression in normal epithelia, tumors and cultured cells, *Cell* **31**:11–24.
19. Tseng, S. C. G., Jarvinen, M. J., Nelson, W. G., Huang, J.-W., Woodcock-Mitchell, J., and Sun, T.-T., 1982, Correlation of specific keratins with different types of epithelial differentiation: Monoclonal antibody studies, *Cell* **30**:361–372.
20. Pruss, R. M., Mirsky, R., Raff, M. C., Thorpe, R., Dowding, A. J., and Anderton, B. H., 1981, All classes of intermediate filaments share a common antigenic determinant defined by a monoclonal antibody, *Cell* **27**:419–428.

21. Nadakavukaren, K. K., Summerhayes, I. C., Salcedo, B. F., Rheinwald, J. G., and Chen, L. B., 1984, A monoclonal antibody recognizing a keratin filament protein in a subset of transitional and glandular epithelia, *Differentiation* **27**:209–220.
22. Debus, E., Weber, K., and Osborn, M., 1982, Monoclonal cytokeratin antibodies that distinguish simple from stratified squamous epithelia: Characterization on human tissues, *EMBO J.* **1**:1641–1647.
23. Gown, A. M., and Vogel, A. M., 1982, Monoclonal antibodies to intermediate filament proteins of human cells: Unique and cross-reacting antibodies, *J. Cell Biol.* **95**:414–424.
24. Lane, E. B., 1982, Monoclonal antibodies provide specific intramolecular markers for the study of epithelial tonofilament organization, *J. Cell Biol.* **92**:665–673.
25. Summerhayes, I. C., and Chen, L. B., 1982, Localization of a MW 52,000 keratin in basal epithelial cells of the mouse bladder and expression throughout neoplastic progression, *Cancer Res.* **42**:4098–4109.
26. Summerhayes, I. C., Cheng, Y.-S., Sun, T.-T., and Chen, L. B., 1981, Expression of keratin and vimentin intermediate filaments in rabbit bladder epithelial cells at different stages of benzo(*a*)pyrene induced neoplastic progression, *J. Cell Biol.* **90**:63–69.
27. Sun, T.-T., and Green, H., 1978, Immunofluorescent staining of keratin fibers in cultured cells, *Cell* **14**:469–476.
28. Lin, J. J. C., and Feramisco, J. R., 1981, Disruption of the *in vivo* distribution of the intermediate filaments in fibroblasts through the microinjection of a specific monoclonal antibody, *Cell* **24**:185–193.

Chapter 16

Monoclonal Antibodies as Molecular Probes of the Nervous System

COLIN J. BARNSTABLE

1. Introduction

The central nervous system (CNS) has been studied intensively using anatomic and electrophysiological methods such that an overall concept of the structure and function of the various neural cell types has been obtained. In spite of the large body of information about the CNS, the molecular differences among the different subclasses of neural cells and the ways in which these differences account for the observed differences in morphology and synaptic interactions are understood poorly if at all.

The retina provides a number of advantages for molecular studies of the mammalian CNS. It has a laminated structure and is composed of a relatively small number of cell types. A drawing of a human retina is shown in Fig. 1. Light is absorbed by the outer segments of the rod (low-light-intensity) and cone (color) photoreceptors. The cell bodies of these cells lie in a separate layer, the outer nuclear layer. The photoreceptors form synapses in the outer plexiform layer with other neurons whose cell bodies make up the inner nuclear layer. Bipolar cells convey information to the inner plexiform layer. They can be divided into subclasses according to whether they receive input from rods or cones and whether they respond to the beginning of illumination (ON-bipolars) or its end (OFF-bipolars). Horizontal cells also make and receive synaptic contacts in the outer plexiform layer. The exact function of these cells is not known, but they probably modulate the response of the photoreceptor–bipolar pathway according to the illumination falling on adjacent areas of the retina. In the inner plexiform layer synapses are made onto the ganglion cells, which conduct the information to other CNS visual areas through their axons, which make up the optic nerve. Ganglion cells also consist of several subtypes, including ON and OFF subclasses and various subclasses that vary in their responses, such as whether they give a transient or a sustained response to

COLIN J. BARNSTABLE • Laboratory of Neurobiology, Rockefeller University, New York, New York 10021.

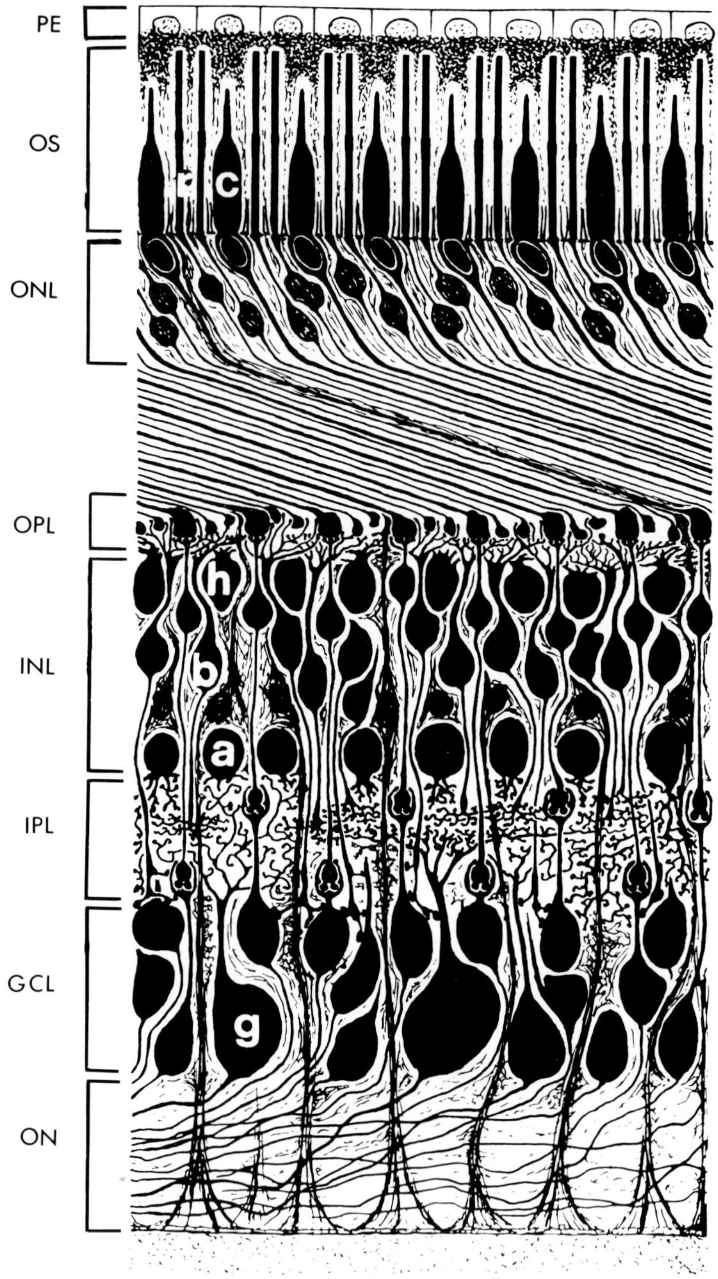

Figure 1. Drawing of a human retina showing the cell types, layered structure, and synaptic connections. PE, Pigment epithelium; OS, photoreceptor outer segments; ONL, outer nuclear layer; OPL, outer plexiform layer; INL, inner nuclear layer; IPL, inner plexiform layer; GCL, ganglion cell layer; ON, optic nerve fiber layer. c, Cone; r, rod; h, horizontal cell; b, bipolar cell; a, amacrine cell; g, ganglion cell. (Adapted from Ref. 1.)

illumination. Amacrine cells mediate a set of lateral connections in the inner plexiform layer. The degree of information processing carried out by this layer varies among species. Different species have different proportions of the various cell types. A more detailed discussion of retina structure and function can be found in recent reviews and books.[2–4]

A further advantage of the retina as a model for the CNS is that much of its maturation is postnatal in experimental animals such as rats and mice. It is accessible and the eye has often been used as a convenient chamber for the application of drugs and radioactive tracers to the retina. These advantages have led to the use of the retina for many studies of neural properties, such as cell adhesion, migration, and neurite outgrowth.

Traditional biochemical methods do not suggest any way of studying most molecules important for neural structure and function. The complexity of the nervous system makes it almost impossible to isolate any but the most abundant of them. In an attempt to overcome these problems a number of groups have turned to immunologic methods, since antibodies can provide a link between biochemistry and the more traditional methods of neurobiology.

Neurons are highly polarized cells and many neuronal molecules are found only in certain parts of the cell. For example, some cytoskeletal proteins are found in dendrites but not axons, some neurotransmitter receptors are clustered at discrete spots on the postsynaptic membrane, and some photoreceptor molecules are found in only the outer segments.[5–8] This discrete localization, which has important implications for understanding the functions of the molecules, can be revealed by immunocytochemical methods.

Given the complexity of neural tissue available as immunogens, it is perhaps not surprising that many antisera have been multispecific and have only begun to show specificity after extensive absorption. The approach of Köhler and Milstein,[9] by which antibody-secreting spleen cells are converted into cloned hybrid cell lines, has overcome many of the problems of the immunologic analysis of the nervous system. It is now possible to use the available heterogeneous immunogens and still derive monospecific (because they are monoclonal) antibodies. In theory, monoclonal antibodies could be produced against every immunogenic molecule in the nervous system. In practice, however, the range of antibodies that can be produced will be limited by the immunogens available, the sensitivity and discrimination of the assays used to detect them, as well the natural biases in immunogenicity of the immune system.

In this chapter I shall discuss some of the antibodies that have been produced against retinas of a number of species. Although still at an early stage, the work carried out so far has begun to provide some clues concerning the extent of molecular diversity within the retina and the ways in which the tissue develops and forms functional patterns of connections.

2. Immunologic Structure of the Retina

2.1. Photoreceptors

Some of the first specific antisera against any neural antigens were in fact raised against photoreceptor proteins. A number of laboratories have purified the visual pigment protein rhodopsin from mammalian photoreceptors. Antisera against rhodopsin have been used for a variety of studies, including immunocytochemical labeling.[10,11] These labeling studies have suggested both that rhodopsin is a transmembrane protein and that its plasma membrane distribution is limited to the outer and part of the inner segment. It is known that light triggers a conformational change from 11-*cis*- to all-*trans*-retinal, in the pigment moiety bound to the apoprotein opsin. This change affects the opsin structure and leads to an interaction with transducin or G-protein, a GTP-binding protein, which, when activated by photoexcited rhodopsin, mediates the activation of a cGMP phosphodiesterase (see Ref. 12 for a recent review of the biochemistry of phototransduction). Since these events occur at the internal photoreceptor disk membranes, whereas the end result of light excitation in photoreceptors is a closure of plasma membrane Na channels, the signal must be carried by some soluble molecule. cGMP may be one such second messenger, although Ca^{2+} has also been implicated. Some of the proteins involved in these later stages of the visual transduction mechanism have also been partially purified and used as immunogens for monoclonal antibody production by a number of different laboratories. One of these antibodies, which recognizes the α subunit of transducin, has been shown to block the light-stimulated activation of cGMP phosphodiesterase when added to disrupted frog photoreceptor outer segments.[13] The use of monoclonal antibodies as pharmacological agents is likely to play an important role in dissecting complex biochemical pathways mediating both transmission and cell interactions in the nervous system.

Using membranes from adult rat retinas as immunogen, several years ago we produced a series of monoclonal antibodies, some of which were specific for photoreceptors.[14] The antibody called RET-P1 labels the whole photoreceptor cells of rods but not cones (Fig. 2c). It is the earliest biochemical marker of photoreceptor differentiation so far described. It is first detectable on a few cells at birth in rat retinas (Fig. 2a). Over the next few days the number of RET-P1-positive cells increases in a gradient from the center to the periphery, until by postnatal day 4–5 the whole photoreceptor layer is positive (Fig. 2b). This pattern is similar to that of the final mitosis, or birth, of photoreceptor precursors, but the exact relationship between final mitosis and antigen expression is not yet clear. Although the time of appearance and the histological localization of RET-P1 antigen differed from previously published accounts for opsin, we found that RET-P1 antibody could be inhibited by purified bovine opsin.[15] Furthermore, in collaboration with Dr. P. Hargrave, we found that fragments of the opsin molecule, obtained by chemical degradation or chemical synthesis, were equally effective at inhibiting the antibody activity. Such fragments have

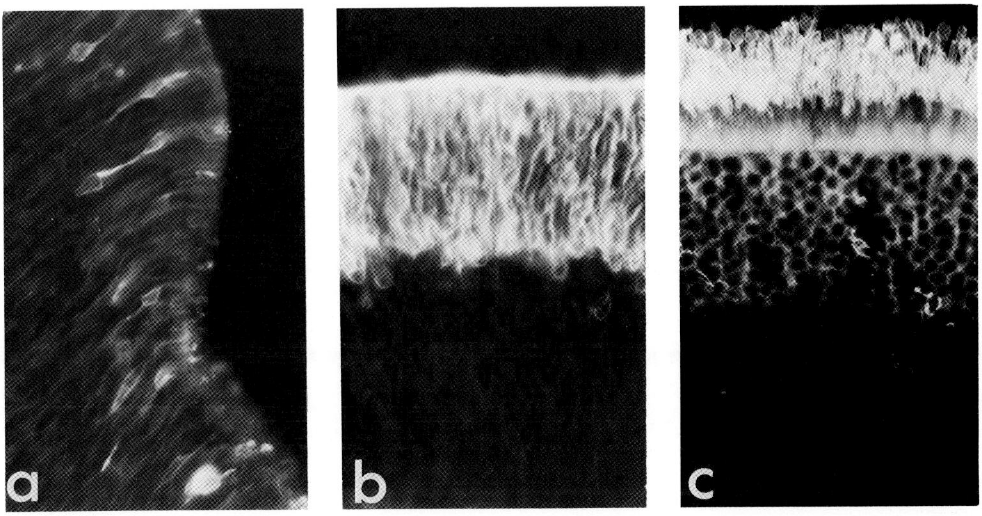

Figure 2. Changing expression of photoreceptor antigen RET-P1 with time in rat retina. (a) Two days postnatal; (b) 8 days postnatal; (c) adult. Fifteen-micrometer cryostat sections were treated with monoclonal antibody and then rhodamine-conjugated goat anti-mouse IgG as described in Ref 14.

allowed us to localize the antigenic site to the NH_2-terminal 30 amino acids of the opsin polypeptide chain.

Other monoclonal antibodies produced against retinal membranes were found to label either just the photoreceptor outer segment or just the phororeceptor cell bodies. An antibody that labels what appears to be only photoreceptor synaptic terminals has also been described.[16] Several groups have now used immunocytochemical procedures to show that the Na/K ATPase is restricted to the inner segments of rod photoreceptors.[17,18] These labeling patterns, as well as indicating the extent of the molecular complexity of photoreceptors, demonstrate that photoreceptor membranes are composed of a number of distinct domains. More recently, monoclonal antibodies have been produced against photoreceptors of *Drosophila* and squid.[19–21] In these very different organisms one of the most striking features has been a similar compartmentalization of the cells into discrete domains. Since electrophysiological studies have indicated that a variety of ion channels are found in either the inner or the outer segment but not both,[7] it is likely that a number of other such molecules will be found. The mechanism by which such domains are set up is by no means clear. One possible model for such compartmentalization is that molecules are routed to a particular domain, are inserted, and are held in place by interactions with cytoplasmic elements.[22] An alternative model for the observed photoreceptor domains is that molecules are inserted in particular domains and are prevented from migration by barriers at the boundaries between the domains.[23]

2.2. Bipolar Cells

In several separate immunizations we have found classes of antibodies that react with bipolar cells.[24,25] Since most, if not all, cells in the bipolar cell layer of the inner nuclear layer were labeled, and several bands of labeling were found across the inner plexiform layer, it is likely that these antibodies are reacting with all subclasses of bipolar cells. One class of antibodies reacts with bipolar cells alone. A second class labels bipolar cells, photoreceptor inner segments, and a very small number of cells in the amacrine cell layer. The exact nature of this last group of cells is not yet clear. It is becoming a common finding that monoclonal antibodies against neural tissue detect antigens on groups of cells not previously known to be related. This was first discussed in the leech, where antibodies recognizing nociceptive neurons in the segmental ganglia also recognized a few other cells in the head ganglion.[26] This prompted the suggestion that some of these antigens may be defining interconnected cells or pathways.

2.3. Ganglion Cells

We and other laboratories have found that in retina Thy-1 antigen is expressed only by ganglion cells.[27–30] The antibody we have used in these studies, 2G12, was produced by immunizing with a glycoprotein fraction of rat cerebral cortex.[30] As well as immunocytochemical labeling of tissue sections,[30] a further property of ganglion cells was used to characterize the antibody specifity. Since ganglion cells are the only retinal neurons to project out of the retina, tracers injected into the superior colliculus or lateral geniculate nucleus are transported retrogradely and label only the ganglion cells. When retinas were labeled with a fluorescent retrograde tracer (a wheat germ agglutinin–lucifer yellow complex), dissociated, and the suspension labeled with antibody 2G12, there was essentially complete coincidence of the two labels.[30] Thus it would appear that 2G12 labels all and only ganglion cells. Using other antibodies, we found that Thy-1 is also restricted to ganglion cells in mouse retina. Thy-1 had been described as a general neuronal marker.[31] The retina is the first area of the central nervous system in which selectivity of Thy-1 expression has been described. The difference in Thy-1 expression is presumably a reflection of functional differences between ganglion cells and other retinal neurons. Ganglion cells differ in that their axons are myelinated, they project a greater distance, and they conduct action potentials. In addition, they are the only retinal cells whose axons are associated with true astrocytes. It is not yet clear which of these properties, if any, is related to the function of Thy-1. Based on its sequence homology with immunoglobulins, it has been suggested that Thy-1 is one of a family of molecules involved in interaction between neurons and astrocytes.[32]

In chick retina, ganglion cell-specific antibodies have also been described and some of these are probably analogous to the rodent Thy-1.[33]

In an effort to enrich for the production of ganglion cell-specific antibodies, we also carried out an immunization with a horizontal section of retina that was primarily the ganglion cell layer. One of the antibodies produced by this procedure turned out to recognize the 200,000-dalton polypeptide of neurofilaments. Neurofilaments consist of three polypeptide subunits of 200,000, 145,000, and 70,000 daltons. It had been generally assumed that all neurons contained all three polypeptides. From our work in retina and other independent studies elsewhere in the rodent CNS it has become apparent that this is not the case.[34,35] In retina only ganglion cells and some of the horizontal cells express neurofilaments (Fig. 3a). Within ganglion cells, although all three subunits are present in the axons that bundle together to form the optic nerve, there appears to be no 200,000-dalton subunit in the dendritic neurofilaments. Thus, the subunit composition of neurofilaments can vary within different areas of the same cell. A further difference between the 200,000-dalton subunit and the 145,000-dalton subunit has been found in developmental studies of the retina. In collaboration with Drs. R. Majocha and C. Marotta (McLean Hospital, Belmont, Massachusetts) we have used monoclonal antibodies in both histological and biochemical analyses to look at the appearance of the two subunits.[36] The 140,000-dalton subunit appears in the ganglion cells of the late embryo rat retina. By immunocytochemical analysis no 200,000-dalton subunit was detectable. Biochemically, however, 200,000-dalton subunit was detectable in neonatal animals. This appeared to be in a soluble protein pool rather than in an insoluble cytoskeleton. This result raises the possibility of two developmental control points for neurofilaments. The first is at the initial synthesis of the 200,000-dalton subunit and the second is at the event that allows this soluble pool of protein to become incorporated into preexisting neurofilament core structures.

2.4. Horizontal Cells

A retinal wholemount labeled with a monoclonal antibody against the 200,000-dalton subunit of neurofilaments is shown in Fig. 3b and indicates the network of horizontal cell processes in the outer plexiform layer. By examining the morphology of individual cells within this network, it became clear that the labeled cells resembled one of the two types of horizontal cells present in most mammalian species, the axonless horizontal cell. In addition, these cells have been shown to share some intermediate filament proteins with glial cells (see below). Although immunocytochemical methods had previously shown the coexistence of both neuronal and glial markers in embryonic cells, this is the first example of such dual properties in the mature nervous system. Interestingly, these findings rekindle an old debate as to whether these cells are glia or neurons.[37] So far no markers unique to horizontal cells have been detected in mammals, although such markers do exist in fish retina.[38]

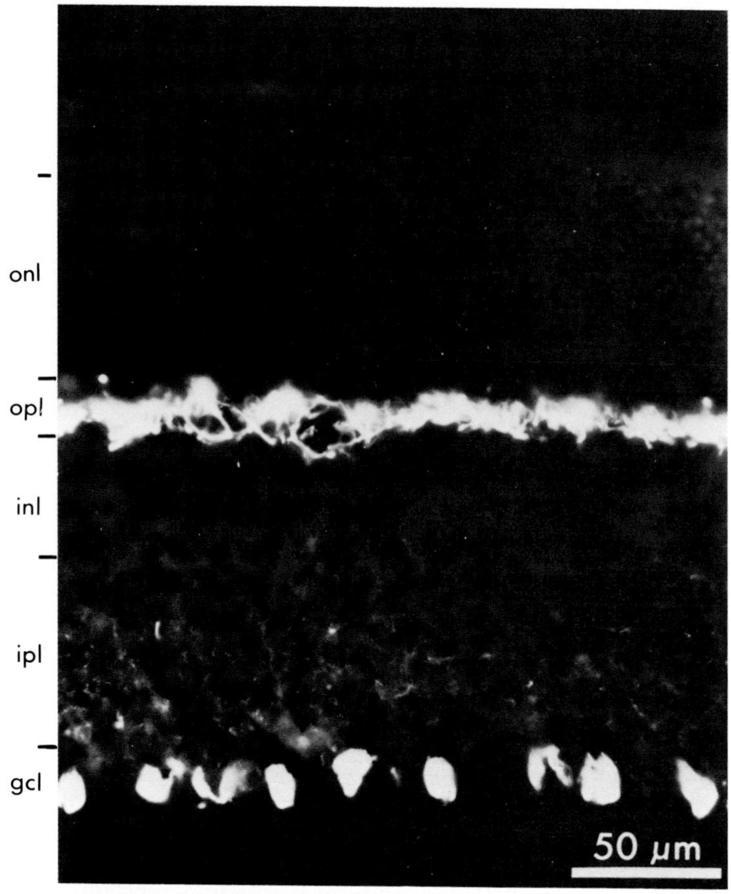
onl
opl
inl
ipl
gcl
50 μm

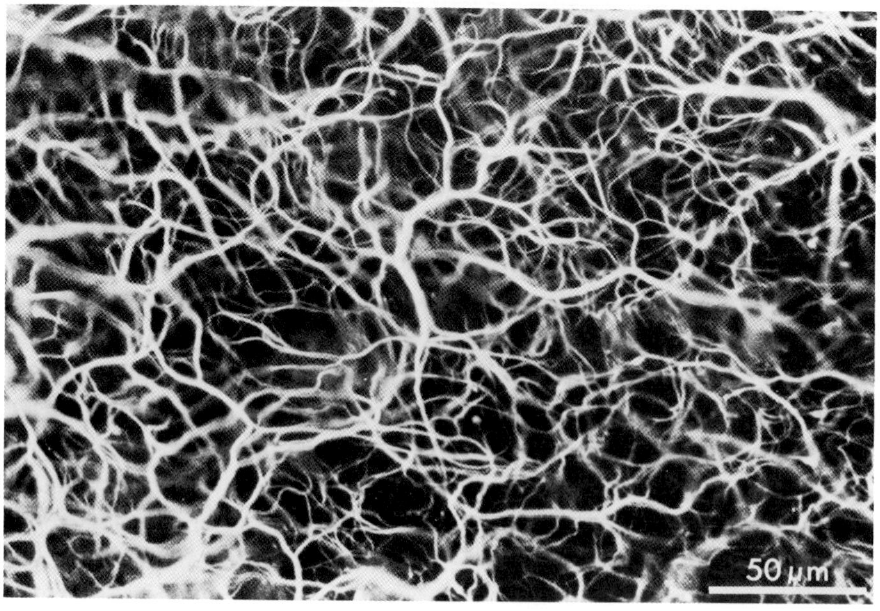
50 μm

2.5. Amacrine Cells

Amacrine cells are defined as those retinal neurons whose processes are entirely confined to the inner plexiform layer and which do not have an identifiable axon. Within this broad definition, however, there are clearly many different subclasses of amacrine cells. These subclasses can be defined morphologically[39] and immunocytochemical studies have confirmed that these subclasses are also molecularly distinct using antisera raised against a whole variety of neuropeptides.[40] In addition to reagents that subdivide amacrine cells into various subsets, we have found a membrane antigen that is common to all amacrine cells and does not appear to be expressed by any other retinal neuron.[41] The antigen is a 35,000-dalton polypeptide, but whether the molecule is glycosylated and the true subunit structure of the antigen have yet to be determined. It is interesting to consider what the function of such an antigen might be. Since it reacts with all amacrine cells rather than any neurochemically defined subset, its function is unlikely to be related to any particular neurotransmitter system (unless of course all amacrine cells share a second, common transmitter system). Since some amacrine cells synapse with bipolar cells and others synapse with ganglion cells, the antigen is also unlikely to play a role in detailed cell interactions. It is possible that the function of the molecule is in some grosser aspect of amacrine function, such as formation of the inner plexiform layer or some other retinal layer. It is certainly expressed by developing amacrine cells as they migrate into the inner nuclear layer and begin to form the inner plexiform layer (see below).

2.6. Retinal Glial Cells

Two classes of glia have been defined in the retina. Muller glia are radial cells that span the whole thickness of the retina. They isolate the retina from other tissues by forming the outer and inner limiting membranes and also insulate neuronal processes in the plexiform layers. Astrocytes are confined to the optic nerve fiber layer and only interact with the ganglion cell axons. The functions and relationships of the two glial cell types have not been defined either in molecular terms or from the point of view of their cell lineages.

2.6.1. Muller Glia

Two classes of antigens have been defined that are to some extent specific for Muller cells. The first class consists of a variety of cytoplasmic antigens.

Figure 3. Labeling of retina by antineurofilament antibody R3. (a) A 15-μm cryostat section. Labeling is confined to the outer plexiform layer and optic nerve fiber bundles. Abbreviations as in Figure 1. (b) Retinal wholemount. The focus is on the outer plexiform layer and shows the network of horizontal cell processes. (From Ref. 35.)

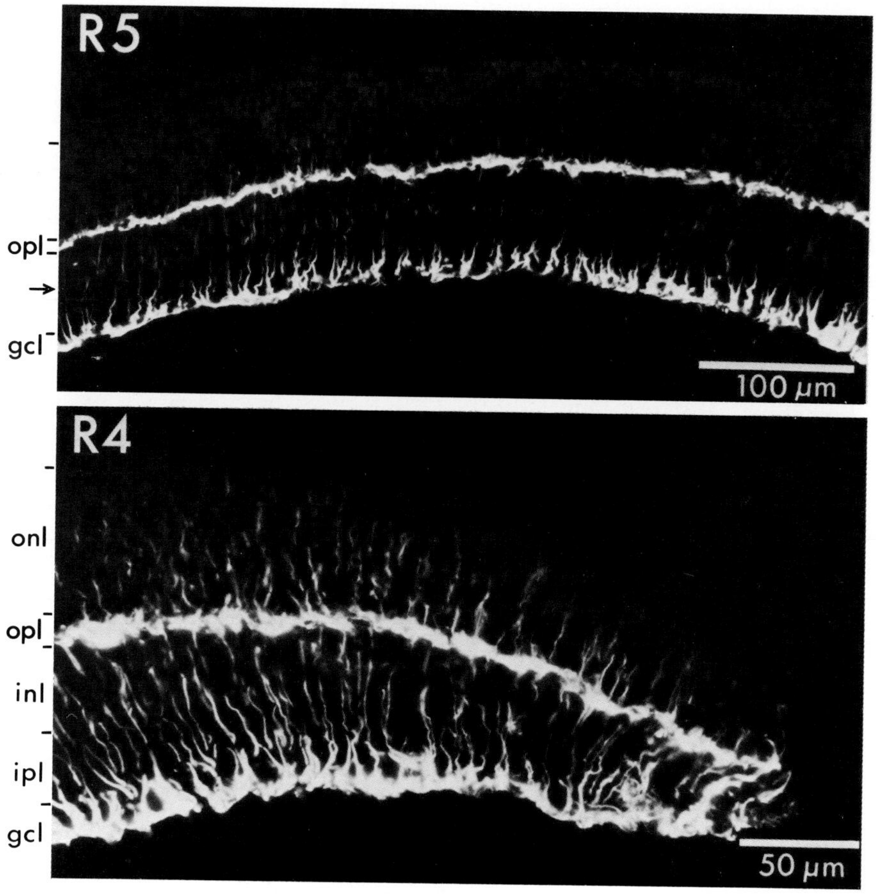

Figure 4. Labeling of retina with antibodies (upper) R5 and (lower) R4. Both antibodies label radial Muller fibers and horizontal cells in the outer plexiform layer. The location of the cell bodies of the Muller glia is shown by the arrow in the upper panel. Abbreviations as in Fig. 1. (From Ref. 35.)

The enzymes carbonic anhydrase and glutamine synthetase both seem to be selectively localized to the Muller cells when studied immunocytochemically with a variety of antisera.[42,43] The other cytoplasmic antigens seem to be related to intermediate filaments. The filament protein vimentin has been described in Muller cells but not neurons, although it now appears that it is also present in horizontal cells.[44] We have also described a number of other filamentous proteins that have a similar distribution (Fig. 4). Several of these differ in molecular weight from vimentin and appear to be filament "associated-proteins."[35]

The second class of Muller cell antigens are a series of membrane molecules that we detected with monoclonal antibodies.[14] These have not yet been char-

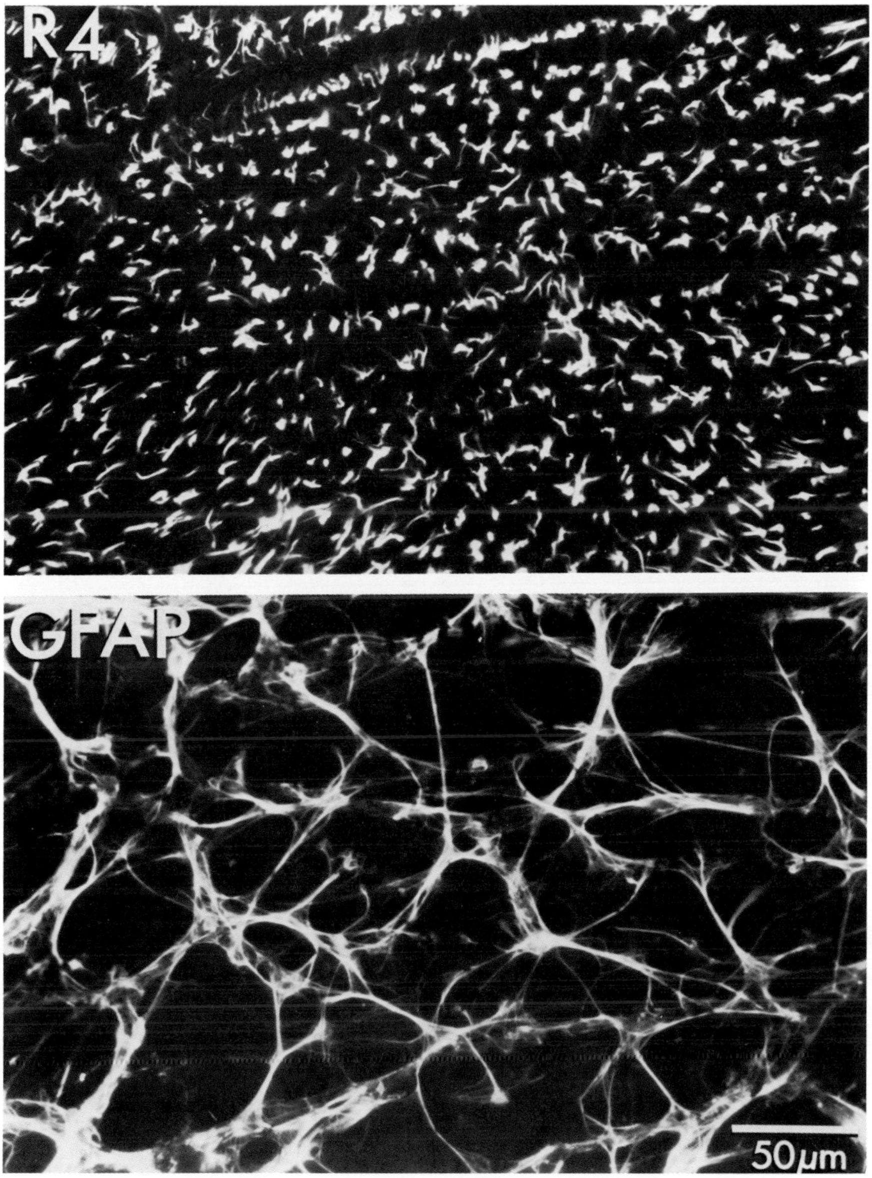

Figure 5. Horizontal section through the Muller endfeet and the optic fiber layer double-labeled with antibody R4 (fluorescein optics) and anti-GFAP (rhodamine optics); R4 does not react with astrocytes. (From Ref. 35.)

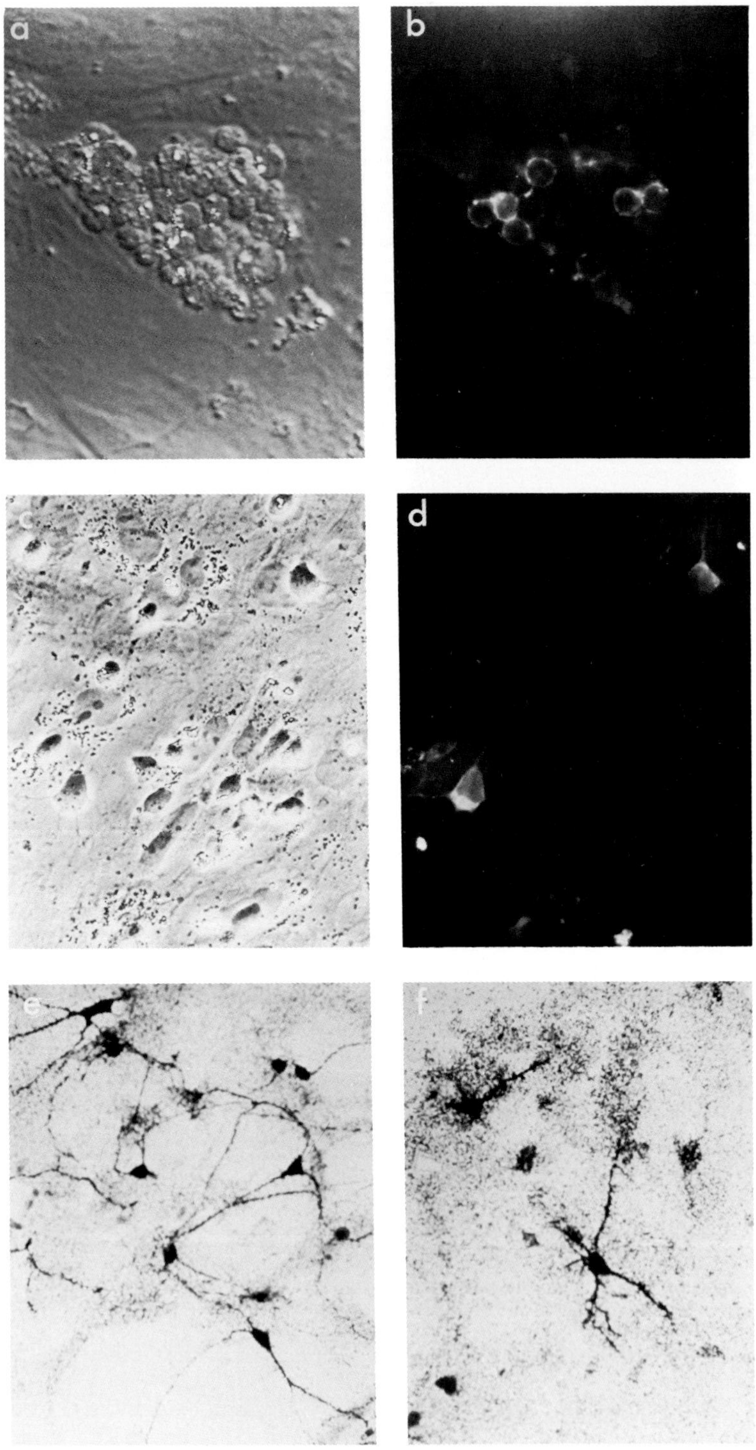
a
b
c
d
e
f

acterized biochemically, but are clearly different, since they appear at distinct periods during rat retinal development.[45]

2.6.2. Astrocytes

Both Muller cells and astrocytes express some markers, such as vimentin and several of the filament associated proteins. There are, however, several clear antigenic distinctions that can be made between the two cell types. We have found one filament associated protein that is expressed by Muller cells but not astrocytes (Fig. 5). Similarly, only one of the six membrane antigens that we have described appears to be common to the two glial cell types. Astrocytes have been defined in part by the expression of an intermediate filament protein, glial fibrillary acidic protein (GFAP). In retina this protein is expressed by the astrocytes in the optic nerve fiber layer and just a few Muller cells at the peripheral edge of the retina.

3. *In Vitro* Studies of Retinal Cells

One of the major goals of cellular neurobiology has been to study the properties of neural cells in a controlled environment free from many of the influences of other cells. Monolayer cultures provide such an environment but create another problem. Once placed in culture, it is no longer possible to identify cells by positional or morphological cues. Since the antibodies described above have enabled us to identify each of the major subclasses of cells in the rat retina, we were able to examine the cell types present in monolayer cultures set up from retinas of neonatal rats.[24,46]

3.1. Expression of Retinal Antigens in Monolayer Cultures

Photoreceptors, identified with antibody RET-P1, appeared in these cultures as small cells with at most a single process (Figs. 6a and 6b). No outer segment formation was found in these monolayer cultures under a variety of culture conditions.

A different restriction on development was found for retinal ganglion cells. We found Thy-1-positive ganglion cells only in dense cell clusters, never in sparse cultures. There is still some doubt as to whether this result indicates an effect of cell density upon cell differentiation or upon cell survival.

Figure 6. Appearance of retinal cells in monolayer cultures. (a) Cluster of small cells resting on a glial monlayer; (b) the same cells labeled with antibody RET-P1. (c) Phase contrast view of a culture; (d) the same cells labeled with antibody R3 to reveal horizontal cells; (e) autoradiograph of culture labeled by tritiated GABA uptake; (f) autoradiography of culture labeled by tritiated glycine uptake. (From Ref. 24.)

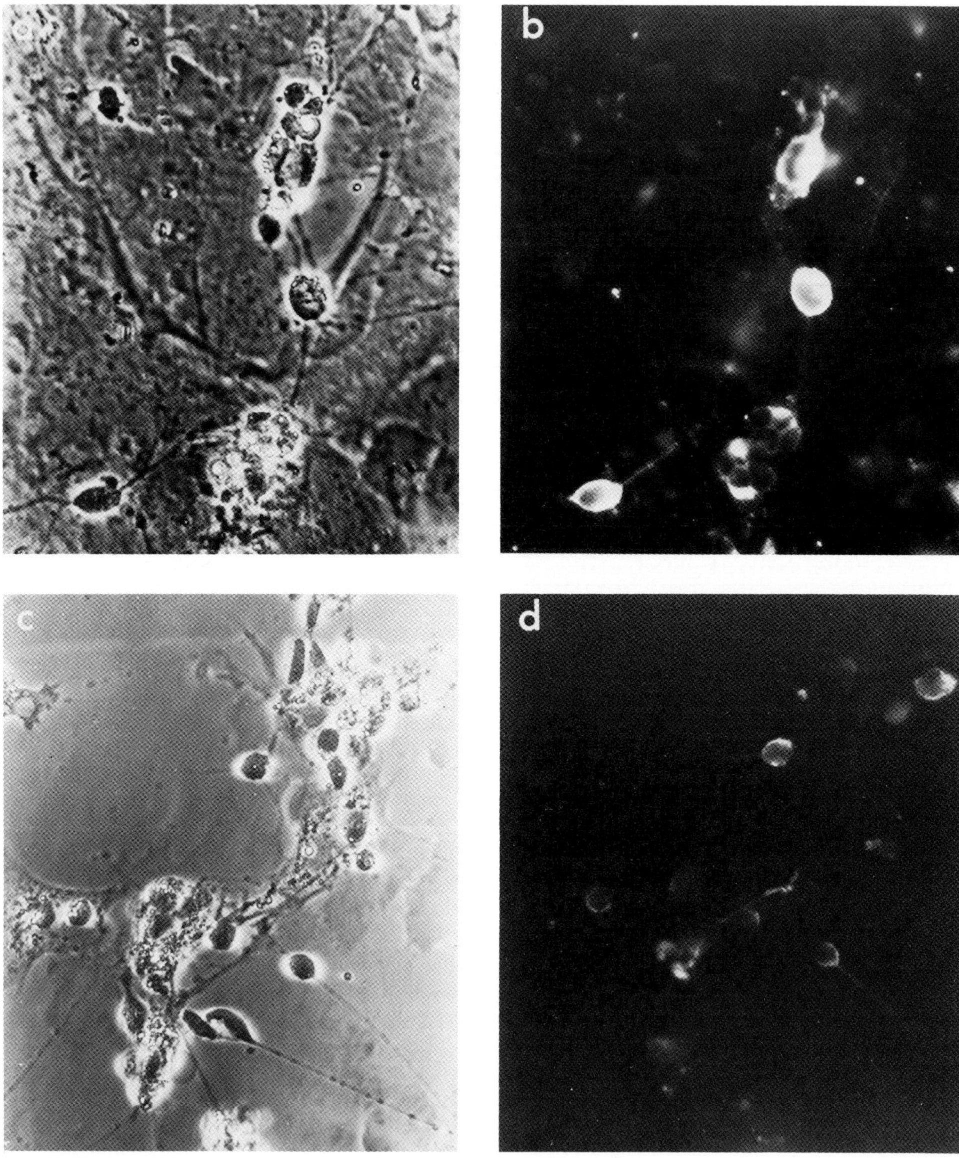

Figure 7. Retinal cultures labeled with (a,b) antibodies RET-B2 and (c,d) HPC-1. (a,c) phase contrast; (b,d) fluorescence. (From Ref. 24.)

Bipolar cells could be identified with antibodies such as RET-B2 (Figs. 7a and 7b). One interesting feature of this labeling was that it was only detectable after the cells had been in culture for 7 days. It is not clear whether this delay represents the progress of some internal clock within these cells or some interactions between cells in the cultures that take this long to develop.

Three subclasses of retinal cells were routinely found in the cultures. Amacrine cells comprised about 30–40% of the neuronal cells in most cultures as defined by labeling with HPC-1 antibody. Horizontal cells (defined as neurofilament-positive, glial filament-positive, Thy-1-negative cells) were a rare but characteristic cell type present (Figs. 6c and 6d). Finally, glial cells could be identified with several of the glial-specific intermediate filament antibodies. Because of the changed expression of some of these molecules upon retinal disruption, it has not been possible to label separately Muller cells and astrocytes in culture.

3.2. Morphology of Cells *in Vitro*

Some of our observations in culture suggest that at least some aspects of cell morphology are an intrinsic property. As already mentioned, RET-P1-positive photoreceptors are always small cells without extensive processes. Horizontal cells invariably appeared as large multipolar cells that are unlike any other cell that can be identified. On the other hand, there appears to be more heterogeneity in the morphology of the HPC-1-positive amacrine cells. Some of this is due to the different subclasses of amacrine cells present in the cultures. Subpopulations of amacrine cells can be double-labeled in culture with HPC-1 and either GABA or glycine, two putative amacrine cell transmitters. Almost all the GABAergic amacrine cells had two or three long primary processes that showed little branching. Most glycine cells, on the other hand, were multipolar, with short, densely branched processes (Figs. 6e and 6f). Thus, at least four cell types assume characteristic morphologies even in the artificial environment of monolayer cultures. The mechanisms determining the process outgrowth and branching are unknown, but culture systems such as those described here will allow examination of the role of features such as cytoskeletal organizing centers.

3.3. The Extent of Differentiation of Neural Cells *in Vitro*

As already mentioned, we have not found photoreceptor outer segment formation in monolayer cultures of neonatal retinas, and ganglion cell survival (or differentiation) is dependent upon cell density in the cultures. In addition, a number of Muller cell antigens that appear between days 5 and 10 postnatally have not been found in culture.[45] These results can be contrasted with some normal features of amacrine and bipolar differentiation that take place in the same cultures. It is clear that monolayer cultures do not represent an ideal environment for the differentiation of all neural cells.

As an alternative culture system, we have used aggregate cultures.[24] In these cultures there is considerable morphological differentiation. Layers of cell bodies form and are separated by neuropil layers. In the center of the aggregates small, darkly staining cells become arranged in rosette structures.

These can be labeled by antibody RET-P1, suggesting that they are photoreceptors. In the central lumen of the rosettes membranous structures are found that can be labeled with outer segment-specific antibodies. Thus, it would appear that in these cultures further differentiation of photoreceptors can occur. By comparing the differences between the two culture systems, it may be possible to learn something of the mechanisms controlling normal photoreceptor differentiation.

3.4. Survival and Regeneration of Mature Neurons

Some of the problems of cell differentiation in low-density monolayer cultures would be avoided if identified neurons from the mature nervous system were used. A persistent problem in such an approach has been to provide a suitable substrate for the dissociated neurons that would allow them to adhere and survive. The substrates used for embryonic or neonatal neurons, such as collagen or polylysine, do not seem to be effective for mature neurons. A possible solution to this problem was suggested by the observations of Dr. P. MacLeish. As part of a collaborative project we had produced a series of monoclonal antibodies against cells of the salamander retina. One of these antibodies, Sal-1, reacted with surface antigens on almost all salamander tissues. When mature dissociated retinal cells were plated onto glass coverslips coated with purified Sal-1 antibody virtually all the cells adhered within seconds.[47] Processes present at the time of dissociation were maintained and over a period of several weeks many cells elaborated a dense network of processes. Binding to the antibody did not disrupt the cell structure or properties as judged by both electron microscopic analysis and electrophysiological recording. In an extension of this work we have analyzed the survival of mature rat retinal ganglion cells when plated on a substrate of 2G12 (anti-Thy-1) antibody.[48] Like other neurons of the CNS, mammalian ganglion cells do not regenerate their axons after transection and indeed many of the cells degenerate. Ganglion cells were labeled by fluorescent retrograde tracers and plated on 2G12 substrates. The cells plated on the 2G12 substrate grew more and longer processes than cells plated on collagen, glass, polylysine, fibronectin, or a variety of other monoclonal antibodies. Electrophysiological recordings showed that these cells had healthy resting potentials and were capable of firing action potentials.

The mechanism by which these antibody substrates promote neurite outgrowth is unknown. It either could be a function of the strength of adhesion, which may be related to antigen density, or may be the result of binding to specific receptor molecules on the cell surface. Whatever the mechanism, the finding that certain antibodies promote cell survival and process regeneration in mammalian CNS neurons that would normally degenerate has important clinical implications and suggests an extremely important role for such reagents in the future.

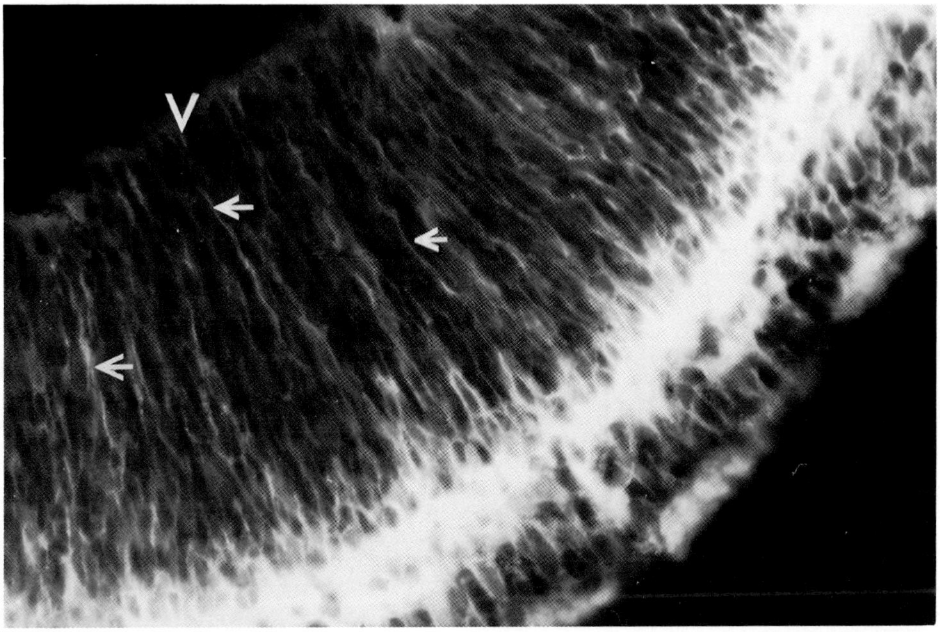

Figure 8. Labeling of day 17–18 rat embryo retina by antibody HPC-1. Arrowheads mark HPC-1-positive radial fibers of migrating amacrine cells. Some of these fibers can be traced up to the ventricular surface of the retina (V). (From Rev. 41.)

4. Layers, Gradients, and Positional Information

4.1. Layer Formation in the Developing Retina

An important aspect of neural development concerns features that are related to the three-dimensional structure of the CNS. In the retina, for example, all mitoses of the neuronal precursors take place at the ventricular surface (outer limiting membrane). After their final mitosis cells migrate from this region to their correct layers. Layer formation could be due to either recruitment of undifferentiated neuroblasts or homing of already differentiated cells. For amacrine cells we believe that the latter mechanism operates. Antibody HPC-1 labels cells in retinas of day 17–18 embryos.[41] At this stage the ganglion cell and inner plexiform layers are not fully formed. One finds HPC-1-positive cells not only in the forming amacrine cell layer, but also at the ventricular surface and positions in between (Fig. 8). This suggests that the cells begin to differentiate before they migrate. The migrating cells retain a radial process attached to the ventricular surface as they migrate. Such processes may be used by the cells to sense the depth to which they have migrated. Different layers would form if different cell types had different maximum radial process lengths. This speculation was reinforced by the observation that some horizontal cells also maintain a radial process as they migrate during the late embryonic stages of retinal development. This process is probably important because these cells seem to stop and form a layer in an otherwise uniform layer of undifferentiated neuroblasts. The reason for the development of these horizontal cells before other elements of the outer retina is not at all clear, but they may in some way form a scaffold that delineates the future outer plexiform layer and thus influences photoreceptor and bipolar cell differentiation.

4.2. Gradients and Positional Information

Besides the laminar development of cell types in the retina, each cell forms a characteristic network of processes and connections. The distribution of some of these cells and processes is not uniform across the retina, which implies that cells within the tissue require some positional sense. Retinal ganglion cells form topographic patterns in other visual areas, such as the superior colliculus (optic tectum) and lateral geniculate nucleus. Although the mechanism of map formation is still quite controversial, it remains a reasonable hypothesis that specification of position has a molecular correlate. Two molecular mechanisms of specification are a qualitative mechanism, where each cell or group of cells expresses a unique molecule, and a quantitative mechanism, where cells express varying levels of a single molecule. No firm evidence currently exists for a qualitative mechanism. Graded levels of molecules have been postulated for some time and within the retina monoclonal antibodies have now detected two such molecular gradients. The first was detected by immunizing with a dorsal segment of chick retina and then screening the resulting antibodies on dorsal and ventral retina. An antibody (named TOP) was found that preferentially bound to dorsal retina.[49] The difference between dorsal and ventral edges is difficult to define, but TOP is probably at least 50-fold more abundant in dorsal parts of the tissue. Biochemical studies of TOP have suggested that it is a cell surface protein of apparent molecular weight 46,000–49,000.

We have recently found a second molecular gradient in rat retina using apparently equivalent antibodies raised against embryonic rat retina (JONES)[50] and adult retinal membranes (3.1E).[25] In embryonic and early postnatal retina these antibodies detect a molecule that is expressed in high levels in all layers of dorsal retina and decreases to almost negligible levels in ventral regions. The exact gradient is difficult to quantitate because there is a thin strip of enhanced antigen expression at the ventral edge of the retina. Unlike TOP, JONES/3.1E appears to be a ganglioside, although the exact chemical composition of the molecule is still under investigation. Although neither gradient has yet been shown to biologically important in retinal pattern formation, it is clear that monoclonal antibody techniques can allow the detection of such gradients, provide the reagents with which to test their function, and aid experiments that investigate the mechanisms by which such gradients are set up and maintained.

5. Discussion

This chapter has discussed briefly some of the monoclonal antibodies that we have produced against one part of the mammalian CNS, the retina. A great deal of work from our own and many other laboratories is providing similar reagents with which to study other parts of the CNS. From our work on retina certain generalizations can be made and these seem to be valid for these other regions. One of the most important points is that it is possible to take part of the CNS and, even with fairly crude immunogens, generate monoclonal antibodies against each of the major subclasses of cells present. These monoclonal antibodies can be used to study neural tissue *in vitro* to define the cell types in various culture systems and to monitor the extent of their differentiation. Not only will this aid studies of the patterns of cell interactions *in vitro*, but it also will allow experiments designed to identify factors directly influencing neural differentiation. It is possible to use cell subclass-specific antibodies to isolate cells and cell fragments that can be used as a more restricted immunogen to produce antibodies of even more refined specificity, for example, against the subclasses of ganglion or bipolar cells. This sequential approach to defining neural molecular heterogeneity is likely to be of increasing importance in the future.

The use of antibiotics as culture substrates for adult neurons will allow the study of cells that have matured in their natural environment. This is likely to be of great importance in studies of neurodegenerative diseases such as Huntington's disease, amyotropic lateral sclerosis, and Alzheimer's disease. In these conditions neurons appear normal for many years and thus the disease may well only be manifested in adult cells.

In summary, monoclonal antibodies have aleady become important tools for the molecular study of the nervous system. With increasingly sophisticated immunogens, methods of immunization, and assay systems they are certain to bring about a revolution in our understanding not only of individual cell types, but also of the mechanisms governing patterning in the nervous system and perhaps in biology in general.

ACKNOWLEDGMENTS. Work from my laboratory described in this article was supported by NIH grants EY05206 and NS20483 and a grant from the Hereditary Disease Foundation. The author is an Alfred P. Sloan Research Fellow. The contributions of K. Akagawa, D. Fekete, and R. Hofstein, and the technical assistance of E. Silvestro and W. Louie are gratefully acknowledged.

References

1. Polyak, S., 1941, *The Retina*, University of Chicago Press, Chicago.
2. Rodieck, R. W., 1973, *The Vertebrate Retina*, Freeman, San Francisco.
3. Ehinger, B., 1982, Neurotransmitter systems in the retina, *Retina* **2**:305–321.
4. Kaneko, A., 1979, Physiology of the retina, *Annu. Rev. Neurosci.* **2**:169–191.

5. Matus, A., Huber, G., and Bernhardt, R., 1983, Neuronal microdifferentiation, *Cold Spring Harbor Symp. Quant. Biol.* **48**:775–782.
6. Frank, E., and Fischbach, G. D., 1979, Early events in neuromuscular junction formation *in vitro*, *J. Cell Biol.* **83**:143–159.
7. Bader, C. R., Bertrand, D., and Schwartz, E. A., 1982, Voltage-activated and calcium-activated currents studied in solitary rod inner segments from the salamander retina, *J. Physiol.* **331**:253–284.
8. Bridges, C. D. B., and Fong, S.-L., 1980, Lectins as probes of glycoprotein and glycolipid oligosaccharides in rods and cones, *Neurochem. Int.* **1**:255–267.
9. Köhler, G., and Milstein, C., 1975, Continuous cultures of fused cells secreting antibody of predefined specificity, *Nature* **256**:495–497.
10. Dewey, M. M., Davis, P. K., Blasie, J. K., and Barr, L., 1969, Localisation of rhodopsin antibody in the retina of the frog, *J. Mol. Biol.* **39**:395–405.
11. Papermaster, D. S., Schneider, B. G., Zorn, M. A., and Kraehenbuhl, J. P., 1978, Immunocytochemical localization of opsin in outer segments and Golgi zones of frog photoreceptor cells, *J. Cell Biol.* **77**:196–210.
12. Stryer, L., 1983, Transducin and the cyclic GMP phosphodiesterase amplifier protein in vision, *Cold Spring Harbor Symp. Quant. Biol.* **48**:841–852.
13. Hamm, H., and Bownds, D., 1984, A monoclonal antibody to guanine nucleotide binding protein inhibits the light-activated cyclic GMP pathway in frog rod outer segments, *J. Gen. Physiol.* **84**:265–280.
14. Barnstable, C. J., 1980, Monoclonal antibodies which recognise different cell types in the rat retina, *Nature* **286**:231–235.
15. Fekete, D. M., and Barnstable, C. J., 1983, The subcellular localisation of rat photoreceptor-specific antigens, *J. Neurocytol.* **12**:785–803.
16. Balkema, G. W., and Drager, U. C., 1984, Monoclonal antibodies against components of the mouse retina, *Soc. Neurosci. Abstr.* **10**:21.
17. Stirling, C. E., and Lee, A., 1980, [^{3}H]Ouabain autoradiography of frog retina, *J. Cell Biol.* **85**:313–324.
18. Stahl, W. L., and Baskin, D. G., 1984, Immunocytochemical localisation of Na,K adenosine triphosphatase in the rat retina, *J. Histochem. Cytochem.* **32**:248–250.
19. Fujita, S. C., Zipursky, S. L., Benzer, S., Ferrus, A., and Shotwell, S. L., 1982, Monoclonal antibodies against the *Drosophila* nervous system, *Proc. Natl. Acad. Sci. USA* **79**:7929–7933.
20. Zipursky, S. L., Venkatesh, T. R., Teplow, D. B., and Benzer, S., 1984, Neuronal development in the *Drosophila* retina: Monoclonal antibodies as molecular probes, *Cell* **36**:15–26.
21. Kremer, N. E., Stewart, G. H., and Wong, F., 1982, Photoreceptor specific antigens: Localisation and identification by monoclonal antibodies, *Soc. Neurosci. abstr.*, **8**:688.
22. Lazarides, E., Nelson, W. J., and Kasamatsu, T., 1984, Segregation of two spectrin forms in the chick optic system: A mechanism for establishing restricted membrane-cytoskeletal domains in neurons, *Cell* **36**:269–278.
23. Kelly, R. B., Buckley, K. M., Burgess, T. L., Carlson, S. S., Caroni, P., Hooper, J. E., Katzen, A., Moore, H.-P., Pfeffer, S. R., and Schroer, T. A., 1983, Membrane traffic in neurons and peptide-secreting cells, *Cold Spring Harbor Symp. Quant. Biol.* **48**:697–705.
24. Barnstable, C. J., Akagawa, K., Hofstein, R., and Horn, J. P., 1983, Monoclonal antibodies that label discrete cell types in the mammalian nervous system, *Cold Spring Harbor Symp. Quant. Biol.* **48**:863–876.
25. Akagawa, K., and Barnstable, C. J., 1984, Monoclonal antibodies that detect cell type and laminar differences in the rat retina, *Soc. Neurosci. Abstr.* **10**:21.
26. Zipser, B., and McKay, R. D., 1981, Monoclonal antibodies distinguish identifiable neurones in the leech, *Nature* **289**:549–554.
27. Barnstable, C. J., 1982, Analysis of retina and other neural tissues using cell-specific antibodies, in: *Molecular Genetic Neuroscience* (F. O. Schmitt, S. J. Bird, and F. E. Bloom, eds.), Raven Press, New York, pp. 137–146.
28. Beale, R., and Osborne, N. N., 1982, Localisation of the Thy-1 antigen to the surfaces of rat retinal ganglion cells, *Neurochem. Int.* **4**:587–595.

29. Sarthy, P. V., Curtis, B. M., and Catterall, W. A., 1983, Retrograde labelling, enrichment and characterisation of retinal ganglion cells from the neonatal rat, *J. Neurosci.* **3**:2532–2544.
30. Barnstable, C. J., and Drager, U. C., 1984, Thy-1 antigen: A ganglion cell specific marker in rodent retina, *Neuroscience* **11**:847–855.
31. Fields, K. L., Brockes, J. P., Mirsky, R., and Wendon, L. M. B. L., 1978, Cell surface markers for distinguishing different types of rat dorsal root ganglion cells in culture, *Cell* **14**:43–51.
32. Williams, A. F., 1982, Surface molecules and cell interactions, *J. Theor. Biol.* **98**:221–234.
33. Lemmon, V., and Gottlieb, D. I., 1982, Monoclonal antibodies selective for the inner portion of the chick retina, *J. Neurosci.* **2**:531–535.
34. Shaw, G., and Weber, K., 1984, The intermediate filament complement of the retina: A comparison between different mammalian species, *Eur. J. Cell Biol.* **33**:95–104.
35. Drager, U. C., Edwards, D. L., and Barnstable, C. J., 1984, Antibodies against filamentous components in discrete cell types of the mouse retina, *J. Neurosci.* **4**:2025–2042.
36. Hofstein, R., Majocha, R. E., Barnstable, C. J., and Marotta, C. A., 1985, Non-uniform distribution of neurofilament epitopes in the CNS during development, *Ann. N. Y. Acad. Sci.* (in press).
37. Villegas, G. M., and Villegas, R., 1963, Neuron–glia relationship in the bipolar cell layer of the fish retina, *J. Ultrastruct. Res.* **8**:89–106.
38. Young, L. H. Y., and Dowling, J. E., 1983, Monoclonal antibodies associated with H1 horizontal cells in the carp retina, *Soc. Neurosci. Abstr.* **9**:801.
39. Ramon y Cajal, S., 1972, *The Structure of the Retina* (S. A. Thorpe and M. Glickstein, transl.), Thomas, Springfield, Illinois.
40. Brecha, N. C., and Karten, H. J., 1983, Identification and localization of neuropeptides in the vertebrate retina, in: *Brain Peptides* (D. Kreiger, M. Brownstein, and J. Martin, eds.), Wiley, New York, pp. 437–462.
41. Barnstable, C. J., Hofstein, R., and Akagawa, K., 1985, A marker of early amacrine cell development in rat retina, *Dev. Brain Res.* (in press).
42. Linser, P. J., 1983, Glial specific markers in the horizontal neurons of teleost neural retina, *Soc. Neurosci. Abstr.* **9**:339.
43. Linser, P. J., and Moscona, A. A., 1981, Induction of glutamine synthetase in embryonic neural retina: Its suppression by the gliotoxic agent a-aminoadipic acid, *Dev. Brain Res.* **1**:103–119.
44. Drager, U. C., 1983, Coexistence of neurofilaments and vimentin in a neuron of the adult mouse retina, *Nature* **303**:169–172.
45. Barnstable, C. J., 1982, Immunological studies of the retina, in: *Neuroimmunology* (J. Brockes, ed.), Plenum Press, New York, pp. 183–214.
46. Akagawa, K., and Barnstable, C. J., 1985, Identification and characterisation of cell types in monolayer cultures of rat retina using monoclonal antibodies, Submitted.
47. MacLeish, P. R., Barnstable, C. J, and Townes-Anderson, E., 1983, Use of a monoclonal antibody as a substrate for mature neurons *in vitro*, *Proc. Natl. Acad. Sci. USA* **80**:7014–7018.
48. Leifer, D., Lipton, S. A., Barnstable, C. J., and Masland, R. H., 1984, Monoclonal antibody to Thy-1 enhances regeneration of processes by rat retinal ganglion cells in culture, *Science* **224**:303–306.
49. Trisler, G. D., Schneider, M. D., and Nirenberg, M., 1981, A topographic gradient of molecules in retina can be used to identify neuron position, *Proc. Natl. Acad. Sci. USA* **78**:2145–2149.
50. Constantine-Paton, M., and Barnstable, C. J., 1984, Monoclonal antibodies with developmentally varying binding distributions in the rat nervous system, *Soc. Neurosci. Abstr.* **10**:787.

Chapter 17

Application of Monoclonal Antibodies to Issues of Plasma Lipoprotein Structure and Function

LINDA K. CURTISS

1. Introduction

An understanding of the role of plasma lipoproteins in biology and in diverse pathophysiologic states is expanding rapidly. The ability of these supramolecular complexes to transport smaller hydrophobic molecules, including cholesteryl esters, triglycerides, fat-soluble vitamins, and hormones, places them in the limelight as important mediators of molecular traffic *in vivo*. However, much remains obscure regarding the organization of these protein–lipid complexes as well as the structure and the function of the individual molecular constituents that make up the lipoproteins. Immunochemical approaches to studies of apoprotein structure and analyses of lipoproteins *per se* have been utilized for many years. These studies have facilitated both identification and quantitation of the protein constituents of the plasma lipoproteins. However, not until monoclonal antibodies of defined specificity were available in significant numbers did immunochemical approaches gain the popularity they hold today. The striking degree of specificity inherent in a monoclonal antibody has been successfully applied to relevant issues of lipoprotein biology, including the identification of receptor binding domains, genetic polymorphisms, and putative atherogenic lipoproteins. These advances will be discussed in detail following a brief description of the important participants in these studies, the antibodies and the lipoproteins.

2. Background. Plasma Lipoprotein Structure and Function

Plasma lipoproteins are lipid–protein complexes that are heterogeneous with respect to a variety of physiochemical properties, including composition,

LINDA K. CURTISS • Department of Immunology, Research Institute of Scripps Clinic, La Jolla, California 92037.

Table I. Classification and Properties of the Human Plasma Lipoproteins

Properties	Chylomicrons	VLDL	LDL	HDL
Solvent density range for isolation g/m	<0.95	0.95–1.006	1.006–1.063	1.063–1.21
Electrophoretic mobility	Origin	Pre-beta	Beta	Alpha
Molecular weight	$>4 \times 10^8$	$(5–10) \times 10^6$	$(2.7–4.8) \times 10^6$	$(1.8–3.9) \times 10^5$
Diameter, Å	>750	250–750	200–250	40–140
Percent protein by weight	0.5–2.5	10–13	20–27	45–50

size, density and charge. The most commonly used and universally applicable nomenclature is based upon buoyant density. On this basis the plasma lipoproteins are grouped into four major classes: chylomicrons, very low-density lipoproteins (abbreviated VLDL), low-density lipoproteins (LDL), and high density-lipoproteins (HDL) (Table I). Paralleling advances in the technology of ultracentrifugal separations, such as the use of zonal rotors, there has been a further subdivision of the LDL and HDL density classes into subclasses. The LDL class of density 1.006–1.063 g/ml can be resolved into an LDL_1 or intermediate-density lipoprotein (IDL) and an LDL_2 subclass. Similarly, HDL can be subdivided into more homogeneous subclasses of HDL_2, and HDL_3, and very high-density lipoprotein (VHDL). However, even these subclasses are composed of functionally heterogeneous populations of lipoprotein particles. Table I lists the average composition and properties of the major density classes, and serves to illustrate the concept that normal lipoproteins represent a diverse spectrum of noncovalently linked protein–lipid complexes that differ with respect to size, density, and charge.

The composition of a lipoprotein is a direct reflection of its specific function. Therefore, the contribution of total lipid to the mass of a lipoprotein varies from greater than 98% for the chylomicrons to about 50% for HDL. Although all lipoproteins contain triglyceride, free and esterified cholesterol, and phospholipid, the relative amounts of each of these lipids differ. The buoyant density of a lipoprotein is a direct function of the amount of lipid in each particle. For example, triglyceride-rich lipoproteins (chylomicrons and VLDLs) are large particles in the molecular weight $(5–800) \times 10^6$, and float, forming a cloudy or milky layer when plasma or serum is stored. These particles, which can be of either intestinal or hepatic origin, serve as important vehicles for delivery of triglycerides to the peripheral tissues. During this process, the progressive loss of triglyceride from the lipoprotein results predominantly in the formation of a more dense, cholesterol-rich LDL. The LDLs, serve to transport the cholesterol to all tissues of the body. HDLs, which are less than 50% lipid, play an important role in the retrieval of cholesterol from peripheral tissues.

All plasma lipoproteins contain protein (referred to as apoproteins) and polar lipids that are organized in the surface film that surrounds the neutral lipid (triglycerides and cholesteryl ester) core. The apoproteins constitute as little as 1% to as much as 50% of the lipoprotein particle mass. Eight major apoproteins have been isolated and characterized, and the list of minor apoproteins continues to grow. The most commonly used nomenclature for the apoproteins is the ABC nomenclature of Alaupovic *et al.*,[1] which is outlined in Table II. Specific apoproteins can be recovered in larger amounts from certain density classes; however, most can be found also in other density classes. Thus, most LDL particles contain only apoprotein B (apo B); however, a few particles also contain other apoproteins, and this accounts for the trace amounts of apo C-I, apo C-II, C-III, and apo E present in this density class. Similarly, just as the HDLs contain predominantly apo A-I and apo A-II, they also contain trace amounts of other apoproteins, suggesting again particle heterogeneity. Furthermore, whereas some apoproteins, such as apo B, serve as integral surface components of the lipoprotein, other apoproteins are exchanged readily between different lipoproteins and this leads to additional heterogeneity. In some cases specific functions have been assigned to particular apoproteins. For example, apo A-I, which is found predominantly in the HDL, activates lecithin:cholesterol acyltransferase (LCAT)[2]; and apo C-II, which is found predominantly in the VLDL, is a cofactor for triglyceride hydrolysis by lipoprotein lipases of extrahepatic origin.[3] Additional functional roles of specific apoproteins will be discussed below.

3. Monoclonal Antibodies That Bind Lipoproteins

3.1. Apoprotein B-Specific Antibodies

By far the largest number of apoprotein-specific monoclonal antibodies generated to date are those that bind apo B. A major reason for this stems from the fact that very little is known about the structure of apo B. Neither the size nor the primary structure of apo B is known, and one can only guess at how it is organized on a lipoprotein particle. Additional reasons for the popularity of apo B as a molecule for study are probably related to its availability and relative ease of isolation, the fact that apo B is a potent immunogen and consistently elicits high-titer antibody responses with all immunization regimens, and the notoriety that apo B has earned as a contributing factor to atherosclerosis and coronary heart disease.

At least seven research groups[5–11] have generated and characterized one or more apo B-specific antibodies (Table III). The number of likely antigenic determinants or epitopes on a protein can be predicted from sequence data by assigning charge and hydrophilic values to separate amino acids.[12,13] However, because neither the molecular weight nor the primary amino acid sequence of apo B is known, the total number of unique antigenic epitopes that may be expressed by apo B still cannot be estimated. The number could be quite high. Therefore, the 36 different apo B-specific antibodies listed in Table III could represent anywhere from 10 to 20 unique epitopes.

Table II. Apoproteins of Human Plasma Lipoproteins

	Apo A-I	Apo A-II	Apo B	Apo C-I	Apo C-II	Apo C-III	Apo D	Apo E
Molecular weight	28,300	17,000 (dimer)	—[a]	6331	8837	8700	22,700	34,000
NH_2 terminal	Asp	PCA[b]	Glu	Thr	Thr	Ser	(Blocked)	Lys
COOH terminal	Gln	Gln	(Blocked)	Ser	Glu	Ala	Ser	Ala
Carbohydrate	+	+	+	0	0	+	+	+
Distribution (% of total protein)								
Chylomicrons	7.4	4.2	22.5	15	15	36	0	+
VLDL	Trace	Trace	36.9	3.3	6.7	39.9	Trace	13
LDL	0	0	98	Trace	Trace	Trace	Trace	Trace
HDL	67	22	Trace	1–3	1–3	3–5	1–2	+

[a] Molecular weight estimates of the monomeric unit have been reported by different laboratories to range from 8000 to 550,000.
[b] Pyrrolidone carboxylic acid.

Table III. Apo B- and LDL-Binding Monoclonal Antibodies

Antibody or hybridoma designation	Special properties	Ref.
L1C6F2	Binds only 20% of LDL	4, 5, 27, 30
LP-22	Discriminates CAD[a]	
LP-34	Binds 100% of LDL	
LP-47	Binds 40% of LDL	
1a, 457C4D1	Lipolysis decreases binding	6, 29, 35, 47, 52
1b, 457C4D1	Lipolysis decreases binding	
2a, 464B1B3	Inhibits LDL receptor binding	
2b, 464B1B6	Inhibits LDL receptor binding	
3, 465B6C3	Binds apo B-48	
4, 465C3D1	Lipolysis increases binding	
5, 465D3D5	Lipolysis increases binding	
1D1	Binds apo B-48	7, 37, 48, 49, 51
2D8	Binds apo B-48	
3A8 or 3A10	Inhibits LDL receptor binding	
3F5	Binds delipidated LDL	
4G3	Inhibits LDL receptor binding	
5E11	Inhibits LDL receptor binding	
TRW-1	SDS decreases binding	8, 36
TRW-3	No effect of SDS	
TRW-5	SDS increases binding	
TRW-6	SDS increases binding	
TRW-8	SDS abolishes binding	
TRW-13	SDS abolishes binding	
B3 or A	Equal affinity for VLDL, IDL, LDL	9, 28, 38, 40
B24 or B	Decreased binding of an apo B allotype	
B14 or C	Equal affinity for VLDL, IDL, LDL	
B19 or D	Binds 100% of LDL	
B1 or E	Decreased binding of an apo B allotype	
B2 or F	Decreased binding of an apo B allotype	
B11, G	Equal affinity for VLDL, IDL, LDL	
B16, H	Binds 94% of LDL	
B20, I	Binds 45% of LDL	
B17, J	SDS abolishes binding	
B18, K	SDS abolishes binding	
18C4	Inhibits LDL receptor binding	10
3OC2	Inhibits LDL receptor binding	11

[a] Coronary heart disease.

While investigators have used different types of assays to characterize the binding properties of their antibodies, characterizations have for the most part centered around three important properties: (1) the influence of lipids on antibody binding; (2) the ability of the antibody to identify either all or a subpopulation of apo B-containing lipoprotein; and (3) the ability of these anti-

Table IV. Apoprotein-Binding Monoclonal Antibodies

Apoprotein	Hybridoma or antibody designation	Special properties	Ref.
Apo E	1D7	Inhibits receptor binding	14, 17
	3B7	No inhibition of binding	
	6C5	No inhibition of binding	
	6H7	No inhibition of binding	
	7C9	No inhibition of binding	
Apo E	Emab-1	Binds COOH terminal	15
	Emab-2	Binds COOH terminal	
	Emab-3	Binds NH_3 terminal	
Apo E	1E	Binds COOH terminal	16
	2E	Binds COOH terminal	
	3E	Binds COOH terminal	
	4E	Binds COOH terminal	
	5E	Binds COOH terminal	
	6E	Binds soluble apo E	
Apo A-I	AI-4	Binds 60% of HDL	20
	AI-7	Binds 60% of HDL	
	AI-9	Binds 20% of HDL	
Apo A-II	AII-1	Binds 100% of apo A-II	20
Apo A-II	2-22	Binds apo A-II	21
Apo C-I	CI-1	Binds apo C-I	23
Apo C-III	AC6	Binds apo C-III	22

bodies to interfere with cellular receptor interactions that are mediated by apo B.

3.2. Apoprotein E-Specific Antibodies

Apo E plays a major role in the hepatic uptake of lipoprotein particles. It is a protein of 35,000 molecular weight and, as illustrated in Table II, is found in all density classes of lipoproteins. However, it is found predominantly in the chylomicron and VLDL density classes, where it directs the rapid clearance of these lipoproteins by the liver. Use of the computer-based predictive program of Hopp and Woods[12,13] suggests that apo E should contain at least two major antigenic determinants or epitopes. Although at least 14 antibodies have been generated (Table IV),[14–16] it is not known whether each is directed toward a unique epitope on apo E. As will be outlined in subsequent sections, one of these apo E antibodies has been particularly useful in delineating the structural domain of apo E that is involved in binding to cellular receptors.[17]

3.3. Apoprotein AI- and AII-Specific Antibodies

The major apoproteins of HDL are apo A-I and apo A-II (Table II). The biological function of apo A-II has not been established, but apo A-I has been identified as an important activator of lecithin:cholesterol acyltransferase (LCAT), the plasma enzyme that catalyzes the esterification of free cholesterol as it is collected from the peripheral tissues and transported back to the liver.[18] Elevated levels of plasma HDL and its associated apoproteins have been shown to exhibit an inverse correlation with the risk of atherosclerotic disease.[19] Therefore the measurement of plasma levels of HDL can provide important risk information for coronary heart diease. One apo A-II-specific antibody and three apo A-I-specific monoclonal antibodies recently have been generated and characterized (Table IV).[20] In addition, a commercial assay for plasma apo A-I using a monoclonal antibody is available (Ventrex, Portland, Maine), and a second apo A-II-specific antibody has been used to measure plasma levels of apo A-II[21] (Table IV).

3.4. Apoprotein C-Specific Antibodies

Apoproteins C-I, C-II, and C-III are found predominantly in VLDL; however, as illustrated in Table II, they can be found in all lipoprotein density classes. The apo C-specific monoclonal antibodies are listed in Table IV. Although a couple of antibodies have been generated, neither has been rigorously characterized.[22,23]

4 Application of Monoclonal Antibodies to Issues of Lipoprotein Structure and Function

4.1. Immunodiagnostic Assays for Plasma Apo A-I and Apo B in Coronary Heart Disease

Atherosclerotic vascular disease and its complications, including cerebral and coronary infarction and pulmonary obstruction, are the leading cause of death and delibitation in Western society. Although the exact cause of the development of atherosclerotic plaques is not known, plasma lipids have been shown to be related directly to the rate and severity of plaque formation. Epidemiologic studies have identified that elevated levels of LDL are a risk factor for the development of coronary artery and peripheral vascular disease.[24] In some cases elevated plasma levels of apo B also have been directly implicated as a risk factor.[25] The opposite is true for plasma levels of HDL or its associated apoprotein, apo A-I. High levels of HDL or apo A-I are considered to be protective and therefore are associated with a decreased risk of coronary heart disease.[26] For this reason, plasma ratios of LDL (apo B) to HDL (apo A-I) may prove to be a more useful indicator, because the ratio takes into account both positive and negative risk factors.

The application of immunoassays to measurements of total plasma levels of apo B and apo A-I has had limited success. In spite of a great deal of work, many problems remain. Most can be directly related to the physical and chemical properties peculiar to lipoproteins and apoproteins. Assays employing polyclonal antibodies have encountered problems with: (1) differences in the physical states of apoprotein standards and samples: (2) differences in the immunoreactivity of apoproteins present as either apoproteins or associated with lipoproteins; (3) the masking of antigenic determinants; (4) the polymorphism of the apoproteins; and (5) striking variations in antibody populations.

A major "stumbling block" to the development of immunoassays with monoclonal reagents for total plasma levels of apo A-I or apo B is the observation that neither apo A-I nor apo B represents immunochemically homogeneous proteins. Many apo B-specific monoclonal antibodies do not bind 100% of plasma LDL[4,27,28] and similar observations recently have been made with the binding of HDL by the apo A-I antibodies.[20] This problem is perhaps best illustrated with the apo A-I-specific antibodies. When each of three unique apo A-I-specific antibodies (Table IV) was characterized with respect to its ability to bind radioiodinated HDL in a fluid phase radioimmunoassay, none of the antibodies were found to bind greater than 60% of HDL.[20] Such heterogeneity of HDL is further supported by the demonstration that increased binding of HDL occurs when the antibodies are combined to form oligoclonal mixtures, and that 100% binding of HDL can be achieved only by mixing two apo A-I-specific antibodies with a single apo A-II-specific antibody.[20] The data suggest that if all HDL is to be quantitated in plasma, oligoclonal antibody mixtures composed of selected monoclonal antibodies may be more useful.

The preceding use of monoclonal antibodies for immunodiagnostic purposes is based on the premise that all lipoproteins are involved either positively or negatively in atherosclerosis, and that the important determining factor is the amount of each lipoprotein. However, some studies have used monoclonal antibodies to quantitate plasma levels of certain lipoprotein subsets. This approach is based on the hypothesis that rather than an overabundance of "normal" LDL, a particular subpopulation of LDL particles is atherogenic and that this lipoprotein subpopulation can be distinguished immunochemically from other, nonatherogenic lipoproteins. To this end Tikkanen *et al.*[29] have measured the binding of five different monoclonal antibodies to the LDL isolated from 17 individuals, and observed a large variation in the expression of some epitopes (epitopes that represented anywhere from 30 to 400% of that expressed by a "standard" LDL). Thus, individual immunochemical differences in epitope expression have been observed. The association of a specific apo B epitope with angiographically documented coronary artery disease has been described.[30] The available data suggest that patients with coronary artery disease have a significant increase in a form of atherogenic plasma apo B that can be distinguished by increased binding to a particular antibody.[4,5,30] Further documentation should establish the usefulness of this antibody as a diagnostic reagent for atherogenic LDL. In addition, with the development of additional apo A-I- or A-II-specific antibodies, perhaps a similar HDL antibody can be found that specifically identifies a protective HDL subpopulation.

4.2. Molecular Weight of Apoprotein B

The pioneering work of Smith *et al.*[31] demonstrated that human apo B isolated from LDL was a high-molecular-weight protein. However, other studies[32–34] have suggested that apo B has a much smaller molecular weight, and this issue continues to be debated. Proponents of a large molecular weight for apo B argue that isolated small-molecular-weight apo B fragments are generated by proteolytic or oxidative degradation, whereas proponents of a low molecular weight for apo B argue that a large-molecular-weight apo B is observed because of the strong tendency of apo B to form aggregates even in the presence of denaturants. Apo B-specific monoclonal antibodies provide an independent approach to resolving this issue. The existence of multiple low-molecular-weight apo B subunits would be supported by finding in stoichiometric binding assays that the total number of identical antibodies bound per LDL particle was greater than one. The existence of a single high-molecular-weight apo B polypeptide in LDL would be supported by observing that the molar ratio of antibody per LDL was equal to or less than one.

Hahm *et al.*,[35] in studies to determine if limited proteolysis of LDL with a staphylococcal protease would selectively affect the expression of specific apo B epitopes, found that one of their antibodies bound apo B material that could be recovered in both an LDL-core fraction as well as a released soluble peptide fraction. They interpreted this observation as support for the possibility that this particular apo B epitope occurs more than once per LDL particle. However, no quantitative estimate of the total number of epitopes per LDL particle could be assigned. Also, because complete proteolytic digestion was not verified, the data are not considered conclusive.[35] Further evidence that antibody per LDL molar ratios of greater than 1.0 may exist for some epitopes was obtained by Watt and Watt.[36] In their studies of the stoichiometric binding of the Fab′ fragments of a single apo B-specific antibody to LDL (TRW-8, Table III), curvilinear Scatchard binding parameters that suggested the presence of at least two epitopes on LDL were observed. One epitope was a lower affinity epitope present at a molar ratio of Fab′ per LDL of 1.36.[36] In sharp contrast to the above observations, the binding data for three different monoclonal antibody Fab fragments reported by Milne and Marcel[37] are consistent with the presence of only a single apo B epitope per LDL particle. Furthermore, the binding of these three antibodies differs from the binding of the TRW-8 antibody, in that each antibody displays linear Scatchard binding (a parameter that suggests the presence of a single class of epitopes per LDL). Further support for the presence of only single copies of at least eight apo B epitopes on LDL has come from our own studies of the stoichiometric binding of apo B-specific antibodies to LDL.[38] Binding studies analyzed with the aid of the LIGAND program of Munson and Rodbard[39] using both single- and multiple-site models consistently verified the existence of a single site per LDL.[38] By assigning a molecular weight of 550,000 to apo B, molar ratios of antibody per LDL of 0.50–1.21 were obtained with all eight antibodies with an overall mean of 0.75 ±

0.19. This data lend good support to the notion that a single very large-molecular-weight peptide of apo B is present per LDL particle.

4.3. Genetic Polymorphism of Apoprotein B

Because of the apparent large size and extreme hydrophobicity of apo B, the application of electrophoretic techniques to the identification of genetic polymorphisms have had very limited success. Immunochemical approaches have been more successful. Whereas some investigators have looked for and not found allotypic variation using certain apo B-specific monoclonal antibodies,[27] allotypic differences have been documented.[40] With the use of a large panel of apo B-specific monoclonal antibodies,[20,28] at least two allelic forms of human apo B were identified by Schumaker *et al.*[40] This was accomplished using a binding assay that simultaneously compares the binding of 11 different monoclonal antibodies to LDL from a test individual with LDL from a single standard donor. When LDL isolated from a large number of individuals is tested, two types of binding patterns are observed. One pattern is characterized by a consistent binding ratio of amount bound to test LDL vs. standard LDL of 1.0 for all 11 antibodies, whereas the other pattern gives reduced binding with three of the 11 antibodies to the test LDL relative to the standard.

Proof that the observed immunologic polymorphism reflects a true genetic polymorphism consisting of two codominant autosomal alleles has been supported with family studies.[41] Furthermore, additional studies have verified that the allelic variation identified with these monoclonal antibodies is not a property of either the lipids or the carbohydrate moieties of LDL, but can be expressed by the delipidated apoprotein.[42] Thus, by their ability to detect changes in primary amino acid sequence, monoclonal antibodies have provided an alternative approach to the identification of apoprotein polymorphisms.

4.4. Identification of a Receptor Binding Domain on Apoprotein B

A major role for cellular lipoprotein receptors has been identified in the plasma transport of cholesterol. Recent reviews summarizing the important advances in this area are available.[43,44] The LDL receptor expressed by fibroblasts and most extrahepatic tissues binds cholesterol-carrying LDL in plasma and serves to facilitate the transport of cholesterol from the liver to all tissues of the body (Table V). A second cholesterol transport pathway serves to transport dietary cholesterol from the intestine to the liver via a chylomicron/remnant receptor system. The binding of lipoproteins to these cellular receptors is mediated by the apoproteins. The LDL receptor recognizes a species of apo B, termed apo B-100, that is synthesized by the liver. Another species of apo B, termed apo B-48, is not recognized by the LDL receptor. This apo B species, which is only 48% as large as apo B-100, is synthesized in humans only by the intestine.[45] Lipoproteins containing apo B-48, such as chylomicrons and

Table V. Apoprotein B-Lipoproteins and Cholesterol Transport

	Apo B-100	Apo B-48
Lipoprotein	VLDL and LDL	Chylomicrons and remnants
Cellular origin (humans)	Liver	Intestine
Target tissue	All extrahepatic cells	Liver
Receptor on target tissue	LDL receptor	Remnant receptor

chylomicron remnants, do not bind to the LDL receptor, whereas other lipoproteins, such as LDL, that contain apo B-100, do bind.[43]

Although these two species of apo B appear to be under separate genetic control (a single patient has been described who makes apo B-48, but not apo B-100),[46] immunochemical identity among apo B-100 and apo B-48 has been observed. At least three laboratories have generated a total of seven different monoclonal antibodies that bind both apo B-100 and apo B-48.[7,9,47] The data strongly suggest that apo B-48 and apo B-100 are structurally related proteins (i.e., that apo B-48 may represent a portion of the apo B-100 protein). Good evidence also has been obtained, using monoclonal preparative immunoadsorbents, that apo B-48 and apo B-100 are not found on the same lipoprotein particle.[48] Thus, separate apo B particles exist (Table V). However, a further question arises concerning the structural identity between apo B-48 and apo B-100. Whereas it is generally accepted that apo B-48 and apo B-100 probably share large regions of structural homology, it is not known whether all portions of apo B-48 are present also on apo B-100, i.e., whether apo B-48 is a true fragment of apo B-100. This could be tested immunochemically by generating antibodies with apo B-48 as the immunogen and then determining if all of these antibodies bind apo B-100. To date this has not been done. All available antibodies that bind apo B-48 were generated with apo B-100 as the immunogen, and of course all of these antibodies bind both apo B-100 and apo B-48.

The LDL receptor binding properties of apo B-100 suggest that the portion of apo B-100 that is represented also in apo B-48 should not contain the region of apo B-100 that is recognized by the LDL receptor (Table V). This supposition has been tested with the six antibodies generated by Marcel *et al.*[7,49] None of the apo B-specific antibodies that bind apo B-48 block the binding of ^{125}I-LDL to its receptor on fibroblasts; and none of the antibodies that interfere with LDL receptor binding, binds to apo B-48. Another recently generated apo B-specific antibody, specifically selected after fusion for its ability to totally block the cellular degradation of ^{125}I-LDL in fibroblasts,[11] further supports this observation. This high-affinity antibody,[11] which blocks LDL receptor interactions, binds to delipidated apo B-100, but does not bind to delipidated chylomicron apo B-48.

Because primary sequence data are not available for apo B, structural information concerning the region of apo B that is recognized by the LDL receptor is limited. However, some information can be deduced from a comparison of the binding characteristics of those apo B-antibodies that interfere with receptor interaction with the binding characteristics of those apo B-antibodies that do not interfere with LDL receptor binding. Three apo B-binding characteristics are of particular significance.

The functional importance of certain lysine and arginine residues on apo B has been established by demonstrating that chemical modification of these amino acid residues will abolish the ability of apo B to bind to the LDL receptor.[50] It follows that chemical modification of these same residues on LDL also may interfere with the binding of some, but not all, apo B-specific antibodies. Furthermore, among the antibodies whose binding might be altered by blocking lysine or arginine residues, one would expect to find antibodies that would block LDL receptor binding. In fact, this has been demonstrated. One of the apo B-specific antibodies generated by Tikkanen *et al.*[6] that inhibits the cellular degradation of ^{125}I-LDL does not bind acetylated LDL. However, another antibody that was obtained from the same fusion and does not inhibit cellular degradation of ^{125}I-LDL actually displays increased binding to acetylated LDL. Thus, the important role of free lysine residues in the domain of apo B that specifies LDL receptor binding can be extended to include the role of free lysines in the binding of antibodies that are specific for similar or identical domains of apo B.

Further structural information about the LDL receptor binding domain of apoprotein B has been obtained by studying the binding of a panel of apo B-antibodies to isolated and solubilized apo B that was reconstituted to differing degrees with lipids and detergents.[51] In these studies, three types of antigenic determinants or epitopes were identified on apo B. One type of determinant was conformational, in that it was expressed by unfolded soluble and delipidated apo B. A second type was a conformational determinant that was expressed by delipidated apo B only when it was refolded in the presence of amphipathic lipids such as lecithin and free cholesterol, or detergent micelles. A third type of complex conformational determinant was defined by its requirement for the association of apo B with lipid structures that formed a hydrophobic core, such as cholesteryl esters. The association of this latter type of determinant with the region of apo B on LDL that binds to the receptor was confirmed by identifying that each of three antibodies that bound this complex conformational determinant on apo B also inhibited binding to the LDL receptor.[51]

The third binding characteristic concerns the striking interspecies cross-reactivity of some of the apo B antibodies. In competitive radioimmunoassays, the binding to human LDL of an apo B-specific mouse monoclonal antibody that binds to a region of apo B that blocks binding to the LDL receptor was inhibited by LDL isolated from 23 different mammalian species and one marsupial.[52] In contrast, the binding of other apo B antibodies of higher or comparable affinity for human LDL that do not interfere with LDL receptor binding was not inhibited by LDL isolated from the other species. Similar observations have been obtained with separate apo B antibodies that block LDL receptor binding.[11] These data suggest that the region of apo B that is involved in LDL receptor binding is an evolutionarily conserved region of apo B.

Therefore, while neither the primary sequence nor the conformational structural requirements for apo B cellular receptor interactions are known, immunochemical studies employing monoclonal antibodies have established that the domain of apo B that is recognized by the LDL receptor is: (1) a highly conserved antigenic determinant or domain of apo B that is expressed very similarly in the apo B of all species so far tested; (2) a complex conformational determinant that is expressed predominantly by apo B that is folded onto a spherical particle containing core lipids; (3) a region that contains the amino acids lysine and arginine, which probably participate in an ionic interaction between apo B and the cellular receptor; and (4) a region of apo B that is expressed by the apo B-100 species derived from the liver, but is not expressed by the apo B-48 portion of apo B synthesized by the intestine.

4.5. Identification of a Receptor Binding Domain on Apoprotein E

In contrast to the striking lack of information about the molecular weight, genetic polymorphism, and receptor binding domain of apoprotein B, much of this information is available for apo E. Apo E plays a central role in exogenous cholesterol transport and mediates the normal hepatic removal of chylomicron remnants via the chylomicron remnant receptor.[43,44] The primary structure of apo E is known and studies aimed at identifying the region of apo E that is involved in receptor binding have successfully identified a lysine- and arginine-rich region of 66 amino acid residues (residues 126–191) that is critical for receptor binding.[53] An immunochemical approach to further characterization of this region using monoclonal antibodies has further refined the available information.[17] Of five apo E-specific antibodies tested,[14] only one was found to interfere with the receptor binding activity of apo E. When the binding of this antibody to proteolytic or synthetic apo E fragments was tested, binding to a synthetic fragment that spanned residues 139–169 was observed. The results suggest that this apo E epitope, which is contained within the receptor binding domain, is probably a simple nonconformational determinant that is contained solely within residues 139–169.[17]

A review of the preceding sections would suggest that the apo B and apo E ligand/receptor systems are separate. However, these lipoprotein receptor systems are in fact much more complex. First, as pointed out earlier, lipoproteins are present in plasma (such as VLDL) that contain both apoproteins B and E. This suggests that some particles can theoretically bind to either the LDL receptor or the remnant receptor.[43] Second, it has been clearly demonstrated that lipoproteins containing only apo B or only apo E can bind with high affinity to one of the receptors, the LDL receptor. Thus, the molecular specificities of these lipid transport systems are more complex than originally thought. Monoclonal antibodies have been used to understand the molecular traffic patterns *in vivo* and to identify the apoprotein specificities involved.

Because both apo B and apo E (which are biochemically distinct ligands) can bind to the LDL receptor, it has been suggested that they might possess a similar structural region. If so, this region could conceivably also be immunochemically similar. However, to date neither the eight apo B-specific antibodies nor the single apo E-specific antibody that have demonstrable capacities to block LDL receptor binding have shown any cross-reactivity.[11,14,51] That is, none of the apo B-specific antibodies bind either soluble apo E or apo E-lecithin vesicles, and the apo E-specific antibody does not bind apo B or apo E-free LDL. Instead, the data suggest that the domains of apo E and apo B that mediate LDL receptor binding are distinct. If so, it follows that the structural region of the LDL receptor that binds apo B is distinct from the region that binds apo E, and this may soon be verified.[54]

All available data suggest that the structural portions of apoproteins B and E that interact with receptors are distinct. However, it does not immediately follow that lipoproteins containing both apoproteins can be recognized and bound by either receptor system. In fact, the value of monoclonal antibodies in identifying the specific apoprotein determinant responsible for the receptor-binding activity of a particular lipoprotein has been aptly demonstrated in recent studies by Hui *et al.*[10] The quantitative contribution of apo B-100 and apo E to the binding of both normal and abnormal VLDL was determined by assessing the ability of apo B- and apo E-specific antibodies with demonstrable capacity to inhibit cellular binding to block VLDL binding to both hepatic remnant receptors and LDL receptors. The binding of VLDL to the remnant receptor (which binds only apo E) or the LDL receptor (which binds both apo B-100 and apo E) was inhibited by the apo E-specific antibody and not the apo B-specific antibody.[10] The data indicate that apo E is the dominant apoprotein in specifying the interaction of VLDL with both remnant and LDL receptors.

5. Future Applications and Summary

Plasma lipoproteins represent a physically and chemically diverse set of regulatory and transport macromolecules, and they continue to present a unique challenge to our efforts to understand structure–function relationships. Although much remains to be done, monoclonal antibodies have made significant contributions to the elucidation of the molecular weight of apo B, the apoproteins that specify cellular binding, the apoprotein polymorphisms, and finally the role of these lipoproteins in atherosclerosis and coronary heart disease. Just as they have in the past, monoclonal antibodies will continue in the future to be applied to issues of lipoprotein metabolism. Many exciting potential applications exist and the possibilities are perhaps best illustrated with the following final example.

Cholesterol, an essential constituent of all tissues of the body, can be synthesized by most cells in the body; however, it cannot be degraded by most cells. Cholesterol is obtained also from ingested foods via adsorption in the gut. Exit of cholesterol from the tissues and the body occurs only after it is transported via lipoproteins to the liver for excretion into the bile. Therefore, to ensure low levels of cholesterol in plasma, hepatic clearance of cholesterol-carrying lipoproteins must occur. When hepatic clearance of cholesterol-rich lipoproteins is impaired, dangerously high plasma levels of potentially damaging atherogenic lipoproteins can result. The recent observations of Bernini *et al*,[55] indicate that apoprotein-specific monoclonal antibodies may some day be very useful in enhancing the specific hepatic clearance of certain cholesterol-rich lipoproteins. These investigators have demonstrated that antibody Fab fragments modified by conjugation with lactose are cleared by a specific hepatic receptor that recognizes neoterminal galactose residues, termed the galactose receptor.[55] Their studies show that lactosamination of the Fab fragments promotes their plasma clearance by the liver and that the clearance exceeds that of the kidney. The data suggest that lactosamination of the Fab fragments of apo B- or apo E-specific monoclonal antibodies could facilitate or enhance the hepatic uptake of the specific endogenous cholesterol-containing lipoproteins containing these apoproteins. If successful, this manipulation could prove to be an extremely powerful method for specifically directing the hepatic clearance of discrete and potentially damaging lipoprotein particles.

References

1. Alaupovic, P., Lee D. M., and McConathy, W. J., 1972, Studies on the composition and structure of plasma lipoproteins (distribution of lipoprotein families in major density classes of normal human plasma lipoproteins), *Biochim. Biophys. Acta* **260**:689–707.
2. Fielding, C. J., and Fielding, P. E., 1977, in: *Cholesterol Metabolism and Lipolytic Enzymes* (J. Blonovski, ed.), Massen, New York, pp. 165–172.
3. Sparrow, J. T., and Gotto, Jr., A. M., 1981, Apolipoprotein/lipid interactions: Studies with synthetic peptides, *CRC Crit. Rev. Biochem.* **13**:87–107.
4. Mao, S. J. T., Kazmar, R. E., Silverfield, J. C., Alley, M. C., Kluge, K., and Fathman, C. G., 1982, Immunochemical properties of human low density lipoproteins as explored by monoclonal antibodies. Binding characteristics distinct from those of conventional serum antibodies, *Biochim. Biophys. Acta* **713**:365–374.
5. Patton, J. G., Alley, M. C., and Mao, S. J. T., 1982, Evaluation of monoclonal antibodies to human plasma low density lipoproteins. A requirement for lipids to maintain antigenic structures, *J. Immunol. Meth.* **55**:193–203.
6. Tikkanen, M. J., Dargar, R., Pfleger, B., Gonen, B., Davle, J. M., and Schonfeld, G., 1982, Antigenic mapping of human low density lipoprotein with monoclonal antibodies, *J. Lipid Res.* **23**:1032–1038.
7. Marcel, Y. L., Hogue, M., Theolis, J. R., and Milne, R. W., 1982, Mapping of antigenic determinants of human apolipoprotein B using monoclonal antibodies against low density lipoproteins, *J. Biol. Chem.* **257**:13165–13168.
8. Watt, T. S., and Watt, R. M., 1983, Detection of unique antigenic determinants on human plasma low density lipoprotein and on delipidated apolipoprotein B, *Proc. Natl. Acad. Sci. USA* **80**:124–128.
9. Curtiss, L. K., and Edgington, T. S., 1982, Immunochemical heterogeneity of human plasma apolipoprotein B. I. Apolipoprotein B binding of mouse hybridoma antibodies, *J. Biol. Chem.* **257**:15213–15221.

10. Hui, D. Y., Innerarity, T. L., and Mahley, R. W., 1984, Defective hepatic lipoprotein receptor binding of β-very low density lipoproteins from Type III hyperlipoproteinemic patients. Importance of apolipoprotein E, *J. Biol. Chem.* **259**:860–869.
11. Young, S., Witztum, J. L., and Curtiss, L. K., 1985, Evidence for evolutionary conservation of the LDL receptor recognition domain on apolipoprotein B using monoclonal antibodies, *Clin. Res.* **33**:68A.
12. Hopp, T. P., and Woods, K. R., 1981, Prediction of protein antigenic determinants from amino acid sequences, *Proc. Natl. Acad. Sci. USA* **78**:3824–3828.
13. Hopp, T. P., and Woods, K. R., 1983, A complete program for predicting protein antigenic determinants, *Mol. Immunol.* **20**:483–489.
14. Milne, R. W., Douste-Blazy, P. H., Marcel, Y. L., and Retequi, L., 1981, Characterization of monoclonal antibodies against human apolipoprotein E, *J. Clin. Invest.* **68**:111–117.
15. Voyta, J. C., Via, D. P., and Sparrow, J. T., 1982, Monoclonal antibodies to human apolipoprotein E, *Fed. Proc.* **41**:931.
16. Pepe, M. G., and Curtiss, L. K., 1985, A sensitive radioimmunoassay for monitoring cellular synthesis and secretion of apolipoprotein E. In press.
17. Weisgraber, K. H., Innerarity, T. L., Harder, K. J., Mahley, R. W., Milne, R. W., Marcel, Y. L., and Sparrow, J. T., 1983, The receptor-binding domain of human apolipoprotein E. Monoclonal antibody inhibition of binding, *J. Biol. Chem.* **258**:12348–12354.
18. Fielding, P. E., Fielding, C. J., Havel, R. J., Kane, J. P., and Tun, P., 1983, Cholesterol net transport, esterification and transfer in human hyperlipidemic plasma, *J. Clin. Invest.* **71**:449–460.
19. Fager, C., Wiklund, O., and Olofsson, S., 1980, Serum apolipoprotein levels in relation to acute myocardial infarction and its risk factors, apolipoprotein A-I levels in male survivors of myocardial infarction, *Atherosclerosis* **36**:67–74.
20. Curtiss, L. K., and Edgington, T. S., 1985, Heterogeneity of human plasma high density lipoproteins. I. Identification with apolipoprotein AI- and AII-specific monoclonal antibodies, *J. Biol. Chem.* **260**:2982–2993.
21. Stein, E. A., and Pesce, A. J., 1983, Enzyme linked immunoassays for apolipoproteins: Advantages, problems and prototype assay, in: *Proceedings Workshop on Apolipoprotein Quantification*, NIH Pub. No. 83-1266, pp. 319–328.
22. Marhaug, G., Gaudernack, G., Bogen, B., and Husby, G., 1982, Monoclonal hybridoma antibodies to human amyloid related protein SAA, *Clin. Exp. Immunol.* **50**:390–396.
23. Curtiss, L. K., and Plow, E. F., 1984, Interaction of plasma lipoproteins with human platelets, *Blood* **64**:365–374.
24. Whayne, T. F., Alaupovic, P., Curry, M. D., Lee, E. T., Anderson, P. S., and Schecter, E., 1981, Plasma apolipoprotein B and VLDL-, LDL-, and HDL-cholesterol as risk factors in the development of coronary artery disease in male patients examined by angiography, *Atherosclerosis* **39**:411–424.
25. Sniderman, A., Shapiro, S., Marpole, D., Skinner, B., Teng, B., and Kwiterovich, P. O., Jr., 1980, Association of coronary atherosclerosis with hyperapobetaalipoproteinemia [increased protein but normal cholesterol levels in human plasma low density lipoproteins], *Proc. Natl. Acad. Sci. USA* **77**:604–608.
26. Gordon, T., Castelli, W. P., and Hjortland, M. C., 1977, High density lipoprotein as a protective factor against coronary heart disease, The Framingham Study, *Am. J. Med.* **62**:707–714.
27. Mao, S. J. T., Patton, J. G., Badimon, J., Kottke, B. A., Alley, M. C., and Cardin, A. D., 1983, Monoclonal antibodies to human plasma low density lipoproteins. I. Enhanced binding of ^{125}I-labeled low density lipoproteins by combined use of two monoclonal antibodies, *Clin. Chem.* **29**:1890–1897.
28. Tsao, B. P., Curtiss, L. K., and Edgington, T. S., 1982, Immunochemical heterogeneity of human plasma apolipoprotein B. II. Expression of apolipoprotein B epitopes on native lipoproteins. *J. Biol. Chem.* **257**:15222–15228.
29. Tikkanen, M. J., Cole, T. G., and Schonfeld, G., 1983, Differential reactivity of human low density lipoproteins with monoclonal antibodies, *J. Lipid Res.* **24**:1494–1499.

30. Patton, J. G., Badimon, J., and Mao, S. J. T., 1983, Monoclonal antibodies to human plasma low density lipoproteins. II. Evaluation for use in radioimmunoassay for apolipoprotein B in patients with coronary artery disease, *Clin. Chem.* **29**:1898–1903.
31. Smith, R., Dawson, J. R., and Tanford, C., 1972, The size and number of polypeptide chains in human serum low density lipoprotein, *J. Biol. Chem.* **247**:3376–3381.
32. Socorro, L., Lopez, F., Lopez, A., and Camejo, G., 1982, Apo LDL: Evidence for an aggregating system of heterogeneous subunits, *J. Lipid Res.* **23**:1283–1291.
33. Olofsson, S. O., Bostrom, K., Svanberg, U., and Bondjers, G., 1980, Isolation and partial characterization of a polypeptide belonging to Apolipoprotein B from low density lipoproteins of human plasma, *Biochemistry* **19**:1059–1064.
34. Bradley, W. A., Rohde, M. F., Gotto, Jr., A. M., and Jackson, R. L., 1978, The cyanogen bromide peptides of the apoprotein of low density lipoprotein (ApoB): Its molecular weight from a chemical view, *Biochem. Biophys. Res. Commun.* **81**:928–935.
35. Hahm, K., Tikkanen, M. J., Dargar, R., Cole, T. G., Davie, J. M., and Schonfeld, G., 1983, Limited proteolysis selectively destroys epitopes on apolipoprotein B in low density lipoproteins, *J. Lipid Res.* **24**:877–885.
36. Watt, T. S., and Watt, R. M., 1984, Probing the antigenic structure of human serum low density lipoproteins (LDL) with monoclonal antibodies. *Fed. Proc.* **43**:1642.
37. Milne, R. W., and Marcel, Y. L., 1982, Monoclonal antibodies against human low density lipoprotein. Stoichiometric binding studies using Fab fragments, *FEBS Lett.* **146**:97–100.
38. Wiklund, O., Dyer, C. A., Tsao, B. P., and Curtiss, L. K., 1985, Studies of the stoichiometric binding of apolipoprotein B-specific monoclonal antibodies to low density lipoproteins, *J. Biol. Chem.* In press.
39. Munson, P. J., and Rodbard, D., 1980, LIGAND: A versatile computerized approach for characterization of ligand-binding systems, *Anal. Biochem.* **107**:220–239.
40. Schumaker, V. N., Robinson, M. T., Curtiss, L. K., Butler, R., and Sparks, R. S., 1984, Anti-apoprotein B monoclonal antibodies detect human low density lipoprotein polymorphism, *J. Biol. Chem.* **259**:6423–6430.
41. Balla, M. A., Schumaker, V. N., and Curtiss, L. K., 1985, Demonstration of apolipoprotein B genetic polymorphism using the Western blot technique, *J. Lipid, Res.* In press.
42. Schumaker, V. N., Balla, M. A. Robinsen, M., Spence, A., Sparks, R., and Curtiss, L. K., 1985, The use of monoclonal antibodies to detect genetic polymorphism: Application to apolipoprotein B, in: *Genetic Disorders Medical Genetics: Past, Present and Future*, Alan Liss, New York.
43. Brown, M. S., and Goldstein, J. L., 1983, Lipoprotein receptors in the liver. Control signals for plasma cholesterol traffic, *J. Clin. Invest.* **72**:743–747.
44. Brown, M. S., Kovanen, P. T., and Goldstein, J. L., 1981, Regulation of plasma cholesterol by lipoprotein receptors, *Science* **212**:628–635.
45. Kane, J. P., Hardman, P. A., and Paulus, H. E., 1980, Heterogeneity of apolipoprotein B: Isolation of a new species from human chylomicrons, *Proc. Natl. Acad. Sci. USA* **77**:2365–2369.
46. Malloy, M. J,. Kane, J. P. Hardman, D. A., Hamilton, R. L., and Dalal, K. B., 1981, Normotriglyceridemic abetalipoproteinemia: Absence of the B-100 apolipoproteins, *J. Clin. Invest.* **67**:1441–1450.
47. Tikkanen, M. J., Cole, T. G., Hahm, K., Krul, E. S., and Schonfeld, G., 1984, Expression of apolipoprotein B epitopes in very low density lipoprotein subfractions. Studies with monoclonal antibodies, *Arteriosclerosis* **4**:138–146.
48. Milne, R. W., Weech, P. K., Blanchette, L., Davignon, J., Alaupovic, P., and Marcel, Y. L., 1984, Isolation and characterization of apolipoprotein B-48 and B-100 very low density lipoproteins from Type III hyperlipoproteinemic subjects, *J. Clin. Invest.* **73**:816–823.
49. Milne, R. W., Theolis, J. R., Verdery, R. B., and Marcel, Y. L., 1983, Characterization of monoclonal antibodies against human low density lipoprotein, *Arterioclerosis* **3**:23–30.
50. Weisgraber, K. H., Innerarity, T. L., and Mahley, R. W., 1978, Role of the lysine residues of plasma lipoproteins in high affinity binding to cell surface receptors on human fibroblasts, *J. Biol. Chem.* **253**:9053–9062.

51. Marcel, Y. L., Hogue, M., Weech, P. K., and Milne, R. W., 1984, Characterization of antigenic determinants on human solubilized apolipoprotein B. Conformational requirements for lipids, *J. Biol. Chem.* **259:**6952–6957.
52. Nelson, C. A., Tasch, M. A., Tikkanen, M,. Dargar, R., and Schonfeld, G., 1984, Evolution of low density lipoprotein structure probed with monoclonal antibodies, *J. Lipid Res.* **25:**821–830.
53. Innerarity, T. L., Friedlander, E. J., Rall, Jr., S. C., Weisgraber, K. H., and Mahley, R. W., 1983, The receptor-binding domain of human apolipoprotein E. Binding of apolipoprotein E fragments, *J. Biol. Chem.* **258:**12341–12347.
54. Russell, D. W., Schneider, W. J., Yamamoto, T., Luskey, K. L., Brown, M. S., and Goldstein, J. L., 1984, Domain map of the LDL receptor: Sequence homology with the epidermal growth factor precursor, *Cell* **37:**577–585.
55. Bernini, F., Tanenbaum, S. R., Sherrill, B. C., Gotto, A. M., Jr., and Smith, L. C., 1985, Enhancement of Fab fragment uptake in the rat liver by lactosamination, In press.

Chapter 18

Enzyme Active Sites

SANDRA J. SMITH-GILL

1. Introduction

Monoclonal antibodies (MAbs) have provided powerful new tools for analysis of enzyme function. MAbs directed at specific subsites of the enzyme active site allow analysis of catalysis at a new level of resolution even for relatively simple, monomeric enzymes. Because many different MAbs can be prepared to a given enzyme protein or polypeptide complex, and each will be exquisitely specific for a given antigenic determinant or epitope, multiple subunits and associated catalytic functions become potentially separable. In addition, because the binding of MAbs to protein antigens is sensitive to even single residue changes in the antigenic determinant, it is possible to discriminate between very closely related but structurally distinct multiple molecular forms of enzymes.[1] This discussion reviews several unique studies in which MAbs have been used to examine catalysis in ways not previously approachable by conventional biochemical methods.

1.1. Relationship of Catalytic Sites to Antigenic Structure

In general, there does not appear to be any special immunogenicity associated with catalytic sites of enzymes; enzymes, like other proteins, appear to be potentially antigenic on their entire surface.[2] For example, out of a total of 40 characterized MAbs recognizing influenza virus neuraminidase, 29 MAbs (73%) did not inhibit catalysis, and only two strongly inhibited enzyme activity when tested with a small substrate.[3] Similarly, only 4.2% of 177 anti-β-D-galactosidase[4] and 41% of anticarboxypeptidase[5] MAbs inhibited enzyme activity; in the latter case, two out of three MAbs that were examined in detail showed noncompetitive inhibition of catalysis, indicating that the MAbs were not directly binding the catalytic site.

One property of catalytic sites that has been elegantly demonstrated utilizing MAbs is the strong conservation of sequences associated with catalytic activity.

SANDRA J. SMITH-GILL • Laboratory of Genetics, National Cancer Institute, National Institutes of Health, Bethesda, Maryland 20205; and Department of Zoology, University of Maryland, College Park, Maryland 20742.

Thus, for a number of enzymes, polyclonal antibodies recognizing portions of the protein distinct from the catalytic center show cross-reactivity that is proportional to the degree of evolutionary relatedness, and MAbs to the same regions frequently do not cross-react among different species at all.[6] In contrast, MAbs directed against catalytic centers of enzymes frequently are highly cross-reactive with homologous enzymes isolated form widely divergent species, indicating a strong conservation.[7] Such conservation may even make the active site appear to be *less* immunogenic than the rest of the molecule.

A dramatic example of active site conservation is found in influenza virus neuraminidase; residues associated with neuraminidase catalytic function are completely invariant.[8] The antigenic structure of this protein in relation to its catalytic function has been investigated extensively utilizing large panels of MAbs, and is examined in detail below.

1.2. Influenza Virus Neuraminidase

Influenza virus neuraminidase (NA) (EC 3.2.1.18) is a tetrameric glycoprotein with a box-shaped head, approximately 100 × 100 × 60 Å, attached to a slender stalk buried in the membrane of the virus. The enzyme catalyzes the cleavage of the α-ketosidic linkage between the terminal sialic acid and an adjacent sugar residue, thus destroying the hemagglutinin (HA) receptor and presumably facilitating several functions: transport of virus through the mucin of the host cell, elution of progeny virus particles from infected cells, and prevention of self-aggregation of the virus by removing sialic acid from the carbohydrate moiety of newly synthesized HA and NA.[9] Each monomer contains six topologically identical β-sheets arranged in a propellar formation to form a large pocket on the distal surface which binds the product of catalysis, sialic acid.[9] This pocket is surrounded by highly conserved charged or hydrophobic residues (Fig. 1A). NA and HA occur in close association on the surface of the influenza virus; MAb specific for one of those molecules frequently will inhibit activity of the other, although there is some variation, which may relate to among-strain variation in the number or grouping of NA molecules on viruses.[3,11,12]

Based on the crystal structure of NA, a very complex antigenic structure has been proposed to consist of seven families of potential determinants, each associated with one of seven variable segments clustered preferentially into distal surface loops of the β-sheets[8,9] (Fig. 1B). These potential antigenic regions form a nearly continuous surface encircling the pocket that forms the catalytic site of each monomer. Sequence analyses have revealed that amino acid changes in antibody-selected variants, as well as during natural antigenic drift (which presumably is also antibody-selected), are clustered preferentially on the distal surface loops of the β-sheets[10,12–14] (Figs. 1B and 1C). Antigenic drift in NA has been less rapid than that in HA, perhaps because anti-HA antibodies are much more effective at neutralizing infectivity than are anti-NA antibodies.[13]

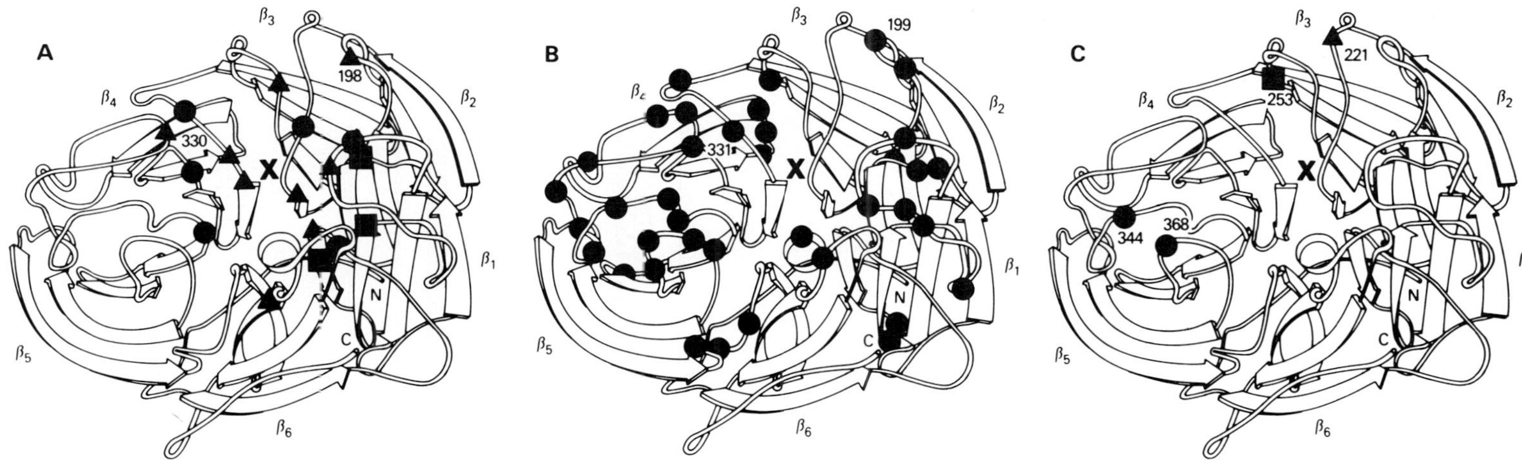

Figure 1. Diagrams of subunit folding of N2 neuraminidase, adapted from Ref. 9, to show position occupied by sialic acid (×), and: (A) Invariant residues associated with catalytic center. (▲) Acid residues; (●) basic residues; (■) other, hydrophobic residues. Positions of two invariant residues that are immediately adjacent to variable residues are numbered. (Based on Refs. 8 and 9.) (B) Positions of variable residues during antigenic drift; positions of two residues immediately adjacent to invariant residues are numbered. (Based on Refs. 8, 10, and 13.) (C) Positions of substitutions in antigenic variants selected by neutralizing MAbs in panel A. (●) Variants selected by MAbs in group I generated to Tokyo H_2N_2; (■) Variant selected by MAb 113/2 in group Ii generated to Jap H_2N_2; (▲) variant selected by MAb 18/1 in group II generated to Tex H_3N_2. (Based on Ref. 14.) Diagrams are adapted from Ref. 9.

Two panels of MAbs have been utilized in a series of elegant studies to elucidate the relationship of the enzyme active center to its antigenic structure. One panel (A) consisted of neutralizing MAbs that had been generated against six different N2 virus strains and had been selected on the basis of their ability to inhibit catalytic activity.[12–14] High titers of all these anti-NA MAbs were able to effectively neutralize all parental viruses and to select for antigenic variants in a single passage *in vitro* in chick embryos. However, there was little cross-reactivity between MAbs generated to H_2N_2 strains and those generated to later H_3N_2 strains.[12]

A second, broader panel (B) consisted of MAbs that all had been generated against a single H_2N_2 viral strain (A/RI/5$^+$/57) and were selected by their ability to bind crystalline NA in ELISA.[3] This panel included MAbs that would specifically bind NA in ELISA, but did not inhibit NA activity, confirming earlier conclusions based on polyclonal antisera that NA contains antigenic sites distinct from the enzyme active site. There was a good correlation between the ability to neutralize catalysis and neutralization of infectivity; although all MAbs were able to inhibit viral release in an *in vitro* plaque assay, only those capable of inhibiting catalysis were able to neutralize infectivity or select antigenic variants in embryonated eggs.

In order to probe the position of the enzyme active center relative to antigenic sites, the interactions of selected MAbs from both panels with two different-sized substrates were examined.[3,11] The rationale of the studies was that MAbs with determinants close to the catalytic site would inhibit hydrolysis of sialic acid from a relatively small substrate, such as neuraminyl lactose (NAL, molecular weight 600), while those antibodies binding further from the catalytic site might inhibit only hydrolysis of a larger substrate, such as fetuin (molecular weight 50,000). Only half of the antibodies from panel A inhibited hydrolysis of both substrates, while the other half inhibited hydrolysis of fetuin but not NAL.[11] Only two out of 24 neutralizing MAbs from panel B strongly inhibited catalysis of the smaller substrate, while the majority did not interact at all with NAL.[3] These results with both panels suggest the majority of neutralizing MAbs do not interact directly with the catalytic center, but presumably inhibit catalysis by other, noncompetitive, mechanisms.

MAbs from panel A were used to select antigenic variants of Tokyo H_2N_2 strain.[12] MAbs that were originally generated against any given viral strain were only sensitive to substitutions selected by MAbs against the same strain. Sequence analyses[13,14] of those antigenic variants identified four residues, which were located on the loops of different β-sheets; all the MAbs generated to the Tokyo H_2N_2 strain selected substitutions on the loops of β-5, while the MAbs generated against Jap H_2N_2 and Tex H_3N_2 selected substitutions on the opposite side of the catalytic center (Fig. 1C). These results suggest that as the NA molecule changes due to antigenic drift, different regions apparently become immunodominant, and the apparent antigenic structure of NA may therefore differ depending upon the strain of virus utilized for generation of the MAbs used for analysis.

Three types of substitutions were selected by the anti-Tokyo H_2N_2 MAbs. One MAb, S10/1, selected for a substitution at position 368 (V-368) on a loop of the β-5 sheet, while five other MAbs selected a total of nine variants with substitutions at position 344 (V-344), which is on an adjacent loop between the β-4 and β-5 sheets (Fig. 1C). While the S10/1 MAb did not bind or neutralize with the V-344's, the MAbs that had selected the 344 substitutions varied in their reactivity with V-368, even though the substitution involved a charge change. Three MAbs that inhibited catalysis of the small substrate NAL selected a total of four variants, all of which had an Arg-344 → Ile substitution. These MAbs could neither neutralize nor bind in ELISA any V-344, and two also did not react with V-368. In contrast, two MAbs that did not inhibit catalysis of NAL selected for all possible substitutions at position 344, which could result from a single nucleotide change; although they could not neutralize the V-344's, they could still bind V-344's in ELISA, and all neutralized V-368. These results suggest that the two sets of MAbs recognize different overlapping subregions, including Arg-344, and that they exert different selective pressures on the viral NA. It is also apparent that there is more than one mechanism by which the virus may escape neutralizing antibodies, and that total abrogation of antibody binding is not necessary to escape antibody neutralization; several variants that had escaped neutralization but could still be bound in ELISA were also found among variants selected by neutralizing MAbs from panel B.[3] An understanding of the structural bases of these important complex functional interactions will require further investigation.

Detailed analysis of the MAbs from panel B revealed an equally complex antigenic structure for the NA molecule as a whole.[3] Competitive binding RIAs defined four overlapping antigenic regions. The largest region, hypothesized to localize on the front of the NA molecule, could be further subdivided into four overlapping areas based on patterns of reactivity with antigenic variants of NA, chemically modified NA, and inhibition of the smaller substrate NAL. It was concluded that these subregions overlap those that had been defined in the studies with neutralizing panel A,[11–14] and that selection of only MAbs capable of neutralizing NA had selected a subset of the total specificities possible in the anti-NA response and of those represented by panel B.[3]

What is remarkable about the antigenic structure of NA as it relates to the catalytic function is the very close proximity of the variable segments containing the antigenic determinants to the completely invariant residues associated with catalytic function. In fact, some of these invariant residues are contained within variable segments and may even be within the epitopes recognized by the MAbs; two invariant residues are directly adjacent to variable residues (Figs. 1A and 1B). Despite this close proximity, antibodies apparently cannot select for modification of those residues.

2. Enzymes with Multiple Interacting Sites

Many intracellular enzymes are composed of subunits, and enzymes with multiple functions may be complexed together as "holoenzymes." The functional interactions among polymeric enzyme subunits as well as their structural interrelationships are frequently complex. Subunit complexation often makes understanding of a particular catalytic function difficult, because subunits can be separated and purified in active form only with great difficulty. The utilization of MAbs to identify particular enzymatic functions and subunit interactions has proven particularly useful for enzyme complexes, because it allows unambiguous separation of activities that could not previously be resolved. The discussion below reviews four enzymes with multiple interacting sites: a relatively simple, well-characterized enzyme, two very complex holoenzymes, and an enzyme cascade complex. In each of these systems, MAbs have been used in very different ways to analyze various aspects of enzyme subunit structure and function.

2.1. Carboxypeptidase A

Carboxypeptidase A (CPA) (EC 3.4.17.1) is a zinc-containing enzyme having two catalytic activities: it catalyzes the hydrolysis of the carboxy-terminal peptide bonds in protein and peptide substrates, and in addition catalyzes esterase reactions. In order to examine the interrelationships of these two enzymatic functions and the structure of CPA, a panel of MAbs was prepared against purified enzyme.[5] Twenty-six clones were examined for their inhibition of peptidase and esterase activities. The results indicated that the two catalytic centers are physically separable; MAbs inhibiting only peptidase or only esterase catalysis were identified, as well as MAbs that inhibited both activities and neither, respectively.

The kinetics of peptidase inhibition by three MAbs was examined in detail. One MAb was found to inhibit catalysis competitively, and circular dichroism studies revealed an interaction between the MAb and Tyr-246, a catalytically essential residue. This MAb therefore could be considered to be interacting directly with the peptidase catalytic site. The fact that this MAb did not inhibit esterase activity demonstrated that the two catalytic centers are structurally separate.

Two other MAbs that partially inhibited only peptidase activity were shown to inhibit noncompetitively. The authors hypothesized that the noncompetitive inhibition resulted from an antibody-induced conformational change in the enzyme, which did not change the substrate affinity but lowered the V_{max} of the reaction. Again, the lack of an effect of these MAbs on esterase activity indicated that the two catalytic sites are structurally as well as functionally separate.

2.2. Eukaryotic RNA Polymerase

DNA-dependent RNA polymerase (EC 2.7.7.6) catalyzes the transcription of DNA into RNA using the four ribonucleoside triphosphates as substrates.

Three distinct classes of the enzyme exist in eukaryotic nuclei, referred to as I, II, and III, that transcribe 18S and 28S rRNA, hn and mRNA, and 5S rRNA and tRNA, respectively. Each of these forms has a complex subunit structure, and subunits may be shared by the various forms (reviewed in Ref. 15). Although elucidation of the subunit structure of these enzymes is critical to an understanding of transcription, the complexity of the enzymes and limited success in isolating purified subunits in workable quantities have hampered investigation of RNA polymerase structure and function. Several recent studies utilizing MAbs have begun to provide specific reagents for studying these complex enzymes.

Two MAbs, C171 and C168, from mouse spleens immunized with rat hepatoma polymerase I, inhibited RNA polymerase I activity as well as polymerase III but not polymerase II activity *in vitro*.[16] When partially purified MAb was added to polymerase I that was already initiated on a DNA template, elongation was inhibited. In all cases, the presence of MAb increased k_{M}UTP and k_{M}ATP, although the kinetics of inhibition was not that of classic competitive inhibition. In contrast, altering DNA concentration did not affect kinetics. These results suggested that the MAbs were directed against a determinant in close proximity to the nucleotide binding site for RNA chain elongation. The results also suggested that the centers for chain elongation of polymerases I and III are closely related, but that of polymerase II is distinct. Subunit analysis using Western blots indicated that the MAbs C171 and C168 bound the largest (molecular weight 190,000) polypeptide, suggesting that this subunit probably contains the chain elongation catalytic center of eukaryotic RNA polymerase I.

Another MAb, HC-18a, generated against RNA polymerase I from the silk glands of the silkworm moth, was shown by Western blot analysis to be specific for the second largest (molecular weight 132,000) of the subunits of polymerase I.[17] This MAb also neutralized polymerase I activity, and preincubation studies with DNA demonstrated that it was not interacting with the DNA recognition site. In contrast to the MAbs recognizing the chain elongation site, this MAb showed only slight cross-reactivity with either polymerase II or III. Thus, the recognition or catalytic function abrogated by this MAb may not be structurally conserved among the various polymerase classes.

A MAb (G11) specific for RNA polymerase II from calf thymus was shown to inhibit transcription by inhibiting DNA binding.[18] The inhibitory ability depended upon preincubation of the MAb with the enzyme; the MAb did not affect elongation if added after the enzyme was bound to the DNA, except in long incubations of 15 min, where there was a net inhibition, perhaps due to inhibition of reinitiation.[18] Western blot analyses showed that the G11 antigenic site was on the largest subunit; the DNA binding site of eukaryotic RNA polymerase II therefore is located on the largest subunit.[7]

There are three forms of eukaryotic RNA polymerase II enzymes, which differ in their abilities to be phosphorylated. They are termed RNA polymerase II_O, II_A, and II_B, and are classified by the apparent molecular weight of their largest subunits, II_o, II_a, II_b, respectively (discussed in Ref. 19). The MAb G11 was found to bind specifically to the largest subunit of all three forms, II_o

(molecular weight 240,000), II_a (215,000), and II_b (180,000), suggesting that the DNA binding site is conserved among the polymerase II forms.[7] Furthermore, the MAb reacted with the II_a and II_b subunits of all the eukaryotic RNA polymerase II enzymes tested, but not with that of *Escherichia coli*. In contrast, cross-reactivity of nonneutralizing polyclonal antiserum was proportional to the evolutionary relatedness of the polymerases; among the subunits, the largest was the most conserved.[7]

The *in vivo* transcriptional specificities of RNA polymerases II_O, II_A, and II_B are not known, although both polymerases II_A and II_B appear to be active in nonspecific transcription systems. Another MAb was utilized to demonstrate that the transcriptional properties of polymerases II_O, II_A, and II_B are not equivalent.[19] The MAb was shown to bind specifically to the subunits II_a and II_o, but not II_b, and to remove the holoenzymes II_A and II_O in immunoaffinity purification.[20] The MAb did not cross-react with either polymerase I or III, except for a very low level of cross-reactivity with two small subunits common to polymerases I and II. The MAb was shown not to inhibit nonpromotor-directed transcription under a variety of conditions, suggesting that the MAb does not interfere with DNA binding and RNA chain initiation at nonpromotor sites nor with chain elongation. However, selective transcription *in vitro* of conalbumin, ovalbumin, and adenovirus-2 major late promotor by polymerase II was completely inhibited by the MAb, suggesting that at least some specific promotor-directed transcription is catalyzed by RNA polymerases II_A and/or II_O, but not by polymerase II_B.[19] Further studies will be necessary to determine whether RNA polymerase II_B, which lacks the MAb-inhibited promotor/recognition site, is active in the transcription of other promotor-regulated genes or whether the promotors examined in the *in vitro* study can be transcribed *in vivo*.

2.3. DNA Polymerase-α

DNA polymerase-α (EC 2.7.7.7) has a key role in the replication of nuclear DNA in eukaryotes, representing 90–95% of the total DNA polymerase activity in mammalian cells.[21] It is very heterogeneous, consisting of a number of subunits, with molecular weights that range from 50,000 to 70,000, in association with one or more major catalytic polypeptides of molecular weight about 150,000. Unlike RNA polymerases, DNA polymerases cannot start a chain, but frequently elongate short oligoribonucleotide primers, which may be synthesized *de novo* by only two classes of enzymes: RNA polymerases, and a class of polymerases classified as "primases." DNA primases have been found in apparent association with DNA polymerase-α's, but investigations of the molecular bases of these associations have been hampered by lack of highly purified complexes (discussed in Ref. 22).

Recently, a panel of 16 MAbs specific for DNA polymerase-α from cultured mammalian KB cells allowed a detailed investigation of the interaction between KB DNA primase and polymerase-α activities.[23] These MAbs did not cross-react with either DNA polymerases-β or -γ, and recognized epitopes on a family

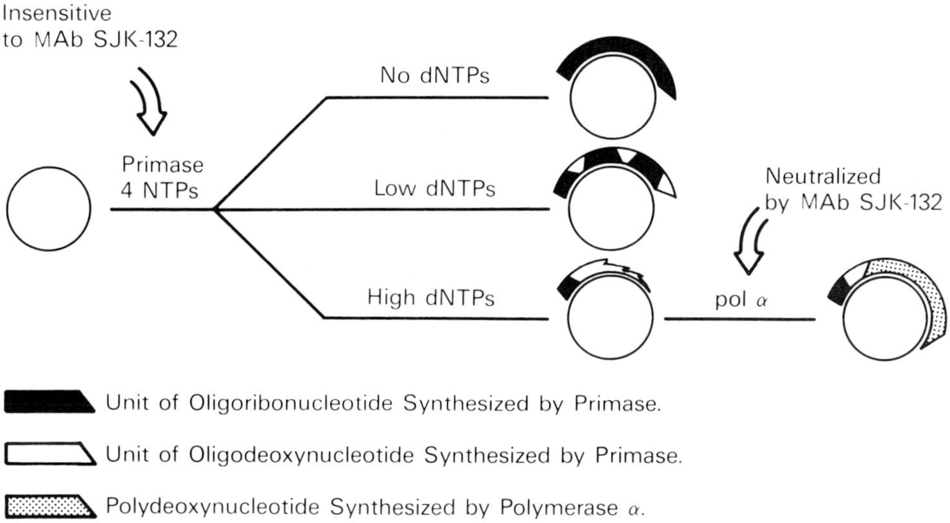

Figure 2. Model for regulation of KB DNA primase, and proposed effects of MAb SJK-132 on the catalytic activity of the KB DNA polymerase-α holoenzyme complex. (Adapted from Ref. 24.)

of large polypeptides (p180, p165, p140, and p125) that contained polymerase-α activity.[22] Three of the 16 MAbs neutralized polymerase-α activity, and one of these, SJK-132, has been utilized to affinity-purify DNA polymerase-α from KB cells and to examine the molecular mechanism of chain initiation and elongation by the enzyme complex.[22,23]

The MAb SKJ-132 was used to immunoaffinity-purify DNA polymerase-α from cultured KB cells. The fraction also contained DNA primase activity, which was not detectable in biochemically purified KB cell polymerase-α fractions.[22] The primase and polymerase-α activities could not be separated by biochemical procedures that preserved both activities, yet the two activities could be distinguished by a variety of physical, chemical, and immunologic means. The kinetics of the RNA-dependent DNA synthesis reaction suggested the cooperative participation of at least two distinct catalytic entities. The two activities also differed significantly in thermostability and in sensitivity to the inhibitor N-ethylmaleimide. Finally, while the polymerase-α activity could be neutralized by only 10–30 ng of SJK-132, a 100-fold excess (1 μg) of antibody neutralized only 30–50% of the primase activity.

Experiments performed in the presence of excess SJK-132 allowed examination of the products of primase activity.[22,24] These experiments could not have been performed without specific inactivation of the polymerase-α, which would otherwise have displaced the primase in the course of the normal reaction (see Fig. 2). In the complete absence of dNTPs, with purified rNTPs as substrate, the primase synthesized a family of distinctively banding oligoribonucleotides (~20–35 nucleotides). The same results were obtained in the presence or absence of SJK-132, except there was a slight reduction in size in the presence of SJK-132, reflecting the partial inhibitory effect of the MAb on the primase activity. However, when dNTPs were added to the reaction mixture in any concentration, smaller and relatively homogeneous oligomeric (~10–14 mers) primase products were synthesized, both in the presence and absence of SJK-132. These observations suggested that qualitatively different primer products were made depending on the presence or absence of dNTPs, but independent of the dNTP concentration. Additionally, these experiments demonstrated that KB primase activity was independent of the DNA polymerase-α activity.

In contrast to primase activity, the subsequent incorporation of the dNTP-dependent oligoribonucleotide primer units was dependent upon the concentration of dNTPs in the reaction mixture. In the presence of low levels (0.05 μM) of dNTPs the primers were incorporated into longer and more heterogeneous chains (~25–40 nucleotides) whether or not excess SJK-132 was present. These chains were found to be composed of tandemly alternating oligoribo- and oligodeoxynucleotide units with an average length of ~10–25 nucleotides. However, when high levels (1.2–50 μM) of dNTPs were added to the reaction mixture in the absence of SJK-132, the primer products were incorporated into long DNA sequences, while in the presence of neutralizing MAb, the primers were recovered as a heterodisperse population of oligomers similar to the reaction in the presence of low levels of dNTPs. These results clearly demonstrated that the extension of the primers into long chains was specifically due to the polymerase-α activity, and that the DNA polymerase-α was only activated in the presence of high levels of dNTPs.

In conclusion, the authors[24] proposed that KB primase is a complex enzyme with bifunctional catalytic capacity, capable of synthesizing both oligoribunucleotide and oligodeoxynucleotide products in an alternating and synchronous manner, and that the level of dNTPs regulates the transition between the two modes of catalysis as illustrated in Fig. 2. Furthermore, although both the DNA primase and DNA polymerase-α activities are closely physically linked and copurified as an immune complex recognized by a highly specific MAb, the experiments performed in the presence of excess SJK-132 clearly indicated that the tightly regulated oligodeoxynucleotide polymerase activity is operationally and perhaps structurally distinct from the conventional polymerase-α activity. Additional experiments, utilizing combinations of immunologic and biochemical techniques, will be necessary to determine which of the polypeptides recognized by the MAbs contain each of the catalytic activities, and the functional and physical interrelationships among them.

More recently, a complex of DNA polymerase-α and DNA primase was isolated from yeast by both conventional biochemical and immunologic methods.[25] The primase was physically associated with, but not part of, the 78- and 140-kD peptides of DNA polymerase-α, as shown by immunopurification of the complex with a MAb against yeast DNA polymerase-α. It was of interest that recovery of an active complex from the immunoaffinity column was Mg-dependent, suggesting a complex interaction between primase and polymerase that may involve binding through a third protein.

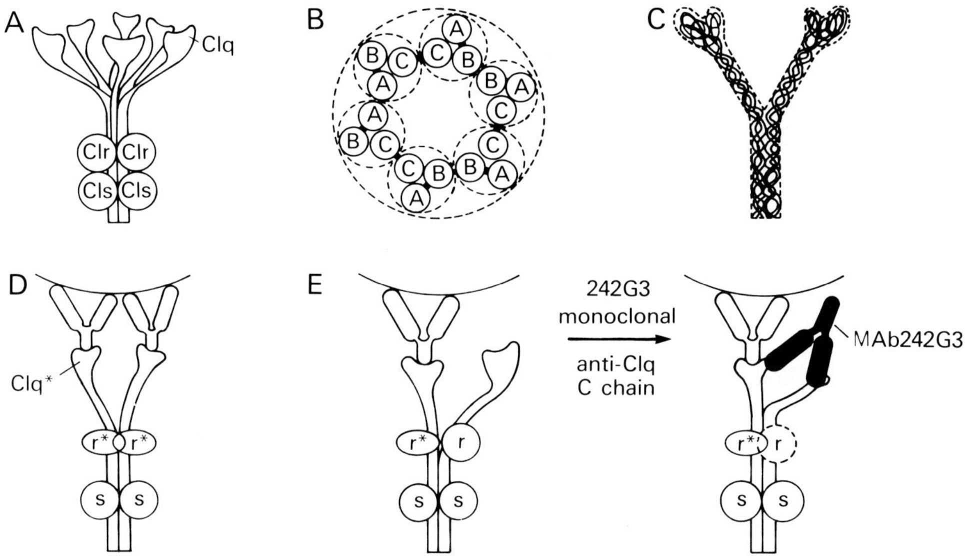

Figure 3. Structure of mammalian C1, and model for activation by cross-linking. (A) C1 complex containing one C1q, two C1r, and two C1s molecules. The C1q is often referred to as a "bouquet of tulips," with each "tulip" consisting of three polypeptide chains designated A, B, and C. (B) Cross-section through "stalk" region of the C1q bouquet showing the three polypeptide chains of each "tulip," which are cross-linked via disulfide bridges (solid, connecting lines). (C) Helical arrangement of polypeptide chains in one double "tulip." (D) Hypothetical activation of C1q* and C1r* through cross-linking via Fc binding. (E) Hypothetical mechanism for activation of C1q* by MAb 242G3 when C chains of an Fc-bound "tulip" and C chains of an adjacent, unactivated "tulip" are cross-linked by the dimeric MAb. (Parts A–C are from Ref. 26; Parts D–E are after Ref. 28.)

2.4. The First Component of Complement

Another enzyme complex whose molecular mechanism of action and activation has been difficult to study, due to the transient nature of many of the active states, is the first component of complement, C1. The C1 component includes three high-molecular-weight glycoprotein subcomponents, C1q, C1r, and C1s, which are activated to initiate the complement cascade that ultimately results in cell lysis (Figs. 3A–3C). All components of activation complex are enzymes, with the exception of C1q; C1q initiates the cascade by interaction with an Ig molecule, undergoing a conformational change, and converting to activated C1q*. The C1q* in turn activates one of the monomers of the C1r to C1r*, presumably by conformation alteration that exposes an enzyme active site that in turn cleaves the second C1r monomer to $C1\bar{r}$, which cleaves the first single-chain to C1r* to $C1\bar{r}$ as well as C1s to $C1\bar{s}$. This leads to the activated form $C\bar{1}$, which then activates further components in the cascade (discussed in Refs. 27 and 28).

The molecular mechanisms underlying the initial activation of C1q and C1r are still poorly understood. Functional analyses have indicated that activation is accompanied by conformational changes, and recent immunochemical studies utilizing the MAb directed at C1 components have provided direct evidence for such changes. A series of MAbs generated against purified human C1q were tested for reactivity with fluid phase C1q, C1q bound to immune complexes, activated C1 ($\overline{C1}$), or native serum C1.[27] The results indicated that binding of C1q to immune complexes exposes new antigenic determinants, or neoantigens, while other determinants are no longer detectable. The neoantigen recognized by one MAb could be formed either by binding of C1q or to immune complexes or by binding of C1r and C1s to the collagen part of C1q. Binding of most anti-C1q MAb to serum C1 inhibited the hemolytic function of C1, but fluid phase C1 was not inhibited, demonstrating that the MAbs were interfering with internal activation of the macromolecular C1, rather than inhibiting the esterolytic activity of C1s. One MAb, 242G3, which was specific for the C chain of C1q, inhibited the hemolytic function of fluid phase C1q and serum C1, but activated immune-complex-bound serum C1, as measured by cleavage of serum C4. In contrast, the univalent Fab fragment could no longer activate immune-complex-bound C1, but could inhibit activation of C1q.[28] It was postulated that the MAb 242G3 cross-linked two C1q stalks via the C chain, resulting in a closer approximation of the second C1r to the C1r,* thus facilitating cleavage of C1r → C1$\bar{r}$. A proposed mechanism of this facilitation is diagrammed in Figs. 3D and 3E.

3. Molecular Mechanisms of Catalysis

3.1. Introduction

Highly specific, well-characterized MAbs provide tools for probing molecular mechanisms underlying enzyme catalysis. To date only a few systems have been thus analyzed in detail. One category of enzymes whose catalytic mechanisms have been probed with MAbs are those whose activation and/or inactivation involve conformational changes, such as *E. coli* β-galactosidase or calmodulin; these enzymes and their study with MAbs have recently been reviewed elsewhere.[29] I discuss below the interaction of avian lysozyme with its oligosaccharide substrates as studied with MAbs specific for various subregions of the lysozyme catalytic site.

3.2. Substrate Binding by Lysozyme

Avian lysozyme (EC 3.2.1.17) has long served as a model protein in antigenic studies (reviewed in Ref. 6), and recently its antigenic structure has been investigated with MAbs.[2,30,31] It is a relatively small protein (molecular weight 14,300), particularly well suited for structural and functional studies, whose three-dimensional structure has been determined[32,33] to include three distinct structural domains (Fig. 4A) (discussed in Ref. 31). These structural domains have been shown to correspond to antigenic regions operationally defined by overlapping specificities of MAbs; structural domains can essentially interact independently with MAbs[31] (Figs. 4A and 4B).

The enzyme cleaves oligomers of β-D-N-acetylglucosamine, and activity is generally measured by the lysis of *Micrococcus lysodeikticus* cells. The active site is a deep cleft between two domains, bordered by a β-sheet in domain II on the left side, and a helical structure extending from residue 101 to 114 of domain III on the right side (Figs. 4A–4C). The catalytic site interacts with six saccharide units, and the amino acids making contact with the sugar in each position have been designated by a letter in order from A (at residue 101) to F at the reducing end[32,33] (Figs. 4C and 4D). Cleavage of the hexasaccharide is between sites D and E[34,35] (Fig. 4D).

X-ray diffraction analysis allowed placement of sugar residues A–D in the catalytic cleft, but the crystal packing did not accommodate the full hexasaccharide substrate.[32,33] Furthermore, in the crystal model, saccharide units A–C could be placed in the cleft in chair positions, but the D unit required distortion to a high-energy "half-chair" conformation,[32,33] a distortion that has been proposed to make a major contribution to catalysis.[34,35] Model-building studies incorporated the distorted ring at site D, and placed the six-saccharide substrate with positions E and F on the right side of the cleft contacting Arg-114 in site F[32,33] (Fig. 4D, right). However, energy minimization studies predicted a preferred, lower energy binding site on the other (left) side of the cleft formed by the β-sheet of domain II, including residues 45–47[36] (Figs. 4C and 4D, left).

Recently antilysozyme MAbs with defined specificities were used in combination with biochemical techniques to examine experimentally the initial binding mode of the hexasaccharide to lysozyme, particularly residues involved in sites E and F, which could not be directly observed in crystal studies.[37] The MAbs HyHEL-5 and HyHEL-9 each recognize a different structural domain (domains II and III, respectively), and they can bind the antigen simultaneously.[31] HyHEL-5 recognizes an epitope including Arg-45, Asn-46, Thr-47, Asp-48, and Arg-68,[30] all on the left side of the cleft. HyHEL-9 recognizes an epitope that includes Asn-113/Arg-114,[31] on the right side of the cleft. Thus, each interacts with a different side of the F site in the catalytic cleft in nonoverlapping manner (Figs. 4A–4C).

The MAb HyHEL-5 efficiently inhibited lysis of *M. lysodeikticus*, was competitively displaced by the dye Biebrich scarlett, which interacts exclusively with the F site, but was not competitively displaced by either the monosaccharide N-acetylglucosamine or the disaccharide substrate.[30] These results suggested that the MAb was interacting with the F site of the catalytic cleft. At low temperatures (-20°C) (where no catalysis occurs, but binding is actually stronger) HyHEL-5 was competitively displaced by the penta- and hexasaccharide substrates, but not by the tetrasaccharide.[37] These results confirmed that HyHEL-5 was interacting with the E and/or F sites; since HyHEL-5 was

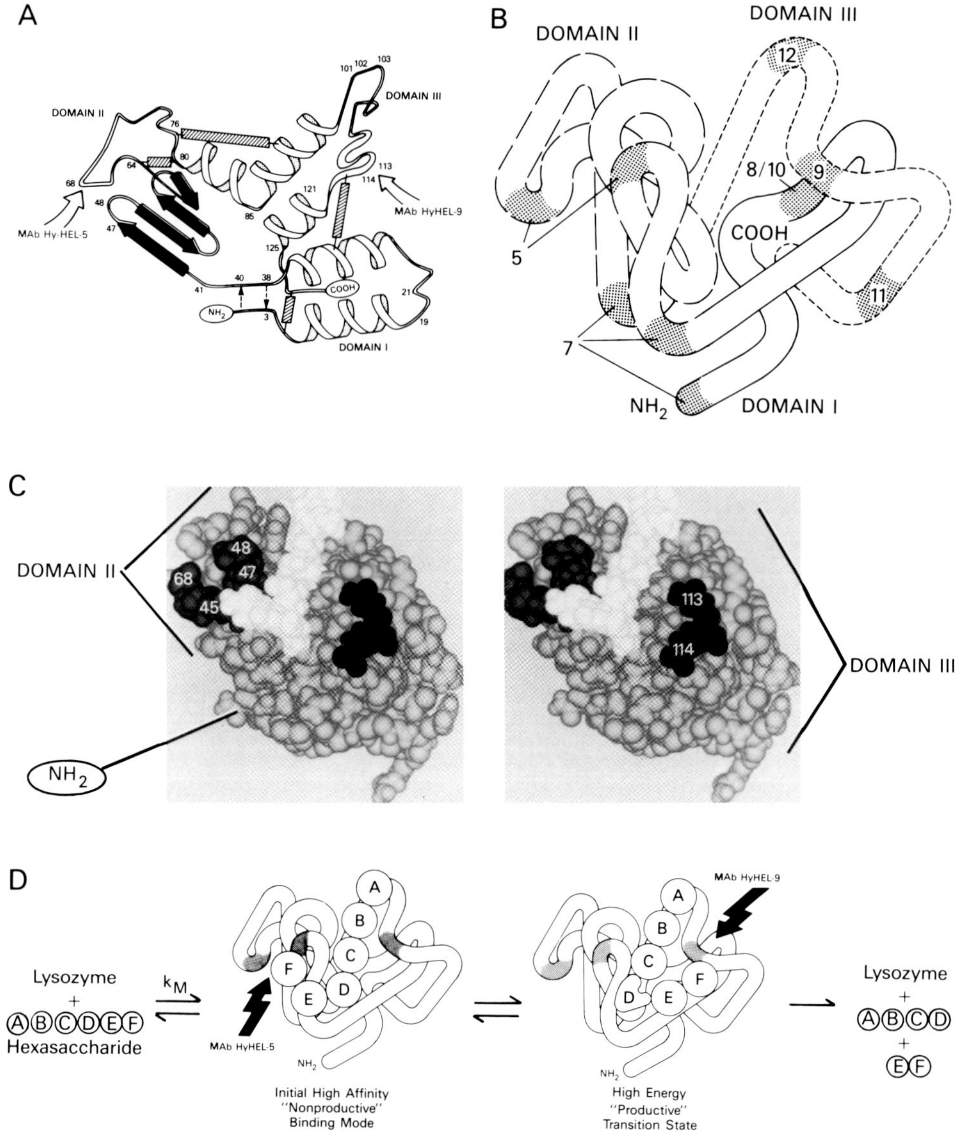

Figure 4. Antigenic and catalytic structures of avian lysozyme. (A) Diagrammatic representation of tertiary structure of lysozyme, showing topographic relationships of the three structural domains. Positions of residues recognized by characterized MAbs are numbered, and location of HyHEL-5 and -9 epitopes are indicated. (Adapted from Ref. 31.) (B) Secondary structure of lysozyme, showing positions of residues recognized by seven MAbs on structural domains. (C) Stereo view of space-filling model of lysozyme facing toward the catalytic cleft at approximately the same orientation as diagrammatic representations in (A) and (B). Numbered residues in left panel indicate the location of HyHEL-5 epitope on domain II; numbered residues in right panel are part of the HyHEL-9 epitope on domain III. White molecule represents $(GlcNac)_6$ in predicted energy-minimized, left-sided binding mode. (Adapted from Ref. 37 by permission). (D) Model for initial binding and cleavage of $(GlcNac)_6$, showing interaction of substrate with MAbs HyHEL-5 and -9.

known to recognize residues on the left side of the cleft and *not* to recognize residues on the right side of the cleft,[30,31] these results further confirmed that the penta- and hexasaccharides were binding in the "left"-sided mode predicted by theoretical studies[36] (Fig. 4C).

Parallel biochemical studies examined steady-state kinetics of binding of the hexasaccharide substrate to chicken lysozyme and to ring-necked pheasant lysozyme, which has substitutions of Asn-113 → Lys and Arg-114 → His. The K_M values of these two enzymes did not differ significantly, while the K_{cat} of the pheasant lysozyme was about three times lower than that of chicken lysozyme. These results indicated that right-sided binding was *not* involved in the formation of the equilibrium complex, but may contribute to catalysis.[37] Furthermore, the pentasaccharide and hexasaccharide substrates can competitively displace HyHEL-9 binding,[31] indicating that right-sided binding *can* also occur.

Extensive previous studies based on the cleavage patterns, kinetics, and thermodynamics of interactions of various substrates with lysozyme had predicted two modes of binding, an initial ("nonproductive") complex in which cleavage does not occur, and which is the primary contributor to equilibrium properties, and a second ("productive") binding mode in which D-ring distortion and cleavage are thought to occur, but which is weak and does not contribute to the equilibrium properties.[35,38] Previously, the initial binding step was thought to involve only sugars A–C. However, the kinetic and immunochemical studies discussed above suggest that the initial binding mode consists of the left-sided binding of all six sugars, while the "productive" mode would involve interaction with the right-sided residues and an associated "transition state" distortion of the D ring (Fig. 4D).

It is interesting that MAbs that recognize epitopes not directly associated with the catalytic cleft can efficiently inhibit lysis of *M. lysodeikticus*, including MAbs HyHEL-8 and -10, whose epitopes are on domain I, which is totally independent of the catalytic site[31] (Fig. 4B). The inhibition could reflect steric hindrance of the large bacterial cells used as substrate, or, alternatively, antibody-induced conformational alterations of lysozyme. These results are reminiscent of those with neuraminidase, where the majority of MAbs inhibited catalysis of a large but not a small substrate, and point out that effects of MAbs on catalysis must be interpreted with caution. Understanding the mode of inhibition of these antilysozyme antibodies will require kinetic studies with the smaller saccharide substrates.

4. Conclusions

The studies reviewed above demonstrate a number of very different applications of MAbs as direct probes of catalytic function and/or active site structure. In each study, the conclusions reached would not have been possible without the exquisitely specific and sensitive MAb probes. The application of MAb analysis of enzyme active sites has only begun, and the potentials of this powerful technology as a tool for enzymology are apparent from the studies performed to date.

References

1. Harris, H., 1983, Applications of monoclonal antibodies in enzyme genetics, *Annu. Rev. Genet.* **17**:279–314.
2. Benjamin, D. C., Berzofsy, J. A., East, I. J., Gurd, F. R. N., Hannum, C., Leach, S. J., Margoliash, E., Michael, J. G., Miller, A., Prager, E. M., Reichlin, M., Sercarz, E. E., Smith-Gill, S. J., Todd, P. E., and Wilson, A. C., 1984, The antigenic structure of proteins: A reappraisal, *Annu. Rev. Immunol.* **2**:67–101.
3. Webster, R. G., Brown, L. E., and Laver, W. G., 1984, Antigenic and biological characterization of influenza virus neuraminidase (N2) with monoclonal antibodies, *Virology* **135**:30–42.
4. Frackelton, A. R., Jr., and Rotman, B., 1980, Functional diversity of antibodies elicited by bacterial β-D-galactosidase, *J. Immunol.* **255**:5286–5290.
5. Solomon, B., Moav, N., Pines, G., and Katchalski-Katzir, E., 1984, Interaction of carboxypeptidase A with monoclonal antibodies, *Mol. Immunol.* **21**:1–11.
6. Arnon, R., 1977, Immunochemistry of lysozyme, in: *Immunochemistry of Enzymes and Their Antibodies* (M. R. J. Salton, ed.), Wiley, New York, pp. 1–28.
7. Carroll, S. B., and Stollar, B. D., 1983, Conservation of a DNA-binding site in the largest subunit of eukaryotic RNA polymerase II, *J. Mol. Biol.* **170**:777–790.
8. Colman, P. M., Varghese, J. N., and Laver, W. G., 1983, Structure of the catalytic and antigenic sites in influenza virus neuraminidase, *Nature* **303**:41–44.
9. Varghese, J. N., Laver, W. G., and Colman, P. M., 1983, Structure of the influenza virus glycoprotein antigen neuraminidase at 2.9 Å resolution, *Nature* **303**:35–40.
10. Laver, W. G., Colman, P. M., Ward, C. W., Varghese, J. M., Air, G. M., Webster, R. G., Hinshaw, V., Brown, L., and Jackson, D., 1984, Influenza virus neuraminidase: Structure and variation, in: *The Molecular Virology and Epidemiology of Influenza* (C. Stuart-Harris and C. W. Potter, eds.), Academic Press, New York, pp. 77–91.
11. Jackson, D. C., and Webster, R. G., 1982, A topographic map of the enzyme active center and antigenic sites on the neuraminidase of influenza virus A/Tokyo/3/67 (H2N2), *Virology* **123**:69–77.
12. Webster, R. G., Hinshaw, V. S., and Laver, W. G., 1982, Selection and analysis of antigenic variants of the neuraminidase of N2 influenza viruses with monoclonal antibodies, *Virology* **117**:93–104.
13. Laver, W. G., Air, G. M., Webster, R. G., and Markoff, L. J., 1982, Amino acid sequence changes in antigenic variants of type A influenza virus N2 neuraminidase, *Virology* **122**:450–460.
14. Lentz, M. R., Air, G. M., Laver, W. G., and Webster, R. G., 1984, Sequence of the neuraminidase gene of influenza virus A/Tokyo/3/67 and previously uncharacterized monoclonal variants, *Virology* **135**:257–265.
15. Lewis, M. K., and Burgess, R. R., 1982, Eukaryotic RNA polymerases, in: *The Enzymes*, Volume 15 (P. D. Boyer, ed.) Academic Press, New York, pp. 109–153.
16. Rose, K. M., Maguire, K. A., Wurpel, J. N. D., Stetler, D. A., and Marquez, E. D., 1983, Monoclonal antibodies directed against mammalian RNA polymerase I. Identification of the catalytic center, *J. Biol. Chem.* **258**:12976–12981.
17. Gowda, S., and Sridhara, S., 1983, Monoclonal antibody to RNA polymerase I of the silkworm, *J. Biol. Chem.* **258**:14532–14538.
18. Carroll, S. B., and Stollar, B. D., 1982, Inhibitory monoclonal antibody to calf thymus RNA polymerase II blocks formation of enzyme–DNA complexes, *Proc. Natl. Acad. Sci. USA* **79**:7233–7237.
19. Dahmus, M. E., and Kedinger, C., 1983, Transcription of adenovirus-2 major late promoter inhibited by monoclonal antibody directed against RNA polymerases II_0 and II_A, *J. Biol. Chem.* **258**:2303–2307.

20. Christmann, J. L., and Dahmus, M. E., 1981, Monoclonal antibody specific for calf thymus RNA polymerases II_0 and II_A, *J. Biol. Chem.* **256:**11798–11803.
21. Weissbach, A., 1982, Cellular and viral-induced eukaryotic polymerases, in: *The Enzymes*, Volume 14 (P. D. Boyer, ed.), Academic Press, New York, pp. 67–86.
22. Wang, T. S.-F., Hu, S.-Z., Korn, D., 1984, DNA primase from KB cells. Characterization of a primase activity tightly associated with immunoaffinity-purified DNA polymerase-α, *J. Biol Chem.* **259:**1854–1865.
23. Tanaka, S., Hu, S.-Z., Wang, T. S.-F., and Korn, D., 1982, Preparation and preliminary characterization of monoclonal antibodies against human DNA polymerase-α, *J. Biol. Chem.* **257:**8386–8390.
24. Hu, S.-Z., Wang, T. S.-F., and Korn, D., 1984, DNA primase from KB cells. Evidence for a novel model of primase catalysis by a highly purified primase/polymerase-α complex, *J. Biol. Chem.* **259:**2602–2609.
25. Plevani, P., Badaracco, G., Augl, C., and Chang, L. M. S., 1984, DNA polymerase I and DNA primase complex in yeast, *J. Biol. Chem.* **259:**7532–7539.
26. Klein, J., 1982, *Immunology. The Science of Self–Nonself Discrimination*, Wiley, New York.
27. Golan, M. D., Burger, R., and Loos, M., 1982, Conformational changes in C1q after binding to immune complexes: Detection of neoantigens with monoclonal antibodies, *J. Immunol.* **129:**445–447.
28. Heinz, H.-P., Burger, R., Golan, M. D., and Loos, M., 1984, Activation of the first component of complement, C1, by a monoclonal antibody recognizing the C chain of C1q, *J. Immunol.* **132:**804–808.
29. Celada, F., and Rotman, B., 1984, Monoclonal antibodies in enzymology, in: *Handbook of Monoclonal Antibodies. Applications in Biology and Medicine* (S. Ferrone and M. P. Dierich, eds.), Noyes Publications, New Jersey (in press).
30. Smith-Gill, S. J., Wilson, A. C., Potter, M., Feldmann, R. J., and Mainhart, C. R., 1982, Mapping the antigenic epitope for a monoclonal antibody against avian lysozyme, *J. Immunol.* **128:**314–322.
31. Smith-Gill, S. J., Lavoie, T. B., and Mainhart, C., 1984, Antigenic regions defined by monoclonal antibodies correspond to structural domains of avian lysozyme, *J. Immunol.* **133:**384–393.
32. Blake, C. C. F., Johnson, L. N., Mair, G. A., North, T. A., Phillips, D. C., and Sarma, V. R., 1967, Crystallographic studies of the activity of hen egg white lysozyme, *Proc. R. Soc. Lond. B* **167:**378–388.
33. Phillips, D. C., 1974, Crystallographic studies of lysozyme and its interactions with inhibitors and substrates, in: *Lysozyme* (E. F. Osserman, R. E. Canfield, and S. Beychok, eds.), Academic Press, New York, pp. 9–30.
34. Rupley, J. A., 1967, The binding and cleavage by lysozyme of *N*-acetylglucosamine oligosaccharides, *Proc. R. Soc. Lond. B* **167:**416–428.
35. Rupley, J. A., and Gates, V., 1967, Studies on the enzymic activity of lysozyme II. The hydrolysis and transfer reactions of *N*-acetylglucosamine oligosaccharides, *Proc. Natl. Acad. Sci. USA* **57:**496–510.
36. Pincus, M. R., and Sheraga, H. A., 1979, Conformation energy calculations of enzyme–substrate and enzyme–inhibitor complexes of lysozyme. 2. Calculation of the structures of complexes with a flexible enzyme, *Macromolecules* **12:**633–644.
37. Smith-Gill, S. J., Rupley, J. A., Pincus, M. R., Carty, R. P., and Sheraga, H. A., 1984, Experimental identification of a theoretically predicted "left-sided" binding mode for $(GlcNac)_6$ in the active site of lysozyme, *Biochemistry* **23:**993–997.
38. Holler, E., Rupley, J. A., and Hess, G. P., 1975, Productive and unproductive lysozyme chitosaccharide complexes. Equilibrium measurements, *Biochemistry* **14:**1088–1094.

Chapter 19

Studies of the Hong Kong Influenza Hemagglutinin

JOHN J. SKEHEL and DONALD C. WILEY

1. Introduction

An influenza virus consists of a transcriptase complex surrounded by a lipid membrane. Each complex contains eight RNA molecules, which make up the virus genome in association with polypeptides of five different types, members of at least three of which participate in transcriptase activity. The virus membrane is derived from the surface membrane of the infected cells, from which the assembled virus is released by a process of membrane budding. During infection, this membrane is modified to contain two types of virus-specified glycoproteins, the hemagglutinins (about 500–1000 per virus) and the neuraminidase molecules (about 100–500 per virus). The more abundant hemagglutinin is the glycoprotein that interacts with infectivity-neutralizing antibodies.[1] Because of the hemagglutinin's consequent importance in antigenic variation, its structure and antigenicity have been analyzed in detail. In this chapter, we will describe a number of the applications of antihemagglutinin monoclonal antibodies in these studies. We will concentrate on the hemagglutinins of viruses of the H3 antigenic subtype, the Hong Kong influenza viruses, primarily because detailed information on the three-dimensional structure of a hemagglutinin is at present only available for the hemagglutinin of the 1968 Hong Kong virus.

2. The X-31 Hong Kong Hemagglutinin

X-31 virus is a reassortant, produced for use as a high-yielding vaccine strain,[2] which contains the hemagglutinin of a 1968 prototype virus, A/Aichi/2/68. The hemagglutinin of X-31 is a 220,000-dalton trimer of identical subunits, each made up of two disulfide-linked glycopolypeptide chains, HA1 and HA2. HA1 contains 328 amino acids and six asparagine-linked carbohydrate

JOHN J. SKEHEL • National Institute for Medical Research, London NW7 1AA, England. DONALD C. WILEY • Department of Biochemistry and Molecular Biology, Harvard University, Cambridge, Massachusetts 02138.

side chains, and HA2 contains 221 amino acids and a single carbohydrate side chain.[3] The molecule is associated with the virus membrane through a region of uncharged amino acids (residues HA2 185–210) near the COOH terminus of each HA2 glycopolypeptide and can be released from this association by detergent extraction or proteolytic digestion. Digestion with the protease bromelain at a single site, HA2 residue 175, releases the soluble trimer BHA (bromelain-released hemagglutinin), crystals of which have been used to solve the structure of the molecule. X-ray crystallographic analyses indicate that the amino terminus of HA1 as well as the carboxyl terminus of HA2 is near the membrane of the virus (Fig. 1). The HA1 chain extends from this position through a fibrous region into a peripheral β-structure-rich region and then returns to terminate about 30 Å from the virus membrane. The most prominent features of the part of the subunit composed of HA2 residues are two antiparallel α-helices, one 29 Å long, which proceeds distally from the membrane end of the molecule to connect through an extended chain with the other helix, the major component of the central fibrous stem of the molecule, which stretches 76 Å back toward the membrane.[4]

Hemagglutinins have two functions in virus infection; they bind virus particles to sialic acid-containing receptors, and following endocytosis, they appear to mediate fusion between virus and endosomal membranes, which results in transfer of the genome transcriptase complex into the cytoplasm and initiation of virus replication. Probably as a consequence of inhibiting these functions, antibodies neutralize virus infectivity and impose selection pressures that lead to the emergence of antigenic variants. In the Hong Kong viruses following the initial pandemic of 1968, pandemics occurred in 1972 and 1975 and more limited epidemics in 1977 and 1979. On each occasion, the viruses responsible were antigenically distinct from previous isolates and consequently were able to infect individuals in what had become a nonimmune population. Routinely in influenza surveillance studies of such epidemics, antigenic differences between viruses are detected in hemagglutination inhibition tests using postinfection ferret antisera. Antihemagglutinin monoclonal antibodies have also been used in similar tests.[5] Table I demonstrates that monoclonal antibodies can distinguish between early Hong Kong viruses which react similarly with reference antisera. As yet, however, because of the effort required to define the specificities of the antibodies, because of the difficulty in assessing the epidemiologic significance of the observed antigenic differences, and because new preparations of antibodies are frequently required to discriminate between collections of viruses isolated in different years, antihemagglutinin monoclonal antibodies have not been used extensively for the routine identification of influenza isolates.

3. Antibody Binding Sites

The majority of experiments with monoclonal antibodies against hemagglutinins have been concerned with defining the regions of the molecule to

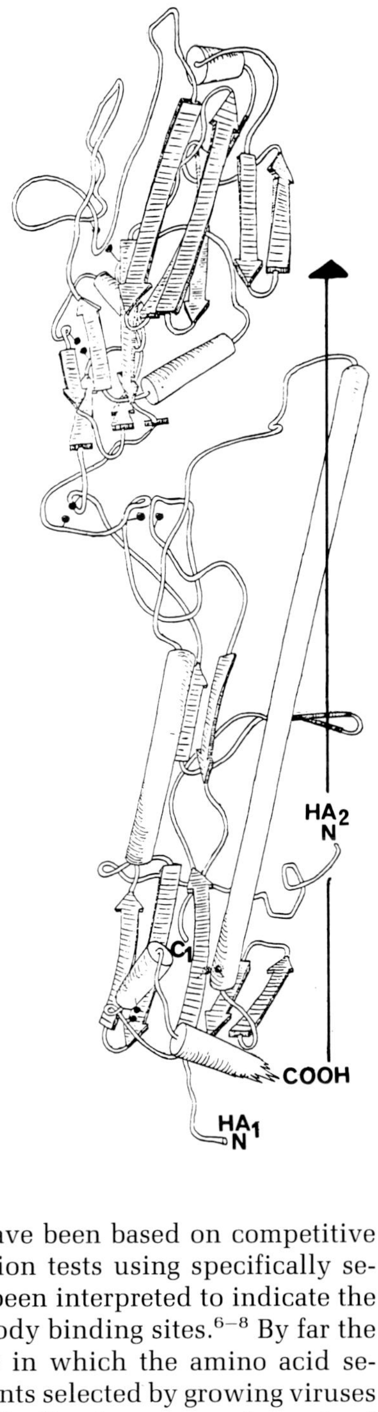

Figure 1. Drawing of the three-dimensional structure of the influenza virus HA. The terminal residues of HA1 and HA2 are labeled. The threefold symmetry axis relating monomers in the trimer is shown. α-Helices and β-pleated sheets are represented by cylinders and arrows, respectively. Lollipops represent disulfide bonds.

which antibodies bind. A number of studies have been based on competitive binding, or ELISA or hemagglutination inhibition tests using specifically selected antigenic variants as antigens, and have been interpreted to indicate the existence of three or four nonoverlapping antibody binding sites.[6–8] By far the most informative, however, have been studies in which the amino acid sequences of the hemagglutinins of antigenic variants selected by growing viruses in the presence of individual monoclonal antibodies have been determined and compared with the wild-type hemagglutinin sequence. Such studies have

Table I. Inhibitory Titers of Anti-HA Monoclonal Antibodies[a]

Virus \ MAb	3(144)	19(157)	21(198)	67(156 + 193)	68(193)	73(134 + 145)	100(63)	126(189)	159(14)
A/HK/1/68	6400	6400	6400	6400	6400	6400	3200	6400	6400
A/England/878/69	<	6400	6400	3200	6400	<	<	6400	<
A/Hong Kong/107/71	<	1600	<	<	<	<	<	200	<
A/England/42/72	<	<	6400	1600	6400	<	<	6400	<
A/Hong Kong/15/72	<	<	<	<	<	<	3200	<	<
A/P.Chalmers/1/73	<	1600	<	<	<	<	<	<	<
A/Scotland/840/74	<	<	<	<	<	<	<	<	<

[a] Monoclonal antibodies were produced as follows. BALB/c mice were immunized by intraperitoneal injection of 8000 HA units of purified virus. Eight weeks later, they received 32,000 HA units of virus intraperitoneally and intravenously. Three days later their spleens were removed and the cells fused with SP2/0-Ag14 myeloma cells[33] as described by Köhler and Milstein.[34,35] Hybrid cell culture conditions were based on those described by Fazekas de St. Groth and Scheidegger.[36] The specificity of the antibodies is given in parentheses by the position of the amino acids substituted in the variant hemagglutinins that they select, and appears after the monoclonal clone number. Thus, for example, 3(144) indicates that antibodies from clone 3 recognize amino acid 144. Influenza virus-induced agglutination of erythrocytes is inhibited by antisera that react with the HA molecule. The inhibition of influenza hemagglutination by monoclonal and polyclonal sera were measured by standard procedures and the results are presented as the reciprocals of the highest dilutions of the antibodies at which hemagglutination was inhibited. The symbol < signifies <100.

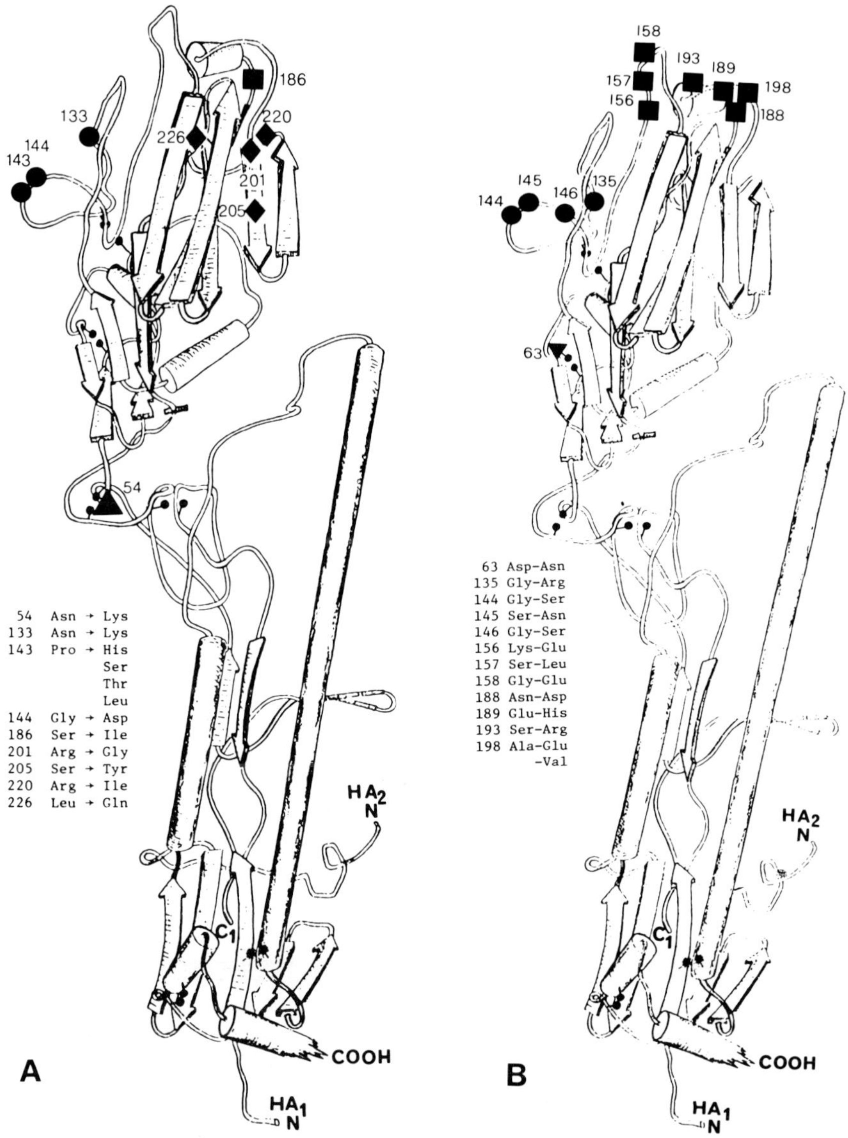

Figure 2. Schematic drawing of a monomer of the A/Aichi/2/68 hemagglutinin showing the location of laboratory-selected antigenic variants from growth in monoclonal sera. α-Helices, β-pleated sheets, and disulfides are depicted as described in the legend to Fig. 1. The proposed antigenic regions A–E are denoted as follows: (●) A, (■) B, (▲) C, (◆) D, (▼) E. Each symbol represents a single amino acid substitution that is sufficient for the virus to escape neutralization by one of the monoclonal antibodies used to select the variants. (A) Variants selected from the MEM/102/72 H3 strain. (B) Variants selected from the X-31 A/Aichi/2/68 strain.

yielded the information shown in Fig. 2.[9–15] There appear to be five regions of the distal HA1 globular domains of early Hong Kong virus hemagglutinins in which amino acid substitutions prohibit the binding of defined antibodies[16] (Fig. 2). The majority of antibodies that have been analyzed recognize amino acids in one of three regions: a prominently protruding loop between amino acids HA1 140 and 147 and amino acids in that vicinity, (site A); a loop and short α-helix, residues HA1 156–159 and 186–199, which form the distal tip of the molecule (site B), and the interface between HA1 domains, e.g., residues HA1 201, 205, 220, (site D)[7] (also A. R. Douglas, M. L. Wang, J. J. Skehel and D. C. Wiley, unpublished results). In addition, antigenic variants have been obtained with amino acid substitutions at HA1 63 (site E)[15] and HA1 54 (site C),[9] which define two other regions of antigenicity (Fig. 2). The nature of the amino acid substitutions in all five regions is listed in Fig. 2. Changes in amino acid side-chain charge and size are observed in different mutants, the majority of which (43 out of 45 in our studies) contain single amino acid substitutions. In the case of substitutions at HA1 residue 63 a number of mutants contain asparagine instead of aspartic acid in the sequence Asn-Cys-Thr and as a consequence the asparagine residue is glycosylated. It has been shown by binding antibodies to the nonglycosylated variant hemagglutinin produced in cells incubated in the presence of tunicamycin that glycosylation is required to prevent antibody binding. Modulation of antigenicity by glycosylation in this way also occurs in a number of antigenically distinct Hong Kong viruses (see below) and may be a factor in determining differences in the antigenic importance of structurally equivalent regions of the hemagglutinins of different antigenic subtypes.[15–17]

In general, the contributions of particular amino acid substitutions to the mechanism of antigenic change are not known. In this last case, direct hindrance of antibody binding as a result of the addition of a bulky carbohydrate side chain seems most likely. In others, the introduction of a charged residue, for example, in the site of antibody binding, may make the antibody–hemagglutinin complex unstable or may allow additional contacts with other residues in the vicinity that render the site less favorable for antibody binding. In most studies, it has certainly been assumed that the sites of amino acid substitutions indicate the sites of antibody binding, although there is strong evidence to support the assumption in only one case.[18] This concerns an antigenic mutant in which glycine-146 of HA1 is substituted by an aspartic acid. The three-dimensional structure of the mutant hemagglutinin has been determined and compared with that of the wild-type hemagglutinin to show that the addition of the aspartic acid side chain and minor displacement of neighboring HA1 arginine-141 are the only detectable structural modifications (Fig. 3). These results clearly show that the binding site of wild-type hemagglutinin for this antibody includes residue 146. They do not precisely indicate which structural feature is responsible for the decreased affinity of the antibody for the mutant hemagglutinin, since this may be influenced simply by the charged nature of the substituted amino acid or by the formation of the salt bridge with HA1 arginine-141, which may stabilize the conformation of this exposed loop and

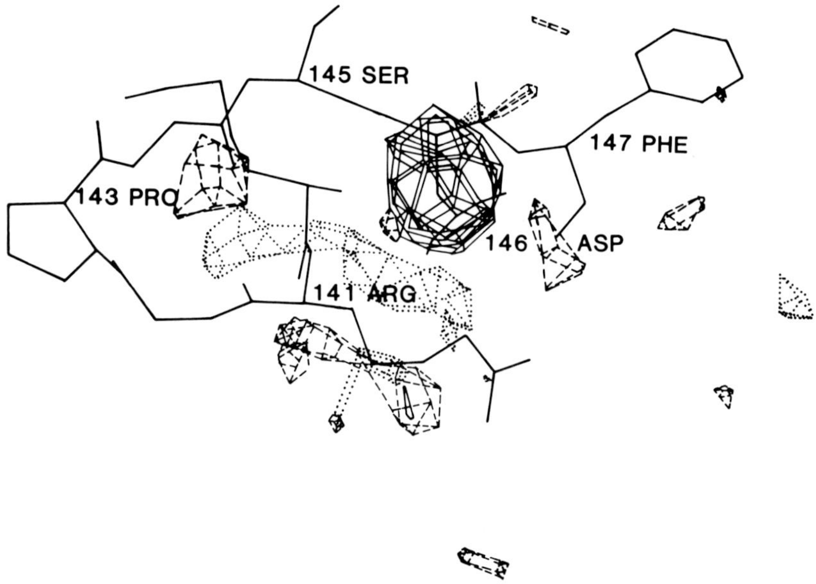

Figure 3. A difference electron density map calculated from the Gly to Asp 146 antigenic variant, showing a large peak at amino acid 146, the only significant difference between the variant and wild-type HA (polyhedron with solid lines at position 146). Less significant peaks (dashed and dotted lines) indicate a slight (<1 Å) movement of the side chain of Arg-141, presumably to allow hydrogen bonding to the Asp-146 side chain. No other significant changes are seen in the remainder of the molecule. Thus the monoclonal antibody used to select this antigenic variant must bind at this location on the HA structure.[18]

may as a consequence modify the overall structure recognized in the wild-type molecule by the antibody.

Less definitive but consistent evidence that amino acid substitutions in antibody-selected antigenic variant hemagglutinins are located in the sites of antibody binding has been obtained by electron microscopy of antibody–hemagglutinin complexes.[19] Monoclonal antibodies recognizing residues 63 (site E), 144 (site A), 157 (site B), and 198 of HA1 have been examined in this way (Fig. 4), which are representative of three of the five regions shown in Fig. 2. Concerning the other two sites, C and D, little is known. Site C is defined by an antibody that recognizes HA1 54, which, like the residues recognized by antibodies at sites A, B, and E, is on the surface of the molecule. Some of the substitutions in site D, however, are in the interface between subunits of the trimer and whether these residues form part of an antibody binding site or influence antibody binding to a separate position on the molecular surface is not known.

4. Antigenic Variation

An important application of this information on the locations of antibody binding sites is in the assessment of the antigenic significance of changes in

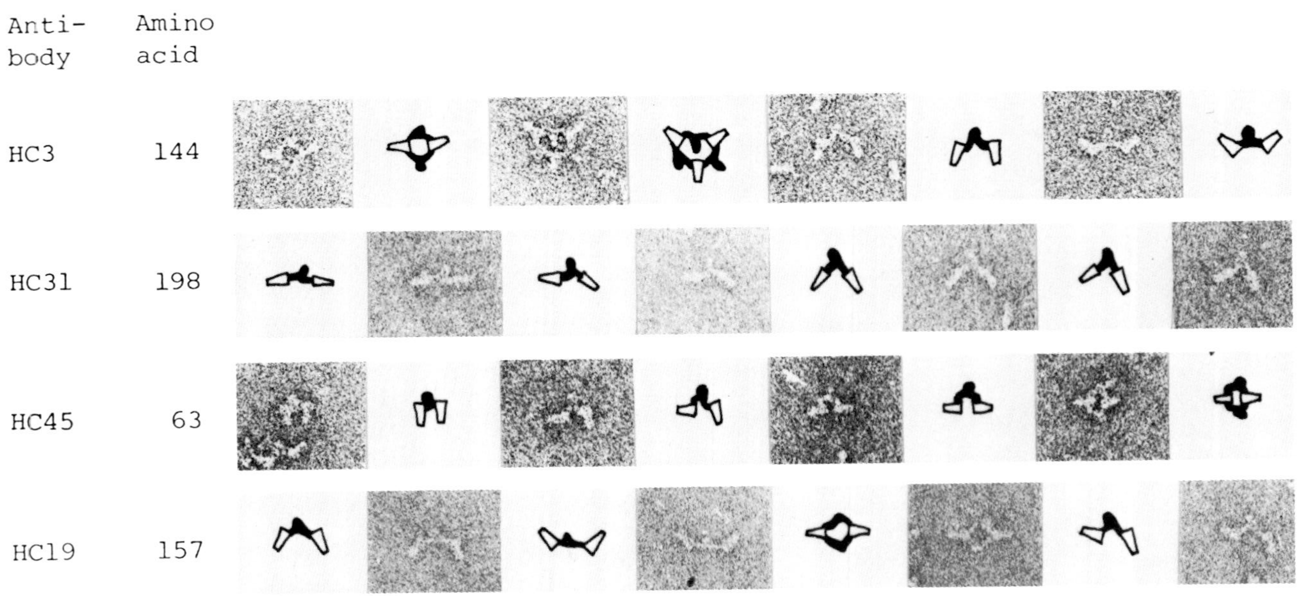

Figure 4. Complexes of BHA (bromelain-released hemagglutinin) with (from top to bottom in rows) antibodies 3(144), 31(198), 45(63), and 19(157) from Table I. BHA was diluted in PBS (pH 7.2) to 50 μg/ml for optimum spreading on carbon support films. Antibody was added until only a few molecules remained unbound to BHA after 5 min. Complexes were adsorbed to thin carbon films, floated on a 1% w/v solution of sodium silicotungstate (pH 7.0), and air-dried. Magnification ×200,000. To aid interpretation, sketches of the sample complexes shown are included. In the sketches the two-armed dark objects represent IgG molecules, and the elongated open structures represent hemagglutinin trimers, which are widest at the top (Fig. 1) of the molecule. The expected location of binding (from Fig. 2) compares well with that observed in these micrographs.

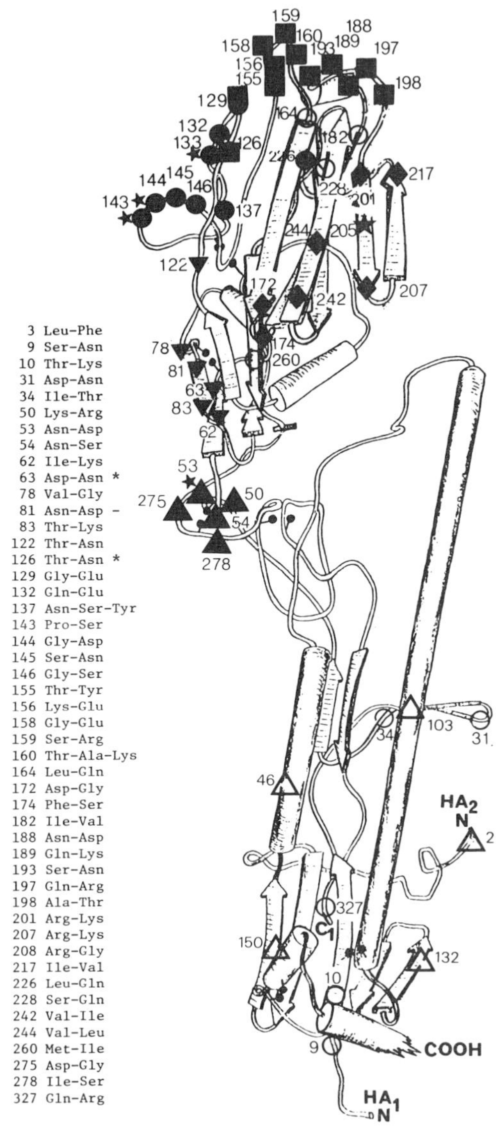

Figure 5. Natural sequence variation of the 1968 hemagglutinin observed between 1968 and 1979. Proposed antigenic regions A–E (see text) are denoted as follows: (●) A, (■) B, (▲) C, (◆) D, (▼) E. Stars denote MAb variants. Open symbols mark changes that appear stereochemically unimportant. In the list of amino acid substitutions, asterisks denote new potential N-glycosylation sites.

amino acid sequence that occur in the hemagglutinins of viruses isolated from epidemics of influenza. As noted above, a number of distinct epidemics caused by viruses of the Hong Kong (H3) subtype have been recorded since 1968 and the hemagglutinins of the antigenic variants isolated at the time have been sequenced.[20–23] The molecular locations of the amino acid differences detected in the hemagglutinins of viruses isolated between 1969 and 1983 are shown in Fig. 5. They are almost exclusively found in the distal HA1 region of the molecule and because of this and the correspondence of their locations with those of the substitutions found in monoclonal antibody-selected variants, the majority probably contribute to the differences in antigenicity detected among the viruses. For some substitutions, such as those at 63, 143–145, 156, 158, 188, and 198, which correspond in both location and in the nature of the amino acid involved to those in monoclonal antibody-selected variant hemagglutinins, this conclusion is firmly based. Among these is the asparagine substitution at position 63, which leads to the addition of a carbohydrate side chain, and it may be noted that the amino acid sequence changes at HA1 124, 126, and 248 in epidemic viruses also introduce potential sites for glycosylation.

5. Analysis of Hemagglutinin Functions

5.1. The Antigenic Properties of Hemagglutinins with Different Receptor-Binding Specificities

In a study to determine the location of the receptor binding site by which the hemagglutinin binds the virus to sialic acid-containing receptors on target cells, mutant viruses with altered receptor specificity were isolated.[28] Sequence analysis revealed that single amino acid substitutions at position HA1 226 were responsible for altering receptor specificity from oligosaccharides with α2–6-linked sialic acid to those with α2–3-linked sialic acid. Recently, some of the monoclonal antibodies binding to defined sites have been found to distinguish between HA molecules with different receptor binding specificity.[27] Whereas the majority of antihemagglutinin monoclonal antibodies react equally well with the hemagglutinins of both receptor-binding specificities, a number that specifically recognize residues 193, 199, 219, and 229 of HA1 of the α2–6 linkage-binding mutant fail to recognize the α2–3 linkage-binding hemagglutinins. Amino acids 193, 219, and 229 are close to the sialic acid-binding pocket and residue 226. Binding by antibodies to sites that include these residues therefore could be directly modified by changes in the receptor binding pocket. Amino acid 199 is over 12 Å away from 226, but a clear path by which it could affect the binding of an antibody near 226 is apparent on the HA molecular model.[27]

It has been known for some time (e.g., Ref. 24) that influenza virus isolates, when passaged in cells of different species, may yield viruses with antigenically distinguishable hemagglutinins. Recently, antihemagglutinin monoclonal antibodies have been used to study this phenomenon.[25,26] The location of some of the antigenic changes indicates that the antigenically distinct HAs selected by growth of virus on different types of cells have alterations in the vicinity of their sialic acid receptor binding sites, suggesting that antigenic selection can derive from different cell receptors in the absence of immune pressure.

5.2. The Antigenicity of Hemagglutinin at the pH Optimum of Virus-Mediated Membrane Fusion

The initial events in infection by influenza viruses involve binding of virus to sialic acid receptors, endocytosis, and fusion of the membranes of virus and endosome. *In vitro*, membrane fusion mediated by influenza viruses is maximal at about pH 5.0, a pH close to that in endosomes, and at this pH the conformation of hemagglutinin differs from that at neutrality. The changes in conformation have been analyzed by circular dichroism, sedimentation, electron microscopy, and proteolytic susceptibility studies[23] and monoclonal antibodies have also been used to obtain information on low-pH-induced modification of antigenicity[12] and immunogenicity.[29] The results obtained indicate that the structures of antigenic sites A, C, and E (Fig. 2) are maintained on acidification to pH 5, or, more precisely, since antigen conformation may be influenced by antibody interaction, that the structures of these sites are not irreverisbly modified at this pH. On the other hand, antibodies that recognize amino acids in site B close to the trimer interface or in site D were found not to bind to hemagglutinin in the low-pH conformation. Such antibodies may recognize epitopes that span the monomer–monomer boundary; for example, only 15 Å separates residue 198 in site B in one monomer from 198 in another monomer of the trimer, and a single antibody might contact both residues simultaneously. It is more likely, however, that disorientation of the residues at this site occurs as a result of monomer–monomer contact breakage and the consequent loss of structural constraints unique in the trimer. Such trimer dissociation in the distal region of the molecule is reasonably concluded from a number of other observations,[13,30] and is supported by these studies with monoclonal antibodies.

Finally, there are two areas of research in which antihemagglutinin monoclonal antibodies play an important role. First, they provide powerful tools for studying the mechanisms of antigenic drift, by which new, antigenically distinct viruses reoccur in the human population to spawn respiratory disease epidemics. A series of observations on (1) the frequency of isolation of antigenic variants in the presence of monoclonal antibodies,[31] (2) the observed variation in the antibody repertoire of individual mice,[7] and (3) the existence of certain antigenic variants containing single amino acid substitutions that can react significantly differently with complete antisera,[10] suggest two not necessarily exclusive hypotheses concerning the process involved in antigenic drift. The first suggests that different individuals possess different antibody repertoires and the antigenic drift occurs at a rate that reflects these individual differences; the second proposes that certain epitopes of the hemagglutinin are antigenically dominant and that the rate at which they change dictates the overall rate of antigenic drift. Using radiolabeled Fab fragments prepared from monoclonal antibodies of defined specificity in competitive hemagglutinin-binding assays with postinfection human sera, support has been obtained for the former proposal (M. L. Wang, J. J. Skehel, and D. C. Wiley, in preparation). Information such as this should provide knowledge of the mechansim of antigenic drift in the human population.

Second, the availability of monoclonal antibodies has made possible studies of the three-dimensional structures of antibodies of selected specificity[32] and of antibody–antigen complexes. Similar studies of antihemagglutinin monoclonal antibodies and fragments are in progress to complement structural analyses of monoclonal antibody-selected antigenic variant hemagglutinins such as that described here (Fig. 3).

ACKNOWLEDGMENTS. We gratefully acknowledge the colleagues in our laboratories who have been involved in this work, especially Dr. R. S. Daniels, M. L. Wang, I. A. Wilson, and M. Knossow, and the excellent technical assistance of D. Stevens, R. Gonsalves, G. White, and A. Douglas; we thank N. G. Wrigley and E. Brown for Fig. 4. We also acknowledge support from NIH grant AI-13654 to D.C.W. We are grateful to Rod Hubbard, York University, for allowing us to use his unpublished graphics program, HYDRA.

References

1. Webster, R. G., and Laver, W. G., 1975, Antigenic variation of influenza viruses, in: *Influenza Viruses and Influenza* (E. D. Kilbourne, ed.), Academic Press, New York, pp. 270–314.
2. Kilbourne, E. D., 1969, Future influenza vaccines and the use of genetic recombinants, *Bull. WHO* **41**:643–645.
3. Ward, C. W., 1981, Influenza haemagglutinin, *Curr. Top. Microbiol. Immunol.* **94**:1–74.
4. Wilson, I. A., Skehel, J. J., and Wiley, D. C., 1981, Structure of the haemagglutinin membrane glycoprotein of influenza virus at 3 Å resolution, *Nature* **289**:366–373.
5. Skehel, J. J., Daniels, R. S., Douglas, A. R., and Wiley, D. C., 1983, Antigenic and amino acid sequence variations in the haemagglutinins of type A influenza viruses recently isolated from human subjects, *Bull. WHO* **61**:671–676.
6. Webster, R. G., and Laver, W. G., 1980, Determination of the number of nonoverlapping antigenic areas on Hong Kong (H3N2) influenza virus HA with monoclonal antibodies and the selection of variants with potential epidemiological significance, *Virology* **104**:139–148.
7. Underwood, P. A., 1984, An antigenic map of the haemagglutinin of the influenza Hong Kong subtype (H3N2) constructed using mouse monoclonal antibodies, *Mol. Immunol.* **21**:663–671.
8. Breschkin, A. M., Ahern, J., and White, D. O., 1981, Antigenic determinants of influenza virus haemagglutinin. VIII. Topography of the antigenic regions of influenza virus haemagglutinin determined by competitive radioimmune assay with monoclonal antibodies, *Virology* **113**:130–140.
9. Laver, W. G., Air, G. M., Webster, R. C., Gerhard, W., Ward, C. W., and Dopheide, T. A. A., 1979, Antigenic drift in type A influenza virus: Sequence differences in the haemagglutinin of Hong Kong (H3N2) variants selected with monoclonal hybridoma antibodies, *Virology* **98**:226–237.
10. Laver, W. G., Air, G. M., and Webster, R. G., 1981, Mechanism of antigenic drift in influenza virus. Amino acid sequence changes in an antigenically active region of Hong Kong (H3N2) influenza virus haemagglutinin, *J. Mol. Biol.* **145**:339–361.
11. Newton, S. E., Air, G. M., Webster, R. G., and Laver, W. G., 1983, Sequence of the haemagglutinin gene of influenza virus A/Memphis/1/71 and previously uncharacterized monoclonal antibody-derived variants, *Virology* **128**:495–501.
12. Daniels, R. S., Douglas, A. R., Skehel, J. J., and Wiley, D. C., 1983, Analyses of the antigenicity of influenza haemagglutinin at the pH optimum for virus mediated membrane fusion, *J. Gen. Virol.* **64**:1657–1662.
13. Daniels, R. S., Douglas, A. R., Skehel, J. J., Waterfield, M. D., Wilson, I. A., and Wiley, D. C., 1983, Studies of the influenza virus haemagglutinin in the pH5 conformation, in: *The Origin of Pandemic Influenza Viruses* (W. G. Laver, ed.), Elsevier, New York, pp. 1–8.
14. Moss, B. A., Underwood, P. A., Bender, V. J., and Whittaker, R. G., 1980, Antigenic drift in the haemagglutinin from various strains of influenza virus A/Hong Kong/68 (H3N2), in: *Struc-*

ture and Variation in Influenza Virus (W. G. Laver and G. M. Air, eds.), Elsevier, New York, pp. 329–338.
15. Skehel, J. J., Stevens, D. J., Daniels, R. S., Douglas, A. R., Knossow, M., Wilson, I. A., and Wiley, D. C., 1984, A carbohydrate side-chain on haemagglutinins of Hong Kong influenza viruses inhibits recognition by a monoclonal antibody, *Proc. Natl. Acad. Sci. USA* **81:**1779–1783.
16. Wiley, D. C., Wilson, I. A., and Skehel, J. J., 1981, Structural identifications of the antibody-binding sites of Hong Kong influenza haemagglutinin and their involvement in antigenic variation, *Nature* **289:**373–378.
17. Caton, A. J., Brownlee, G. G., Yewdell, J. W., and Gerhard, W., 1982, The antigenic structure of the influenza virus A/PR/8/34 haemagglutinin (H1 subtype), *Cell* **31:**417–427.
18. Knossow, M., Daniels, R. S., Douglas, A. R., Skehel, J. J., and Wiley, D. C., 1984, Three dimensional structure of an antigenic mutant of influenza virus haemagglutinin, *Nature* **311:**678–680.
19. Wrigley, N. G., Brown, E. B., Daniels, R. S., Douglas, A. R., Skehel, J. J., and Wiley, D. C., 1983, Electron microscopy of influenza haemagglutinin–monoclonal antibody complexes. *Virology* **131:**308–314.
20. Laver, W. G., Air, G. M., Dopheide, T. A., and Ward, C. W., 1980, Amino acid sequence changes in the haemagglutinin of A/Hong Kong (H3N2) influenza virus during the period 1968–1977, *Nature* **283:**454–457.
21. Both, G. W., Sleigh, M. J., Cox, N. J., and Kendal, A. P., 1983, Antigenic drift in H3 influenza haemagglutinin from 1968–1980: Multiple evolutionary pathways and sequential amino acid changes at key antigenic sites, *J. Virol.* **48:**52–60.
22. Sleigh, M. J., Both, G. W., Underwood, P. A., and Bender, V. J., 1981, Antigenic drift in the haemagglutinin of the Hong Kong influenza subtype: Correlation of amino acid changes with alterations in viral antigenicity, *J. Virol.* **37:**845–853.
23. Skehel, J. J., Bayley, P. M., Brown, E. B., Martin, S. R., Waterfield, M. D., White, J. M., Wilson, I. A., and Wiley, D. C., 1982, Changes in the conformation of influenza virus haemagglutinin at the pH optimum of virus-mediated membrane fusion, *Proc. Natl. Acad. Sci. USA* **79:**968–972.
24. Jensen, K. W., Minuse, E., and Francis, T., Jr., 1957, Serologic comparisons with lines of influenza virus isolated and serially transferred in different experimental hosts, *J. Immunol.* **787:**356–364.
25. Schild, G. C., Oxford, J. S., de Jong, J. C., and Webster, R. G., 1983, Evidence for host-cell selection of influenza virus antigenic variants, *Nature* **303:**706–709.
26. Rott, R., Orlich, M., Klenk, H.-D., Wang, M. L., Skehel, J. J., and Wiley, D. C., 1984, Studies on the adaptation of influenza viruses to MDCK cells, *EMBO J.* **3:**3329–3332.
27. Daniels, R. S., Douglas, A. R., Skehel, J. J., Wiley, D. C., Naeve, C. W., Webster, R. G., Rogers, G. N., and Paulson, J. C., 1984, Antigenic analyses of influenza virus haemagglutinins with different receptor-binding specificities, *Virology* **138:**174–177.
23. Rogers, G. N., Paulson, J. C., Daniels, R. S., Skehel, J. J., Wilson, I. A., and Wiley, D. C., 1983, Single amino acid substitutions in influenza haemagglutinin change receptor binding specificity, *Nature* **304:**76–78.
29. Webster, R. G., Brown, L. E., and Jackson, D. C., 1983, Changes in the antigenicity of the haemagglutinin molecule of H3 influenza virus at acidic pH, *Virology* **126:**587–599.
30. Daniels, R. S., Downie, J. C., Hay, A. J., Knossow, M., Skehel, J. J., Wang, M. L., and Wiley, D. C., 1985, Fusion mutants of the influenza virus haemagglutinin, *Cell* (in press).
31. Yewdell, J. W., Webster, R. G., and Gerhard, W. U., 1979, Antigenic variation in three distinct determinants of an influenza type A haemagglutinin molecule, *Nature* **279:**246–248.
32. Amit, A. G., Mariuzza, R. A., Saludjian, P., Poljak, R. J., Lamoyi, E., and Nisonoff, A., 1983, Preliminary crystallographic study of the Fab fragment of a monoclonal anti-phenylarsonate antibody possessing a major idiotypic specificity, *J. Mol. Biol.* **169:**637–638.
33. Schulman, M., Wilde, C. D., and Köhler, G., 1978, A better cell line for making hybridomas secreting specific antibodies, *Nature* **276:**269–270.

34. Köhler, G., and Milstein, C., 1975, Continuous cultures of fused cells secreting antibody of predefined specificity, *Nature* **256**:495–497.
35. Köhler, G., and Milstein, C., 1976, Derivation of specific antibody-producing tissue culture and tumor lines by cell fusion, *Eur. J. Immunol.* **6**:511–519.
36. Fazekas de St. Groth, S., and Scheidegger, D., 1980, Production of monoclonal antibodies: Strategy and tactics, *J. Immunol. Meth.* **35**:1–21.

Chapter 20

Virus Receptors on Somatic and Immune Cells

MAN SUNG CO, GLEN N. GAULTON, NOBORU MATSUZAKI, and MARK I. GREENE

1. Introduction

The susceptibility of cells to viral infection is often determined during the early stages of interaction.[1] This is particularly evident in the mammalian viruses, where infection and virus disease are largely determined by the ability of viruses to bind to the cells of a particular species. Even within a given species, the expression of different genes in different cell types or within the same cell type at different stages of development can result in the formation of different sets of specific virus receptors. The identification of virus receptors and the study of their interactions with ligands are therefore of critical importance in understanding viral tropism and subsequent disease patterns.[2,3]

Over the last few years, there have been a number of studies attempting to identify the nature of the cellular membrane proteins that several viruses have used as receptors. For example, it has been speculated that Semliki Forest virus binds to histocompatibility antigens in humans and mice.[4] However, although binding studies have supported this association, Semliki Forest virus can grow in cells devoid of histocompatibility antigens, raising questions as to the significance of the role of histocompatibility antigens as receptors.[5] Lactate dehydrogenase virus has been found to interact with mouse Ia antigens, suggesting a role of Ia in targeting virus to a subset of macrophage.[6] Rabies virus has been reported to bind in close association with the acetylcholine receptors[7] and Epstein–Barr virus has been shown to recognize the complement receptor type 2 (CR2) of human B lymphocytes.[8]

Work in our laboratory has centered on the utilization of anti-idiotypic antibodies in the study of the reovirus type 3 cellular receptor.[9–11] We have used the mammalian reovirus as a model system to determine if structures

MAN SUNG CO and NOBORU MATSUZAKI • Department of Pathology, Harvard Medical School, Boston, Massachusetts 02115. GLEN N. GAULTON and MARK I. GREENE • Departments of Medicine and Pathology, Tufts University School of Medicine, Boston, Massachusetts 02111.

responsible for virus binding and recognition by the immune system are shared by non-immune cell surface receptors for reovirus. Syngeneic monoclonal and xenogeneic polyclonal anti-idiotypic antibodies with specificity for the reovirus receptor have been constructed and successfully used to isolate the reovirus receptors on both transformed and normal cells.[12] We have further shown that the mammalian reovirus receptor shares extensive structural homology with the mammalian β-adrenergic receptor.[13]

2. Reovirus as a Model System for Studying Viral Receptor Interactions

2.1. Role of Reovirus Hemagglutinin

The mammalian reoviruses consist of three serotypes (1, 2, and 3). The virions have a double-capsid structure with an internal core, which contains the segmented, double-stranded RNA genome, and a closely applied inner capsid, which is surrounded by a second outer capsid shell.[14] Each RNA segment transcribes a unique mRNA which is in turn translated into a primary polypeptide. The outer capsid is composed of the viral polypeptides σ1, μ1C, and σ3.

Following entry into the mammalian host, reoviruses induce a potent immune response. Two types of antibody activities are generally detected: neutralization antibodies and hemagglutination (HA)-inhibiting antibodies. Using a variety of recombinant reovirus clones in which genetic segments of one serotype have been imposed on a genetic background of another, it has been revealed that the σ1 polypeptide is the type-specific antigen responsible for determining specificity in both neutralization and HA inhibition.[15–17] The viral HA also serves as the viral attachment protein[18,19] and is immunodominant for both B-cell- and T-cell-mediated immune responses.[20–23]

2.2. Anti-idiotype as Antireceptor Antibody

Based on the observations that the immune response to reovirus is dominated by anti-HA, and that anti-HA antibodies are themselves relatively restricted in their clonal diversity, we reasoned that a substantial natural enrichment would exist for the generation of internal image anti-idiotypic antibodies. The theoretical and experimental verification of internal image antibodies, which mirror the binding patterns of the primary ligand (in this instance HA3), is the topic of a recent review.[11]

The generation of rabbit anti-idiotypic antibodies has been previously reported.[24] Briefly, BALB/c mice (Charles River Breeding Laboratories, Wilmington, Massachusetts) were repeatedly inoculated with 10^9 particles of purified reovirus type 3 virions, and sera obtained were twice precipitated with 40% saturated ammonium sulfate followed by Sephracryl-200 gel filtration. To enrich for anti-HA antibody, serum was absorbed on type 1 and the 3HA1 recombinant reovirus that differs only in the gene encoding the σ1 protein. The enriched antibodies (500 μg) in complete Freund's adjuvant were injected intramuscularly and in the footpads into outbred New Zealand rabbits (Microbiological Associates, Walkersville, Maryland). Rabbits were immunized at 3 and 5 weeks with the same emulsion, and were bled 7 days after the last injection. Sera were purified by precipitation twice in 40% saturated ammonium sulfate, then absorbed with normal mouse sera. The binding specificity of these purified antisera was demonstrated by affinity for HA3-specific Ig using a solid phase radioimmunoassay. The rabbit anti-idiotypic antibodies were also shown to bind the anti-HA3-specific monoclonal antibody 9BG5 and to block the binding of 9BG5 to ^{125}I-labeled HA3.

The generation and screening of syngeneic monoclonal anti-idiotypic antibodies has also been described.[25] BALB/c mice were immunized repeatedly with 5×10^6 irradiated (1500 R) idiotype-bearing 9BG5 hybridoma cells. The final immunization was given 72 hr before fusion. Cells were fused according to the method of Köhler and Milstein and the resulting antibodies were screened for their ability to bind to the 9BG5 monoclonal. One such syngeneic monoclonal antibody, 87.92.6 (IgM, κ), was shown to specifically inhibit binding of 9BG5 to purified ^{125}I-labeled reovirus type 3 hemagglutinin.

We have found that both monoclonal and a subset of polyclonal anti-idiotypic antibodies appear to represent effective "internal images" of the reovirus hemagglutinin domain that interacts with cellular receptors for the virus. The evidence supporting this claim is as follows: (1) anti-idiotype binding parallels the cellular tropism of reovirus type 3[24]; (2) the anti-idiotype and reoviruses have similar biological effects in limiting conconavalin A-induced stimulation of murine lymphocytes[26]; (3) anti-idiotype specifically inhibits reovirus 3 binding to target cells[27] (4) anti-idiotype prevents isolated HA protein from binding to monoclonal anti-HA antibodies[24,25]; and (5) anti-idiotype specifically stimulates both T- and B-cell immunity to reovirus *in vivo*.[28] Based on these observations we have utilized anti-idiotypic antibodies in studying the function and isolation of the cell surface receptors for reovirus, which is described in the following sections.

3. Studies of Reovirus Receptors with Anti-idiotypic Antibody

3.1. Cytoskeletal Association, Modulation, and Quantitation

Reovirus anti-idiotypic antibodies have been shown to specifically recognize the reovirus type 3 cell surface viral receptor.[24,25] Both xenogeneic polyclonal and syngeneic monoclonal anti-idiotypic antibodies mimic the tropism of reovirus type 3 and specifically inhibit the binding of reovirus type 3 to cellular and immune targets.[27] Incubation of R1.1 thymoma cells with monoclonal anti-idiotypic antibodies prior to reovirus exposure resulted in a 62% decrease in the binding of reovirus as determined by measuring the peak mean channel fluorescence in a fluorescence activated cell sorter. In comparison, anti-idiotype failed to alter the binding of either anti-H-2 or anti-Thy-1.2 immunoglobulins.

The linkage of reovirus receptors to cytoskeletal elements was established by the induction of receptor patching and capping in the presence of anti-receptor antibodies and secondary anti-immunoglobulin. Capping occurred rapidly at 37°C, in a manner indistinguishable from that seen upon the addition of anti-immunoglobulin to B cells.[28,29] Viral receptors progressed from evenly dispersed, to patched, to capped distribution within 10 min. Capping was inhibited by the addition of 0.2% sodium azide, 0.5 M glucose, 10 μg/ml cytochalasin B, or by incubation at 4°C, but was not affected by the addition of either colchicine or 1 μg/ml cytochalasin B. Thus, capping of reovirus receptors is rapid, energy dependent, and requires the presence of intact microfilament organization.

Clearing of viral receptors from the cell surface by antireceptor-antibody-mediated capping was also utilized to determine the timing of receptor reexpression. Following clearing, low levels of receptors first reappeared within 4 hr. By 12 hr approximately 50% of receptors were reexpressed and by 24 hr receptor density was equivalent to initial levels.[28,29] No effect of viral receptor capping on the expression of either H-2, Thy-1.2, or Lyt-1,2,3 surface markers was seen. Clearing of receptors was also achieved by enzymatic treatment. Exposure of cells to either pronase or trypsin significantly reduced the amount of surface viral receptor. Reexpression of receptor following enzymatic digestions followed the same time course as that seen with antireceptor-induced capping, suggesting that capped receptors are enzymatically degraded following internalization.

These results indicate that the turnover of viral receptors on lymphoid cells follows a pattern seen with a number of other lymphocyte surface markers.[30] Receptor reexpression was sensitive to tunicamycin and thus appears to require the synthesis of new glycoprotein rather than a rapid membrane reshuttle process as seen with the transferrin receptor.[31] This is consistent with the observation that internalized reovirus particles are processed through lysosomes prior to initiating the infective cycle.

Antireceptor antibodies have also proven useful in determining, with low background, the number of viral receptors present on target cells. Purified monoclonal anti-idiotype iodinated to high specific activity using the chloramine T methodology was used to quantitate receptors on a variety of reovirus-binding and -nonbinding cell lines. Table I presents a summary of some of these binding data obtained by Scatchard plot analysis of iodinated antireceptor binding. As expected from our previous data, only cells that bound reovirus were shown to express significant levels of viral receptors.

3.2. Purification

Our initial experiments indicated that the most effective reovirus receptor purification was achieved utilizing polyclonal rabbit anti-idiotypic antibodies

Table I. Number and Affinity of Anti-idiotypic Antibody Receptors on Reovirus High-Binding and Low-Binding Cells[a]

Cell	Number of binding sites	K_d ($\times 10^{10}$)
Reovirus type 3 high-binding		
R1.1 thymoma	67,000	9.6
B104 neuroblastoma	78,000	9.2
Splenic T	64,500	7.9
Splenic B	49,500	8.6
Reovirus type 3 low-binding		
YAC thymoma	<2,000	—

[a] Increasing amounts of purified monoclonal ^{125}I-anti-id were added to 2×10^5 cells in 50 μl PBS containing 1% BSA and 0.2% NaN_3. Following labeling, cells were pelleted through phthalate oils and cell bound ^{125}I determined. The results presented were obtained by Scatchard analysis of binding data.[12]

rather than monoclonal anti-idiotypic antibodies.[12] Following surface iodination the solubilized membrane extracts of R1.1 thymoma cells were incubated with antireceptor antibodies and precipitated with Sepharose–protein A. The precipitate was analyzed by two-dimensional PAGE under reduced conditions. The immunoprecipitate has a single molecule weight of 67,000 with a heterogeneous pI around 5.9.

Confirmation that the 67,000-dalton structure is the reovirus receptor was achieved using Western blot analysis. The R1.1 cell membranes were first purified using differential and equilibrium gradient centrifugation. Membrane extracts were then run under reduced conditions on 10% SDS–PAGE and blotted onto nitrocellulose paper. Identification of the reovirus receptor was achieved by independent hybridization with either ^{125}I-labeled reovirus or anti-idiotype. Results showed that both radiolabeled virus and anti-idiotype bound to a single band of 67,000 daltons.[12] Control hybridization with radiolabeled anti-BSA did not detect the same band. Thus, recognition of the 67,000-dalton structure is specific for reovirus type 3 particles and anti-idiotypic antibodies.

We have also demonstrated directly that the 67,000-dalton receptor on R1.1 is a glycoprotein. This was achieved by treatment of immunoprecipitates with neuraminidase, which catalyzes the release of sialic acid residues from glycoproteins before analysis on SDS–PAGE gels. Results indicate that neuraminidase treatment generates an additional band of 62,000 daltons, the latter being the partially deglycosylated product.

Using polyclonal antireceptor antibody for immunoprecipitation, we have identified a similar 67,000-dalton structure on a variety of cell lines, including rat neuroblastoma, human lymphoma, monkey kidney, and several other lymphoid lines.[12] The presence of the 67,000-dalton structure on such diverse cell lines and its occurrence across species strongly suggests that it is a common cell surface structure, perhaps in association with normal cellular functions.

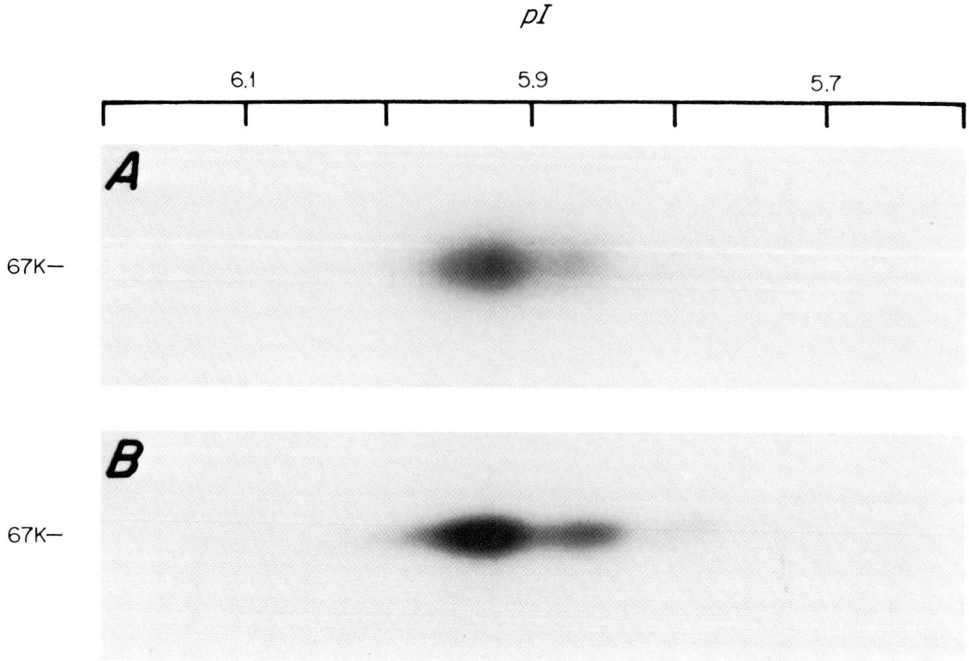

Figure 1. Two-dimensional gel electrophoresis of immunoprecipitated reovirus type 3 receptor and calf lung β-adrenergic receptor. (A) Reovirus receptor was purified from murine thymoma cells R1.1 following iodination. Membrane proteins were solubilized following incubation in phosphate-buffered saline containing detergents, the debris was cleared by centrifugation, and aliquots containing 300,000 cpm were immunoprecipitated with polyclonal anti-id3. Pellets were adjusted to IEF sample buffer: 9.5 M urea, 2% (w/v) NP40, 1.6% pH 5–8 Pharmalyte (Pharmacia), 0.4% pH 3–10 Pharmalyte (Pharmacia), and 5% 2-mercaptoethanol. The sample (50 μ) was loaded into the basic end of 120-mm × 2.8-mm-diameter tube gels containing 9.5 M urea, 4% acrylamide, 2% NP40, and 2% Pharmalyte, and run at 500 V for 16 hr before being placed on top of 10% SDS–PAGE slab gel run at 30 mA for 5 hr. The gels were fixed, dried, and exposed to a Kodak X-OMAT AR film for 2 days at −70°C. (B) β-Adrenergic receptor was purified from calf lung as described.[13]

We noted that several membrane proteins with molecular weights similar to the purified reovirus receptor have been reported. One of these proteins, the mammalian β-adrenergic receptor, also shows a coincident distribution in reovirus binding tissues. To examine the possibility that the mammalian reovirus and β-adrenergic receptors are related structurally, we obtained a sample of purified β-adrenergic receptor isolated from calf lung tissues and tested its ability to bind the anti-reovirus receptor antibody.[13] Results indicated that anti-idiotypic antibody bound to and precipitated the purified β-adrenergic receptor. Two-dimensional gel analysis of the purified reovirus and β-adrenergic receptors (Fig. 1) showed that the two receptors are structurally similar, suggesting that mammalian reoviruses may utilize the β-adrenergic receptor on the host cell surface for binding and entry.

Table II. Lysis by Reovirus-Specific CTL Lines of Anti-idiotypic Hybridoma Cells[a]

Target	Line	Percent specific lysis at given effector/target ratio	
		40:1	10:1
Uninfected P815	1	10.8	3.5
	2	14.1	5.9
	3	16.6	4.9
	4	20.3	8.1
Reovirus 3-infected P815	1	54.7	36.0
	2	48.8	34.0
	3	46.6	34.0
	4	46.6	30.9
87.92.6 Hybridoma cells	1	23.8	18.6
	2	35.6	24.6
	3	50.0	27.7
	4	35.0	17.3

[a] Reovirus-specific CTL lines were generated by giving 10^7 PFU virus ip and harvesting spleen cells at 7 days. Cells were restimulated *in vitro* by incubation with 10^7 PFU virus/well (7×10^6 cells/1.6 ml) for 5 days prior to conducting a 5-hr ^{51}Cr-release assay on 10^3 target cells.[39]

4. Similarities of Somatic and Immune Cell Viral Receptors

4.1. Cytolytic T Cells Specific for Reovirus Type 3 Recognize Anti-idiotype

The observation that anti-idiotypic antibodies made to anti-viral HA antibodies bind to viral receptors indicated that a proportion of anti-HA antibodies share an idiotype with the viral receptor, and in a like manner that the anti-idiotype and viral HA share a common recognition epitope. In light of multiple demonstrations of common idiotypic determinants on immune B and T cells specific for the same antigen,[32] we investigated whether reovirus type 3-specific cytolytic T cells would bind anti-idiotype. The addition of syngeneic monoclonal anti-idiotypic (antireceptor) antibody was first shown to bind and block the lytic activity of reovirus-specific CTLs.

Interestingly, reovirus-specific CTLs were found to lyse the anti-idiotypic hybridoma cells in an H-2-restricted fashion.[33,34] Table II presents the results of studies conducted in a series of cloned lines of reovirus-specific CTL cells. As shown, CTL clones that lyse reovirus-infected targets lyse 87.92.6 hybridomas with varying degrees of effectiveness. Forty percent of reovirus-specific CTLs were found to lyse the hybridoma targets. The immunodominance of this T-cell response by the viral binding epitope is consistent with previous ob-

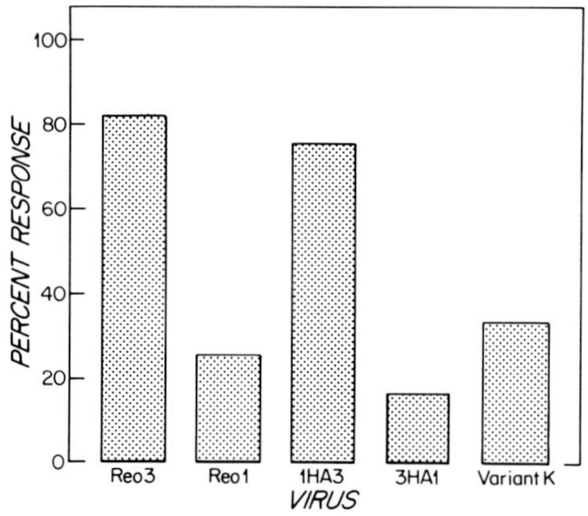

Figure 2. Specificity of the DTH response elicited by the monoclonal anti-idiotype. BALB/c mice were immunized subcutaneously with 100 μg of anti-idiotype, boosted with an additional 100 μg 2 days later, and challenged in the footpad on day 6 with either reovirus type 3, type 1 reassortant 1HA3, reassortment 3HA1, variant virus K, or saline. Footpad swelling was measured 24 hr. later. Results are expressed as a percentage of the DTH response (±SEM) in mice primed and challenged with reovirus type 3. For Reo 1, 3HA1, variant K, and saline, $p < 0.001$. For Reo 3 and 1HA3, $p < 0.01$. (From Ref. 34 by permission).

servations of a restricted anti-HA immunoglobulin response.[24] More recently, we have demonstrated that anti-idiotype can stimulate anti-HA3-specific antibody production.[35]

These studies indicate that the configurations of the binding domains of somatic receptors for reovirus, the receptors used by immune T cells, and immune B cells (exemplified by the 9BG5 hybridoma) appear to be quite similar. Our results are also consistent with the hypothesis that recognition by CTLs of antigen receptors on virally infected targets occurs by a dual antigen–H-2 recognition process.

4.2. Induction of Viral Immunity by Anti-idiotype

The previous studies clearly indicated that reovirus idiotype–anti-idiotype networks involve the regulation of both T- and B-cell populations. The use of anti-idiotypic antibodies to stimulate antigen-specific immunity dates to the work of Eichman.[36] More recently, xenogeneic and syngeneic anti-idiotypic antibodies have been utilized to enhance hepatitis[37] and sendai virus immunity.[38] Using a similar rationale, we investigated the ability of a purified monoclonal anti-idiotypic antibody to induce T- and B-cell-mediated immunity in a syngeneic system.

Immunization with purified anti-idiotype or hybridoma cells, in the absence of adjuvant, was successful in the induction of both CTL and DTH classes of T-cell immunity.[34] The specificity of this immunity is depicted in Fig. 2. Mice immunized with anti-idiotype specifically responded only to subsequent challenge with virus that bears the type 3 HA. Induction of specific immunity was dose dependent for anti-idiotypic protein (Fig. 3), enabling a direct comparison of the number of viral particles to that of anti-idiotype required for establishing immunity (approximately one vs. 10^4, respectively).

These studies further confirm the conformational similarities of immune T- and B-cell receptors to those found on nonimmune and somatic cells. They

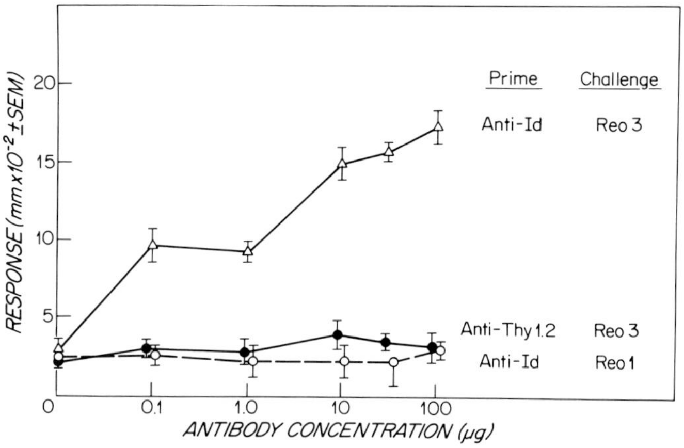

Figure 3. Dose response of anti-idiotype with regard to magnitude of DTH response. BALB/c mice were immunized subcutaneously with varying amounts of purified monoclonal anti-idiotype or control and challenged in the footpad 6 days later with reovirus type 3 or type 1. (From Ref. 34 by permission.)

also provide an attractive means for inducing or augmenting immunity to virus without direct exposure to the pathogen.

5. Conclusion

This chapter summarizes our recent work on the biochemical and functional characterization of the cellular receptors for the mammalian reovirus type 3. The approach we adopted has been to utilize both polyclonal and monoclonal anti-HA3 anti-idiotypic antibodies as specific probes of the viral receptor. The activities of these two antibody preparations were of identical specificity, although polyclonal anti-idiotype has proven more effective in immunoprecipitation analyses.

Anti-idiotypic antibodies have been utilized to purify extensively the reovirus type 3 receptor and have allowed comparative analysis of similarities between the mammalian reovirus and β-adrenergic receptors. Purified anti-idiotypic antibodies have also been employed as vaccines to stimulate antiviral immunity of both T- and B-cell classes.

These results clearly demonstrate the usefulness of monoclonal antibodies in receptor research and particularly in the generation of anti-idiotypic antibody receptor probes.

References

1. Dimmock, N. J., 1982, Initial stages in infection with animal viruses, *J. Gen. Virol.* **59**:1–22.
2. Meager, A., and Hughes, R. C., 1977, Virus receptors, in: *Receptors and Recognition*, Series A, No. 4 (P. Cuatrecasas and M. F. Greaves, eds) Chapman and Hall, London, pp. 143–195.

3. Tardieu, M., Epstein, R. E., and Weiner, H. L., 1983, Interaction of viruses with cell surface receptors, *Int. Rev. Cytol.* **80:**27–61.
4. Helenius, A., Morein, B., Fries, E., Simons, K., Robinson, P., Schirrmacher, V., Terhorst, C., and Strominger, J. L., 1978, Human [HLA-A and HLA-B] and murine [H-2K and H-2D] histocompatability antigens are cell surface receptors for semliki forest virus, *Proc. Natl. Acad. Sci. USA* **75:**3846–3850.
5. Oldstone, M. B. A., Tishon, A., Dutko, F. J., Kennedy, S. I. T., Holland, J. J., and Lampert, P. W., 1980, Does the major histocompatibility complex serve as a specific receptor for semliki forest virus, *J. Virol.* **34:**256–265.
6. Inada, T., and Mims, C. A., 1984, Mouse Ia antigens are receptors for lactate dehydrogenase virus, *Nature* **309:**59–61.
7. Lentz, T. L., Burrage, T. G., Smith, A. L., Crick, J., and Tignor, G. H., 1982, Is the acetylcholine receptor a rabies virus receptor, *Science* **215:**182–184.
8. Fingeroth, J. D., Weis, J. J., Tedder, J. F., Strominger, J. L., Biro, P. A., and Fearon, D. T., 1984, Epstein–Barr virus receptor of human B lymphocytes is the C3d receptor CR2, *Proc. Natl. Acad. Sci. USA* **81:**4510–4514.
9. Fields, B. N., and Greene, M. I., 1982, Genetic and molecular mechanisms of viral pathogenesis: Implications for prevention and treatment, *Nature* **300:**19–23.
10. Noseworthy, J. H., and Greene, M. I., 1984, Studies on idiotypes shared by neuronal and lymphoid cells, in: *Idiotypy in Biology and Medicine* (P. A. Cazenue and J. A. Urbain, eds.), Academic Press, New York, pp. 303–328.
11. Gaulton, G. N., Co, M. S., Royer, H. D., and Greene, M. I., 1984, Anti-idiotypic antibodies as probes of cell surface receptors, *Mol. Cell Biochem.* **65:**5–21.
12. Co, M. S., Gaulton, G. N., Fields, B. N., and Greene, M. I., 1984, Isolation and biochemical characterization of the mammalian reovirus type 3 cell surface receptor, *Proc. Natl. Acad. Sci. USA* **82:**1494–1498.
13. Co, M. S., Gaulton, G. N., Tominaga, A., Homcy, C. J., Fields, B. N., and Greene, M. I., 1985, Structural similarities between the mammalian beta-adrenergic and reovirus type 3 receptors, *Proc. Natl. Acad. Sci.* (in press).
14. Fields, B. N., 1982, Molecular basis of reovirus virulence, *Arch. Virol.* **71:**95–107.
15. Weiner, H. L., and Fields, B. N., 1977, Neutralization of reovirus: The gene responsible for the neutralization antigen, *J. Exp. Med.* **146:**1305–1310.
16. Spriggs, D. R., Kaye, K., and Fields, B. N., 1983, Topological analysis of the reovirus type 3 hemagglutinin, *Virology* **127:**220–224.
17. Burstin, S. J., Spriggs, D. R., and Fields, B. N., 1982, Evidence for functional domains on the reovirus type 3 hemagglutinin, *Virology* **117:**145–155.
18. Weiner, H. L., Ramig, R. F., Mustoe, T. A., and Fields, B. N., 1978, Identification of the gene coding for the hemagglutinin of reovirus, *Virology* **86:**581–584.
19. Lee, P. W. K., Hayes, E. C., and Joklik, W. K., 1981, Protein σ1 is the reovirus cell attachment protein, *Virology* **108:**156–163.
20. Weiner, H. L., Greene, M. I., and Fields, B. N., 1980, Delayed hypersensitivity in mice with reovirus. I. Identification of host and viral gene products responsible for the immune response, *J. Immunol.* **125:**278–282.
21. Greene, M. I., and Weiner, H. L., 1980, Delayed hypersensitivity in mice infected with reovirus. II. Induction of tolerance and suppressor T cells to viral specific gene products, *J. Immunol.* **125:**283–287.
22. Fontana, A., and Weiner, H. L., 1980, Interaction of reovirus with cell surface receptors. II. Generation of suppressor T cells by the hemagglutinin of reovirus type 3, *J. Immunol.* **125:**2660–2664.
23. Rubin, D., Weiner, H. L., Fields, B. N., and Greene, M. I., 1981, Immunologic tolerance after oral administration of reovirus: Requirement for two viral gene products for tolerance induction, *J. Immunol.* **127:**1697–1701.
24. Nepom, J. T., Weiner, H. L., Dichter, M. A., Tardieu, M., Spriggs, D. R., Gramm, C. F., Powers, M. L., Fields, B. N., and Greene, M. I., 1982, Identification of a hemagglutinin-specific idiotype

associated with reovirus recognition shared by lymphoid and neuronal cells, *J. Exp. Med.* **155**:155–167.

25. Noseworthy, J. H., Fields, B. N., Dichter, M. A., Sobotka, C., Pizer, E., Perry, L. L., Nepom, J. T., and Greene, M. I., 1983, Cell receptors for the mammalian reovirus. I. Syngeneic monoclonal anti-idiotypic antibody identifies a cell surface receptor for reovirus, *J. Immunol.* **131**:2533–2538.
26. Nepom, J. T., Tardieu, M., Epstein, R. L., Noseworthy, J. H., Weiner, H. L., Gentsch, J., Fields, B. N., and Greene, M. I., 1982, Virus-binding receptors: Similarities to immune receptors as determined by anti-idiotypic antibodies, *Surv. Immunol. Res.* **1**:255–261.
27. Kauffman, R. S., Noseworthy, J. H., Nepom, J. T., Finberg, R., Fields, B. N., and Green, M. I., 1983, Cell receptors for the mammalian reovirus. II. Monoclonal anti-idiotypic antibody blocks viral binding to cells, *J. Immunol.* **131**:2539–2941.
28. Gaulton, G. N., Co., M. S., and Green, M. I., 1985, Anti-idiotypic antibody identifies the cellular receptor of reovirus type 3, *J. Cell. Biochem.* (in press).
29. Gaulton, G. N., Co., M. S., and Greene, M. I., 1985, Cell receptors for the mammalian reovirus. V. Receptor number, modulation and isolation using anti-idiotypic antibody, *Virology*, submitted for publication.
30. Schreiner, G. F., and Unanue, E. R., 1976, Membrane and cytoplasmic changes in B lymphocytes induced by ligand–surface immunoglobulin interaction, *Adv. Immunol.* **24**:37–165.
31. Yamashiro, D. J., Tycko, B., Fluss, S. R., and Maxfield, F. R., 1984, Segregation of transferrin to a mildly acidic (pH 6.5) paragolgi compartment in the recycling pathway, *Cell* **37**:789–800.
32. Hart, D. A., Wang, A.-L., Pawlak, L. L., and Nisonoff, A., 1972, Suppression of idiotypic specificities in adult mice by administration of anti-idiotypic antibody, *J. Exp. Med.* **135**:1293–1300.
33. Ertl, H. C., Green, M. I., Noseworthy, J. H., Fields, B. N., Nepom, J. T., Spriggs, D. R., and Finberg, R. W., 1983, Identification of idiotype receptors on reovirus specific cytolytic T cells, *Proc. Natl. Acad. Sci. USA* **75**:7479–7483.
34. Sharpe, A. H., Gaulton, G. N., McDade, K. K., Fields, B. N., and Greene, M. I., 1984, Syngeneic monoclonal anti-idiotype can induce cellular immunity to reovirus, *J. Exp. Med.* **160**:1195–1205.
35. Gaulton, G. N., Sharpe, A. H., McDade, K. K., Fields, B. N., and Greene, M. I., 1985, Immunization with syngeneic monoclonal anti-idiotypic antibody induces type specific anti-reovirus antibodies, submitted for publication.
36. Eichman, K., 1975, Idiotypic suppression. II. Amplification of a suppressor T cell with anti-idiotypic activity, *J. Immunol.* **5**:511–517.
37. Kennedy, R. C., Sparrow, J. T., Sanchez, Y., Melnick, J. L., and Dreesman, G. R., 1984, Enhancement of viral hepatitis B antibody (anti-HBS) response to a synthetic cyclic peptide by priming with anti-idiotype antibodies. *Virology* **136**:247–252.
38. Ertl, H. C. J., and Finberg, R. W., 1984, Sendai virus-specific T-cell clones: Induction of cytolytic T cells by an anti-idiotypic antibody directed against a helper T-cell clone, *Proc. Natl. Acad. Sci. USA* **81**:2850–2854.
39. Sharpe, A. H., Gaulton, G. N., Ertl, H. C. J., Finberg, R. W., McDade, K. K., Fields, B. N., and Greene, M. I., 1985, Cell receptors for the mammalian reovirus: IV. Reovirus specific cytolytic T cell lines which have idiotypic receptors recognize anti-idiotypic B cell hybridomas, *J. Immunol.* (in press).

Part III

Uses of Antibodies in Recombinant DNA Technology

Chapter 21

Designing and Using Site-Specific Antibodies to Synthetic Peptides

BRIAN S. SCHAFFHAUSEN

1. Introduction

Over the past 4 years synthetic peptides have become widely used as "determinants in search of antibodies." The production of antibodies to small peptides is now common laboratory practice. As with hybridoma technology, the method yields site-specific immunologic reagents. However, the isolation of a monoclonal against any particular determinant is a matter of chance. The identification of the determinant that is recognized by a given monoclonal is a laborious or even impossible task. By starting with a small peptide, the potential determinants are narrowly defined.

The production of antibodies to peptides is by no means new. In the 1960s Anderer[1,2] used COOH-terminal hexapeptide derived from the tobacco mosaic virus (TMV) coat protein to develop an antibody that could recognize the virus. Furthermore, antibodies to the synthetic peptide could be used to inactivate the virus. In the 1970s, a synthetic peptide was used to elicit neutralizing antibody to coliphage MS-2.[3] Working with a decapeptide from TMV coat protein, Fearney and colleagues developed an antibody that would bind the protein, but not TMV itself.[4] X-ray diffraction subsequently showed that the sequence was not accessible in the virion. Furie and his colleagues used purified cyanogen bromide fragments to develop antibodies that could be used to probe structural transitions in staphylococcal nuclease.[5,6] Prothrombin activation was analyzed with antibodies to peptide fragments.[7]

The examples just cited represented individual cases and did not immediately give rise to a commonly used technology. The reason for this lies in the traditional view of antigenic determinants in proteins (see Benjamin *et al.*[8] for a current view). In cases such as myoglobin where the determinants were worked out, they were found to be few in number and dependent upon the conformation of the protein.[9] The chance of randomly selecting a peptide from the protein sequence that would be part of such a determinant would be small.

BRIAN S. SCHAFFHAUSEN • Department of Biochemistry and Pharmacology, Tufts University School of Medicine, Boston, Massachusetts 02111.

Further, the amino acid sequence would not be able to assume the same conformation in the small peptide as in the protein. The work of Schechter and colleagues supported this view.[10] They raised antibodies to Tyr-Ala-Glu polymers that are α-helical in solution. Shorter blocks of the tripeptide inhibited poorly because they were not α-helical. The study of the loop peptide (residues 60–83) of lysozyme is perhaps the best known demonstration of the effect of conformation on the antigenicity of a sequence.[11,12] There is an internal disulfide bridge between residues 64 and 80. The antigenicity of the loop depends upon this disulfide bridge remaining intact; antibodies to the closed loop did not bind the open chain peptide. Another very discouraging observation for the prospect of using peptides as antigens was that determinants could be made up of amino acids from noncontiguous portions of the sequence. For example, Atassi and colleagues characterized one antigenic site of lysozyme made up of residues 33, 34, 113, and 114.[13] All these kinds of experiments implied that making antibodies to peptides would be a futile endeavor.

Beginning around 1980 the efforts of Gernot Walter and Richard Lerner and their respective colleagues demonstrated that antibodies to small peptides could be readily obtained. In particular, peptides as short as six amino acids could be used to derive antibodies that would recognize the proteins containing the peptide sequence. The peptides chosen could come from widely varying regions of the protein. Most importantly, the peptides do not have to be derived from portions of the protein involved in determinants recognized by antisera against the protein, i.e., it is not necessary to know anything about the immunology of the protein. The detailed work on the influenza virus hemagglutinin (HA) makes this point quite clearly.[14,15] Twenty peptides spanning 75% of the HA molecule were synthesized. From X-ray diffraction data, it was known that some of the peptides come from α-helical regions, other from β-sheets, and others from coils, so the choice of peptides was not restricted to "flexible" domains of the protein molecule. Eighteen of these peptides gave rise to antibodies that would react with the hemagglutinin molecule. The peptides were not restricted to sequences thought to be immunogenic in the intact molecule; in fact, antibody to HA did not react with the peptides. The results obtained making antibodies to synthetic peptides have been part of the stimulus in reevaluating the view of the nature of the antigenic structure of proteins. The current view suggests that, while there are immunodominant sites, most if not all of the protein surface is immunogenic and can include multiple overlapping determinants.

Following the lead of Lerner, Walter, and their colleagues, a large number of other investigators have used peptide antibodies in diverse areas for a wide variety of purposes. There are two principal advantages to the approach. One is selectivity. Since the investigator controls the determinant by the choice of the peptide, it is possible to prepare antisera to peptides differing by as little as a single amino acid to develop site-specific reagents. The second advantage is that there is no need to isolate the protein to use as antigen. In its most extreme application, proteins can be identified using antibodies to peptides chosen on the basis of nucleic acid sequences.

The purpose of this chapter is to describe briefly examples of how peptide antibodies have been used and then to describe briefly how to prepare them. It is hoped that the reader will be encouraged to try this technology in his or her own work. For more information, there are several recent reviews.[16–19]

2. How Can Antibodies to Synthetic Peptides be Used?

Table I summarizes some of the recent applications of antibodies to synthetic peptides. The most important application is certainly the identification of previously unknown gene products for which DNA sequencing information is available. Papkoff and colleagues were able to identify the 37K product of the Moloney murine sarcoma virus using an antibody against the COOH terminus of the protein.[20,21] This protein is present as only 0.0002% of the total cell protein in the transformed cell. It had remained undetected when sera from tumor-bearing animals were used to try to find it. The list of gene products identified using this approach is now quite substantial. Ironically, even a protein of TMV, the virus originally used by Anderer, has recently been detected with peptide antisera.[24] The study of human T-cell leukemia virus has been aided considerably by this approach. The products of the *gag* and *env* genes have been identified using several different peptides.[25,26] Most recently the product of the transforming gene of HTLV has been demonstrated.[27] While many of the gene products detected in this way are encoded by viruses, other proteins have also been analyzed. Sutcliffe and his colleagues, after studies on mRNAs specific to brain, identified a tissue-specific protein.[28] A protein involved in the maturation of mRNA in yeast[29] and a human mitochondrial protein[30] have also been detected in this way. Alternatively, it is possible to use a peptide antiserum to decide which gene has been cloned.[31] Another variation occurred in the analysis of v-*sis* and the platelet-derived growth factor (PDGF).[32] Nucleic acid sequencing suggested that the oncogene v-*sis* and PDGF are very similar. This similarity was confirmed by the preparation of a peptide antibody to a common sequence; the antibody recognized both proteins. There are two potential concerns in the detection of proteins predicted by nucleic acid sequencing. The first is that the protein detected might not be the one expected. In fact, one of the earliest efforts of this sort, the analysis of murine leukemia virus proteins, gave somewhat misleading results.[33,34] The second problem is inherent in immunologic purification of polypeptides. Unlike purifications based on activity, the researcher is often faced with protein to which no function can yet be ascribed.

Peptide antibodies can be used to answer questions about processing. This processing can occur at the level of the protein or in variations in exon usage in the DNA. The classic example is the processing of poliovirus proteins.[38–40] The polyprotein NCVPOO yields a 63K replicase and a genome linked protein (VPg) through processing. A number of intermediates can be identified because they react with antibody to peptides with VPg sequence and to antibody to peptides of 63K sequence. The *gag* gene product of HTLV is one recent example

Table I. Applications of Anti-peptide Antibodies

In identification of proteins predicted by nucleic acid sequence
1. Murine sarcoma virus-transforming gene product[20,21]
2. Adenovirus E1A and E1B products[43–46]
3. Simian sarcoma virus (SSV)-transforming gene product[22,23]
4. MC29 v-*myc* and cellular homologue c-*myc*[36,37]
5. Avian myeloblastosis virus (AMV) leukemogenic protein
6. AMV pp32/Rous sarcoma virus (RSV) polymerase β subunit[94]
7. Human T-cell leukemia virus (HTLV) *gag/env*[25,26] and transforming gene product[27]
8. Tobacco mosaic virus (TMV) 30K protein[24]
9. Measles phosphoprotein[31] (identification of cloned gene)
10. Epstein-Barr virus nuclear antigen[123]
11. "Brain-specific" proteins[28]
12. Yeast mRNA maturase[29]
13. Human mitochondrial protein[30]

For discrimination among proteins of similar sequence
1. Actins[52]
2. Keratins[53]
3. Hu-*ras*^{T24} vs. Hu-*ras*^{HA}[51]
4. SV40 T antigens[89,120]
5. Murine leukemia virus glycopolypeptide[88]
6. Hepatitis B surface antigen subtypes[75]

For demonstration of similarities between related proteins
1. Platelet-derived growth factor and v-*sis*[32]
2. Herpes simplex virus type 1 and type 2 glycopeptides[110]

For analysis of proteolytic processing
1. Poliovirus polyprotein[38–40]
2. HTLV *gag/env* proteins[25,26]
3. v-*sis*[42]
4. MuLV polyprotein[34]
5. Enkephalins[41]
6. Fibrinogen[122]

For analysis of tissue or intracellular localization
1. RSV p60^{src}[47–49]
2. SV40 large T antigen[50]
3. Adenovirus E1A[43]
4. v-*myc*[36]
5. Y73 and Esh sarcoma virus-transforming gene products[49]
6. Hu-*ras*[51]
7. Actin[52]
8. Keratin[53]

For analysis of protein–protein association
1. RSV pp60^{src}[48,57,58]
2. Histones H3 and H4[54–56]
3. HLA[59]
4. SV40 large T/p53[60] (p53[121])

As probes of protein function
1. Poliovirus replicase[40]
2. Polyoma virus middle T[61]
3. pp60^{src}[48,65]
4. Transforming protein Abelson murine leukemia virus[64]
5. Transforming protein of feline sarcoma virus[63]
6. v-*myc*[66]

Table I. *(Continued)*

As immunogens to develop neutralizing sera or to protect against disease

1. TMV[1,2]
2. *Streptococcus pyogenes*[67]
3. Diptheria[68,69] or cholera[70] toxin
4. Foot and mouth disease virus[71,72]
5. Influenza virus[73,74]
6. Hepatitis virus[75,93,98]
7. Poliovirus[76]

Miscellaneous

1. Purification[77]
2. Radioimmunoassay[79]
3. Idiotype analysis[80–84]

of this. Based on analogy to other retroviruses, it would be predicted that a 48K precursor would be processed into polypeptides of 14K, 24K, and 9K. Antibodies were prepared to peptides predicted for each of the three products. As expected, each of the individual polypeptides could be detected in cell lines producing HTLV. Furthermore, the antibody recognizing the 24K product also detected a larger protein; pulse-chase experiments showed a precursor–product relationship between the two polypeptides.[28] Recently enkephalin-containing peptide has been analyzed using this approach.[41] Experiments on the processing of v-*sis* have strengthened the analogy to PDGF.[42] Studies on the adenovirus early regions E1A and E1B illustrate the possible use of peptide antibodies to sort out reading frames.[43–46] The E1B region, for example, gives rise to multiple, overlapping mRNAs and protein products. Green and co-workers have synthesized six peptides targeted against the NH_2 and COOH termini of both the presumptive 19K and 53K gene products.[45] Each antiserum precipitates the appropriate polypeptide, confirming the genome location and reading frame for each protein. The same study showed that the E1B 20K product shared common peptide determinants with the NH_2 terminus of the 53K protein.

Some of the uses of peptide antisera parallel those of traditional antisera. Immunochemical localization, for example, has been carried out frequently with such sera. For example, pp60^{src} has been shown to concentrate in remaining adhesion plaques and in cell–cell contact area.[47–49] One of the advantages of the antipeptide sera is that specificity can be easily demonstrated. There is a loss of fluorescence staining of pp60^{src} when the reaction is carried out in the presence of excess peptide. Very recently, monoclonal antibodies prepared toward Hu-*ras*^{T24} have been shown to stain human colon and mammary carcinomas.[51] This might make possible direct analysis of clinical material. A second advantage of the peptide antibody stems from the specificity conferred by the choice of peptide. Bulinski and colleagues prepared an antibody specific for the amino terminus of skeletal muscle α-actin after isolation of the 18-amino acid NH_2-terminal fragment.[52] The antiserum did not react with smooth muscle or brain isozymes. The antibody was then used to follow the appearance of the α-actin in developing myoblasts. The preparation of specific peptides has provided antisera for the staining of specific keratins.[53]

Increasingly, antibodies to synthetic peptides are being used to probe the topology and the activities of proteins. Work from van Regenmortel's laboratory has used antisera to peptides from H3 and H4 to probe the structure of the nucleosome.[54–56] For example, the COOH terminus of H3 seems to be equally exposed in free histone, nucleosomes, or chromatin subunits. By contrast, the association of pp60*src* with the cellular proteins pp50 and pp80 seems to prevent recognition of the protein by peptide antibodies.[48,57,58] Antibodies directed against HLA heavy chain sequences bind free heavy chains on nitrocellulose, but not heavy chains associated with β_2-microglobulin in solution.[59] A very striking result was obtained by Paucha and co-workers using peptide antibodies against SV40 large T.[60] Only large T complexed to the cellular protein p53 could be detected, but not free large T itself. This suggests that the conformation recognized by the peptide antiserum is one that is stabilized as the result of association with the cellular protein. The tyrosine kinase activities of several tumor viruses can be inhibited by antipeptide sera. The phosphorylation of polyoma virus middle T,[61,62] v-*fes* and v-*fps*,[63] and v-*abl*[64] are all drastically reduced when appropriate peptide antisera are used. Phosphorylation of exogenous substrates by v-*abl*[64] and v-*src*[48,65] are similarly reduced. Antibody to the COOH terminus of the poliovirus replicase inhibits both replicase and polyuridylic acid polymerase activities.[38] The DNA binding activity of v-*myc* can be inhibited by antibodies specific to 16 amino acids from residues 239–254.[66]

The hope that peptides could be used as immunogens to protect against disease has led to quite a large number of experiments.[18] While a detailed discussion of this work is not possible here, some results are worth noting. In a variety of cases synthetic peptides have been used to elicit antibodies that will neutralize viruses, bacteria, or toxins. Beachey and co-workers reported that a peptide from *Streptococcus pyogenes* M protein could induce antibodies in rabbits that could be used to protect mice against streptococcal challenge.[67] Active immunization can protect animals against the effects of diptheria toxin[68,69] or cholera toxin.[70] Effective protection in animals against foot and mouth disease virus has been demonstrated after immunization with peptides.[71,72] Other virus systems have been more difficult. However, significant progress has been achieved in the influenza/mouse[73,74] and hepatitis/chimpanzee[75] systems. Priming the immune response to virus by prior immunization with peptide has shown promise in studies on poliovirus.[76]

There are additional applications of peptide antibodies that should be mentioned, but do not fall into broad categories. In the long term the most important may be in affinity purification, as has been applied to the isolation of middle T antigen of polyoma virus.[77] The technique offers the potential advantage that the protein being purified can be released from the antibody by incubation with excess peptide. The harsher conditions often used in eluting proteins from affinity gels can be avoided by this methodology. As in the case of erythropoietin, peptides and antisera can be used to establish a radioimmunoassay.[78,79]

The difficulty in obtaining antigen to set up the assay is thereby avoided. Quite recently synthetic peptides have been used to probe the nature of idiotypes.[80–84]

3. Preparations of Antibodies to Synthetic Peptides

The preparation of antibody to a synthetic peptide is not really different than preparation of antibody to any hapten. The peptide sequence to be used is selected and synthesized. Very often the peptide is purchased commercially; two commonly used suppliers are Peninsula Labs (San Carlos, California) and Bachem (Torrance, California and Bubendorf, Switzerland). The peptide is coupled to a carrier protein. The animals are immunized and boosted with conjugate. Serum is then screened for antibody to the immunizing peptide or the protein containing its sequence. The next paragraphs will consider each of these steps more closely.

3.1. Selection of the Peptide

When the peptide antibody is needed to probe a specific protein sequence, the experimental problem dictates the choice of sequence. For example, the sequence around the principal phosphorylation site was used to prepare an antibody that could inhibit the phosphorylation of the polyoma virus middle T antigen. However, if all that is needed is an antibody that recognizes the protein, then the entire sequence becomes a potential target. The investigator must choose a peptide sequence with the greatest chance of success in eliciting an immune response.

There are several considerations in choosing a sequence. The sequence should be exposed on the surface of the protein. This means that a hydrophilic sequence is a likely choice. Hopp and Woods have shown that naturally occurring antigen determinants can be predicted based on hydrophilicity values calculated from the amino acid sequence.[84] Hydrophilic sequences have the practical advantage that the peptide will be soluble and easier to manipulate. Inspection of the peptides actually used in different studies indicates that every one has at least one charged residue; about three-fourths have either lysine or arginine residues and about two-thirds have acidic residues. A program written in BASIC has been published and can be used to calculate the Hopp–Woods hydrophilicity value of any protein.[85] Kyte and Doolittle have provided a method for calculating hydropathicity that gives a similar series of values.[86] Another consideration is conformational. Chou and Fasman, for example, have developed programs to predict protein secondary structure.[87] The work of Bayer and colleagues on the murine leukemia virus glycopolypeptide provides an example of the contribution of structure calculation in the selection of peptide sequence.[88] β-Turns are almost always found on the surface of proteins; recognition of proteins, for example, by enzymes involved in postsynthetic modifications such as phosphorylation and glycosylation, seems to very often involve sequences of β-turns. Proline is one amino acid very often associated with turns, and both the Hopp–Woods and Kyte–Doolittle programs include adjustments for proline. Surveying the peptides that people have actually used, about two-thirds contain at least one proline. The peptides lacking proline were generally chosen because a specific target was involved. The conclusion from this analysis is that a peptide containing charged amino acids as well as proline is a very likely candidate to be used as an immunogen. Very often the sequences at the ends of proteins have been chosen. As pointed out very early by Walter and colleagues,[89] the ends of the molecule may be less restricted in their conformation and by coupling at the COOH terminus of an NH_2-terminal peptide or at the NH_2-terminus of a COOH-terminal peptide it is possible to mimic the attachment in the native protein.

Once the decision has been made about which region of the protein to attack, the next question is, How long should the peptide be? For the most part this question is a practical one relating to cost or ease of synthesis. The shortest sequence routinely used is a hexapeptide. The COOH termini of middle T of polyoma virus[90] or of $pp60^{src}$ [57] are examples of sequences that have been used to elicit antibodies that recognize the corresponding proteins. A survey of the peptides used in a sample of the papers discussed here shows that out of 80 peptides, 18 were 6–9 residues long, 14 were 10–12 residues long, 20 were 13–15 residues long, and 28 were longer than 15 residues. Looking at the literature as a whole, it appears that somewhat longer peptides might be expected to be better. To quote, for example, the comment of Paucha and colleagues on a series of peptides to SV40 large T, "In general, the longer peptides elicited a stronger anti large T activity than the shorter ones."[60] In some instances investigators have compared the effectiveness of overlapping peptides. A clear conclusion from such results is difficult, because the variation from animal to animal immunized with the same peptide can be quite large and the numbers of animals used are usually small. Studies on overlapping peptides of the hepatitis envelope protein showed instances where a shorter peptide failed to elicit a response while a larger one worked well.[91] Pfaff and colleagues compared the effectiveness of a 16-amino acid peptide from foot and mouth disease virus protein with the effectiveness of the two octapeptides making up the larger sequence.[72] The longer sequence gave antibodies that were significantly higher titer against the immunizing peptide and that were strikingly better in the recognition of the protein. It should be noted, however, that in constrast to sequences usually chosen, this sequence was chosen from an α-helical region of the protein. The longer sequence in this case would be able to assume a configuration matching that in the protein much more easily. *A priori* a longer sequence might be expected to contain a larger number of possible antigenic determinants, since even very short sequences can exhibit multiple determinants. Green and colleagues showed that antisera to some of the influenza hemagglutinin peptides could react with different overlapping peptides that did not themselves share common sequence.[14]

Beyond the choice of peptide sequence, two technical considerations arise. Since the peptide is almost always coupled to a carrier protein, additional amino acids are sometimes added to simplify the coupling process. Cysteine permits easy coupling with sulfhydryl cross-linking agents such as *m*-maleimidobenzoyl *N*-hydroxysuccinimide ester (MBS).[14,92] Occasionally cysteines have been placed at both ends to permit the formation of a cyclic peptide. In some instances such a cyclic peptide is helpful.[93] In others, it has been less effective. Grandgenett and co-workers compared a linear and cyclic peptide for the avian retrovirus pp32 protein; they found the cyclic peptide was not as effective in inducing a response as the keyhole limpet hemocyanin (KLH)-coupled form.[94] Tyrosine is routinely added at the end of a sequence so that the peptide can be coupled with bis-diazobenzidine.[89] Occasionally linker amino acid(s) have been inserted between the peptide sequence and the carrier in analogy to the spacer arms used in affinity chromatography. There is no reason to believe that this is routinely necessary. For labeling purposes either a radioactive amino acid can be added during synthesis or a tyrosine can be included to permit labeling with ^{125}I.

3.2. Conjugation with Carrier Proteins

The peptides are almost always conjugated to a carrier protein. Comparison of immunizations with conjugated and unconjugated erythropoietin, for example, showed that the conjugated form worked better.[78] An interesting exception to this is recent work from Atassi's laboratory, in which small peptides from myoglobin have been used for immunization.[95–97] The usual variety of carrier proteins have been employed. Keyhole limpet hemocyanin and bovine serum albumin have been used with approximately equal frequency in about 80% of the work reviewed here. Thyroglobulin, edestin, and tetanus toxoid were also used in some instances. In rarer cases, synthetic copolymers were chosen. One very recent application describes the covalent coupling of hepatitis virus protein sequences to liposomes.[98] The choice of a carrier sometimes depends upon the application envisioned. As pointed out by Walter and Doolittle,[19] when studying intracellular localization in cells grown in serum-containing medium, antibody to bovine serum albumin used as a carrier could potentially cause difficulties. Sutcliffe and colleagues encountered problems in immunolocalization experiments because antibodies to the KLH carrier stained brain samples.[28] Switching to thyroglobulin or edestin carriers alleviated the problem.

The choice of cross-linker is ordinarily made to avoid unusual internal linking between carrier and peptide. However, it should be noted that some laboratories have successfully produced peptide antibodies using cross-linking agents with the potential to form internal links. Presumably the resulting product consists of an ensemble of the possible configurations.

Any of the standard methods available for protein–protein cross-linking can be applied. The book edited by Jaffe and Behrman is the traditional source of many of the techniques.[99] Glutaraldehyde is the most commonly used cross-linking agent. It is difficult to imagine a simpler reaction.[100] Glutaraldehyde is added in aliquots to a mixture of carrier and peptide in phosphate buffer. The chemistry of glutaraldehyde is also especially attractive.[101] In neutral solution it consists of a heterologous collection of polymers $\{CHO—(CH_2)_2—CH{=}[{=}C(CHO)—(CH_2)_2—CH{=}]_n{=}C(CHO)—(CH_2)_2—CHO\}$. This means that the peptide is linked to the carrier with variable spacing; the peptide antigen is presented to the host in a number of configurations. *m*-Maleimidobenzoyl-*N*-hydroxysuccinimide ester (MBS) is commonly used to couple cysteine residues that have been added at the ends of sequences.[14,92] MBS and glutaraldehyde account for about two-thirds of all peptide–carrier conjugations. Water-soluble carbodimides are zero-length cross-linkers, which offer one significant advantage. Depending on the reaction conditions, the peptide can be coupled to the carrier through either the NH_2 terminus or the COOH terminus. This is desirable where a peptide is being chosen from one end of the protein sequence; the antigen should also be presented in the same configuration. The procedure, published by Tamura and colleagues,[58] involves first reacting the peptide or carrier protein at pH 3.0 and then adding the second component at pH 9.0. Diaminobenzidine is commonly used for cross-linking through added tyrosine residues.[102]

3.3. Immunization

The great majority of the antisera to synthetic peptides have been derived by immunizing rabbits. No one has reported systematic studies on the effects of different immunization protocols. An "average" protocol might be the immunization with 500 μg conjugate in complete Freund's adjuvant, followed by boosts of conjugate in incomplete Freund's at intervals of 3 weeks to 1 month. Persistence is important because several boosts may be necessary to obtain the best response. Also, Patschinsky and colleagues have pointed out that even though boosting may not increase titer, it may be useful in preventing a loss of titer.[37] It is clearly important to immunize a number of animals. Sometimes not all animals will respond to the immunizing peptide to give a good titer serum. Assay of titer of different sera toward the same peptide shows differences of as much as a factor of 16.[91] There is potentially a more significant problem. Antisera that have similar titers toward the peptide antigen will differ strikingly in their ability to recognize the protein containing the sequence. Neurath and colleagues observed an equilibrium constant of $4 \times 10^5\ M^{-1}$ for the association of antibody with hepatitis surface antigen.[98] By comparison, the equilibrium constant for the interaction with peptide was greater than $10^7\ M^{-1}$. For peptide antisera against MuLV glycopeptides, sera with the same titer toward the peptide could also differ by two logs in their reactivity with the protein.[88] There has been a recent suggestion that priming the animal with anti-idiotype antibodies may be of some use in improving the response.[104]

Recently reports have begun to characterize the preparation of monoclonal antibodies toward synthetic peptides. Monoclonals to peptides of HLA,[102] pp60^{src}, [106]*ras*,[51] v-*fes*,[102] myoglobin,[96] and the influenza hemagglutinin[98] have all been reported. Such reagents are intriguing from both a practical and theoretical point of view. From a practical point of view, monoclonals should be of value in purification. Efforts to purify proteins such as polyoma middle T antigen have been hampered by difficulties in elution of the protein with the peptide. By the choice of an appropriate affinity-class monoclonal it should be possible to establish rapid mild purification techniques.

The recognition of proteins by antipeptide monoclonals seems to be a high-frequency event.[15,105] This is quite a startling result. Originally it was presumed that only the fraction of antibody directed against the conformational state of the peptide matching that of the protein would react with the intact protein. The results obtained with the monoclonals suggest that there may be flexibility in structure of the antigen, antibody, or both. Work from Sela's laboratory showed some time ago that antibody binding can have the potential to shift the conformational equilibrium of a copolymer.[107] Antibodies to the α-helical form of Tyr-Ala-Glu could bind to intermediate-length copolymers, inducing a transition to an α-helical state.

3.4. Analysis of the Peptide Response

The standard method of analyzing the response to the peptide is the enzyme-linked immunoabsorbant assay (ELISA).[108,109] The peptide can either be adsorbed to the well directly, or a conjugate prepared using a heterologous carrier can be used instead. The extent of the reaction under the two circumstances may be different.[88] Also, because recognition of the protein and the peptide may not be identical, it is desirable to screen the antisera for activity toward the protein. Prudence dictates screening the samples both by Western blotting and by direct immunoprecipitation. In the case of herpes simplex virus glycoprotein C, peptide antibody would react with the protein in an ELISA assay, in immunofluorescence tests on fixed cells, and on Western blots, but not in solution.[110] For the oligopeptide from murine leukemia virus, recognition of the protein target was successful on plates but not in solution.[88] Such observations suggest that the process of preparing the ELISA plates may result in the exposure of the determinant. In all cases, confirmation of the specificity of the reaction is made by demonstrating that the peptide efficiently inhibits the reaction.

The possibility of cross-reactivities must be evaluated for each antiserum, since cross-reactions have been frequently reported. Like the homologous reactions, these cross-reactions can be blocked by incubation in the presence of peptide. The simplest form of cross-reaction is between similar proteins of different virus strains. The HSV type 1 and HSV type 2 glycoprotein Cs will both react with a peptide antibody directed against type 1.[110] Cross-reactivities occur sometimes between homologous proteins of different viruses. For example, the antiserum directed against the NH_2-terminus of SV40 large T will react with the large T antigen of polyoma virus.[111] Sometimes this can be put to practical application. Gentry and Rohrschneider have used an antiserum directed against the pp60*src* sequence (Cys-Tryp-**Arg**-Lys-Asp-Pro-**Glu**-Glu-Arg-Pro-Thr-Phe-**Lys**-Thr-**Leu**) to study the Y73 *yes* gene products.[49] P90 and P80 are expected to differ from pp60*src* at the four amino acids indicated in boldface: Arg to Lys, Glu to Asp, Lys to Glu, and Leu to Ileu. When antisera are used in higher concentrations, more distant cross-reactivities can be demonstrated. Nigg and colleagues noticed that their antiserum directed against pp60*src* would also react with structures in normal cells, such as the microtubules.[112] This reactivity was especially prominent when the antiserum was used at higher concentration. These workers suggested that the cross-reaction might have arisen from a sequence in β-tubulin that showed some similarity to the sequence of the pp60*src* peptide. Different antisera against the same peptide do not always detect the same cross-reacting species. Ito and colleagues detected a 130K cellular protein that cross-reacted with a nonapeptide sequence from polyoma virus middle T,[113] which was not observed with different antisera[61] against the same peptide. The appearance of cross-reactions is hardly surprising, since they have often been observed with monoclonal antibodies. Monoclonals directed against large T antigen of SV40 have encountered a number of different cross-reacting cellular proteins.[114] In the SV40 case the monoclonal antibodies that reacted with cellular proteins were all against determinants that were insensitive to denaturation. Peptide antibodies are generally of this sort. The less common occurrence of interference by antibodies in the serum directed against the carrier protein has been discussed earlier. In a number of instances antiserum has been freed of antibody to the carrier by passage through an affinity column to which the carrier has been coupled (e.g. Ref. 47).

4. A Specific Example of the Use of Antipeptide Antibody: Polyoma Middle T Antigen

To show how the points discussed generally in the previous sections can be applied specifically, it is worth describing the application of this methodology to a specific experimental situation, the study of the polyoma middle T antigen. The early region of the polyoma virus genome encodes three proteins: large T, middle T, and small T antigen.[115] Because of the patterns of mRNA splicing, middle T shares a common NH_2-terminal sequence with the other two proteins, but has its own COOH-terminal sequence. Ordinarily middle T is detected by antitumor serum that recognizes all three proteins. The middle T antigen is required for viral transformation. It has an associated tyrosine kinase activity that arises as a result of association with the cellular homologue of pp60*src*.[116] This tyrosine kinase results in the phosphorylation of middle T antigen; the major phosphorylation site is tyrosine-315, but tyrosine-322 and to a limited extent tyrosine-250 are labeled.[61,117,118]

The availability of an immunologic reagent specific for middle T but unreactive with large T antigen and small T antigen was highly desirable. Two different sequences have been used to generate antibodies. Walter and colleagues used the COOH-terminal amino acids to raise an antibody specific for middle T.[90] The antibody has been used for the rapid 2500-fold purification of the protein in limited amounts.[77] Cellular proteins cross-react with the antibody. In this instance, this is perhaps expected. The COOH-terminal region of the protein is involved in anchoring middle T into the membrane; its sequence is similar to that of other membrane proteins.[118]

The approach taken by us[61] and more recently in other laboratories[62,113] focuses on sequences around the major phosphorylation site.[61,62,113] The nonapeptide Glu-Glu-Glu-Glu-Tyr-Met-Pro-Met-Glu (residues 311–319) spans the major phosphorylation site at tyrosine residue 315. Since there are no internal lysine residues, the peptide was coupled to bovine serum albumin using glutaraldehyde or dimethylsuberimidate.[61] Antibody was raised with the glutaraldehyde-coupled material in rabbits that is specific for middle T. No response was observed with the dimethylsuberimidate cross-linked material. However, only one animal was used, so the significance of this observation is uncertain. Interestingly, the antibody is sensitive to the state of phosphorylation at tyrosine-315. It does not recognize the protein if tyrosine-315 is phosphorylated prior to binding. The antibody will recognize a mutant middle T in which the tyrosine has been replaced by a phenylalanine.[119] The phosphorylation of middle T in immunoprecipitates made with the antipeptide serum is inhibited approximately 20-fold compared to those made with anti-T serum. This was expected because the antibody binds at or very near the phosphorylation site. Both the phosphorylation at residue 315 and the phosphorylation at residue 322 are affected. The results of Ito and colleagues with the same peptide show that different antisera may have different properties.[113] Their serum will recognize middle T that is phosphorylated prior to antibody binding. Also, their serum cross-reacts with a 130K cell protein not detected with the earlier serum.

5. Conclusion

The ability to create immunologic reagents sensitive to specific amino acid sequences is now within the reach of every laboratory. The work of the past few years shows that it is possible to discriminate between proteins of very similar sequence. There will certainly be instances where the need for conformation-dependent antibodies renders this approach unsuitable. However, it is now possible to probe the functions and interactions among proteins in calculated fashion. The value of the method will be limited only by our ingenuity in its use.

Acknowledgments. I would like to thank Dr. Beverly Bockus for a critical reading of the manuscript. I am an Established Investigator of the American

Heart Association. The work in my laboratory is supported by a grant from the National Cancer Institute, RO1-CA-34722.

References

1. Anderer, F., 1963, Preparation and properties of an artificial antigen immunologically related to tobacco mosaic virus, *Biochim. Biophys. Acta* **71**:246–248.
2. Anderer, F., and Schlumberger, H., 1965, Properties of artificial antigens immunologically related to tobacco mosaic virus, *Biochim. Biophys. Acta* **97**:503–509.
3. Langbeheim, H., Arnon, R., and Sela, M., 1976, Antiviral effect of MS2 coliphage obtained with a synthetic antigen, *Proc. Natl. Acad. Sci. USA* **73**:4636–4640.
4. Fearney, F., Leung, C., Young, J. D., and Benjamini, E., 1971, The specificity of antibodies to a peptide determinant of TMV protein induced by immunization of the peptide conjugate, *Biochim. Biophys. Acta* **243**:509–514.
5. Furie, B., Schechter, A., Sachs, D., and Anfinsen, C., 1974, Antibodies to the unfolded form of a helix rich region in staphylococcal nuclease, *Biochemistry* **13**:1561–1566.
6. Furie, B., Schechter, A., Sachs, D., and Anfinsen, C., 1975. An immunological approach to the conformational equilibrium of staphyloccocal nuclease, *J. Mol. Biol.* **92**:497–506.
7. Lau, H., Rosenberg, J., Beeler, D., and Rosenberg, R., 1979, The isolation and characterization of specific antibody population directed against prothrombin activation fragments F2 and F1,2*, *J. Biol. Chem.* **254**:8751–8761.
8. Benjamin, D., Berzofsky, J., East, I., Gurd, F., Hannum, C., Leach, S., Margoliash, E., Michael, J., Miller, A., Prager, E., Reichlin, M., Sercarz, E., Smith-Gill, S., Todd, P., and Wilson, A., 1984, The antigenic structure of proteins: A reappraisal, *Annu. Rev. Immunol.* **2**:67–101.
9. Atassi, M., 1975, Antigenic structure of myoglobin: The complete immunochemical anatomy of a protein and conclusions relating to antigenic structures of proteins, *Immunochemistry* **12**:423–438.
10. Schechter, B., Schechter, I., Ramachandran, J., Conway-Jacobs, A., Sela, M., Benjamin, E., and Shimizu, M., 1971, Synthetic antigens with sequential and conformation-dependent determinants containing the same L-tyr-L-ala-L-glu sequence, *Eur. J. Biochem.* **20**:309–320.
11. Arnon, R., 1977, Immunochemistry of lysozyme, in: *Immunochemistry of Enzymes and Their Antibodies* (M. Salton, ed.), Wiley, New York, pp. 1–19.
12. Ibrahimi, I., Eder, J., Prager, E., Wilson, A., and Arnon, R., 1980, The effect of a single amino acid substitution on the antigenic specificity of the loop region of lysozome, *Mol. Immunol.* **17**:37–46.
13. Atassi, M., and Lee, C., 1978, The precise and entire antigenic structure of native lysozyme, *Biochem. J.* **171**:429–434.
14. Green, N., Alexander, H., Olson, A., Alexander, S., Shinnick, T., Sutcliffe, J., and Lerner, R., 1982, Immunogenic structure of the influenza virus hemagglutinin, *Cell* **28**:477–487.
15. Wilson, I., Niman, H., Houghten, R., Cherenson, A., Connolly, M., and Lerner, R., 1984, The structure of an antigenic determinant in a protein, *Cell* **37**:767–778.
16. Lerner, R., 1982, Mapping the immunologic repertoire to produce antibodies of predetermined specificity, *Nature* **299**:592–596.
17. Sutcliffe, J., Shinnick, T., Green, N., and Lerner, R., 1983, Antibodies that react with predetermined sites on proteins, *Science* **219**:660–666.
18. Shinnick, T., Sutcliffe, J., Green, N., and Lerner, R., 1983, Synthetic peptide immunogens as vaccines, *Annu. Rev. Microbiol.* **37**:425–446.
19. Walter, G., and Doolittle, R., 1983, Antibodies against synthetic peptides, *Genet. Eng.* **5**:61–91.
20. Papkoff, J., Lai, L., Hunter, T., and Verma, I., 1981, Analysis of transforming gene products from Moloney murine sarcoma virus, *Cell* **27**:109–119.
21. Papkoff, J., Verma, I., and Hunter, T., 1982, Detection of a transforming gene product in cells transformed by Moloney murine sarcoma virus, *Cell* **29**:417–426.

22. Robbins, K., Devare, S., Reddy, E., and Aaronson, S., 1982, *In vivo* identification of the transforming gene product of simian sarcoma virus, *Science* **218:**1131–1133.
23. Devare, S., Reddy, E., Law, J., Robbins, K., and Aaronson, S., 1983, Nucleotide sequence of the simian sarcoma virus genome: Demonstration that its acquired cellular sequences encode the transforming gene product $p28^{sis}$, *Proc. Natl. Acad. Sci. USA* **80:**731–735.
24. Ooshika, I., Watanabe, Y., Meshi, T., Okada, Y., Igano, K., Inoue, K., and Yoshida, N., 1984, Identification of the 30K protein of TMV by immunoprecipitation with antibodies directed against a synthetic peptide, *Virology* **132:**71–78.
25. Hattori, S., Imagawa, K., Shimizu, F., Hashimura, E., Seiki, M., and Yoshida, M., 1983, Identification of envelope glycoprotein encoded by *env* gene of HTLV, *Gann* **74:**790–793.
26. Hattori, S., Kiyokawa, T., Imagawa, K., Shimizu, F., Hashimura, E., Seiki, M., and Yoshida, M., 1984, Identification of *gag* and *env* products of HTLV, *Virology* **136:**338–347.
27. Slamon, D., Shimotohno, K., Cline, M., Golde, D., and Chen, I., 1984, Identification of the putative transforming protein of human T-cell leukemia viruses HTLV-I and HTLV-II, *Science* **226:**61–64.
28. Sutcliffe, J., Milner, J., Shinnick, T., and Bloom, F., 1983, Identifying the protein products of the brain-specific genes with antibodies to chemically synthesized peptides, *Cell* **33:**671–682.
29. Guiso, N., Dreyfus, M., Siffert, O., Danchin, A., Spyridakis, A., Gargouri, A., Claisse, M., and Slonimski, P., 1984, Antibodies against synthetic oligopeptides allow identification of the yeast mRNA-maturase encoded by the second intron of the yeast *cob–box* gene, *EMBO J.* **3:**1769–1772.
30. Mariottini, P., Chomyn, A., Attardi, G., Trovato, D., Strong, D., and Doolittle, R., 1983, Antibodies against synthetic peptides reveal that the unidentified reading frame AGL, overlapping the ATPase 6 gene is expressed in human mitochondria, *Cell* **32:**1269–1277.
31. Bellini, W., Englund, G., Richardson, C., and Rozenblatt, S., 1984, Positive identification of a measles virus cDNA clone encoding a region of the phosphoprotein, *J. Virol.* **50:**939–942.
32. Niman, H., 1984, Antisera to a synthetic peptide of the *sis* viral oncogene product recognize human platelet-derived growth factor, *Nature* **307:**180–183.
33. Sutcliffe, J., Shinnick, T., Green, N., Liu, F., Niman, H., and Lerner, R., 1980, Chemical synthesis of a polypeptide predicted from nucleotide sequence allows detection of a new retroviral gene product, *Nature* **287:**801–805.
34. Green, N., Shinnick, T., Witte, O., Ponticeli, A., Sutcliffe, J., and Lerner, R., 1981, Sequence-specific antibodies show that maturation of Moloney leukemia virus envelope polyprotein involves removal of a COOH-terminal peptide, *Proc. Natl. Acad. Sci. USA* **78:**6023–6028.
35. Boyle, W., Lipsick, J., Reddy, E., and Baluda, M., 1983, Identification of the leukemogenic protein of avian myeloblastosis virus and of its normal cellular homologue, *Proc. Natl. Acad. Sci. USA* **80:**2834–2838.
36. Hann, S., Abrams, H., Rohrschneider, L., and Eisenman, R., 1983. Proteins encoded by v-*myc* and c-*myc* oncogenes: Identification and localization in acute leukemia virus transformants and bursal lymphoma cell lines, *Cell* **34:**789–798.
37. Patschinsky, T., Walter, G., and Bister, K., 1984, Immunological analysis of v-*myc* gene products using antibodies against a *myc*-specific synthetic peptide, *Virology* **136:**348–358.
38. Baron, M., and Baltimore, D., 1983, Antibodies against the chemically synthesized genome-linked protein of poliovirus react with native virus-specific proteins, *Cell* **28:**395–404.
39. Semler, B., Anderson, C., Hanecak, R., Dorner, L., and Wimmer, E., 1982, A membrane-associated precursor to poliovirus VPg identified by immunoprecipitation with antibodies directed against a synthetic heptapeptide, *Cell* **28:**405–412.
40. Baron, M., and Baltimore, D., 1982, Antibodies against a synthetic peptide of the poliovirus replicase protein: Reaction with native, virus-encoded proteins and inhibition of virus-specific polymerase activities *in vitro*, *J. Virol.* **43:**969–978.
41. Lahm, H., Gerber, L., Brink, L., Kilpatrick, D., and Udenfriend, S., 1983, Specific polyclonal antibodies to the carboxyl terminus of [Met] enkephalin-Arg^6-Gly^7-Leu^8, *Arch. Biochem. Biophys.* **225:**422–429.

42. Robbins, K., Antoniades, H., Devare, S., Hunkapiller, M., and Aaronson, S., 1983, Structural and immunological similarities between simian sarcoma virus gene products and human platelet-derived growth factor, *Nature* **305**:605–608.
43. Feldman, L., and Nevins, J., 1983, Localization of the adenovirus E1A_a protein, a positive-acting transcriptional factor, in infected cells, *Mol. Cell. Biol.* **3**:829–838.
44. Yee, S., Rowe, D., Tremblay, M., McDermott, M., and Branton, P., 1983, Identification of human adenovirus early region 1 products by using antisera against synthetic peptides corresponding to the predicted carboxyterminus, *J. Virol* **46**:1003–1013.
45. Green, M., Brackmann, K., Lucher, L., and Symington, J., 1983, Antibodies to synthetic peptides of the transforming genes to human adenoviruses: An approach to understanding early viral gene function, *Curr. Top. Microbiol. Immunol.* **109**:167–191.
46. Lucher, L., Kimelman, D., Symington, J., Brackmann, K., Cartas, M., Thornton, H., and Green, M., 1984, Identification of Ad 12-encoded E1A tumor antigens synthesized in infected and transformed mammalian cells and in *E. coli*, *J. Virol.* **52**:136–144.
47. Nigg, E., Sefton, B., Hunter, T., Walter, G., and Singer, J., 1982, Immunofluorescent localization of the transforming protein of Rous sarcoma virus with antibodies against a synthetic peptide, *Proc. Natl. Acad. Sci.* **79**:5322–5326.
48. Gentry, L., Rohrschneider, L., Casnellie, J., and Krebs, E., 1983, Antibodies to a defined region of $pp60^{src}$ neutralize the tyrosine-specific kinase activity, *J. Biol. Chem.* **258**:11219–11228.
49. Gentry, L., and Rohrschneider, L., 1984, Common features of the *yes* and *src* gene products defined by peptide specific antibodies, *J. Virol.* **51**:539–546.
50. Deppert, W., and Walter, G., 1982, Domains of simian virus 40 large T antigen exposed on the cell surface, *Virology* **122**:56–70.
51. Horan Hand, P., Wunderlich, T., Muraro, R., Caruso, A., and Schlom, J., 1984, Monoclonal antibodies of predefined specificity detect activated *ras* gene expression in human mammary and colon carcinomas, *Proc. Natl. Acad. Sci. USA* **81**:5227–5231.
52. Bulinski, J., Kumar, S., Titani, K., and Hauschka, S., 1984, Peptide antibody specific for the amino terminus of skeletal muscle actin, *Proc. Natl. Acad. Sci. USA* **80**:1506–1510.
53. Roop, D., Cheng, C., Titterington, L., Meyers, C., Stanley, J., Steinert, P., and Yuspa, S., 1984, Synthetic peptides corresponding to keratin subunits elicit highly specific antibodies, *J. Biol. Chem.* **259**:8037–8040.
54. Muller, S., Himmelspach, K., and Van Regenmortel, M., 1982, Immunochemical localization of histone H3 at the surface of chromatin subunits, *EMBO J.* **1**:939–944.
55. Muller, S., Soussanieh, A., Bouley, J., Reinbolt, J., and Van Regenmortel, M., 1983, *Biochim. Biophys. Acta* **747**:100–106.
56. Muller, S., Mazen, A., Martinage, A., and Van Regenmortel, M., 1984, Use of histone antibodies for studying chromatin topography and the phosphorylation of chromatin subunits, *EMBO J.* **3**:2431–2436.
57. Sefton, B., and Walter, G., 1982, Antiserum for the carboxy terminus of the transforming protein of Rous sarcoma virus, *J. Virol.* **44**:467–474.
58. Tamura, T., Bauer, H., Birr, C., and Pipkorn, R., 1983, Antibodies against synthetic peptides as a tool for functional analysis of the transforming protein $pp60^{src}$, *Cell* **34**:587–596.
59. Church, W., Walker, L., Houghten, R., and Reisfeld, R., 1983, Anti-HLA antibodies of predetermined specificity: A chemically synthesized peptide induces antibodies specific for HLA-A,B heavy chain, *Proc. Natl. Acad. Sci. USA* **80**:255–258.
60. Paucha, E., Harvey, R., and Smith, A., 1984, Immunoprecipitation of some forms of SV40 large T antigen by antibodies to synthetic peptides, *J. Virol.* **51**:670–681.
61. Schaffhausen, B., Benjamin, T., Pike, L., Casnellie, J., and Krebs, E., 1982, Antibody to the nonapeptide Glu-Glu-Glu-Glu-Tyr-Met-Pro-Met-Glu is specific for polyoma middle T antigen and inhibits *in vitro* kinase activity, *J. Biol. Chem.* **257**:12467–12470.
62. Harvey, R., Oostra, B., Belsham, G., Gillett, P., and Smith, A., 1984, An antibody to a synthetic peptide recognizes polyomarvirus middle T antigen and reveals multiple *in vitro* tyrosine phosphorylation sites, *Mol. Cell. Biol.* **4**:1334–1342.

63. Sen, S., Houghten, R., Sherr, C., and Sen, A., 1983, Antibodies of predetermined specificity detect two retroviral oncogene products and inhibit their kinase activities, *Proc. Natl. Acad. Sci. USA* **80:**1246–1250.
64. Konopka, J., Davis, R., Watanabe, S., Ponticelli, A., Schiff-maker, L., Rosenberg, N., and Witte, O., 1984, Only site directed antibodies reactive with the highly conserved *src*-homologous region of the v-*abl* protein neutralize kinase activity, *J. Virol.* **51:**223–232.
65. Wong, T., and Goldberg, A., 1981, Synthetic peptide fragment of *src* gene product inhibits the *src* protein kinase and cross-reacts immunologically with avian *onc* kinases and cellular phosphoproteins, *Proc. Natl. Acad. Sci. USA* **78:**7412–7416.
66. Bunte, T., Donner, P., Pfaff, E., Reis, B., Greiser-Wilkie, I., Schaller, H., and Moelling, K., 1984, Inhibition of DNA binding of purified $p55^{V\text{-}myc}$ *in vitro* by antibodies against bacterially synthesized *myc* protein and a synthetic peptide, *EMBO J.* **3:**1919–1924.
67. Beachey, E., Seyer, J., Dale, J., Simpson, A., and Kang, A., 1981, Type specific protective immunity evoked by synthetic peptide of *S. pyogenes* M, *Nature* **292:**457–459.
68. Audibert, F., Jolivet, M., Chedid, L., Alouf, J., Boquet, P., Rivaille, P., and Siffert, O., 1981, Active anti-toxic immunization by a synthetic diptheria toxin synthetic oligopeptide, *Nature* **289:**593–594.
69. Audibert, F., Jolivet, M., Chedid, L., Arnon, R., and Sela, M., 1982, Successful immunization with a totally synthetic diptheria vaccine, *Proc. Natl. Acad. Sci. USA* **79:**5042–5046.
70. Jacob, C., Sela, M., and Arnon, R., Antibodies against synthetic peptides of the B subunit of cholera toxin: cross-reaction and neutralization of toxin, *Proc. Natl. Acad. Sci. USA* **80:**7611–7615.
71. Bittle, J., Houghton, R., Alexander, H., Shinnick, T., Sutcliffe, J., and Lerner, R., 1982, Protection against foot-and-mouth disease by immunization with a chemically synthesized peptide predicted from the viral nucleotide sequence, *Nature* **298:**30–33.
72. Pfaff, E., Mussgay, M., Bohm, H., Schulz, G., and Schaller, H., 1982, Antibodies against preselected peptides recognize and neutralize foot-and-mouth disease virus, *EMBO J.* **1:**869–874.
73. Muller, G., Shapira, M., and Arnon, R., 1982, Anti-influenza response achieved by immunization with a synthetic conjugate, *Proc. Natl. Acad. Sci. USA* **79:**569–573.
74. Shapira, M., Jibson, M., Muller, G., and Arnon, R., 1984, Immunity and protection against influenza induced by synthetic peptide corresponding to antigenic sites of hemagglutinin, *Proc. Natl. Acad. Sci. USA* **81:**2461–2465.
75. Gerin, J., Alexander, H., Shih, J., Purcell, R., Dapolito, G., Engle, R., Green, N., Sutcliffe, J., Shinnick, T., and Lerner, R., 1983, Chemically synthesized peptides of hepatitis B surface antigen duplicate the d/y specificities and induce subtype specific antibodies in chimpanzees, *Proc. Natl. Acad. Sci. USA* **80:**2365–2369.
76. Emini, E., Jameson, B., and Wimmer, E., 1983, Priming for and induction of anti-poliovirus neutralizing antibodies by synthetic peptides, *Nature* **304:**699–703.
77. Walter, G., Hutchinson, M., Hunter, T., and Eckhart, W., 1982, Purification of polyoma virus medium T antigen by immunoaffinity chromatography, *Proc. Natl. Acad. Sci. USA* **79:**4025–4029.
78. Sue, J., and Sytkowski, A., 1983, Site-specific antibodies to human erythropoietin directed toward the NH_2-region, *Proc. Natl. Acad. Sci. USA* **80:**3651–3655.
79. Sytkowski, A., and Sue, J., 1984, A novel radioimmunoassay for human erythropoietin using a synthetic NH_2-terminal peptide and anti-peptide antibodies, *J. Immunol. Meth.* **69:**181–186.
80. Alexander, H., Johnson, D., Rosen, J., Jerabek, L., Green, N., Weissman, I., and Lerner, R., 1983, Mimicking the alloantigenicity of proteins with chemically synthesized peptides differing in single amino acids, *Nature* **306:**697–699.
81. Seiden, M., Clevinger, B., McMillan, S., Srouji, A., Lerner, R., and Davie, J., 1984, Chemical synthesis of idiotypes: Evidence that antisera to the same JH1 peptide detect multiple binding site-associated idiotypes, *J. Exp. Med.* **159:**1338–1350.
82. Chen, P., Fong, S., Normansell, D., Houghten, R., Karras, J., Vaughan, J., and Carson, D., 1984, Delineation of a cross-reactive idiotype on human autoantibodies with an antibody against a synthetic peptide, *J. Exp. Med.* **159:**1502–1511.

83. Chen, P., Houghten, R., Fong, S., Rhodes, G., Gilbertson, T., Vaughan, J., Lerner, R., and Carson, D., 1984, Anti-hypervariable region antibody induced by a defined peptide: An approach for studying the structural correlates of idiotypes, *Proc. Natl. Acad. Sci. USA* **81**:1784–1788.
84. Hopp, T., and Woods, K., 1981, Prediction of protein antigenic determinants from amino acid sequences, *Proc. Natl. Acad. Sci. USA* **78**:3824–3828.
85. Hopp, T., and Woods, K., 1983, A computer program for predicting protein antigenic determinants, *Mol. Immunol.* **20**:483–489.
86. Kyte, J., and Doolittle, R., 1982, A simple method for displaying the hydropathic character of a protein, *J. Mol. Biol.* **157**:105–132.
87. Chou, P., and Fasman, G., 1978, Prediction of protein secondary structure, *Adv. Enzymol.* **47**:251–276.
88. Bayer, H., Gruber, W., Schneider, J., and Hunsmann, G., 1984, Structural and immunological characterization of Friend murine leukemia virus glycopeptide using synthetic oligopeptides, *EMBO J.* **3**:1925–1930.
89. Walter, G., Scheidtmann, K., Carbone, A., Laudano, A., and Doolittle, R., 1980, Antibodies specific for the carboxy- and amino-terminal regions of SV40 large T antigen, *Proc. Natl. Acad. Sci. USA* **77**:5197–5200.
90. Walter, G., Hutchinson, M., Hunter, T., and Eckhart, W., 1981, Antibodies specific for polyoma virus middle-sized tumor antigen, *Proc. Natl. Acad. Sci. USA* **79**:4025–4029.
91. Lerner, R., Green, N., Alexander, H., Liu, F., Sutcliffe, J., and Shinnick, T., 1981, Chemically synthesized peptides predicted from the nucleotide sequence of the hepatitis B virus genome elicit antibodies reactive with the native envelope protein of Dane particles, *Proc. Natl. Acad. Sci. USA* **78**:3403–3407.
92. Liu, F., Zinnecker, M., Hamaoka, T., and Katz, D., 1979, New procedures for preparation and isolation of conjugates of proteins and a synthetic copolymer of D amino acids and immunochemical characterization of such conjugates, *Biochemistry* **18**:690–697.
93. Dreesman, G., Sanchez, Y., Ionescu-Matiu, I., Sparrow, J., Six, H., Peterson, D., Hollinger, F., and Melnick, J., 1982, Antibody to hepatitis B surface antigen after a single inoculation of uncoupled synthetic peptide, *Nature* **295**:158–160.
94. Grandgenett, D., Knaus, R., and Hippenmeyer, P., 1983, Antibodies against a synthetic peptide of the avian retrovirus pp32 protein and the β DNA polymerase, *Virology* **130**:257–262.
95. Young, C., Schmitz, H., and Atassi, M., 1983, Antibodies with specificities to preselected protein regions evoked by free synthetic peptides representing protein antigenic sites or other surface locations: Demonstration with myoglobin, *Mol. Immunol.* **20**:567–570.
96. Schmitz, H., Atassi, H., and Atassi, M., 1983, Production of monoclonal antibodies with preselected submolecular binding specificities to protein determinants: Demonstration with sperm whale myoglobin, *Mol. Immunol.* **19**:1699–1702.
97. Schmitz, H., Atassi, H., and Atassi, M., 1983, Production of monoclonal antibodies with preselected submolecular binding specificities to protein antigenic sites: Antibodies to sperm whale myoglobin sites, *Mol. Immunol.* **20**:719–726.
98. Neurath, A., Kent, S., and Strick, N., 1984, Location and chemical synthesis of a pre-S gene coded immunodominant epitope of hepatitis B virus, *Science* **224**:392–395.
99. Jaffe, B., and Behrman, H. (eds), 1979, *Methods of Hormone Radioimmunoassay*, Academic Press, New York.
100. Kagan, A., and Glick, S., 1979, Oxytocin, in: *Methods of Hormone Radioimmunoassay* (B. Jaffe and H. Behrman, eds.), Academic Press, New York, pp. 327–339.
101. Peters, K., and Richards, F., 1977, Chemical cross-linking reagents and problems in studies of membrane structure, *Annu. Rev. Biochem.* **46**:523–551.
102. Bassiri, R., Dvorak, J., and Utiger, R., 1979, Thyrotropin-releasing hormone, in: *Methods of Hormone Radioimmunoassay* (B. Jaffe and H. Behrman, eds.), Academic Press, New York, pp. 45–56.
103. Neurath, A., Kent, S., and Strick, N., 1982, Specificity of antibodies elicited by a synthetic peptide having a sequence in common with a fragment of a virus protein, the hepatitis B surface antigen, *Proc. Natl. Acad. Sci. USA* **79**:7871–7875.

104. Kennedy, R., Sparrow, J., Sanchez, Y., Melnick, J., and Dreesman, G., 1984, Enhancement of viral hepatitis B antibody (anti-Hbs) response to a synthetic cycle peptide by priming with anti-idiotype antibodies, *Virology* **136:**247–252.
105. Niman, H., Houghten, R., Walker, L., Reisfeld, R., Wilson, I., Hogle, J., and Lerner, R., 1983, Generation of protein-reactive antibodies by short peptides is an event of high frequency: Implications for the structural basis of immune recognition, *Proc. Natl. Acad. Sci. USA* **80:**4949–4953.
106. Tamura, T., and Bauer, H., 1982, Monoclonal antibody against the C-terminal peptide of $pp60^{src}$ of Rous sarcoma virus, *EMBO J.* **1:**1479–1485.
107. Schechter, B., Conway-Jacobs, A., and Sela, M., 1971, Conformational changes in a synthetic antigen induced by specific antibodies, *Eur. J. Biochem.* **20:**321–324.
108. Engval, E., and Perlman, P., 1972, Enzyme-linked immunosorbent assay, ELISA III. Quantitation of specific antibodies by enzyme labeled anti-immunoglobulin in antigen-coated tubes, *J. Immunol.* **109:**129–135.
109. Voller, A., Bidwell, D., and Bartlett, A., 1976, Enzyme immunoassays in diagnostic medicine. Theory and practice, *Bull. WHO* **53:**55–65.
110. Zweig, M., Showalter, S., Simms, D., and Hampar, B., 1984, Antibodies to a synthetic oligopeptide that reacts with herpes simplex virus type 1 and type 2 glycoprotein C, *J. Virol.* **51:**430–436.
111. Walter, G., and Werchau, H., 1982, Cross-reactivity of antibodies against synthetic peptides, *J. Cell. Biochem.* **19:**119–125.
112. Nigg, E., Walter, G., and Singer, S., 1982, On the nature of cross-reactions observed with antibodies directed against defined epitopes, *Proc. Natl. Acad. Sci. USA* **79:**5939–5943.
113. Ito, Y., Hamagishi, Y., Segawa, K., Dalianis, T., Appella, E., and Willingham, M., 1983, Antibodies against a nonapeptide of polyoma virus middle T antigen: Cross-reaction with a cellular protein(s), *J. Virol.* **48:**709–720.
114. Crawford, L., Leppard, K., Lane, D., and Harlow, E., 1982, Cellular proteins reactive with monoclonal antibodies directed against SV40 large T, *J. Virol.* **42:**612–620.
115. Schaffhausen, B., 1982, Transforming genes and gene products of polyoma and SV40, *CRC Crit. Rev. Biochem.* **13:**215–286.
116. Courtneidge, S., and Smith, A., 1983, Polyoma virus transforming protein associates with the product of the c-*src* cellular gene, *Nature* **303:**435–439.
117. Hunter, T., Hutchinson, M., and Eckhart, W., 1983, Polyoma middle T antigen can be phosphorylated at multiple sites *in vitro*, *EMBO J.* **3:**73–80.
118. Carmichael, G., Schaffhausen, B., Dorsky, D., Oliver, D., and Benjamin, T., 1982, Carboxy terminus of polyoma middle-sized tumor antigen is required for attachment to membranes, associated protein kinase activities, and cell transformation, *Proc. Natl. Acad. Sci. USA* **79:**3579–3583.
119. Carmichael, G., Schaffhausen, B., Mandel, G., Liang, T., and Benjamin, T., 1984, Transformation by polyoma virus is drastically reduced by substitution of phenylalanine for tyrosine at residue 315 of middle-sized tumor antigen, *Proc. Natl. Acad. Sci. USA* **81:**679–683.
120. Harvey, R., Faulkes, R., Gillett, P., Lindsay, N., Paucha, E., Bradbury, A., and Smith, A., 1982, An antibody to a synthetic peptide that recognizes SV40 small-t antigen, *EMBO J.* **1:**473–477.
121. Luka, J., Sternas, L., Jornvall, H., Klein, G., and Lerner, R., 1983, Antibodies of predetermined specificity for the NH_2-terminus of a cellular p53 react with the native molecule: Evidence for the presence of different p53s, *Proc. Natl. Acad. Sci. USA* **80:**1199–1203.
122. Pacella, B., Hui, K., Haber, E., and Matsueda, G., 1983, Induction of fibrin-specific antibodies by immunization with synthetic peptides that correspond to amino termini of thrombin cleavage sites, *Mol. Immunol.* **20:**521–527.
123. Dillner, J., Sternas, L., Kallin, B., Alexander, H., Ehlin-Henriksson, B., Jorvall, H., Klein, G., and Lerner, R., 1984, Antibodies against a synthetic peptide identify the Epstein–Barr virus-determined nuclear antigen, *Proc. Natl. Acad. Sci. USA* **81:**4652–4656.

Chapter 22

Gene Transfer as a General Approach to Facilitate the Recombinant DNA Cloning of Surface Antigen Genes

FRANK H. RUDDLE

1. Introduction

Flow cytometry and the use of monoclonal antibodies have contributed significantly to a number of somatic cell genetic methodologies involving surface antigens, such as gene mapping using somatic cell hybrids, DNA-mediated transformation of recipient cells using cloned surface antigen genes, and, most recently, surface antigen gene cloning. These topics have been previously reviewed.[1] In this chapter, I shall discuss recent progress involving the recombinant DNA cloning of surface antigen genes, using the transferrin receptor as a model system.[2] The use of eukaryotic cells as host systems for DNA recombinant cloning of non-membrane protein genes has been reviewed recently.[3]

2. The Transferrin Receptor System

The transferrin receptor (TR) is a transmembrane protein consisting of disulfide-linked homodimers of 90,000 molecular weight (Ref. 4 and Trowbridge, this volume, Chapter 10). The TR binds Fe^{3+}-loaded transferrin and delivers it into the cell by endocytosis.[5,6] In addition to the nutrient function of TR, it has also been implicated in growth regulation.[7] It is well suited to the flow cytometry techniques reported here because of the availability of monoclonal antibodies specific for the human TR, and because of the high level of expression of TR on dividing fibroblasts.

3. General Strategy for Gene Cloning

The strategy for human TR gene cloning is as follows (see Fig. 1). Mouse L cells deficient in thymidine kinase activity are used as recipients for DNA-

FRANK H. RUDDLE • Department of Biology and Human Genetics, Yale University, New Haven, Connecticut 06511.

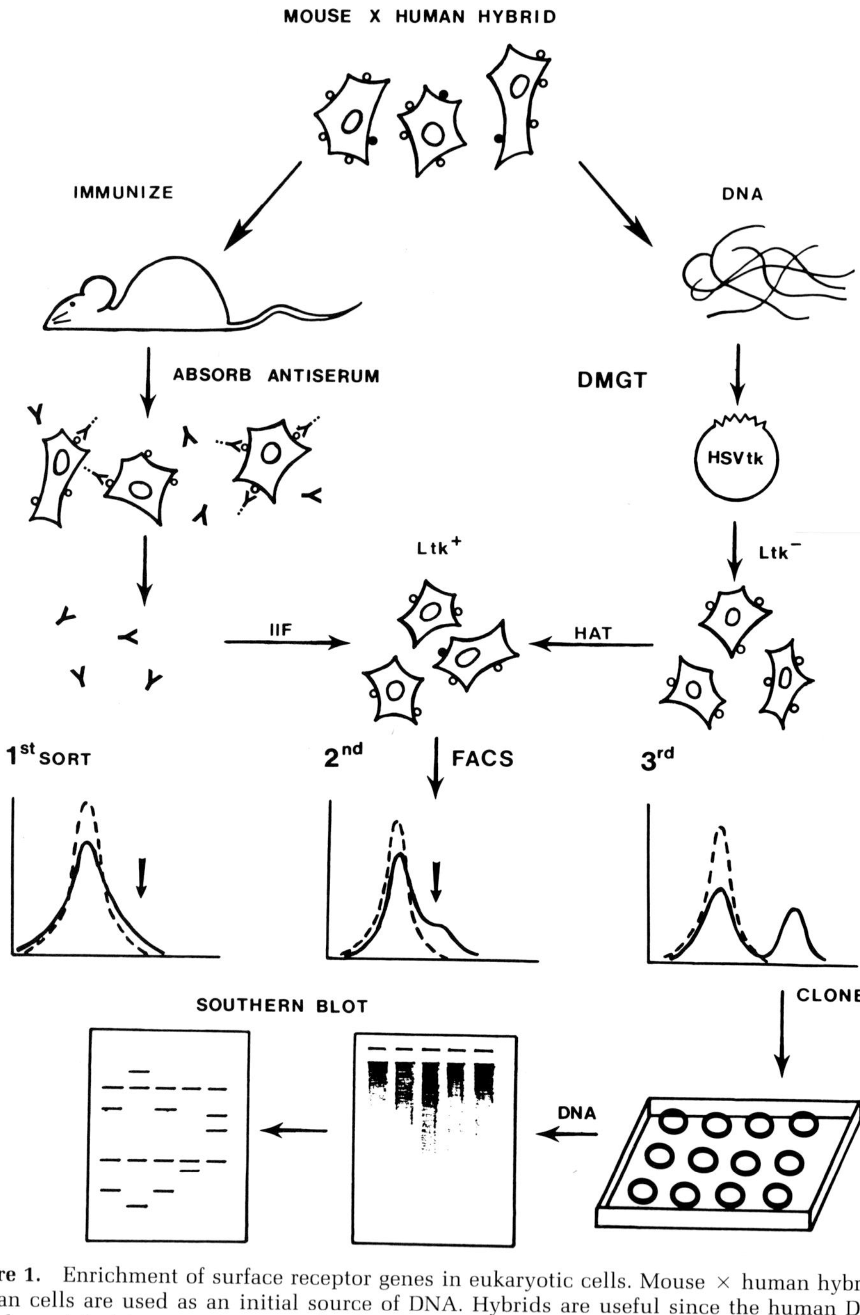

Figure 1. Enrichment of surface receptor genes in eukaryotic cells. Mouse × human hybrids or human cells are used as an initial source of DNA. Hybrids are useful since the human DNA is already enriched to some degree. Hybrid cells can be used to also produce mono- or polyclonal antibody. DNA is extracted from hybrids or primary transformants and cotransferred with HSV *tk* as a selectable marker. TK$^+$ transformants are subsequently sorted by flow cytometry to recover surface antigen-positive transformants. These are sorted to homogenicity. DNA from homogeneous transformed populations is used to produce λ-phage libraries that are screened for human (donor) repetitive sequences. Primary transformants show complex patterns, whereas secondary transformants are simple and evince common restriction fragments between independently derived transformants. (Figure courtesy of Michael Roberts.)

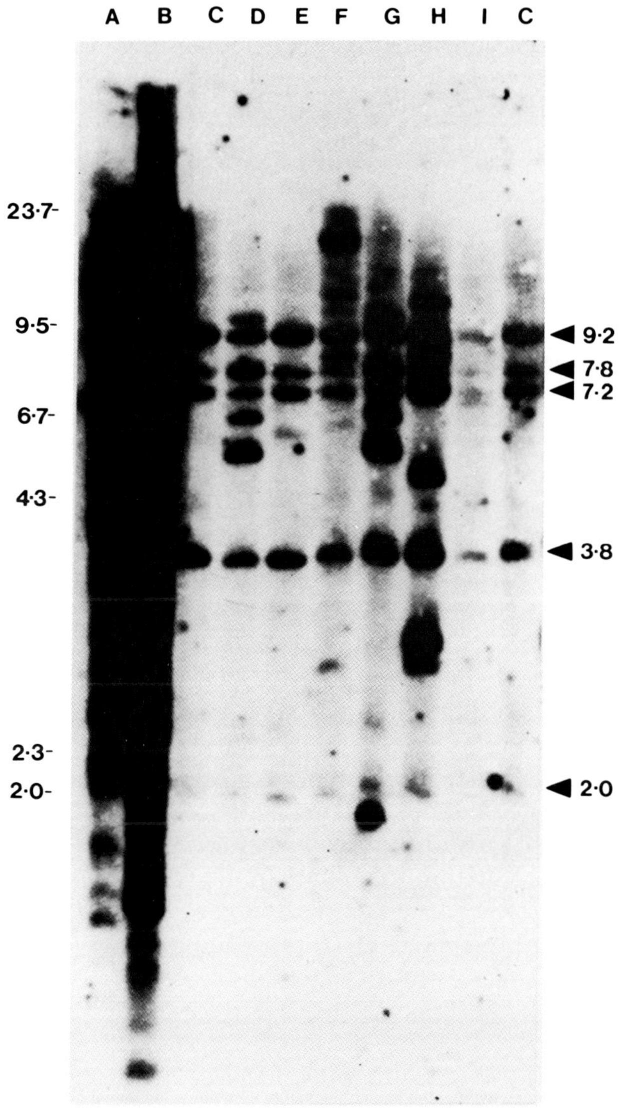

Figure 2. Comparison of primary and secondary transferrin receptor transformants by Southern blotting. (A, B) Primary transformant DNA preparation probed by human middle repetitive DNA. (C–I) Secondary transformant DNA preparations. Note common fragments indicated by molecular size markers (units in kb). (From Ref. 2 by permission).

mediated gene transfer. The recipients are cotransformed with human, high-molecular-weight DNA, and the cloned herpes thymidine kinase gene. The transformants are first selected for the expression of donor TK activity. This population is enriched for cells that have taken up large amounts of human DNA. The TK^+ population is screened for human TR^+ cells using flow cytometry, in combination with an indirect immunofluorescence assay. Positive cells are enriched to homogeneity by repeated sorting. Such cell populations contain an abundance of human DNA fragments, including the TR gene fragments of interest (Fig. 2). Non-TR fragments are purged from the cells by a second round of transformation. Secondary transformants are characterized by only a few human middle repetitive positive fragments when examined by Southern blotting (Fig. 2). Secondary transformant DNA enriched for human TR genes is then used to manufacture a λ recombinant DNA library. Such a library can be probed with human middle repetitive DNA in order to locate the human DNA fragments encoding TR. These fragments are then mapped for restriction enzyme sites in order to establish continuity as a first indication of the actual recovery of TR gene fragments. Validity is more firmly established by transformation, and the subsequent isolation of cDNA cloned fragments from cDNA libraries. This entire process of gene isolation and characterization can be accomplished within 6–12 months.

4. Isolation of Primary Transformants

The production of primary transformants is accomplished by means of calcium phosphate-mediated gene transfer. It is important to use a recipient cell of foreign species origin that has a high frequency of transformation and that takes up large amounts of donor DNA in a stable manner. These characteristics are not only logistically convenient, but essential for success at the cell sorting stage, since one must attempt to maximize the fraction of antigen-positive cells (0.01–0.1% range). We have selected an $L(TK^-)$ cell recipient cell line with a transformation frequency of 0.03%. We also find that a slight, but reproducible increase in transformation can be achieved by a mild sonication of the calcium phosphate–DNA precipitate.

The amount of DNA taken up by recipient cells is also an important variable. We find that the expression of the TK plasmid influences this parameter to some extent.[8,9] If the TK gene is weakly expressed, then one enriches for cells that have taken up larger amounts of DNA. This is presumably related to the number of TK gene copies required for optimal growth. Dot blot estimations of human DNA uptake indicate that the majority of cells incorporate as much as 1×10^6 base pairs of human DNA. Since the human haploid genome consists of approximately 3×10^9 base pairs of DNA, one expects a complete genome to be represented by more than 3000 transformed cells. Taking into account chance cleavage of transformed genes or low expression of intact transformed genes of interest, as well as statistical considerations, one might expect expression of a desired trait at a frequency of approximately 1×10^4. This frequency is actually realized for a number of independent surface antigen systems, including TR. Positive cells present at a frequency of 0.1%–0.01% can be readily isolated by several sequential rounds of cell sorting.

5. Isolation of Secondary Transformants

Primary transformants carry an abundance of human, donor DNA sequences that obscure the identity of the selected gene of interest. This supernumerary DNA can be diluted to a low level by a second round of transformation. Since an average 1×10^6 base pairs of DNA are transformed, the dilution factor is approximately 1/3000, assuming a random distribution of fragments during transformation. This indeed appears to be the case, since the majority of donor fragments observed in the recipient cells represent the donor, selected gene (Fig. 2). In fact, if one carries out Southern blot analysis on independently derived secondary clones using a human middle repetitive DNA probe, then one observes a common set of fragments shared by all expressing clones (Fig. 2). This common set of fragments is assumed to constitute the functional, expressing gene of interest.

6. Recombinant DNA Cloning of Secondary Transformant DNA and Validation of Gene Cloning

*Mbo*1-digested DNA from secondary transformants at a fragment size of 15–24 kb was cloned into λ EMBL3 vector to yield 2.0×10^6 recombinant phages. The library was screened by the method of Benton and Davis using nick-translated whole-cell human DNA as probe.[2] The recombinant, donor DNA fragments recovered by screening were subjected to restriction endonuclease mapping in order to test for overlap between fragments. This was found in the case of six fragments isolated from a selected secondary transformant (see Fig. 3). It could be shown that the common restriction fragments observed in the secondary transformants corresponded to the restriction sites defined by restriction site mapping. The restriction site mapping also made possible an estimate of minimum gene size as approximately 32 kb.

Verification of TR gene cloning was accomplished by returning the cloned gene into recipient L cells and testing for TR expression. Transformation experiments showed that none of the cloned fragments could effect expression by itself, but that certain pairwise combinations of fragments could do so. Transformation with pairs of fragments was carried out in two ways. In the first, the pairs were cut at common restriction sites in regions of overlap, religated, then used for transformation. In the second, the pairs were added directly to recipient cells without treatment. In both instances, expression was obtained. This result provides evidence that the TR gene has been cloned. It is interesting and useful that transformation can be achieved by the simple addition of untreated fragments in combination. This simplifies the transformation test, and indicates that the recipient cells possess mechanisms that allow the precise rejoining of fragments resulting in a functional, expressing gene. We have also observed this splicing phenomenon in the case of the human cytosolic thymidine kinase gene.[10]

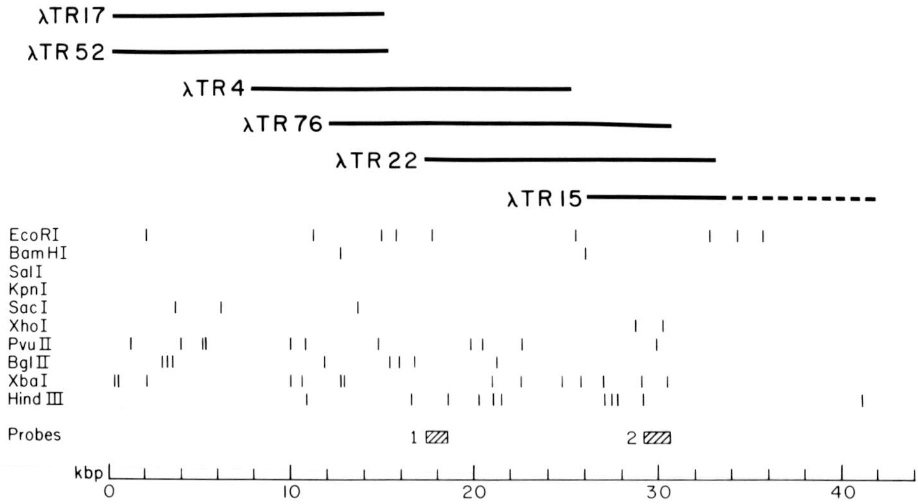

Figure 3. Restriction map of fragments of the human transferrin receptor gene cloned in λ. Fragments show continuity by virtue of overlapping restriction maps. Cotransformation of λ TR17 and λ TR76 produces a positive transformants. None of the fragments alone will do so. Unique fragments were isolated from subregions 1 and 2 (units in kb). Dashed line represents mouse DNA. (From Ref. 2 by permission.)

7. Discussion and Summary

The combined use of gene transfer and recombinant DNA cloning promises to be a general, efficient means to clone surface antigen genes. The method has been developed primarily using TR as a model, but feasibility has also been demonstrated with other human surface antigen genes, such as class 1 HLA genes,[11] the 4F2 gene coding for the high-molecular-weight 4F2 protein,[11] and the S11 gene or genes (M. Roberts, M. E. Kamarck, and F. H. Ruddle, unpublished results). One advantage of the method is that the genomic gene sequences are isolated directly without the necessity of dealing with mRNA or cDNA materials. Another advantage is that the method involves the generation of expression transformants, so that one can begin to study structure–function relationships as they pertain to expression regulation at an early time in the course of experimentation. Possible disadvantages of the approach involve the size of the gene and the possibility that the simultaneous transfer of more than one gene is required to ensure the expression of the selected phenotype. Another complication might involve the epigenetic regulation of the expression of the transformed gene. However, it should be pointed out that Kavathas and Herzenberg have been successful in demonstrating expression of a number of T-cell-specific antigens in transformed fibroblasts (Ref. 12 and Kavathas, this volume, Chapter 23). All in all, considering the advantages and possible disadvantages, it would appear that the transfection/selection methods offer a useful means by which one can clone the genes coding for surface antigens.

As in the case of the transferrin receptor, these can be used to gain insight into a variety of interesting and significant biomedical problems.

ACKNOWLEDGMENTS. This work was supported by NIH grant GM-09966 and by an anonymous gift to Yale University. The author is grateful to Marie Siniscalchi and Suzy Pafka for their help with the manuscript. The author also gratefully acknowledges the use of Fig. 1, which was designed by Michael Roberts.

References

1. Kamarck, M. E., Barbosa, J. A., Kuhn, L., Messer Peters, P., Shulman, L., and Ruddle, F. H., 1983, Somatic cell genetics and flow cytometry, *Cytometry* **4**:99–108.
2. Kuhn, L. C., McClelland, A., and Ruddle, F. H., 1984, Gene transfer expression and molecular cloning of the human transferrin receptor gene, *Cell* **37**:95–103.
3. Ruddle, F. H., Kamarck, M. E., McClelland, A., and Kuhn, L. C., 1984, DNA-mediated gene transfer in mammalian gene cloning, in: *Genetic Engineering*, Volume 6 (J. K. Setlow and A. Hollaender, eds.), Plenum Press, New York, pp. 319–338.
4. Schneider, C., Sutherland, R., Newman, R., and Greaves, M., 1982, Structural features of the cell surface receptor for transferrin that is recognized by the monoclonal antibody OKT9, *J. Biol. Chem.* **257**:8516–8522.
5. Newman, R., Schneider, C., Sutherland, R., Vodinelich, L., and Greaves, M., 1982, The transferrin receptor, *Trends Biochem. Sci.* **1**:397–400.
6. Dautry-Varsat, A., Ciechanover, A., and Lodish, H. F., 1983, pH and the recycling of transferrin during receptor-mediated endocytosis. *Proc. Natl. Acad. Sci. USA* **80**:2258–2262.
7. Neckers, L. M., and Cossman, J., 1983, Transferrin receptor induction in mitogen-stimulated human T lymphocytes is required for DNA synthesis and cell division and is regulated by interleukin 2, *Proc. Natl. Acad. Sci. USA* **80**:3494–3498.
8. Barbosa, J. A., Kamarck, M. E., Biro, P. A., Weissman, S. M., and Ruddle, F. H., 1982, Identification of human genomic clones coding the major histocompatibility antigens HLA-A2 and HLA-B7 by DNA-mediated gene transfer, *Proc. Natl. Acad. Sci. USA* **79**:6327–6331.
9. Barbosa, J. A., Kamarck, M. E., and Ruddle, F. H., 1983, Variation in expression of human major histocompatibility genes in mouse L cells after DNA-mediated gene transfer, in: *Gene Expression in Normal and Transformed Cells* (J. E. Cellis and E. Bravo, eds.), Plenum Press, New York, pp. 379–401.
10. Lin, P.-F., Zhao, S.-Y., and Ruddle, F. H., 1983, Genomic cloning and preliminary characterization of the human thymidine kinase gene, *Proc. Natl. Acad. Sci. USA* **80**:6528–6532.
11. Kuhn, L. C., Barbosa, J. A., Kamarck, M. E., and Ruddle, F. H., 1983, A new approach to the cloning of cell surface protein genes: Selection by cell sorting of mouse L-cells which express HLA or 4F2 antigens after transformation with total human DNA, *Mol. Biol. Med.* **1**:335–352.
12. Kavathas, P., and Herzenberg, L. A., 1983, Stable transformation of mouse L cells for human membrane T-cell differentiation antigens, HLA and β_2-microglobulin: Selection by fluorescence-activated cell sorting, *Proc. Natl. Acad. Sci. USA* **80**:524–527.

Chapter 23

Amplification and Molecular Cloning of Transfected Genes

PAULA KAVATHAS

1. Introduction

The transfection of genes into recipient cells is a very exciting tool because of the diversity of problems that can be attacked and because of the elegance of the answers. For instance, transfer of cloned MHC or immunoglobulin genes has provided important knowledge of the structure, function, and regulation of these genes. Many important genes have been cloned by transfecting with total cellular DNA, selecting transfectants expressing the gene, and then isolating the transferred gene by one of several methods. The identification and cloning of cellular oncogenes, a major breakthrough in the past few years, was an achievement that may not have been possible or have occurred as swiftly without our ability to transfer DNA into mammalian cells and isolate transfectants.

Monoclonal antibodies are extremely useful for selection of transfectants expressing genes coding for cell surface antigens or receptors. Transfectants expressing a variety of mouse and human cell surface molecules can be isolated after staining recipient cells with fluorescein-conjugated monoclonal antibodies and sorting positive cells using a fluorescence activated cell sorter (detailed below). These cell surface molecules include lymphocyte differentiation antigens such as the human T-cell antigen Leu-2 (T8);[2] other cell surface antigens are transferrin receptor,[3,4] and an antigen expressed on human chronic lymphocytic leukemia cells.[5] Genes that code for several of these cell surface antigens can be then isolated from transfected cells.[4,6] It is also possible to select transfectants expressing other types of gene products using monoclonal antibodies and visual selection (see Section 4.3 below).

In this chapter, the process of gene transfer, methods for transfer of DNA into cells, and selection procedures for transfectants will be described. Applications of the technique for gene cloning, for gene amplification, and for analyzing cell surface antigens will also be discussed.

PAULA KAVATHAS • Department of Genetics, School of Medicine, Stanford University, Stanford, California 94305.

2. Movement of DNA from Outside the Cell into the Nucleus: Basic Process

The basic process by which gene transfer is accomplished using total cellular DNA is partially understood. After the DNA is taken up by the recipient cells, most of the DNA is degraded and never reaches the nucleus.[7] DNA that reaches the nucleus may be transiently expressed; however, for stable expression, transfected DNA must be incorporated into the host genome. If the DNA can replicate autonomously, as does bovine papillomavirus DNA[8] or an Epstein–Barr virus plasmid,[9] then integration is not required for stable expression. Transfected DNA fragments that are incorporated into the chromosome are ligated together as a concatamer (also called pekalasome or transgenome) and integrated into an apparently random chromosomal site.[10,11] Rarely does integration of a transferred sequence into homologous site in the host genome occur.[12] Recombination between fragments in the nucleus can occur before integration,[13] as may alterations such as mutation.[14] For human DNA transfected into mouse L cells about $\frac{1}{1000}$ of the genome is incorporated, or about 3×10^3 kb.[10,11] DNA that is incorporated may not be stably expressed. Loss of expression can result from gene loss[1,15] or modulation of expression due to changes in methylation,[16,17] chromatin structure,[18] or other regulatory events.

3. Methods for Transferring DNA into Cells

Various methods exist for transferring DNA into cells.[19] Purified high-molecular-weight DNA (also called "naked" DNA) can be added to cells as a calcium phosphate precipitate,[1,20] as a polyethylene glycol precipitate,[21] by electroporation in high electric fields,[22,23] or by microinjection.[24] Calcium phosphate precipitation has been most widely used with naked DNA and can also be used with chromatin as well as with DNA packaged as bacteriophage.[25] Alternatively, the DNA is enclosed within membrane vesicles, such as bacterial protoplasts[26,27] or liposomes,[28] which are then fused to cells. Viral vectors, such as bacteriophage, or retroviruses,[29,30] which carry foreign genes can transport those genes into cells. When transient expression is to be assayed, naked DNA can be added with DEAE dextran.[31]

The method of choice depends on a variety of factors. Different cell types are transformed with different efficiencies, depending on the method for introducing the DNA. The size of a cell's nucleus and its membrane properties influence the efficiency of transfer by microinjection. Some methods work better with cloned genes than with total cellular DNA. Because cloned genes are often maintained in bacterial cells as part of plasmid vectors, the method of fusing bacterial protoplasts with recipient cells was developed as a convenient method for introducing a cloned gene into a cell.

Although many different cell types are capable of being transfected, the efficiencies vary widely. Some transformed cells, such as mouse L cells,[32] NIH 3T3 cells, and a mouse melanoma line.[33] are transformed at high efficiencies, with frequencies ranging from about 1.0 to 0.1% after transfection with a cloned gene. Normal cells, such as fibroblasts, can also be transformed, although the efficiency is usually less. Therefore, experiments using total cellular DNA usually rely on highly efficient cells as recipients. By contrast, transfer of a cloned gene into a cell line of interest, such as that of an immunoglobulin gene into a hybridoma or myeloma line, can be accomplished even if the frequency of transfer is low.[34,35]

4. Methods of Selection

Because only a small proportion of cells in a given population are competent to take up and express foreign DNA, there must be schemes for selecting transfectants. For cloned genes this is not a problem. A cloned gene can be cotransferred with a gene for which a good selective system exists. A high proportion, in some cases greater than 80%, of transfectants expressing the selected gene also express the cotransferred gene.[1] Alternatively, the cloned gene can be ligated to the selectable gene before transfection. However, for genes that are not cloned, specific selective systems must exist.

4.1. Selection for Complementation of Prototrophic Genes in Mutant Recipient Cells

Initial work in gene transfer relied on the HAT selection method to transfer genes coding for herpes simplex[36,37] or mammalian thymidine kinase[38] into mouse L cells that were deficient in thymidine kinase and were not known to revert. Genes coding for hypoxanthine phosphoribosyltransferase (HPRT) and adenine phosphoribosyltransferase (APRT) could be transferred to mutant cell lines and transfectants similarly selected using HAT medium.[39]

A problem with this approach is that in order to serve as recipients, cells must lack expression of the particular gene product. In cases where a cell line does not have an appropriate mutation, cells can be mutagenized and selection for mutant cells imposed. The revertant frequency, however, must be less than the transfection frequency.

4.2. Dominant Biochemical Selection

Cells expressing a transferred gene normally found in a different species can sometimes be selected. Cells with a particular mutation are not required. Two bacterial genes used for this purpose are: (1) neomycin resistance gene (NEO) coding for the aminoglycoside phosphotransferase that phosphorylates and thus inactivates neomycin and its analogue G418, which block ribosome function,[40] and (2) xanthine-guanine phosphoribosyltransferase (GPT), which utilizes xanthine as a purine source and is not inhibited by mycophenolic acid, in contrast to animal cell HPRT.[41] Cells grown in medium containing mycophenolic acid, aminopterin, xanthine, and thymidine will only survive if they are expressing a transfected GPT gene. A more comprehensive list of selection schemes can be found in Kucherlapati and Skoultchi.[42]

4.3. Visual Selection

Alterations in a visible phenotype can be identified with a microscope. This type of selection was used for isolating transfectants of cellular oncogenes. 3T3 cells transfected with DNA from certain tumor lines formed foci after expressing the cellular oncogene.[43] Besides morphological alterations, histochemical or other cytological procedures can distinguish between cells that have acquired a particular product and those that have not. Unfortunately, the cells are often killed in the process of characterization. However, if the principle of sib selection (see below) is applied, this procedure may be a feasible approach for isolating certain kinds of transfectants.

4.4. Dominant Selection with Monoclonal Antibodies or Ligands

Transfectants expressing a receptor or a cell surface antigen that is not normally expressed by the cells can be selected by staining cells with a monoclonal antibody or a ligand coupled to a fluorochrome. Positive cells are readily detected with a fluorescence activated cell sorter (FACS) if they occur at frequencies of greater than 10^{-4}. Positive cells occurring at a lower frequency can be enriched by several orders of magnitude by a first passage through the FACS. When the culture is sufficiently enriched, positive cells are sorted individually into wells of microtiter plates using the FACS autocloning device. For transfection of mouse and human lymphocyte antigens, cellular DNA from expressing[2] or nonexpressing tissue or cell lines[44] can be cotransferred with the thymidine kinase gene into mouse L cells and TK^+ transfectants selected by growth in HAT medium. This procedure enriches for cells competent to incoporate and express foreign DNA. For most antigens, transfectants expressing a cell surface antigen occur at a frequency of about 10^{-3} of the TK^+ cells. For large genes the frequency is usually reduced tenfold.[37]

5. Cloning Genes

A powerful approach for gene cloning is the transfer of genes into recipient cells by DNA-mediated gene transfer and then isolating the transferred gene by one of several methods. There are many attractive aspects of this approach. First, the success of the approach does not depend on the level of a specific mRNA in a cell. In fact, most genes cloned by this approach encode rare mRNA.

Second, a number of recipient cells (e.g., mouse L cells) that will efficiently incoroporate and express a wide variety of different genes exist. Third, there are multiple ways for isolating the transferred gene (see below) once transfectants are obtained. Fourth, transfection can be used to confirm that a candidate clone is the gene of interest. A genomic clone containing the complete gene or several clones containing parts of the gene should be capable of transfecting for the gene of interest.[4] Fifth, unknown genes responsible for a certain cell phenotype may possibly be cloned by transfection. For instance, a human gene involved in DNA repair was recently cloned from transfectants obtained by first transforming UV-light-sensitive CHO cells with total cellular human DNA and selecting for cells that were no longer sensitive.[45]

A variety of approaches for isolating transferred genes have been developed. Natural linkage of a gene to an identifiable sequence such as a repetitive sequence or linkage by recombinant DNA techniques with a biologically selectable marker allow rescue of the gene. A more recent method relies on cDNA subtraction whereby cDNA made from mRNA of a transfectant is subtracted with mRNA from recipient cells. Since transfectants and recipient cells express the same gene products except for expression of transferred genes, the subtracted cDNA should correspond to those genes. Alternatively, gene libraries can be screened for the gene of interest by transfecting cells and assaying for expression of the gene product. The following describes the methods in greater detail.

5.1. Methods of Isolating Transferred Genes

5.1.1. Plasmid or SupF Rescue

The rescue method was first used by Perucho *et al.*[46] to isolate the chicken thymidine kinase gene. Chicken DNA was digested with an enzyme that did not cleave inside the TK gene and the fragments ligated into pBR322 to construct a plasmid library. After transfection with DNA from the pBR322 plasmid library, TK^+ transfectants were selected. After a second round of transfection to eliminate pBR322 sequences not linked to TK, the DNA from a secondary transfectant was digested with an enzyme that only cut into the plasmid and the DNA was ligated under cyclization conditions. The circular molecules were transferred to *Escherichia coli* and selected for a drug resistance marker carried by the plasmid. The rescued plasmids were then tested for ability to confer the TK phenotype to mouse cells. A variation on the procedure by Lowy *et al.*[47] involved construction of a genomic library from the secondary transfectant and screening it with labeled pBR322 as a probe.

Goldfarb *et al.*[48] developed an alternative strategy because of limitations with plasmid rescue (i.e., insert size). DNA from a human bladder carcinoma cell line was first digested with an enzyme that did not cleave the gene of interest. Restriction fragments were separated by size and fragments in the fraction containing the gene (see Section 5.3) were ligated to a bacterial *SupF* gene. After several rounds of transfection, a phage library was constructed with DNA from a secondary transfectant and a bacterium with a suppressible mutation was infected. Only phage carrying the *SupF* gene would form plaques. A transforming gene was isolated because of its location next to the *SupF* gene.

5.1.2. Search

When DNA from one species is transfected into recipient cells from another species, a repetitive sequence linked to the gene can serve as a marker for gene isolation.[49] There is sufficient divergence between species in repetitive DNA sequences so that most repetitive DNA hybridizes specifically to DNA of the same species. Because the human genome contains at least 300,000 interspersed repetitive sequences, many, though not all, human genes will be closely linked to one or more copies of a repetitive sequence.

The general strategy is to isolate DNA from primary transfectants and retransfect recipient cells for the gene of interest. If human DNA is transferred into mouse cells, then after two or three cycles of transfection the only human DNA likely to be present is the gene of interest and possibly closely linked sequences. Southern blots are then performed with total genomic DNA from a number of independent secondary transfectants and hybridized with ^{32}P-labeled human repetitive or total DNA as a probe. If common bands are observed, then it is likely that the gene of interest contains a repetitive sequence or is closely linked to such a sequence. In some cases a common band may be observed in most but not all transfectants.[50] Since digestion and linkage of transferred DNA occurs (as described above), a new restriction fragment containing the gene may be generated.

5.1.3. Sib Selection

A chicken B cell lymphoma (Blym)-transforming gene[51] and a gene for a cell surface antigen on human chronic lymphocytic leukemia cells[5] were isolated using this procedure. Essentially, a phage library was constructed with DNA from the transfected cells. DNA from pools of phage were tested for the ability to transfect for the gene of interest. If a pool was positive, it was subdivided such that only one or a few subpools were likely to contain the positive phage and the incidence of the phage in that pool would be increased compared with the initial pool. This procedure was continued until a pure phage was isolated. This procedure may require long periods of time, although transfecting and monitoring transient expression may be carried out when the positive phage is sufficiently enriched. In addition, if there is sufficient differential replication between the positive phage and other phage, dilution of the positive phage can occur.

5.1.4. cDNA Subtraction

Because transfectants theoretically contain the same mRNA species as recipient cells as well as mRNA transcribed from the transferred genes, highly specific "subtracted" cDNA probes can be made for identifying transferred genes.[52,53] To make such probes cDNA made from mRNA of transfected cells is depleted of shared sequences by hybridization to mRNA of the recipient cells. Hydroxyapatite columns are used to separate the unhybridizable cDNA which would theoretically correspond to mRNA transcribed from the transferred genes. The "subtracted" cDNA probe can be used for screening cDNA or genomic libraries.

Since primary transfectants typically incorporate about 0.1% of the foreign DNA, the cDNAs specific to the transfectants may correspond to multiple transferred genes if they are expressed. To isolate a specific cDNA corresponding to the gene of interest one of the following approaches can be taken: (1) Selected cDNA made with a secondary transfectant should be quite specific, since the secondary transfectant will only differ from recipient cells by expressing the selected gene as well as possibly linked sequences. (2) Because transfectants only incoporate a small amount of total cellular DNA, several independent transfectants are unlikely to have incorporated the same genes except for the selected gene and perhaps closely linked sequences. Therefore, cDNA clones in a library that hybridize with two subtracted cDNA probes made from different primary transfectants should contain sequences corresponding to the gene of interest. (3) To clone the gene coding for the human T-cell antigen Leu-2,[2] a cDNA library was constructed from a Leu-2 transfectant in which the Leu-2 gene was amplified. Leu-2 cDNA clones were identified by screening with a "subtracted" cDNA probe made from an independent, amplified Leu-2 transfectant.

This technique is probably one of the best for isolating transferred genes. Fewer steps are required compared with some of the other methods. Isolation of genes of any species is possible even when, for instance, a mouse gene has been transferred into a mouse recipient cell. In addition, there is a good chance of success since it is unlikely that the recipient cell will contain an mRNA species highly homologous to the mRNA transcribed from the transferred gene.

5.1.5. Shuttle Vectors and Cosmid Rescue

Cosmids can serve as shuttle vectors between bacteria and mammalian cells since they contain selectable markers for both bacteria and mammalian cells.[54,55] To clone a gene, a cosmid library is constructed, mammalian cells are transfected with DNA from the library, and transfectants are selected. The cosmid DNA is recovered by *in vitro* packaging of the cellular DNA from the transfectant. Cosmid DNA that is packaged is used to transform bacteria. Bacteria now containing the gene of interest are then identified.

One advantage of cosmids is that up to 45 kb of DNA can be inserted per cosmid. Cloning of the gene coding for human thymidine kinase was accomplished by this method.[55] One potential problem is that some cosmids are not always rescued from the mammalian cell by *in vitro* packaging. While cosmids are useful for transferring large genes or closely linked genes to study gene expression, the generality of the approach for gene cloning has yet to be established.

5.2. Transfection with cDNA Expression Vectors

Instead of transfecting cells with DNA from a genomic library and isolating the gene of interest by sib selection, it may be possible in the future to transfect with DNA from a cDNA library constructed in an expression vector. A plasmid vector described by Okayama and Berg[56] contains the simian virus 40 (SV40) early region promoter, a modified SV40 late region intron, and a polyadenylation signal such that cDNA inserts can be transcribed and processed in mammalian cells. Rare cells expressing the gene of interest could then be selected. So far this has not been an approach for cloning genes. However, expression of cloned cDNA in mammalian cells has been used to confirm the identity of specific cDNAs and to isolate full-length cDNA clones.[57]

5.3. Transfection as an Aid in Gene Cloning

Transfection of a gene can provide important information about the gene. For instance, the sensitivity to cleavage by various restriction endonucleases can be determined by transfecting with digested DNA. If no transfectants are obtained, it can be presumed that an endonuclease cuts into the gene. For restriction endonucleases that do not cleave the gene, the size of the restriction fragment containing a complete gene can be determined by fractionating the DNA on gradients and transfecting with the different fractions.

Transfectants can also be useful in helping to identify whether a candidate clone obtained from cDNA or genomic libraries codes for the gene of interest. For instance, if a candidate clone is isolated from a library and is presumed to encode the cell surface antigen for the mouse T-cell antigen Lyt-2, then on Northern blots, the labeled DNA from the clone should hybridize with mRNA from independent Lyt-2 transfectants but not with mRNA from L cells. Hybridization with a number of transfectants would be strong evidence that the candidate clone coded for Lyt-2. The screening of transfectants should be useful for characterizing clones that are isolated from cDNA-selected libraries.

6. Amplification

Gene amplification is one way in which cells can increase expression of a gene product. During normal development, amplification of rRNA genes in amphibian oocytes or chorion genes in *Drosophila* egg chambers occurs to provide abundant amounts of the gene products. Although there are no examples of gene amplification occurring during mammalian cell development, gene amplification occurs in somatic cell lines and in tumor cells. Examples of amplification of specific genes can be found in (1) cells resistant to various drugs (*in vivo* or *in vitro*), (2) tumors such as neuroblastomas or tumors with translocated chromosomes, and (3) transfected cells. Several excellent reviews on gene amplification have recently been written.[58,59] In this chapter, the focus will be on gene amplification occurring after transfection. Such amplification events can be used to (1) study the process of gene amplification, (2) amplify genes that are not normally amplifiable, and (3) improve methods for gene cloning.

Amplification of some genes coding for cell surface antigens can occur spontaneously after transfection and cells with increased expression can be selected using a fluorescence activated cell sorter (FACS). Transfectants expressing a foreign cell surface antigen are first selected by staining with fluorescein-conjugated monoclonal antibodies and sorting and/or cloning with the FACS. If gene amplification has occurred, the staining pattern will be more heterogeneous and the mean fluorescence will be greater than for transfectants in which amplification has not occurred.[60] To select for cells with increased expression, the most brightly staining cells are sorted with the FACS. The cells are grown and the process repeated. Highly amplified mouse L-cell transfectant lines expressing the human T-lymphocyte glycoprotein Leu-2(T8) are obtained in this way.[60] The same is true for transfectants expressing the mouse homologue of Leu-2, Lyt-2, and the nerve growth factor receptor.

About 25–50% of the Leu-2 transfectants spontaneously amplified the Leu-2 gene, but spontaneous amplification for six or seven other antigen transfectants was not observed. It may be that some genes have structural features or sequences that increase their propensity for undergoing gene amplification after transfection. Alternatively, amplification of some genes may not be observed because increased expression is lethal or because increased expression is dependent on increased expression of other unlinked gene products. For instance, the MHC class I gene products must couple to β-microglobulin for expression on the cell surface. Surface expression of MHC class I genes would be limited by the amount of β-microglobulin in the cells.

6.1. Analyzing the Process of Gene Amplification

Genes that can undergo gene amplification in tumor lines, such as dihydrofolate reductase (DHFR), can be transferred into recipient cells, and cells with amplified copies selected in order to study mechanisms of gene amplification. Because transferred genes are integrated in different chromosomal locations and become linked to different sequences, the effect on amplification rates can be examined. Wahl *et al.*[61] found that in three-fourths of CAD gene transfectants the genes were amplified with about the same frequency as observed for the endogenous gene, while those in the remaining transfectant were amplified at a frequency 100 times higher. Examination of linked sequences may provide information on why the frequency was so much greater in the one transfectant.

6.2. Amplification of Normally Nonamplifiable Genes

Selection for amplification of some genes is not possible nor readily feasible. However, by cotransformation with an amplifiable gene such as DHFR, amplification of the nonselected gene can be obtained.[62] Two genes become physically linked after cotransformation. When selection for DHFR amplification is imposed, DHFR gene copies will increase, as will linked sequences. In mammalian cells the amount of DNA coamplified with each gene is large, up to 3000 kb. Therefore, sequences that become linked after transfection will generally be coamplified. 3T3 cells making large amounts of hepatitis B surface antigen can be isolated after cotransformation with the DHFR gene and then selecting for amplification of DHFR.[63] Alternatively, it is possible to insert genes in amplifiable vectors that contain an amplifiable unit.

6.3. Applications for Gene Cloning

Methods for isolating transferred genes would be facilitated if amplification of the gene of interest could be obtained. Cloning of the gene for the human T-cell antigen Leu-2 was aided because of the availability of highly amplified Leu-2 transfectants.[60] In cases where spontaneous amplification may not occur frequently, it still may be possible to obtain amplification for the gene of interest. As described above, an amplifiable gene could be cotransferred with total cellular DNA into recipient cells. After antigen transfectants are selected the cells could be grown in a selective medium to select for amplification of the amplifiable gene. Because the gene of interest has been linked to the amplifiable gene during concatamer formation after transfection, there is a good probability that the linked gene will be coamplified. This approach, originally proposed by Wigler *et al.*,[62] seems promising.

7. Analyzing Cell Surface Antigens

Numerous types of experiments can be performed involving DNA-mediated gene transfer. Some examples are: (1) studying the regulation of gene expression by modifying a cloned gene, transferring the gene into recipient cells, and monitoring expression; (2) structural or functional studies using cells transfected with modified genes; (3) defining the function of cell surface antigens by testing for functional properties acquired by transfectants expressing the antigen and (4) identification of the protein products of cloned genes.

Identification of the products of cloned major histocompatibility genes was possible using gene transfer.[64] For instance, because there are numerous homologous MHC genes in a cell, it is difficult to identify which genes code for the different MHC cell surface antigens. Transfecting with an MHC gene and analyzing the protein product can provide this information. Alternatively, mouse cells transfected with a human gene encoding a cell surface antigen can be used as immunogens in the mouse strain from which the recipient cells were derived in order to generate other specific antibodies to the human cell surface antigen.

ACKNOWLEDGMENT. The author would like to thank Dr. Leonard A. Herzenberg for his many stimulating discussions.

References

1. Wigler, M., Sweet, R., Sim, G. K., Wold, B., Pellicer, A., Lacy, E., Maniates, T., Silverstein, S., and Axel, R., 1979, Transformation of mammalian cells with genes from procaryotes and eucaryotes, *Cell* **16**:777–785.
2. Kavathas, P., and Herzenberg, L. A., 1983, Stable transformation of mouse L cells for human membrane T cell differentiation antigens, HLA and B2-microglobulin: Selection by fluorescence activated cell sorting, *Proc. Natl. Acad. Sci. USA* **80**:524–528.
3. Newman, R., Domingo, D., Trotter, J., and Trowbridge, I., 1983, Selection and properties of a mouse L-cell transformant expressing human transferrin receptor, *Nature* **304**:643–645.
4. Kuhn, L. C., McClelland, A., and Ruddle, F. H., 1984, Gene transfer, expression, and molecular cloning of the human transferrin receptor gene, *Cell* **37**:95–103.
5. Stanners, C. P., Lam, T., Chamberlain, J. W., Stewart, S. S., and Price, G. B., 1981, Cloning of a functional gene responsible for the expression of a cell surface antigen correlated with human chronic lymphocytic leukemia, *Cell* **27**:211–221.
6. Kavathas, P., Sukhatme, V. P., Herzenberg, L. A., and Parnes, J. R., 1984, Isolation of the gene coding for the human T lymphocyte differentiation antigen of Leu-2 (T8) by gene transfer and cDNA subtraction, *Proc. Natl. Acad. Sci. USA* **81**:7688–7692.
7. Loyter, A., Scangos, G. A., and Ruddle, F. H., 1982, Mechanisms of DNA uptake by mammalian cells: Fate of exogenously added DNA monitored by the use of fluorescent dyes, *Proc. Natl. Acad. Sci. USA* **79**:422–426.
8. Law, M. F., Lowy, D. R., Dvoretzky, I., and Howley, P. M., 1981, Mouse cells transformed by bovine papillomavirus contain only extrachromosomal viral DNA sequences, *Proc. Natl. Acad. Sci. USA* **78**:2727–2731.
9. Yates, J., Warren, N., Reisman, D., and Sugden, B., 1984, A *cis*-acting element from the Epstein–Barr viral genome that permits stable replication of recombinant plasmids in latently infected cells, *Proc. Natl. Acad. Sci. USA* **81**:3806–3810.
10. Robins, D. M., Ripler, S., Henderson, A. S., and Axel, R., 1981, Transforming DNA integrates into the host chromosome, *Cell* **23**:29–39.
11. Perucho, M., Hanahan, D., and Wigler, M., 1980, Genetic and physical linkages of exogenous sequences in transformed cells, *Cell* **22**:309–317.
12. Kucherlapati, R. S., Eves, E. M., Song, K. Y., Morse, B. S., and Smithies, O., 1984, Homologous recombination between plasmids in mammalian cells can be enhanced by treatment of input DNA, *Proc. Natl. Acad. Sci. USA* **81**:3153–3157.
13. Anderson, R. A., Krakauor, T., and Camerini-Otero, R. D., 1982, DNA-mediated gene transfer: Recombination between cotransferred DNA sequences and recovery of recombinants in a plasmid, *Proc. Natl. Acad. Sci. USA* **79**:2748–2752.
14. Calos, M. P., Lebkowski, J. S., and Botchan, M. R., 1983, High mutation frequency in DNA transfected into mammalian cells, *Proc. Natl. Acad. Sci. USA* **80**:3015–3019.
15. Wigler, M., Sweet, R., Sim, G. K., Wold, B., Pellicer, A., Lacy, E., Maniatis, T., Silverstein, S., and Axel, R., 1979, Transformation of mammalian cells with genes from procaryotes and eucaryotes, *Cell* **16**:777–785.
16. Christy, B., and Scangos, G., 1982, Expression of transferred thymidine kinase genes is controlled by methylation, *Proc. Natl. Acad. Sci. USA* **79**:6299–6303.
17. Clough, D. W., Kunkel, L. M., and Davidson, R. L., 1982, 5-Azacytidine-induced reactivation of a herpes simplex thymidine kinase gene, *Science* **216**:70–73.

18. Davies, R. L., Fuhrer-Krusi, S., and Kucherlapati, R. S., 1982, Modulation of transfected gene expression mediated by changes in chromatin structure, *Cell* **31**:521–529.
19. Ruddle, F. H., Kamarck, M. E., McClelland, A., and Kuhn, L. C., 1984, DNA-mediated gene transfer in mammalian gene cloning, in: *Genetic Engineering*, Volume 6 (J. K. Setlow and A. Hollaender, eds.), Plenum Press, New York, pp. 319–338.
20. Graham, F. L., and van der Eb, A. J., 1973, A new technique for the assay of infectivity of human adenovirus 5 DNA, *Virology* **52**:456–467.
21. Klebe, R. G., Harriss, J., Hanson, D. P., and Gauntt, C. J., 1984, High efficiency polyethylene glycol mediated transformation of mammalian cells, *Somat. Cell Mol. Genet.* **10**:495–502.
22. Neumann, E., Schaefer-Riddler, M., Wang, Y., and Hofschneider, P. H., 1982, Gene transfer into mouse myeloma cells by electroporation in high electric fields, *EMBO J.* **1**:841–845.
23. Potter, H., Weir, L., and Leder, P., 1983, Enhancer-dependent expression of human K immunoglobulin genes introduced into mouse pre-B lymphocytes by electroporation, *Proc. Natl. Acad. Sci. USA* **81**:7161–7165.
24. Capecchi, M. R., 1980, High efficiency transformation by direct microinjection of DNA into cultured mammalian cells, *Cell* **22**:479–488.
25. Ishiura, M., Hirose, S., Uchida, T., Hamada, Y., Suzuki, Y., and Okada, Y., 1982, Phage particle-mediated gene transfer to cultured mammalian cells, *Mol. Cell Biol.* **2**:607–616.
26. Schaffner, W., 1980, Direct transfer of cloned genes from bacteria to mammalian cells, *Proc. Natl. Acad. Sci. USA* **77**:2163–2167.
27. Sandri-Goldin, R. M., Goldin, A. L., Levine, M., and Glorioso. J., 1983, High-efficiency transfer of DNA into eukaryotic cells by protoplast fusion, *Meth. Enzymol.* **101**:402–411.
28. Straubinger, R. M., and Papahadjopoulos, D., 1983, Liposome-mediated DNA transfer, in: *Techniques in Somatic Cell Genetics* (J. W. Shay, ed.) Plenum Press, New York, pp. 399–413.
29. Cepro, C. L., Roberts, T. E., and Mulligan, R. C., 1984, Construction and applications of a highly transmissible murine retrovirus shuttle vector, *Cell* **37**:1053–1062.
30. Gluzman, Y., 1982, *Eukaryotic Viral Vectors*, Cold Spring Harbor Laboratory, Cold Spring Harbor, New York.
31. McCutchan, J. H., and Pagano, J. S., 1968, Enhancement of the infectivity of simian virus 40 deoxyribonucleic acid with diethylaminoethyl-dextran, *J. Natl. Cancer Inst.* **41**:351–357.
32. Kit, S., Dubbs, P., Pierkarski, L., and Hsu, T., 1963, Deletion of thymidine kinase activity from L cells resistant to bromodeoxyuridine, *Exp. Cell Res.* **31**:297–312.
33. Graf, L. H., Jr., Kaplan, P., and Silagi, S., 1984, Efficient DNA-mediated transfer of selectable genes and unselected sequences into differentiated and undifferentiated mouse melanoma clones, *Somat. Cell Mol. Genet.* **10**:139–151.
34. Oi, V. T., Morrison, S., Herzenberg, L. A., and Berg, P. A., 1983, Immunoglobulin gene expression in transformed lymphoid cells, *Proc. Natl. Acad. Sci. USA* **80**:825–829.
35. Deans, R. J., Denis, K. A., Taylor, A., and Wall, R., 1984, Expression of an immunoglobulin heavy chain gene transfected into lymphocytes, *Proc. Natl. Acad. Sci. USA* **81**:1292–1296.
36. Pellicer, A., Wigler, M., Axel, R., and Silverstein, S., 1978, The transfer and stable integration of the HSV thymidine kinase gene into mouse cells, *Cell* **14**:133–141.
37. Minson, A. C., Wildy, P., Buchan, A., and Darby, G., 1978, Introduction of the herpes simplex virus thymidine kinase gene into mouse cells using virus DNA or transformed cell DNA, *Cell* **13**:581–587.
38. Wigler, M., Pellicer, A., Silverstein, S., and Axel, R., 1978, Biochemical transfer of single copy eukaryotic genes using total cellular DNA as donor, *Cell* **14**:725–731.
39. Lester, S. C., LeVan, S. K., Steglich, C., and DeMars, R., 1980, Expression of human genes for adenine phosphoribosyltransferase and hypoxanthine-guanine phosphoribosyltransferase after genetic transformation of mouse cells with purified human DNA, *Somat. Cell Genet.* **6**:241–259.
40. Southern, P. J., and Berg, P., 1982, Transformation of mammalian cells to antibiotic resistance with a bacterial gene under control of the SV40 early region promotor, *J. Mol. Appl. Genet.* **1**:327–341.
41. Mulligan, R. C., and Berg, P., 1981, Factors governing the expression of a bacterial gene in mammalian cells, *Mol. Cell. Biol.* **1**:449–459.

42. Kucherlapati, R. S., and Skoultchi, A. I., 1984, Introduction of purified genes into mammalian cells, *CRC. Rev. Biochem.* **16**:349–381.
43. Shih, C., Padhy, L. C., Murray, M., and Weinberg, R. A., 1981, Transforming genes of carcinomas and neuroblastomas into mouse fibroblasts, *Nature* **290**:261–264.
44. Hsu, C., Kavathas, P., and Herzenberg, L. A., 1984, Cell-surface antigens in L cells transfected with whole DNA from non-expressing and expressing cells, *Nature* **312**:68–69.
45. Westerveld, A., Hoeijmakers, J. H. J., van Duin, M., de Wit, J., Odijk, H., Patsink, A., Wood, R. D., and Bootsma, D., 1984, Molecular cloning of a human DNA repair gene, *Nature* **310**:425–428.
46. Perucho, M., Hanahan, D., Lipsich, L., and Wigler, M., 1980, Isolation of the chicken thymidine kinase gene by plasmid rescue, *Nature* **285**:207–210.
47. Lowy, I., Pellicer, A., Jackson, I., Sim, O. K., Silverstein, S., and Axel, R., 1980, Isolation of transforming DNA: Cloning the hamster APRT gene, *Cell* **22**:817–823.
48. Goldfarb, M., Shimizu, K., Perucho, M., and Wigler, M., 1982, Isolation and preliminary characterization of a human transforming gene from T24 bladder carcinoma cells, *Nature* **296**:404–409.
49. Gusella, J. F., Keys, C., Varsanyi-Breiner, A., Ikao, F. T., Jones, C., Puck, T. T., and Housman, D., 1980, Isolation and localization of DNA segments from specific human chromosomes, *Proc. Natl. Acad. Sci. USA* **77**:2829–2833.
50. Shih, C., and Weinberg, R. A., 1982, Isolation of a transforming sequence from a human bladder carcinoma cell line, *Cell* **29**:161–169.
51. Goubin, G., Goldman, D. S., Luce, J., Nieman, P. E., and Cooper, G. M., 1983, Molecular cloning and nucleotide sequence of a transforming gene detected by transfection of chicken B-cell lymphoma DNA, *Nature* **302**:114–119.
52. Hedrick, S. M., Cohen, D. I., Nielsen, E. A., and Davis, M. M., 1984, Isolation of cDNA clones encoding T cell-specific membrane-associated proteins, *Nature* **308**:149–153.
53. Alt, F. W., Kellems, R. E., Bertino, J. R., and Schimke, R. T. J., 1978, Selective multiplication of dihydrofolate reductase genes in methotrexate-resistant variants of cultured murine cells, *Biol. Chem.* **253**:1357–1369.
54. Lund, T., Grosveld, F. G., and Flavell, R. A., 1982, Isolation of transforming DNA by cosmid rescue, *Proc. Natl. Acad. Sci. USA* **79**:520–524.
55. Lau, Y.-F., and Kan, Y. W., 1984, Direct isolation of the functional human thymidine kinase gene with a cosmid shuttle vector, *Proc. Natl. Acad. Sci. USA* **81**:414–418.
56. Okayama, H., and Berg, P., 1983, A cDNA cloning vector that permits expression of cDNA inserts in mammalian cells, *Mol. Cell. Biol.* **1983**:280–289.
57. Yokota, T., Lee, F., Rennick, D., Hall, C., Arai, N., Mosmann, T., Nabel, G., Cantor, H., and Arai, K., 1984, Isolation and characterization of a mouse cDNA clone that expresses mast-cell growth factor activity in monkey cells, *Proc. Natl. Acad. Sci. USA* **81**:1070–1074.
58. Schimke, R. T., 1984, Gene amplification in cultured animal cells, *Cell* **37**:705–713.
59. Stark, G. R., and Wahl, G. M., 1984, Gene amplification, *Annu. Rev. Biochem.* **53**:447–491.
60. Kavathas, P., and Herzenberg, L. A., 1983, Amplification of a gene coding for a human T cell differentiation antigen, *Nature* **306**:385–387.
61. Wahl, G. M., deSaint, Vincent, B. R., and DeRose, M. L., 1984, Effect of chromosomal position on amplification of transfected genes in animal cells, *Nature* **307**:516–520.
62. Wigler, M., Perucho, M., Kurtz, D., Dana, S., Pellicer, A., Axel, R., and Silverstein, S., 1980, Transformation of mammalian cells with an amplifiable dominant-acting gene, *Proc. Natl. Acad. Sci. USA* **77**:3567–3570.
63. Christman, J. K., Gerber, M., Price, P. M., Flordellis, C., Edelman, J., and Acs, G., 1982, Amplification of expression of hepatitis B surface antigen in 3T3 cells cotransfected with a dominant-acting gene and cloned viral DNA, *Proc. Natl. Acad. Sci. USA* **79**:1815–1819.
64. Goodenow, R. S., McMillan, M., Orn, A., Nicolson, M., Davidson, M., Frelinger, J. A., and Hood, L., 1982, Identification of a BALB/c H-2L^d gene by DNA-mediated gene transfer, *Science* **215**:677–679.

Chapter 24

Screening λgt11 Expression Libraries with Antibody Probes

MICHAEL SNYDER and RONALD W. DAVIS

1. Introduction

Antibodies can be used as probes to isolate directly a particular gene of interest. A recombinant DNA library is first constructed in an *Escherichia coli* expression vector, and foreign antigens are expressed in *E. coli* from the DNA inserts. The antigens produced are transferred onto nitrocellulose filters and then probed with antibody to detect the desired recombinant. This approach is rapid, and is particularly useful for isolating genes that are expressed at a low level and therefore are difficult to isolate using techniques employing nucleic acid probes (see Ref. 1) or by hybrid/selection methods.[2] This chapter describes methods for isolating eukaryotic genes by constructing and screening *E. coli* expression vector libraries with antibody probes using the bacteriophage expression vector λgt11.[3,4]

2. λgt11

A diagram of λgt11 is shown in Fig. 1.[3] λgt11 contains the structural gene of *E. coli* β-galactosidase (*lac*Z) for expressing foreign DNA inserts. A unique *Eco*RI cloning site is located at the 3′ end of the *lac*Z gene, 53 bp upstream of the translation termination codon. cDNA or genomic DNA inserts are cloned into this site and when introduced in the proper orientation and reading frame will result in the production of exogenous protein fused to β-galactosidase. In several cases[5,6] it has been shown that fusion of a foreign protein to a stable *E. coli* protein enhances the stability of the foreign protein.

Since λgt11 propagates to high copy number during lytic infection of *E. coli*, and since the promotor of the *lac*Z gene is a strong *E. coli* promotor, a significant fraction of the total *E. coli* cellular protein is produced from the *lac*Z gene. In the case of *lac*Z alone (unfused to any other sequences), approx-

MICHAEL SNYDER and RONALD W. DAVIS • Department of Biochemistry, Stanford University School of Medicine, Stanford, California 94305.

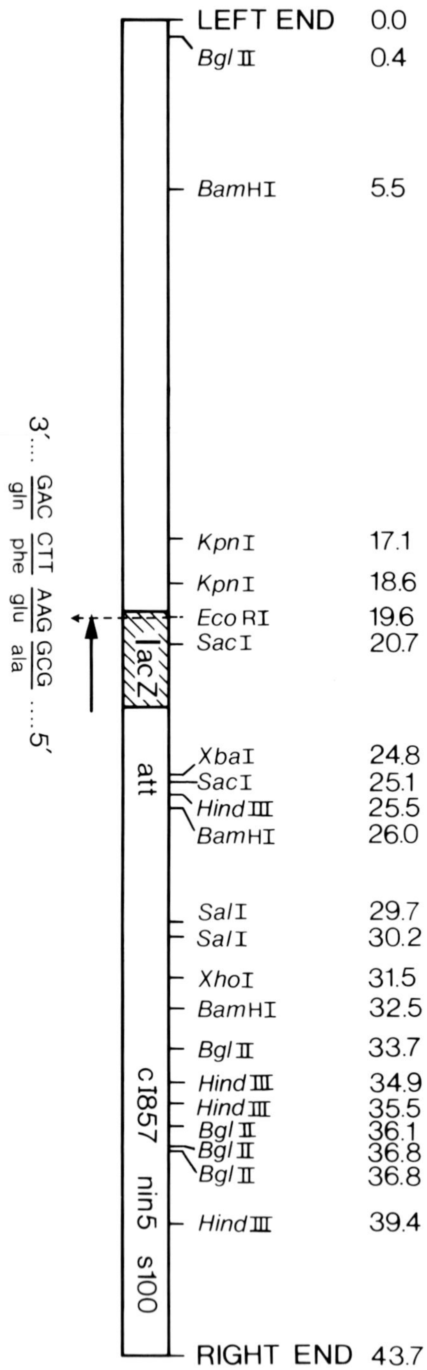

Figure 1. Restriction map and other features of λgt11. Restriction endonuclease sites are shown; the distance in kb from the left end is indicated above each site. The positions of the S100, nin5, and cI857 mutations are shown, as well as the λ attachment site and the *lacZ* gene. The *lacZ* gene is transcribed in the direction of the arrow. The sequence around the *Eco*RI site with the encoded amino acids is also depicted.

imately 5% of the total cellular protein is β-galactosidase (P. Beachy, personal communication). For the λgt11 fusions studied thus far, the fusion proteins comprise from less than 0.1% up to 2% of the total *E. coli* protein (Ref. 3 and P. Beachy, personal communication).

3. *Escherichia coli* Host

The *E. coli* host has three features that are important for immunoscreening λgt11 expression libraries. First, the bacterial strain used is deficient in the *lon* protease. The presence of the *lon* mutation allows the accumulation of β-galactosidase fusion proteins to much higher levels than in wild-type *E. coli* (see Ref. 3).

Second, the bacterial strain carries a pBR322 plasmid (pMC9) containing a *lac*I gene, which codes for *lac* repressor.[7] This allows the regulated expression of β-galactosidase fusion proteins. Expression of these fusion proteins, some of which may be deleterious to growth of the *E. coli* host, is repressed during initial propagation of the phage, but is induced late after infection with isopropyl-β-D-thiogalactoside (IPTG). In the presence of the *lon* mutation and absence of *lac*I plasmids, λgt11 recombinants usually from smaller plaques, and the plaque size varies with the particular recombinant.

The third feature of the *E. coli* host is the presence of the *sup*F suppressor tRNA. The *sup*F is required for forming plaques because λgt11 carries S100, an *amber* mutation in the S lysis gene.

4. Constructing λgt11 Recombinant DNA Libraries

Two types of recombinant DNA libraries can be used for immunoscreening: genomic DNA libraries (M. Snyder and R. W. Davis, unpublished results) and cDNA libraries.[8] The construction of cDNA libraries is detailed elsewhere.[8] Near full-length cDNAs encode the most antigenic determinants and are most useful for screening. For organisms of *Drosophila* genomic size (1.8×10^8 bp) or smaller, genomic DNA libraries can be constructed and screened. Genomic DNA is randomly sheared and cloned into the λgt11 *lac*Z gene. Genomic DNA libraries have the advantage that all sequences can be screened regardless of their level of expression. Genomic DNA libraries differ from cDNA libraries in that the relative probability of having a particular gene fused to *lac*Z depends upon the length of the gene and the size of the organism's genome. For instance, fusion of any portion of a 1-kb yeast gene (yeast genome = 14,000 kb) to *lac*Z will occur one out of 14,000 times and one out of six fusions will present in the proper orientation and reading frame. Therefore, an in-frame fusion will occur an average of once in every 8.4×10^4 recombinants. Fusions nearest the carboxy-terminal protein coding sequences will encode fewer antigenic determinants than amino-terminal protein fusions. In addition, the frequency of identifying a gene within a genomic library will also depend on the number of translational interruptions by intervening sequences. Many organisms of small genome size, such as *Drosophila* and yeast, contain few if any introns within their coding sequences.

A protocol for constructing a random shear genomic DNA library is as follows (M. Snyder and R. W. Davis, unpublished results):

1. Shear genomic DNA (10–20 μg at 100 μg/ml) by forcing DNA through a 27-gauge syringe needle to an average size of 5 kb. The size of the sheared DNA is monitored by agarose gel electrophoresis.[1]
2. Trim the DNA ends with T_4 DNA polymerase using 100 μl of 50 mM Tris-HCl pH 7.8, 5 mM $MgCl_2$, 50 μg/ml BSA, 10 mM β-mercaptoethanol, 20 μM of each dNTP, and 5–10 units of T_4 DNA polymerase. Incubate 30 min at room temperature. Ethanol-precipitate DNA.
3. Methylate DNA using 50 μl of 50 mM Tris-HCl pH, 7.5, 1 mM EDTA, 5 mM DTT, 10 μM S-adenosyl-L-methionine plus 2 μg *Eco*R1 methylase. Incubate 37°C for 15 min, then 10 min at 70°C.
4. (Optional) To ensure flush DNA ends, add 5 μl of 1 M $MgCl_2$ and dNTP to final concentration of 20 μM. Add *E. coli* DNA polymerase I (or Klenow fragment). Incubate 30 min at room temperature. Extract two times with phenol:$CHCl_3$ (50:50), then twice with $CHCl_3$ alone. Ethanol-precipitate DNA and rinse DNA pellet with 70% ethanol.
5. Ligate *Eco*RI linkers on DNA using 50 μl of 70 mM Tris-HCl, pH 7.5, 10 mM $MgCl_2$, 200 μg/ml gelatin, 10 mM DTT, 1 mM rATP, 100 μg/ml phosphorylated *Eco*RI linkers plus 0.5 μl of 1.5 mg/ml T_4 DNA ligase. Incubate at 4°C for 6 hr or longer. Ethanol-precipitate DNA.
6. Dissolve pellet in 100 μl *Eco*RI restriction digest buffer. Add 50 units *Eco*RI and incubate 2 hr at 37°C, then 10 min at 70°C. Ethanol-precipitate DNA twice.
7. DNA purification and size fractionation: The DNA is completely dissolved in electrophoresis buffer and size-fractionated on a 0.8% agarose gel. The 2-to 10-kb DNA is collected as desired. Two methods we use are: (a) Cut an empty well in front of the DNA to be recovered. As the gel is running, remove aliquots from the well every 30–60 sec. The DNA can be recovered by adding NaAcetate, pH 6, to 0.3 M and ethanol-precipitating. (b) Place Schleicher and Schuell NA45 membrane in a gel slot just ahead of the DNA to be collected. Electrophorese DNA into the NA45 membrane at high current. Rinse NA45 membrane in electrophoresis buffer and elute DNA in 1 M NaCl, 0.05 M arginine (free base) at 70°C for approximately 2 hr. Extract the DNA with phenol:$CHCl_3$ and then $CHCl_3$ as in step 4 and recover DNA by ethanol-precipitation. If linker contamination presents a problem, it may be necessary to repeat the gel isolation step.
8. Vector preparation: λgt11 DNA is ligated to form concatamers using the buffer conditions in step 5 (without linkers) at room temperature for 1–2 hr. Incubate at 70°C for 15 min and ethanol-precipitate DNA. Cleave DNA with *Eco*R1. Treat with calf intestine alkaline phosphatase

(CAP) in 50 μl of 50 mM Tris-HCl, pH 9.0, using high-quality CAP enzyme whose activity is well characterized. Extract DNA with phenol:$CHCl_3$ as in step 4 and ethanol-precipitate DNA.

9. Library construction: Ligate genomic insert DNA into λgt11 using mass ratio of insert DNA:vector DNA of 0.5–1:1 using buffer conditions in step 5 and a vector DNA concentration of 400 μg/ml. Incubate at room temperature for several hours to overnight.
10. *In vitro* package DNA and titer according to Ref. 8.
11. Amplify library on Y1088 in the presence of 50 μg/ml ampicillin. Y1088 = Δ*lac*U169 *sup*E *sup*F *hsd*R^- *hsd*M^+ *met*B *trp*R *ton*A21 *pro*C::Tn5 + pMC9. This bacterial strain contains the *lac*I plasmid in order to prevent the expression of proteins that are harmful to *E. coli*.

Using these protocols it has been possible to construct λgt11 genomic DNA libraries containing 2–4 × 10^6 recombinants from yeast and *Mycobacterium leprae* (M. Snyder, R. Young, and R. W. Davis, unpublished results).

5. Preparation of Antibody Probes

The quality of the antiserum is important for successful immunoscreening. In general, antisera that work well on immunoblots or "Westerns" also produce good signals for immunoscreens. Polyclonal antisera have the advantage of recognizing a wide variety of determinants on any given antigen. This is particularly important, since genomic and cDNA inserts often will not be full length and hence only a portion of the polypeptide chain will be expressed. Monoclonal (T. St. John, personal communication) as well as polyclonal antibodies have been successfully used. However, monoclonal antibodies can detect clones other than the particular recombinant of interest (T. St. John, personal communication). Therefore, immunoscreening with polyclonal antisera or with several monoclonal antibodies recognizing different determinants on the same antigen is recommended.

Most rabbit or human sera contain varying amounts of anti-*E. coli* antibodies. These are most easily removed by "pseudoscreening." A general protocol is as follows (M. Snyder and R. W. Davis, unpublished results. Further details can be found in the next section.):

1. Plate out λgt11 phage, 10^5 phage per 150-mm LB plates[10] on strain Y1090 (Y1090 = Δ*lac*U169 *pro*A^+ Δ*lon ara*D139 *str*A *sup*F [*trp*C22::Tn10] + pMC9). Incubate 3 hr at 42°C.
2. Overlay plates with 132-mm nitrocellulose filters that were previously wetted and dried in 10 mM IPTG. Incubate at 37°C for 4 hr or longer.
3. Remove protein-bound filters. Wash in 150 mM NaCl, 50 mM Tris-HCl, pH 8.1 (TBS).
4. Incubate filters in TBS + 20% fetal calf serum (FCS) for 45 min or longer. The TBS + 20% FCS solution can be reused four times or more.

5. Incubate filters with antibody for 2–3 hr. The antibody is diluted in TBS + 20% FCS. For rabbit sera (IgG ~ 2 mg/ml) that we have used, dilutions of 1:100 work well. For human sera (IgG ~ 10 mg/ml) dilutions of 1:300 are used. Use two filters per 25 ml of diluted antibody.
6. Repeat antiserum cleanups (two or three times or as often as appears necessary). The same λgt11 plates can be reused. After removing the first filter, overlay the plate with another IPTG-treated nitrocellulose filter and incubate at 37°C for 2 or more hours.

General methods for plating and handling bacteriophage λ can be found in Refs. 1 and 10.

6. Screening Expression Vector Libraries with Antibody Probes

1. Plate out library: Grow an overnight culture of Y1090 cells in LB media containing 50 μg/ml ampicillin and 0.2% maltose. Infect 0.1 ml of saturated culture with 1×10^5 phage for each 150-mm plate. Adsorb phage at room temperature for 25 min or at 37°C for 15 min. Add 6.25 ml LB top agar, mix, and plate on 150-mm LB plate. Neither top agar nor plates contain ampicillin. Plates work best 2–5 days after preparation.
2. Incubate plates at 42°C for 3.0 hr until lawn just begins to appear.
3. Overlay plates with IPTG-treated nitrocellulose filters. The nitrocellulose filters are previously wetted in 10 mM IPTG in distilled water and air-dried on cellophane wrap. Incubate plates at 37°C for 8–10 hours (overnight). At the end of the incubation period, remove the lid from the plates and incubate an additional 10 min at 37°C. This step prevents top agar from sticking to the filter.
4. Remove plates from incubator, and mark filter position with a syringe needle containing ink. Carefully remove filters from plates. For duplicate screening, overlay plates with a second IPTG-treated filter and return to 37°C for 2–5 hr.

For all subsequent steps, filters are treated two per Petri dish.

5. Rinse filters one to two times in TBS.
6. Treat for 45 min or longer in TBS + 20% FCS (save and reuse this solution several times).
7. Incubate filters in antibody diluted in TBS + 20% FCS for 2–3 hr.
8. Wash 10 min each (a) TBS + 0.1% BSA, (b) TBS + 0.1% BSA + 0.1% NP40, (c) TBS + 0.1% BSA.
9. Incubate with ^{125}I-protein A in TBS + 0.1% BSA for 1.5–2 hr. Use 1 μCi of >30 mCi/mg specific activity ^{125}I-protein A (ICN or Amersham) per 132-mm filter.
10. Wash filters 10 min each (a) TBS + 0.1% BSA, (b) TBS + 0.1% BSA + 0.1% NP40, repeat once, (c) TBS + 0.1% BSA.

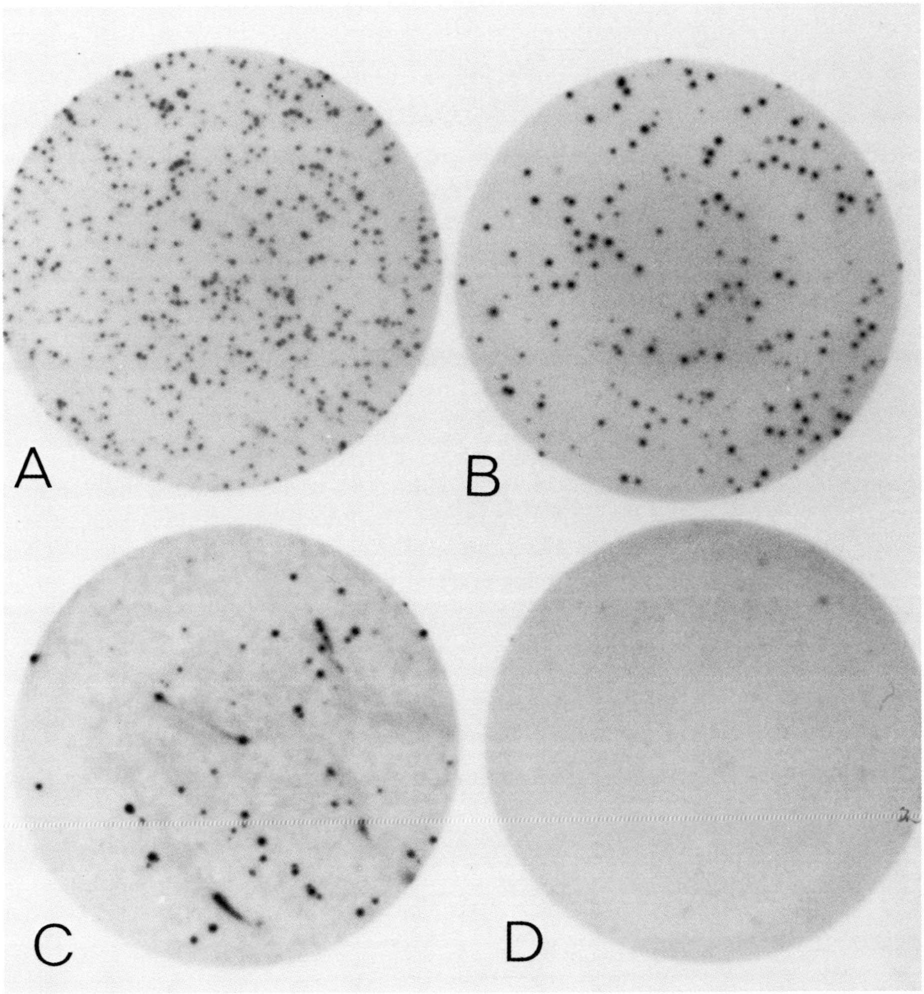

Figure 2. Exemplary positives from immunoscreening. A yeast genomic DNA library was screened with anti-yeast DNA polymerase I antibody[18,19] as described in the text. (A–C) Independent positives were replated and screened at a density of approximately 40–500 positive phage in a background of $0.3–3 \times 10^4$ nonreactive phage. (D) The λgt11 vector alone at the same phage density.

11. Dry and expose to X-ray film.

Exemplary positives for antiserum to yeast DNA polymerase I are shown in Fig. 2 (M. Snyder, L. Johnson, and J. Campbell, unpublished results).

Notes:

1. Incubation of IPTG-treated nitrocellulose filters on the plates for 8–10 hr yields 5–10 times stronger signals than for a 2-hr incubation.

2. The antibody solution can be reused many times. For anti-DNA polymerase I antibodies we have reused the serum 12 times with little reduction in intensity (M. Snyder, L. Johnson, and J. Campbell, unpublished results). Every time the serum is used, the background is reduced, presumably because of the further removal of anti-*E. coli* antibodies from the serum.
3. It is recommended for primary screens that plates be screened in duplicate to avoid false positives, which typically occur at a frequency of one or two per 132-mm filter.
4. Filters can be stored for at least 2 days in TBS + 20% FCS (step 6) prior to treatment with antibody, if desired.
5. Most polyvalent antibodies work fine at room temperature. Signals seem to increase several-fold if antibody treatments and subsequent incubations are performed at 4°C, which is the recommended temperature for low-affinity antibodies.
6. Alternative methods of detection involve using (a) horseradish peroxidase-conjugated second antibody or (b) biotinylated antibody plus avidin-conjugated horseradish peroxidase. The horseradish peroxidase is then detected with a colorimetric substrate directly on the filter. This procedure is described in Ref. 11. It does not offer improved sensitivity.
7. Control experiments (C. Glover and M. Snyder, unpublished results) where known amounts of protein antigen have been spotted onto screening filters and probed with antibody as above indicate that the limit of detection for a given high-titer serum is approximately 100 pg of protein. Actual amounts of antigen in a single plaque range up to approximately 50 times higher than this for the positives thus far isolated.
8. Genes may be expressed in the opposite orientation relative to *lacZ*, presumably because sequences within the foreign DNA insert serve as *E. coli* transcriptional and translational sequences.[9]

7. Confirmation of Gene Identity

The most difficult part of gene isolation by immunoscreening is discerning whether the immunoreactive clones do, in fact, encode the gene of interest. Several useful methods for testing clone identity are as follows.

7.1. Affinity Purification of Antibodies Using λgt11 Clones

A rapid, but not entirely sufficient criterion for testing whether a positive λgt11 recombinant encodes the particular protein of interest is to use the λgt11 clones to affinity-purify antibody from the screening serum, and use the clone-purified-antibody to probe "Western" or immunoblots of a purified or crude preparation of that protein. This is particularly useful if the original antiserum was not made against a homogeneous protein. A protocol is as follows (M. Snyder and R. W. Davis, unpublished results):

1. Plate out the positive recombinants at high density, 2–5 × 10^4 phage/90-mm LB plate. Use 2.5 ml of L top agar and 50 μl of Y1090 cells. Follow steps 1–8 of the immunoscreening protocol for preparing filters, treating with antibody and washes. One plate/clone should be sufficient for most sera.
2. Take the antibody-treated filter, crumple slightly, and put in a capped tube. Add 3.5 ml of 0.2 M glycine-HCl, pH 2.5. Shake tube for 2 min and no longer. Remove filter.
3. Immediately add 1.75 ml of 1.0 M KPO_4, pH 9.0, + 5% FCS and mix.
4. Dilute to lower ionic strength. Add FCS to 20%, and use directly for immunoblots. Immunoblot protocols can be found in Ref. 12.

7.2. DNA Sequencing

The DNA sequence of the λgt11 recombinant insert can be determined and the deduced amino acid sequence compared with the known protein sequence.

7.3. Gene Expression

The λgt11 recombinant can be used as a hybridization probe to recover an intact gene. The intact gene can be overexpressed in *E. coli* or other organisms and assayed for gene activity. Overexpression in *E. coli* has been performed for yeast topoisomerase II.[9] Overexpression in yeast has been performed for yeast DNA polymerase I (M. Snyder, L. Johnson, and J. Campbell, unpublished results).

8. Conclusion

Using the above techniques, clones encoding the following proteins have been isolated and their identity verified: subunits for yeast RNA polymerases I, II, and III (Ref. 4, and J.-M. Buhler and A. Sentenac, unpublished results), yeast DNA polymerase I (M. Snyder, L. Johnson, and J. Campbell, unpublished results), yeast topoisomerase II,[9] *Plasmodium* antigens,[13] human terminal deoxynucleotidyltransferase,[14,15] chicken α- and β-spectrin (R. T. Moon and E. Lazarides, unpublished results), rat fibronectin,[16] and human factor X.[17] These studies have utilized polyclonal[4,9] and affinity-purified polyclonal[13–15,16,17] antibodies.

Acknowledgments. Our thanks to Tom St. John and Rick Young for developing the immunoscreening techniques and to our collaborators, Judith Campbell and Claiborne Glover, for their invaluable help. We are also grateful to Lucy Chang and Frank McKeon for antisera, Steve Elledge for manuscript criticisms, and Juergen Reichardt and many others in our department who provided critical suggestions.

References

1. Maniatis, T., Fritsch, E. F., and Sambrook, J., 1982, *Molecular Cloning*, Cold Spring Harbor Laboratory , Cold Spring Harbor, New York.
2. Ricciardi, R. P., Miller, J. S., and Roberts, B. E., 1979, Purification and mapping of specific mRNAs by hybridization-selection and cell-free translation, *Proc. Natl. Acad. Sci. USA* **76:**4927–4931.
3. Young, R. A., and Davis, R. W., 1983, Efficient isolation of genes by using antibody probes, *Proc. Natl. Acad. Sci. USA* **80:**1194–1198.
4. Young, R. A., and Davis, R. W., 1984, Yeast RNA polymerase II genes: Isolation with antibody probes, *Science* **222:**778–782.
5. Kupper, H., Keller, W., Kurtz, C., Forss, S., Schaller, H., Franze, R., Strommaier, K., Marquardt, O., Zaslavsky, V. G., and Hofschneider, P. H., 1981, Cloning of cDNA of major antigen of foot and mouth disease virus and expression in *E. coli*, *Nature* **289:**555–559.
6. Stanley, K., 1983, Solubilization and immune-detection of β-galactosidase hybrid proteins carrying foreign antigenic determinants, *Nucleic Acids Res.* **11:**4077–4092.
7. Calos, M. P., Lebkowski, T. S., and Botchan, M. R., 1983, High mutation frequency in DNA transfected into mammalian cells, *Proc. Natl. Acad. Sci. USA* **80:**3015–3019.
8. Huynh, T. V., Young, R. A., and Davis, R. W., 1984, Constructing and screening cDNA libraries in λgt10 and λgt11, *DNA Cloning Techniques: A Practical Approach* (D. Glover, ed.), IRL Press, Oxford.
9. Goto, T., and Wang, J. C., 1984, Yeast DNA topoisomerase II is encoded by a single-copy, essential gene, *Cell* **36:**1073–1080.
10. Davis, R. W., Botstein, D., and Roth, J. R., 1980, *Advanced Bacterial Genetics*, Cold Spring Harbor Laboratory, Cold Spring Harbor, New York.
11. Young, R. A., and Davis, R. W., 1984, Immunoscreening λgt11 recombinant DNA expression libraries, *Genetic Engineering* Volume 7 (J. Setlow and A. Hollaender, eds.), Plenum Press, New York.
12. Burnette, W. N., 1981, "Western Blotting": Electrophoretic transfer of proteins from sodium dodecyl sulfate–polyacrylamide gels to unmodified nitrocellulose and radiographic detection with antibody and radioiodinated protein A, *Anal. Biochem.* **112:**195–203.
13. Kemp, D. J., Coppel, R. L., Cowman, A. F., Saint, R. B., Brown, G. V., and Anders, R. F., 1983, Expression of *Plasmodium falciparum* blood-stage antigens in *Escherichia coli*: Detection with antibodies from immune humans, *Proc. Natl. Acad. Sci. USA* **80:**3787–3791.
14. Peterson, R. C., Cheung, L. C., Mattaliano, R. V., Chang, L. M. S., and Bollum, F. J., 1984, Molecular cloning of human terminal deoxynucleotidyltransferase, *Proc. Natl. Acad. Sci. USA* **81:**4363–4367.
15. Landau, N. R., St. John, T. P., Weissman, I. L., Wolf, S. C., Silverstone, A. E., and Baltimore, D., 1984, Cloning of terminal transferase cDNA by antibody screening, *Proc. Natl. Acad. Sci. USA* **81:**5836–5840.
16. Schwarzbauer, J. E., Tamkun, J. W., Lemischka, I. R., and Hynes, R. O., 1983, Three different fibronectin mRNAs arise by alternative splicing within the coding region, *Cell* **35:**421–431.
17. Leytus, S. P., Chung, D. W., Kisiel, W., Kurachi, K., and Davie, E. W., 1984, Characterization of a cDNA coding for human factor X, *Proc. Natl. Acad. Sci. USA* **81:**3699–3702.
18. Badaracco, G., Capucci, L., Plevani, P., and Chang, L. M. S., 1983, Polypeptide structure of DNA polymerase I from *Saccharomyces cerevisiae*, *J. Biol. Chem.* **258:**10720–10726.
19. Chang, L. M. S., 1977, DNA polymerases from bakers yeast, *J. Biol. Chem.* **252:**1873–1880.

Chapter 25

Purification of Low-Abundance Messenger RNAs by Polysome Isolation with Polyclonal Antibodies

JAN P. KRAUS

1. Introduction

Current interest in the isolation and characterization of normal and mutant genes has focused attention on the need for recombinant DNA molecules complementary to low-abundance mRNAs. The low-abundance class of mRNAs (i.e., each constituting <0.5% of total cellular mRNA) comprises approximately 30% of the mRNA of the eukaryotic cell and codes for a majority of its enzymes. Starting with a total unfractionated mRNA, a cDNA library of at least 200,000 independent clones is required to obtain a complete representation of low-abundance mRNAs.[1] A major problem in recovering a cDNA corresponding to a low-abundance mRNA from such a library is the laborious screening required to detect the rare cloned low-abundance sequences. A substantial initial enrichment of a given low-abundance mRNA would simplify dramatically the procedures involved in preparing or identifying recombinant DNA molecules containing complementary nucleotide sequences.

The idea of preparing specific mRNAs by isolating polysomes immunologically by reaction with antibodies directed against their nascent polypeptide chains is now almost 25 years old.[2] Over the years, various immunoprecipitation procedures have been developed, which have generally been used toward purification of abundant mRNAs, i.e., those representing 5–60% of total cellular mRNA.[3–17] The earlier techniques involved formation of insoluble polysome–antibody–antiantibody complexes, which were subsequently isolated by centrifugation through discontinuous sucrose gradients.[3–9] Nonspecific physical trapping of polysomes within the precipitated complex, however, often resulted in contamination of the desired mRNA with other messages.[7,8] Improvement of this immunopurification technique was achieved by binding the polysome–antibody complexes to solid phase reagents, thereby replacing

JAN P. KRAUS • Department of Human Genetics, Yale University School of Medicine, New Haven, Connecticut 06510.

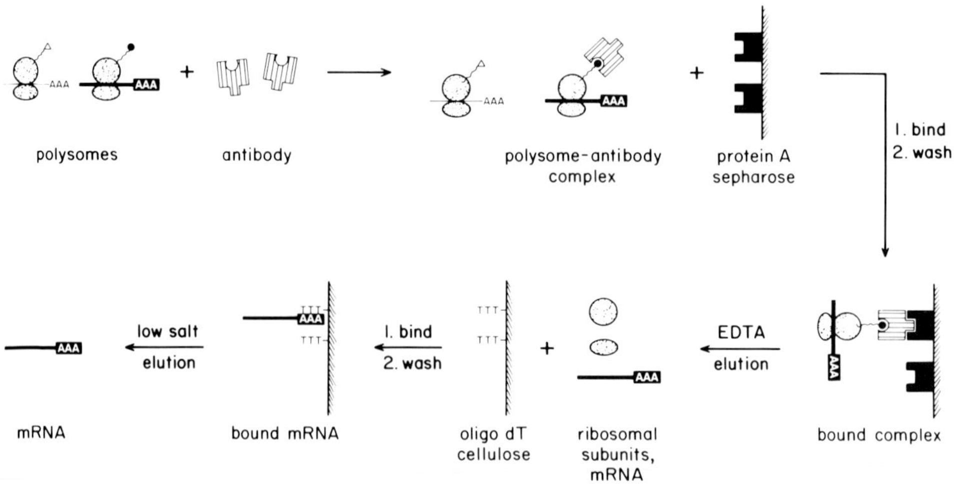

Figure 1. Enrichment of mRNA by immunoadsorption of specific polysomes.

the immunoprecipitation reaction by a binding reaction, lowering the total amount of protein used, and allowing for improved washing of the complexes. The approaches used have included substitution of *Staphylococcus aureus* cells for the second antibody,[11–13] use of cross-linked antigen,[14] and covalent binding of the second antibody[15,16] or additional antigen[17] to derivatized cellulose. With each modification, however, recovery of the polysome–antibody complexes was accomplished by centrifugation. Moreover, most of these procedures used an antigen-purified IgG fraction and therefore required milligram amounts of pure antigen. Whereas this approach sometimes yielded considerable enrichment of abundant mRNA species,[3–17] I have found no mention of its success with low-abundance mRNAs.

Recently, Shapiro and Young[18] reported an impressive purification of a relatively abundant (7–10%) mRNA coding for a trypanosomal surface antigen by immunoadsorption of polysome–antibody complexes to a protein A–Sepharose column. We reasoned that use of such an immunoadsorbent column might facilitate purification of low-abundance mRNAs as well, by permitting more effective removal of extraneous polysomes than could be achieved with centrifugation techniques. We have recently reported[19] purification to near homogeneity of three low-abundance mRNAs from rat liver (representing 0.01–0.05% of total hepatic mRNA) by such specific immunoadsorption. Simultaneously, Korman *et al.*[20] showed that another low-abundance mRNA from human lymphoblastoid cells can be purified using the method of Shapiro and Young.[18] Since then, the mRNA immunopurification protocol has been used successfully to prepare or to identify cDNA clones corresponding to about a dozen[21–31] low-abundance mRNAs from various sources.

The protocol depends on four key steps: purification of an IgG fraction from monospecific polyclonal antiserum on a protein A–Sepharose column;

isolation of intact polysomes bearing nascent polypeptide chains; selective immobilization of the polysome–antibody complexes on a protein A–Sepharose column; and separation of the eluted mRNA from the ribosomal subunits on an oligo-dT cellulose column. An outline of the immunopurification procedure is shown in Fig. 1. Our original purification protocol[19] has been, significantly modified and scaled up in the last 2 years. The most recent version is described below.

2. Materials and Methods

2.1. RNase-Free Techniques

All glassware was heated at 285°C for at least 2 hr. Plasticware was treated with a solution of 0.5% diethylpyrocarbonate (Aldrich) in 70% ethanol, then rinsed with ethanol, and finally rinsed with sterile H_2O. Stock solutions of 0.5 M Tris-HCl, pH 7.5, 4 M NaCl, 0.1 M EDTA, pH 7.5, and H_2O were treated with 0.5% diethylpyrocarbonate for 20 min and then autoclaved. One molar magnesium acetate, 20 mg/ml heparin (Sigma), 1 mg/ml trichodermin (Leo Pharmaceutical Products, DK-2750, Ballerup, Denmark), 10% Nonidet P-40, 10% sodium dodecyl sulfate (SDS), and 2.5 M sucrose were prepared in baked bottles or sterile plastic tubes using autoclaved H_2O and filtered using Nalgene filter units. All buffers and solutions were prepared from these stock solutions using baked glassware. Vanadyl ribonucleoside complexes to inhibit RNase were prepared as described[32] except that the amount of vanadyl sulfate used was doubled. Dialysis tubing was boiled in 10 mM KOH, then boiled in 1 mM EDTA/ 0.5% diethylpyrocarbonate, and rinsed with sterile H_2O.

2.2. Reagents for Polysome Immunopurification

Homogenization buffer: 50 mM Tris-HCl, pH 7.5, 25 mM NaCl, 15 mM magnesium acetate, 0.25 M sucrose, 10 mM vanadyl ribonucleoside complexes, 1 μg/ml trichodermin.

Detergent solution: 10% (w/v) sodium deoxycholate/10% (v/v) Triton X-100.

Sucrose cushion buffer: 25 mM Tris-HCl, pH 7.5, 150 mM NaCl, 5 mM magnesium acetate, 0.4 mg/ml heparin, 1 μg/ml trichodermin.

Polysome buffer: 25 mM Tris-HCl, pH 7.5, 150 mM NaCl, 5 mM magnesium acetate, 0.2 mg/ml heparin, 0.1% Nonidet P-40, 1 μg/ml trichodermin.

Elution buffer: 25 mM Tris-HCl, pH 7.5, 0.2 mg/ml heparin, 20 mM EDTA.

2.3. Antibodies

Antisera against homogeneous bovine hepatic ornithine transcarbamylase,[33] the β subunit of human hepatic propionyl CoA carboxylase,[34] and human hepatic cystathionine β-synthase[35] were raised in rabbits. Each antiserum (3–6 ml) was mixed 1:1 (v/v) with 0.1 M potassium phosphate (pH 7) and applied to 0.7 × 11 cm column of protein A–Sepharose (Pharmacia). The column was washed with 80 ml of 0.1 M potassium phosphate (pH 7) and the IgG fraction was eluted with 0.1 M glycine (pH 3). The eluate was immediately dialyzed against 20 mM sodium phosphate, 150 mM NaCl, pH 7.6. After dialysis, the purified IgG fractions were concentrated to 1.5–3 ml by ultrafiltration (Amicon, XM-50 membrane) and adjusted to 50% (v/v) with glycerol; heparin was added to a final concentration of 0.2 mg/ml. The antibodies were stored at −15°C.

2.4. Isolation of Polysomes

Young male Sprague-Dawley rats (140–160 g) were used in all of the experiments. Livers from six decapitated animals were individually placed in 10–15 ml of homogenization buffer, minced with sharp scissors, and homogenized with a Potter-Elvehjem homogenizer. Sufficient homogenization buffer was added to make a 15% (w/v) homogenate. The homogenate was centrifuged for 10 min at 14,500 rpm in a Sorvall SS 34 rotor. The supernatant was collected and diluted with 0.1 volume of the detergent solution. Aliquots of the supernatant (~ 35 ml) were layered over a discontinuous sucrose gradient (prepared in Beckman polycarbonate bottles) containing 15 ml of 2 M sucrose and 15 ml of 1 M sucrose (both sucrose solutions were prepared in the sucrose cushion buffer). The gradients were centrifuged for 16 hr at 35,000 rpm in the Beckman 35 rotor at 4°C. After centrifugation, the supernatants were carefully aspirated, except for about 1 ml of sucrose cushion on the bottom of the tube. While proceeding to the bottom of the tube, care has to be taken not to disturb the clear polysome pellet on the side of the tube. The polysomes in each tube were resuspended in 1–2 ml of polysome buffer by repeated pipetting with a baked Pasteur pipette. An aliquot was diluted in 100 mM sodium acetate, pH 5, 10 mM EDTA, and 1% SDS, and absorbance at 260 and 280 nm was determined. The typical yield was 50–60 A_{260} units of polysomes per gram of liver with A_{260}/A_{280} ratio of ~1.75. At this point, the polysomes were aliquoted and quickly frozen in a dry ice/ethanol bath and stored at −70°C. The polysomes were fully stable for at least 2 years. The functional integrity and relative yield of the desired mRNA in the isolated polysomes were checked by applying an aliquot of the polysomes (~50 A_{260} units) directly to an oligo-dT cellulose column after disruption by the addition of NaCl, SDS, and EDTA to final concentrations of 0.5 M, 0.5%, and 20 mM, respectively. The eluted poly A^+ RNA was then translated *in vitro* and the presence of the corresponding protein species determined by immunoprecipitation.

2.5. Immobilization of Polysome–Antibody Complexes

Polysomes (800–1000 A_{260} units) were thawed, centrifuged for 10 min at 12,000 × g to remove aggregates, and adjusted with polysome buffer to a concentration of 15 A_{260} units/ml. Polysomes were reacted for 1 hr at 4°C with specific purified IgG at a ratio of 100 A_{260} units of polysomes per milligram of IgG. The mixture was passed through a small (1–2 ml) Sepharose 4B precolumn to remove any nonspecifically binding material. The eluate was then applied to a 1.5 × 3.5 cm column of protein A–Sepharose equilibrated with polysome buffer. During sample application, the flow rate was set at approximately one column volume/hr. The unbound polysomes in the breakthrough fraction were quick-frozen and saved for immunopurification of other mRNA species with different antibodies. After application of the sample the column was washed overnight with polysome buffer (at least 20 column volumes).

2.6. Elution and Isolation of Specific mRNA

After the overnight wash, the ribosomal subunits and the specific mRNA were eluted from the column with two to three column volumes of the elution buffer at a flow rate of one column volume/hr. Elution of the disrupted, immunoselected polysomes was monitored at 254 or 280 nm using a flowthrough UV monitor (Uvicord II, LKB). (Following the elution of RNA, the antibody was recovered by washing the column with 0.1 M glycine, pH 3. The eluted IgG was dialyzed and concentrated as described above.) The RNA eluate was immediately adjusted to 0.5 M NaCl and 0.5% SDS, and applied to a 0.5-ml column of oligo-dT cellulose (type 2, Collaborative Research) using three passes to ensure complete binding. The column was washed with 15 ml of high-salt buffer (0.5 M NaCl, 1 mM EDTA, 0.5% SDS, 10 mM Tris-HCl, pH 7.5), and the bound RNA was eluted with low-salt buffer containing 1 mM EDTA, 0.05% SDS, 10 mM Tris-HCl, pH 7.5 and precipitated at −20°C with two volumes of ethanol and 0.05 volume of 4 M NaCl in the presence of carrier (calf liver tRNA or glycogen, 10 μg/ml). In some instances, in order to remove minor contaminants, the immunoselected mRNA was further purified on a linear sucrose gradient. The entire poly A-selected mRNA sample was loaded on a 5–20% (w/w) gradient of sucrose in 10 mM Tris-HCl, pH 7.4, 1 mM EDTA, 0.5% SDS. Centrifugation was for 16 hr at 20°C in a Beckman SW41 rotor at 28,000 rpm. Gradients were fractionated by using Buchler Auto Densi Flow apparatus, and the RNA in each fraction was precipitated with ethanol as described above. An approximate yield was 30 ng of mRNA from 800 A_{260} units of polysomes (for an mRNA with a relative abundance of 0.01–0.02% of total mRNA). Typically, 2% of the final preparation was checked for purity in a 10-μl translation mixture.

2.7. *In Vitro* Translation and Immunoprecipitation

A rabbit reticulocyte lysate translation kit (Bethesda Research Laboratories) was used according to the supplier's instructions; 25-μl translations were supplemented with 0.18 A_{260} unit of calf liver tRNA (Boehringer Mannheim), 0.05

mCi of [^{35}S]methionine (Amersham), and 0.75 μg of total rat liver mRNA. Ater incubation at 30°C for 60–90 min, ribonuclease A was added (100 μg/ml) and the mixture was incubated for another 10 min at 37°C. Following the incubations, the translated polypeptides were either analyzed directly (2–3 μl) or after immunoprecipitation (10–20 μl) by SDS–polyacrylamide gel electrophoresis. For immunoprecipitation, the sample was diluted to 0.2 ml with NETM buffer (150 mM NaCl, 10 mM EDTA, 0.5% Triton X-100, 2% methionine, pH 7), and 3 μl of normal rabbit serum was added. After 30 min at room temperature, 20 μl of 10% (w/v) fixed *Staphylococcus aureus* cells (Bethesda Research Laboratories) was added, and the mixture was incubated for 10 min and then centrifuged. The supernatant was diluted to 1 ml with NETM buffer, the mixture was adjusted with SDS to 0.1%, 3 μl of antiserum was added, and an additional incubation was carried out overnight at 4°C. A second addition of *S. aureus* cells and subsequent washes were as described.[36] Electrophoresis in SDS/9% polyacrylamide gel was performed as described by Laemmli,[37] and the gels were fluorographed using Autofluor (National Diagnostics).

3. Results and Discussion

3.1. Immunopurification of mRNAs

In the course of these studies, three different low-abundance hepatic mRNAs were purified to near homogeneity.[19] Two of these mRNAs code for proteins ultimately found in the mitochondrial matrix: the precursor to ornithine transcarbamylase[33] and the precursor to the β subunit of propionyl-CoA carboxylase.[35] The third codes for the subunit of the cytosolic enzyme cystathionine β-synthase.[38] A representative result of the purification of the least abundant of the three mRNAs, cystathionine β-synthase mRNA (estimated abundance ~0.015% of total hepatic mRNA), is shown in Fig. 2. Purification of synthase mRNA was begun from the unadsorbed polysomes present in the breakthrough fraction of a protein A–Sepharose column after binding the polysome–anti-ornithine transcarbamylase complexes. Lane 1 of Fig. 2 shows the pattern of polypeptides obtained after translation of total hepatic mRNA. Lane 2 shows the polypeptides obtained after translation of the immunopurified synthase mRNA. Lane 3 contains the polypeptides found when no exogenous RNA was added to the cell-free translation; the major band seen in lane 3 is the [^{35}S]methionine-reticulocyte protein adduct. The absence of translated polypeptides other than synthase in lane 2 documents the powerful purification achievable by this method. Identification of the unique band as the subunit of cystathionine β-synthase (M_r 63,000) was verified by immunoprecipitation of translation mixtures[19] containing purified synthase mRNA and total mRNA with antisynthase antibodies (result not shown). Figure 2 indicates that nearly homogeneous cystathionine β-synthase mRNA was obtained with the described immunoadsorption protocol followed by a density sucrose gradient. This con-

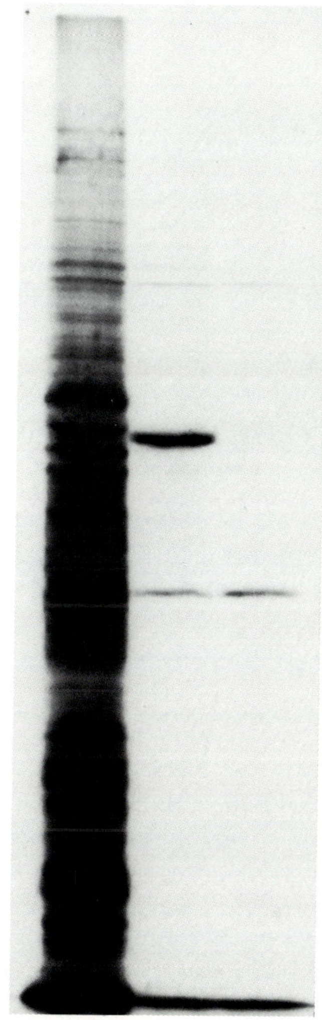

Figure 2. Sodium dodecyl sulfate–polyacrylamide gel analysis of polypeptides translated from total rat liver mRNA and from immunopurified cystathionine β-synthase (CS) mRNA. (1) Translation of total mRNA; (2) translation of purified CS mRNA; (3) translation with no added mRNA. Fluorography was performed for 36 hr.

clusion was supported by liquid scintillation assay of synthase bands excised from gels following immunoprecipitation of translations programmed with either total or purified mRNA. That fraction of total radioactivity, corrected for the acid-precipitable radioactivity in the corresponding translation lacking exogenous mRNA, that localized to the synthase band was 0.015% for total mRNA and 95% for the purified synthase mRNA. This value represents an over 6000-fold purification for cystathionine β-synthase mRNA. Very similar results were obtained when pre-ornithine transcarbamylase mRNA and pre-β-propionyl-CoA carboxylase mRNA were purified.[19]

3.2. Comments on the Procedure

Several features of the method deserve comment. First, purification of the polyclonal antibody need not be carried beyond preparation of an IgG fraction. The mRNA immunopurification protocol is very economical with respect to antibody consumption because, after each column cycle, nearly all of the antibody can be recovered and reused. Immunotitration of twice-used, eluted antibody showed no detectable loss of titer. Surprisingly, polysomes passed over a protein A–Sepharose column containing a preadsorbed IgG fraction did not bind. Therefore, antibody has to be eluted and reacted in solution with each new batch of polysomes. Second, one batch of polysomes can be used at least three times with different antibodies. Alternatively, the polysomes in the breakthrough fraction can be used for preparation of total mRNA specifically depleted of one or more mRNAs. Polysomes stored at −70°C are remarkably stable and can be used for at least 2 years with no apparent difference in results.

3.3. Potential Applications for Enriched mRNAs

Sufficient amounts of mRNA can be obtained from one batch of polysomes to prepare a representative cDNA bank. Using current cloning technology, a cDNA bank of 2500 independent clones can be prepared from the nearly homogeneous mRNA derived from 800 A_{260} units of rat liver polysomes (J. P. Kraus, and L. E. Rosenberg, unpublished results). Alternatively, a highly enriched mRNA and a specifically depleted total mRNA can be used to prepare radioactively labeled cDNAs for a positive and a negative screen of preexisting cDNA library.[21] Using our protocol for immunopurification of mRNA, and either (or both) of the above techniques, more than a dozen cDNAs corresponding to low-abundance mRNAs have been identified in the last two years: preornithine transcarbamylase from rat liver,[21] malic enzyme from rat liver[22] and murine liver,[23] mouse kidney ornithine decarboxylase,[24] canine pancreatic prechymotrypsinogen 2,[25] HeLa cell purine-nucleoside phosphorylase,[26] murine liver ATP-citrate lyase,[27] bovine adrenal low-density lipoprotein receptor,[28] human placental transferrin receptor,[20] type I regulatory subunit of cAMP-dependent protein kinase from bull testes,[30] and rat liver cytochrome c oxidase.[31]

Another potential application for an enriched mRNA that one might envisage is *in vitro* production of a radiolabeled protein that exists *in vivo* only transiently or that is otherwise difficult to obtain—for example, the cytoplasmic precursor of a mitochondrial protein.

4. Conclusions

A method is presented that allows several thousandfold purifications of low-abundance mRNAs to near homogeneity by polysome immunoadsorption.

The following steps are used: interaction of nascent polypeptide chains on the polysomes with an IgG fraction of monospecific polyclonal antiserum; immobilization of polysome–antibody complexes on a protein A–Sepharose column; removal of the bulk of polysomes by extensive washing; dissociation of ribosomal subunits and elution of specific mRNA with EDTA; and isolation of the eluted mRNA by chromatography on an oligo-dT cellulose column. This procedure is widely applicable to polysomes isolated from various species and organs, as well as from tissue culture cells. It has been successful for a number of different low-abundance mRNAs. A single batch of polysomes can be serially reacted with different antibodies, leading to the sequential purification of different mRNAs. Finally, following the elution of the immunoadsorbed polysomes, the antibody can be recovered and reused.

ACKNOWLEDGMENTS. I am grateful to Dr. Frantisek Kalousek for preparations of all antisera used in this work. I also thank Dr. Wayne Fenton for critical reading of the manuscript, Cynthia Williamson for expert technical help, and Connie Woznick for secretarial assistance.

References

1. Williams, J. G., 1981, The preparation and screening of a cDNA clone bank, in: *Genetic Engineering*, Volume 1 (R. Williamson, ed.), Academic Press, New York, p. 2.
2. Cowie, D. B., Spiegelman, S., Roberts, R. B., and Duerksen, J. D., 1961, Ribosome-bound β-galactosidase, *Proc. Natl. Acad. Sci. USA* **47**:114–118.
3. Taylor, J. M., and Tse, T. P. H., 1976, Isolation of rat liver albumin messenger RNA, *J. Biol. Chem.* **251**:7461–7467.
4. Maurer, R. A., 1980, Immunochemical isolation of prolactin messenger RNA, *J. Biol. Chem.* **255**:854–859.
5. Shapiro, D. J., Taylor, J. M., McKnight, G. S., Palacios, R., Gonzalez, C., Kiely, M. L., and Schimke, R. T., 1974, Isolation of hen oviduct ovalbumin and rat liver albumin polysomes by indirect immunoprecipitation, *J. Biol. Chem.* **249**:3665–3671.
6. Lee, D. C., McKnight, G. S., and Palmiter, R. D., 1978, The action of estrogen and progesterone on the expression of the transferrin gene. A comparison of the response in chick liver and oviduct, *J. Biol. Chem.* **253**:3497–3503.
7. Payvar, F., and Schimke, R. T., 1979, Improvements in immunoprecipitation of specific messenger RNA. Isolation of highly purified conalbumin mRNA in high yield, *Eur. J. Biochem.* **101**:271–282.
8. Dugaiczyk, A., Law, S. W., and Dennison, O. E., 1982, Nucleotide sequence and the encoded amino acids of human serum albumin mRNA, *Proc. Natl Acad. Sci. USA* **79**:71–75.
9. Schechter, I., 1974, Use of antibodies for the isolation of biologically pure messenger ribonucleic acid from fully functional eukaryotic cells, *Biochemistry* **13**:1875–1885.
10. Flick, P. K., Chen, J., Alberts, A. W., and Vagelos, P. R., 1978, Translation of rat liver fatty acid synthetase mRNA in a cell-free system derived from wheat germ, *Proc. Natl. Acad. Sci. USA* **75**:730–734.
11. Mueller-Lantzsch, N., and Fan, H., 1976, Monospecific immunoprecipitation of murine leukemia virus polyribosomes: Identification of p30 protein-specific messenger RNA, *Cell* **9**:579–588.
12. Gough, N. M., and Adams, J. M., 1978, Immunoprecipitation of specific polysomes using *Staphylococcus aureus*: Purification of the immunoglobulin K chain messenger RNA from the mouse myeloma MPC11, *Biochemistry* **17**:5560–5566.

13. Lheureux, M., Lheureux, M., Vervoort, T., Van Meirvenne, N., and Steinert, M., 1979, Immunological purification and partial characterization of variant-specific surface antigen messenger RNA of *Trypanosoma brucei brucei*, *Nucleic Acids Res.* **7**:595–609.
14. Palacios, R., Sullivan, D., Summers, N. M., Kiely, M. L., and Schimke, R. T., 1973, Purification of ovalbumin messenger ribonucleic acid by specific immunoadsorption of ovalbumin-synthesizing polysomes and millipore partition of ribonucleic acid, *J. Biol. Chem.* **248**:540–548.
15. Schutz, G., Kieval, S., Groner, B., Sippel, A. E., Kurtz, D. T., and Feigelson, P., 1977, Isolation of specific messenger RNA by adsorption of polysomes to matrix-bound antibody, *Nucleic Acids Res.* **4**:71–84.
16. Groner, B., Hynes, N. E., Sippel, A. E., Jeep, S., Huu, M. C. N., and Schutz, G., 1977, Immunoadsorption of specific chicken oviduct polysomes. Isolation of ovalbumin, ovomucoid, and lysozyme messenger RNA, *J. Biol. Chem.* **252**:6666–6674.
17. Sidorova, E. V., Trudolyubova, M. G., and Lerman, M. I., 1974, Method for isolation of individual polysomes and pure mRNAs by immunoadsorption technique, *Mol. Biol. Rep.* **1**:401–408.
18. Shapiro, S. Z., and Young, J. R., 1981, An immunochemical method for mRNA purification. Application to messenger RNA encoding trypanosome variable surface antigen, *J. Biol. Chem.* **256**:1495–1498.
19. Kraus, J. P., and Rosenberg, L. E., 1982, Purification of low-abundance messenger RNAs from rat liver by polysome immunoadsorption, *Proc. Natl. Acad. Sci. USA* **79**:4015–4019.
20. Korman, A. J., Knudsen, P. J., Kaufman, J. F., and Strominger, J. L., 1982, cDNA clones for the heavy chain of HLA-DR antigens obtained after immunopurification of polysomes by monoclonal antibody, *Proc. Natl. Acad. Sci. USA* **79**:1844–1848.
21. Horwich, A. L., Kraus, J. P., Williams, K., Kalousek, F., Konigsberg, W., and Rosenberg, L. E., 1983, Molecular cloning of the cDNA coding for rat ornithine transcarbamoylase, *Proc. Natl. Acad. Sci. USA* **80**:4258–4262.
22. Magnuson, M. A., and Nikodem, V. M., 1983, Molecular cloning of a cDNA sequence for rat malic enzyme. Direct evidence for induction *in vivo* of rat liver malic enzyme mRNA by thyroid hormone, *J. Biol. Chem.* **258**:12712–12717.
23. Sul, H. S., Wise, L. S., Brown, M. L., and Rubin, C. S., 1984, Cloning of cDNA sequences for murine malic enzyme and the identification of aberrantly large malic enzyme mRNA in MOD-1 null mice, *J. Biol. Chem.* **259**:555–559.
24. Kontula, K. K., Torkkeli, T. K., Bardin, C. W., and Janne, O. A., 1984, Androgen induction of ornithine decarboxylase mRNA in mouse as studied by complementary DNA, *Proc. Natl. Acad. Sci. USA* **81**:731–735.
25. Pinsky, S. D., La Forge, K. S., Luc, V., and Scheele, G., 1983, Identification of cDNA clones encoding secretory isoenzyme forms: Sequence determination of canine pancreatic prechymotrypsinogen 2 mRNA, *Proc. Natl. Acad. Sci. USA* **80**:7486–7490.
26. Goddard, J. M., Caput, D., Williams, S. R., and Martin, D. W., 1983, Cloning of human purine-nucleoside phosphorylase cDNA sequences by complementation in *Escherichia coli*, *Proc. Natl. Acad. Sci. USA* **80**:4281–4285.
27. Sul, H. S., Wise, L. S., Brown, M. L., and Rubin, C. S., 1984, Cloning of cDNA sequences for murine ATP-citrate lyase. Construction of recombinant plasmids using an immunopurified mRNA template and evidence for the nutritional regulation of ATP-citrate lyase mRNA content in mouse liver, *J. Biol. Chem.* **259**:1201–1205.
28. Russell, D. W., Yamamoto, T., Schneider, W. J., Slaughter, C. J., Brown, M. S., and Goldstein, J. L., 1983, cDNA cloning of the bovine low density lipoprotein receptor: Feedback regulation of a receptor mRNA, *Proc. Natl. Acad. Sci. USA* **80**:7501–7505.
29. Schneider, C., Kurkinen, M., and Greaves, M., 1983, Isolation of cDNA clones for the human transferrin receptor, *EMBO J.* **2**:2259–2263.
30. Lee, D. C., Carmichael, D. F., Krebs, E. G., and McKnight, G. S., 1983, Isolation of a cDNA clone for the type I regulatory subunit of bovine cAMP-dependent protein kinase, *Proc. Natl. Acad. Sci. USA* **80**:3608–3612.

31. Parimoo, S., Seelan, R. S., Desai, S., Buse, G., and Padmanaban, G., 1984, Construction of a cDNA clone for a nuclear-coded subunit of cytochrome c oxidase from rat liver, *Biochem. Biophys. Res. Commun.* **118:**902–909.
32. Berger, S. L., Wallace, D. M., Siegal, G. P., Hitchcock, M. J. M., Birkenmeier, C. S., and Reber, S. B., 1981, Preparation of interferon messenger RNAs with the use of ribonucleoside–vanadyl complexes, *Meth. Enzymol.* **79:**59–68.
33. Conboy, J. G., Kalousek, F., and Rosenberg, L. E., 1979, *In vitro* synthesis of a putative precursor of mitochondrial ornithine transcarbamoylase, *Proc. Natl. Acad. Sci. USA* **76:**5724–5727.
34. Kraus, J. P., Kalousek, F., and Rosenberg, L. E., 1983, Biosynthesis and mitochondrial processing of the β subunit of propionyl coenzyme A carboxylase from rat liver, *J. Biol. Chem.* **258:**7245–7248.
35. Kraus, J. P., and Rosenberg, L. E., 1982, Cystathionine β-synthase from human liver: Improved purification scheme and additional characterization of the enzyme in crude and pure form, *Arch. Biochem. Biophys.* **222:**44–52.
36. Kraus, J. P., Conboy, J. G., and Rosenberg, L. E., 1981, Pre-ornithine transcarbamylase. Properties of the cytoplasmic precursor of a mitochondrial matrix enzyme, *J. Biol. Chem.* **256:**10739–10742.
37. Laemmli, U. K., 1970, Cleavage of structural proteins during the assembly of the head of bacteriophage T4, *Nature* **227:**680–685.
38. Skovby, F., Kraus, J. P., and Rosenberg, L. E., 1984, Biosynthesis and proteolytic activation of cystathionine β-synthase in rat liver, *J. Biol. Chem.* **259:**588–593.

Chapter 26

Purification of Messenger RNA by Polysome Isolation with Monoclonal Antibodies

JOSEPH P. BROWN, TIMOTHY M. ROSE, and GREGORY D. PLOWMAN

1. Introduction

In this chapter we discuss the use of monoclonal antibodies to enrich the mRNAs coding for low-abundance proteins by polysome immunopurification. In this technique polysomes (which consist of mRNA, ribosomes, and nascent polypeptide chains) are purified by immunoaffinity chromatography with antibodies that recognize antigenic determinants present on the nascent chains. While there have been numerous reports of the use of polyclonal antisera for this purpose, we are aware of only a few examples of the use of monoclonal antibodies, apart from our own work.[1,2] Since the preceding chapter by Kraus addresses the use of polyclonal antisera, we shall focus on the differences between monoclonal antibodies and polyclonal antisera with respect to this application. Our own experience in cloning the mRNA for p97, a 97,000-dalton cell surface glycoprotein of human melanoma, which we identified by using monoclonal antibodies,[3–5] will be described in some detail. The protein p97 is present in most human melanomas, but it is found in only trace amounts in normal adult tissues.[6–8] It is representative of many other low-abundance cell-surface proteins in that it accounts for only 0.02% of total cell protein even in the cell line expressing the largest amounts of the antigen, and it is reasonable to assume that its mRNA comprises a similar proportion of the cellular mRNA.

2. Monoclonal Antibodies

When monoclonal antibodies are obtained by immunization with intact cells or cell extracts, in most cases they recognize the antigens in their native

JOSEPH P. BROWN, TIMOTHY M. ROSE, and GREGORY D. PLOWMAN • Oncogen, Seattle, Washington 98121.

conformations. Such antibodies may not, however, be appropriate for polysome immunopurification, since there is a significant chance that the antigenic determinants recognized may not be present in nascent chains. Since translation starts at the NH_2 terminus of the polypeptide, epitopes close to the COOH terminus are likely to be absent from the majority of the nascent chains. The problem is easily avoided either by using antibodies that recognize NH_2-terminal epitopes, or by preparing polysomes from cells treated with a protein synthesis inhibitor, such as trichodermin,[1,9,10] that blocks termination, rather than with cycloheximide, which inhibits elongation.

A more serious problem is that mature proteins differ from nascent chains because of posttranslational modifications. This problem is particularly acute for cell surface proteins, which are modified more extensively by removal of the signal peptides, additional of carbohydrate side chains, and formation of disulfide bridges. If a polyclonal antiserum is used for polysome immunopurification, such differences in antigenicity between nascent chains and the mature protein may be of little consequence, since during immunization the rabbit or other animal will have been exposed not only to the native protein, but also to partially or completely denatured forms. Even if these antibodies represent only a minor fraction of the antibody population, there may still be enough to bind the nascent chains. In this regard, antibody monoclonality is a disadvantage. One approach is to use the monoclonal antibody to purify the antigen for further immunizations (see Johnson *et al.*, the volume, Chapter 9 and Springer and Anderson, this volume, Chapter 11).

Another solution is to obtain a monoclonal antibody that recognizes antigenic determinants present in nascent chains, by using denatured antigen as immunogen. Korman *et al.*,[1] for example, immunized with denatured HLA-DR antigen and obtained a monoclonal antibody that recognized not only denatured HLA-DR, but also nascent chains. This antibody was used successfully to purify HLA-DR mRNA. Since we had available a panel of monoclonal antibodies that recognized three distinct epitopes on the NH_2-terminal 40,000-dalton domain of the p97 molecule, our strategy was to use a pool of monoclonal antibodies each with a different specificity in the hope that one or more of them would bind to nascent chains. The antibodies chosen were highly specific for p97, in that each of them immunoprecipitated a single band of p97 from a radiolabeled whole-cell lysate, and they had affinities of approximately 10^{-10} M. For the cloning project we chose one IgG2a antibody specific for each of the three epitopes.

When using monoclonal antibodies the question remains of how one can predict whether a given monoclonal antibody or combination of antibodies will recognize the nascent chains and thus be suitable for use in polysome immunopurification. One approach is to determine whether the monoclonal antibody immunoprecipitates antigen that has been translated *in vitro* in the reticulocyte lysate system, relying on the assumption that the *in vitro* translation product, not being processed, will resemble the nascent chains. An alternative approach is to proceed with the polysome immunoprecipitation on a small scale and then to use *in vitro* translation to determine whether the mRNA species of interest has been enriched. In the next section we describe our experience with both of these approaches.

3. Assaying mRNA Activity

Most cloning strategies require the use of *in vitro* translation at some stage, and the polysome immunopurification procedure is no exception. We used the technique to test unenriched and p97-enriched mRNA preparations for p97 activity, and also to confirm the identity of cDNA clones by the technique of hybrid-selected translation.

When unenriched melanoma mRNA was translated in the micrococcal nuclease-treated rabbit reticulocyte lysate system[11] and the methionine-labeled translation products were analyzed by SDS–PAGE, p97 was too minor a component of the translation products to be seen among the hundreds of more abundant species. Surprisingly, repeated attempts to immunoprecipitate p97 from the translation products were unsuccessful, even though both monoclonal antibodies and a polyclonal antiserum prepared by immunizing mice with denatured p97 were used. Clearly, either the antibodies did not recognize the *in vitro* translation product or the method was not sensitive enough to detect the relatively small amount of p97 synthesized. Since it was difficult to obtain low backgrounds when immunoprecipitating from reticulocyte lysates, we suspected a lack of sensitivity. In either case, we had no assay for p97 mRNA and no evidence that the monoclonal antibodies might recognize nascent chains. We continued to use the reticulocyte assay to monitor the integrity of our mRNA preparations, since the presence of numerous polypeptides with molecular weights greater than 100,000 among the translation products showed that the mRNA preparation as a whole was not degraded.

In order to allow us to monitor the purification, we next turned to the *Xenopus* oocyte translation system,[12] in which proteins are usually processed normally.[13] We hoped that the processed p97 translation product might be recognized by our monoclonal antibodies. One disadvantage of the oocyte assay is that translated proteins cannot be labeled to the same high specific radioactivity as in the reticulocyte translation system. We decided, therefore, to assay the translation products for p97 by using a highly sensitive double determinant immunoassay (DDIA),[7,14] which employs two monoclonal antibodies specific for two different epitopes of p97. Oocytes were injected with mRNA from melanoma cells (50 ng per oocyte), incubated at 20°C for 20 hr, and homogenized in five volumes of 20 mM Tris-HCl, pH 8.0, 100 mM NaCl, 1 mM EDTA, 0.5% Nonidet P-40, 1 mM phenylmethyl sulfonyl fluoride. The lysate was centrifuged at 30,000 × g for 30 min at 0°C and the extracts were tested for p97 as described.[7,14] The first attempt with the oocyte assay was successful: extracts of oocytes that had received melanoma mRNA contained detectable amounts of p97. Since we now had an assay for p97 mRNA, we proceeded with the polysome immunopurification.

4. Polysome Immunopurification

The first attempts to use antibodies to purify polysomes employed an anti-immunoglobulin antibody to form an immunoprecipitate,[15] hence the term "polysome immunoprecipitation." Subsequent studies used formalin-fixed, protein A-bearing *Staphylococcus aureus*, and more recently, protein A bound to Sepharose,[1,2,16,17] and the procedure is now more accurately referred to as "polysome immunopurification." The procedure using protein A–Sepharose gives higher yields and lower backgrounds than its predecessors. The protein A adsorbent has two applications in this procedure. The first is to purify the monoclonal antibodies from the crude ascites fluids, thereby removing contaminating ribonuclease activity.[1,16,17] In our hands, mRNA from polysomes that had been incubated for several hours with protein A-purified antibodies showed no sign of degradation, as judged by translation in the reticulocyte lysate system. The protein A adsorbent is then used in conjunction with the purified antibodies to immunopurify polysomes bearing the specific nascent chain.

To purify polysomes bearing p97 nascent chains, polysomes (100–200 E260 units) prepared from 4 g of SK-MEL 28 melanoma cells by magnesium precipitation[18] were incubated with 1–2 mg of each of the three monoclonal IgG2a antibodies specific for epitopes a, b, and c of p97.[6] The mixture was passed through a 5-ml protein A–Sepharose CL-2B column as described.[1] The p97-enriched mRNA was purified from the adsorbed polysomes by elution with EDTA and affinity chromatography on oligo-dT cellulose. We found that in order to concentrate the recovered mRNA by ethanol precipitation it was necessary to add carrier tRNA. The recovered mRNA was quantitated by measuring incorporation of ^{32}P-TTP into cDNA, since the presence of tRNA carrier precluded simple E260 measurements. In a typical experiment, 140 E260 units of polysomes yielded 0.5 μg of enriched mRNA, which was greatly enriched for p97 activity: oocytes synthesized 80 pg of p97 per ng of p97-enriched mRNA, as opposed to 0.44 pg of p97 per ng of unenriched mRNA. The p97 mRNA activity had thus been enriched 180-fold with 42% yield.

Translation in the reticulocyte lysate system allowed us to characterize the translation product biochemically and to assess the purity of the p97-enriched mRNA. The enriched mRNA coded for a polypeptide with an apparent molecular weight on SDS–PAGE of 84,000, which constituted approximately 10% of the translation products of p97-enriched mRNA.[19] This polypeptide was not detectable in the translation products of unenriched mRNA and was immunoprecipitated by antiserum specific for denatured p97, but not by any of the three monoclonal antibodies obtained by immunization with native p97. We concluded that it was the unglycosylated precursor of p97, and that due to lack of processing in the reticulocyte translation system the epitopes recognized by the monoclonal antibodies were lacking. The apparent paradox that the monoclonal antibodies appeared to have bound to the nascent chains but were unable to bind the reticulocyte translation product will be discussed below.

5. cDNA Cloning

cDNA was cloned as described elsewhere.[19] Briefly, a cDNA library in pBR322 and a ^{32}P-labeled cDNA probe were constructed using the enriched mRNA and standard procedures.[20] Transformants (1.9×10^4) were screened with the ^{32}P-labeled cDNA probe. DNA from the colonies was bound to paper filters as described.[21] The filters were incubated with ^{32}P-labeled cDNA probe (200,000–500,000 dpm/ml) in 5 × NaCl/Cit (1 × NaCl/Cit is 150 mM NaCl, 15 mM sodium citrate, pH 7.0) containing 50% formamide, 25 mM sodium phosphate, and 0.02% bovine serum albumin, Ficoll, polyvinylpyrrolidone, and herring sperm DNA at 42°C, washed at 50°C in 2 × NaCl/Cit, and autoradiographed. Thirty colonies that hybridized at least tenfold more strongly to the p97-enriched probe than to an unenriched probe were selected for further analysis.

6. Characterization of cDNA Clones

It is important to confirm that a recombinant clone that has been identified by differential colony hybridization contains the sequence of interest. The technique of hybrid-selected translation is often used for this purpose. Plasmid DNA is denatured and bound to nitrocellulose filters, which are then incubated with mRNA, and hybridized mRNA is recovered from the filters and translated. To test our p97 clones, plasmid DNA (1–5 μg) was dissolved in 6 μl of 2 M NaCl containing 0.2 M NH_4OH, incubated at 100°C for 1 min, and spotted onto 9-mm-diameter semicircles of nitrocellulose, which were baked overnight at 80°C *in vacuo* and washed as described.[22] The p97-enriched mRNA (200 ng) was dissolved in 30 μl of 65% formamide, 400 mM NaCl, 10 mM PIPES, pH 6.4, 0.1% SDS, and heated at 70°C for 10 min, and 4 μl was spotted on each filter. The filters were sandwiched between glass slides, incubated at 42°C for 2 hr, and then washed. The bound mRNA was recovered as described[22] and translated in the reticulocyte system. The 30 plasmids were tested first as pools of six and then individually. One plasmid, designated p973a2f1, which bound p97 mRNA, was chosen for further study.[19]

Further evidence that clone p973a2f1 contained p97 sequences was obtained by testing it for hybridization to enriched and unenriched mRNA.[19] mRNA was denatured with formaldehyde, bound to nitrocellulose, and hybridized with p973a2f1 cDNA that had been ^{32}P-labeled by nick translation. The probe hybridized more strongly to 5 ng of p97-enriched mRNA than to 500 ng of unenriched mRNA, consistent with their respective p97 mRNA activities in translation assays. Hybridization to 500 ng of fibroblast mRNA was barely detectable, being at least 20-fold weaker than to unenriched melanoma mRNA.

DNA sequence analysis showed that clone p973a2f1 had a poly A stretch at the 3′ terminus, but no open reading frames. The p97 cDNA probe was used to screen additional cDNA and genomic libraries. Thirty-four kilobases of genomic DNA containing the p97 gene was isolated in three overlapping clones in bacteriophage λ (G. D. Plowman, T. M. Rose, C. Estin, D. Teplow, K. E. Hellstroöm, and J. P. Brown, manuscript in preparation). One of these clones contained sequences coding for the known NH_2-terminal sequence of p97,[23] which we consider to be the most convincing demonstration that the polysome immunopurification procedure was successful.

7. Discussion

When we set out to clone p97 cDNA we felt that the best way to obtain a cDNA probe was to use our panel of highly specific monoclonal antibodies to purify polysomes bearing p97 nascent chains. A potential problem with this approach is that many cell surface proteins are posttranslationally modified, and the nascent chains may differ in antigenicity from the mature protein. For example, the monoclonal antibody used to immunopurify HLA-DR polysomes was obtained by immunizing with dissociated HLA-DR heavy chain; it showed no reactivity with the native molecule, although it did bind the cell-free translation product.[1] On the other hand, the monoclonal antibody used to immunopurify murine p53 intracellular tumor antigen polysomes recognized both the native protein and the reticulocyte translation product.[2,24] In the case of p97 we initially had no evidence that our antibodies, which recognized epitopes present on the 40,000-dalton NH_2-terminal domain of mature p97[6] but absent from denatured p97, would also recognize nascent chains. Our success in using these antibodies to immunopurify p97 polysomes implies that at least one of them must bind nascent chains and that p97 nascent chains share antigenic sites with the mature protein. We can draw two general conclusions from the above observations: First, monoclonal antibodies obtained by immunization with native proteins can be used for polysome immunopurification. Second, failure of an antibody to immunoprecipitate a cell-free translation product does not preclude its use for polysome immunopurification.

Translation of mRNA from the immunopurified polysomes, both in oocytes and in a cell-free system, showed that a 180-fold purification had been achieved and suggested that p97 mRNA was a major component of the enriched mRNA. We found that the oocyte assay was the more sensitive of the two (only this assay could detect p97 mRNA activity in unenriched mRNA), possibly because of the longer incubation time and the highly sensitive DDIA used to assay the translation products. The cell-free translation product, which had a molecular weight of 84,000, was precipitated by an antiserum specific for denatured p97, but by none of the monoclonal antibodies. The difference in molecular weight between the cell-free translation product and the protein present at the surface of melanoma cells is probably due to glycosylation of the latter,[5,7] and the difference in antigenicity can be ascribed to lack of appropriate posttranslational modification in the cell-free system. It is interesting to note that the cell-free translation product of p97 is significantly larger than its homologue transferrin, which has a molecular weight of 75,000. This may be due to the presence of transmembranous and cytoplasmic domains.

In retrospect, the greatest difficulty in cloning p97 lay not in the polysome immunopurification or the cloning and screening steps, but in developing translation assays to monitor these steps. With unenriched mRNA we were unable to detect p97 synthesis in the reticulocyte translation system, but we were successful in using monoclonal antibodies to detect p97 translated to oocytes. Both assays worked well with enriched mRNA. The hybrid-selected translation procedure, which we used as a secondary screening procedure, required much more mRNA than was used to prepare and screen the cDNA library. Definitive confirmation of the success of the cloning procedure was obtained by DNA sequencing. We conclude that monoclonal antibodies can be useful for polysome immunopurification and may be the method of choice as a first step toward cloning antigens that have been newly identified by the monoclonal antibody technique.

ACKNOWLEDGMENTS. We are grateful to Drs. Stanley McKnight, Richard Gelinas, Steve McKnight, James Lewis, Diane Durnam, and Greg Barsh for their unstinting advice and encouragement, and to Cynthia Green for her excellent technical assistance. This investigation was supported by PHS grants 34777, 37440, and 38415 awarded by the National Cancer Institute, DHHS.

References

1. Korman, A. J., Knudsen, P. J., Kaufman, J. F., and Strominger, J. L., 1982, cDNA clones for the heavy chain of HLA-DR antigens obtained after immunopurification of polysomes by monoclonal antibody, *Proc. Natl. Acad. Sci. USA* **79**:1844–1848.
2. Oren, M., and Levine, A. J., 1983, Molecular cloning of a cDNA specific for the murine p53 cellular tumor antigen, *Proc. Natl. Acad. Sci. USA* **80**:56–59.
3. Woodbury, R. G., Brown, J. P., Yeh, M.-Y., Hellstrom, I., and Hellstrom, K. E., 1980, Identification of a cell surface protein, p97, in human melanomas and certain other neoplasms, *Proc. Natl. Acad. Sci. USA* **77**:2183–2187.
4. Brown, J. P., Wright, P. W., Hart, C. E., Woodbury, R. G., Hellstrom, K. E., Hellstrom, I., and Wright, P., 1980, Protein antigens of normal and malignant human cells identified by immunoprecipitation with monoclonal antibodies, *J. Biol. Chem.* **255**:4980–4983.
5. Dippold, W. G., Lloyd, K. O., Li, L. T., Ikeda, H., Oettgen, H. F., and Old, L. J., 1980, Cell surface antigens of human malignant melanoma: Definition of six antigenic systems with mouse monoclonal antibodies, *Proc. Natl. Acad. Sci. USA* **77**:6114–6118.
6. Brown, J. P., Nishiyama, K., Hellstrom, I., and Hellstrom, K. E., 1981, Structural characterization of human melanoma-associated antigen p97 using monoclonal antibodies, *J. Immunol.* **127**:539–546.
7. Brown, J. P., Woodbury, R. G., Hart, C. E., Hellstrom, I., and Hellstrom, K. E., 1981, Quantitative analysis of melanoma-associated antigen p97 in normal and neoplastic tissues, *Proc. Natl. Acad. Sci. USA* **78**:539–543.
8. Garrigues, H. J., Tilgen, W., Hellstrom, I., Franke, W., and Hellstrom, K. E., 1982, Detection of a human melanoma-associated antigen, p97, in histological sections of primary human melanoma, *Int. J. Cancer* **29**:511–515.
9. Cundliffe, E., Cannon, M., and Davies, J., 1974, Mechanism of inhibition of eukaryotic protein synthesis by trichothecene fungal toxins, *Proc. Natl. Acad. Sci. USA* **71**:30–34.

10. Wei, C. M., Hansen, B. S., Vaughan, M. H., and McLaughlin, C. S., 1974, Mechanism of action of the mycotoxin trichodermin, a 12,13-epoxytrichothecene, *Proc. Natl. Acad. Sci. USA* **71**:713–717.
11. Pelham, H. R., and Jackson, R. J., 1976, An efficient mRNA-dependent translation system from reticulocyte lysates, *Eur. J. Biochem.* **67**:247–256.
12. Gurdon, J. B., 1974, *The Control of Gene Expression in Animal Development*, Harvard University Press, Cambridge.
13. Miskin, R., and Soreq, H., 1981, Microinjected *Xenopus* oocytes synthesize active human plasminogen activator, *Nucleic Acids Res.* **9**:3355–3363.
14. Plowman, G. D., Brown, J. P., Enns, C. A., Schroder, J., Nikinmaa, B., Sussman, H. H., Hellstrom, K. E., and Hellstrom, I., 1983, Assignment of the gene for human melanoma-associated antigen p97 to chromosome 3, *Nature* **303**:70–72.
15. Palacios, R., Palmiter, R. D., and Schimke, R. T., 1972, Identification and isolation of ovalbumin-synthesizing polysomes, *J. Biol. Chem.* **247**:2316–2321.
16. Kraus, J. P., and Rosenberg, L. E., 1982, Purification of low-abundance messenger RNAs from rat liver by polysome immunoadsorption, *Proc. Natl. Acad. Sci. USA* **79**:4015–4019.
17. Shapiro, S. Z., and Young, J. R., 1981, An immunochemical method for mRNA purification, *J. Biol. Chem.* **256**:1495–1498.
18. Palmiter, R. D., 1974, Magnesium precipitation of ribonucleoprotein complexes. Expedient techniques for the isolation of undegraded polysomes and messenger ribonucleic acid, *Biochemistry* **13**:3606–3615.
19. Brown, J. P., Rose, T. M., Forstrom, J. W., Hellstrom, I., and Hellstrom, K. E., 1985, Isolation of a cDNA for a human melanoma-associated antigen in: *Proceedings Eighth Nobel Conference of the Karolinska Institute*, Raven Press, New York (in press).
20. Efstratiadis, A., and Villa-Komaroff, L., 1979, Cloning of double-stranded cDNA, in: *Genetic Engineering* (J. K. Stelow and A. Hollaender, eds.), Volume 1, Plenum Press, New York, pp. 15–36.
21. Taub, F. and Thompson, B., 1982, An improved method for preparing large arrays of bacterial colonies containing plasmids for hybridization: *In situ* purification and stable binding of DNA on paper filters, *Anal. Biochem.* **126**:222–230.
22. Parnes, J. R., Velan, B., Felsenfeld, A., Ramanathan, L., Ferrini, U., Appella E., and Seidman, J. G., 1981, Mouse β_2-microglobulin cDNA clones: A screening procedure for cDNA clones corresponding to rare mRNAs, *Proc. Natl. Acad. Sci. USA* **78**:2253–2257.
23. Brown, J. P., Hewick, R. M., Hellstrom, I., Hellstrom, K. E., Doolittle, R. F., and Dreyer, W. J., 1982, Human melanoma-associated p97 is structurally and functionally related to transferrin, *Nature* **296**:171–173.
24. Rotter, V., Witte, O. N., Coffman, R., and Baltimore, D., 1980, Abelson murine leukemia virus-induced tumors elicit antibodies against a host cell protein, p50, *J. Virol.* **36**:547–555.

Chapter 27

Expression of Foreign Proteins on the Surface of *Xenopus laevis* Oocytes

JAY C. UNKELESS, DANIEL A. PORTNOY, ANDREW D. LUSTER, and ELLEN PURE

1. Introduction

Xenopus laevis oocytes have been widely used as an *in vitro* translation system for exogenous mRNAs. The utility of the oocyte translation system was first demonstrated by Gurdon and his colleagues,[1] who detected β-globin after injection of reticulocyte mRNA. Subsequently, all eukaryotic mRNAs tested have directed the synthesis of the appropriate protein after injection into oocytes. A major advantage of the system is that the translation by oocytes is as much as 100- to 1000-fold more efficient than wheat germ lysate and rabbit reticulocyte lysate translation systems. This allows detection of translated products by radioimmune assays, ELISA, or biological activity. The efficiency of the translation is due, in part, to the stability of the injected mRNA. The half-life of injected globin mRNA, for example, is greater than 2 weeks.[2]

Xenopus oocytes perform posttranslational modifications, such as cleavage of leader sequences and precursor proteins,[3–6] phosphorylation,[7,8] and glycosylation.[9–14] Colman *et al.*[14] have shown that chicken ovalbumin, guinea pig caseins, and human interferons are synthesized by oocytes and properly glycosylated. Matthews *et al.*[9] have demonstrated that phaseolin, a glycosylated protein, produced by oocytes injected with bean cotyledon mRNA is similar to authentic phaseolin. In addition, Berridge and Lane[7] have shown that vitellogenin synthesized in *Xenopus* oocytes is properly phosphorylated. Thus, it is not surprising that this system is used to study the requirements for synthesis, transport, and processing of proteins.

Recently, it has been shown that secreted proteins produced in *Xenopus* oocytes from heterologous mRNAs are modified, topologically segregated, and subsequently exported from the oocytes.[14–17] The requirements for protein secretion are therefore accessible to study in the *Xenopus* oocyte system. A study

JAY C. UNKELESS, DANIEL A. PORTNOY, ANDREW D. LUSTER, and ELLEN PURE • Laboratory of Cellular Physiology and Immunology, Rockefeller University, New York, New York 10021.

of the synthesis of ovalbumin by oocytes showed that the cytosolic form of chicken ovalbumin, which is synthesized and trapped in the cytosol, is not glycosylated or secreted. Glycosylated ovalbumin was found sequestered in vesicles in the oocyte cytoplasm and secreted. Unglycosylated ovalbumin that is synthesized in the presence of tunicamycin and is indistinguishable by immunoprecipitation, two-dimensional gel electrophoresis, and lectin binding from the unglycosylated cytosolic form of ovalbumin is still transferred across the endoplasmic reticulum (ER) and secreted. Guinea pig caseins and human interferons are also secreted from tunicamycin-treated frog oocytes. Therefore, it has been concluded that the access to the ER, but not glycosylation, is a mandatory intermediate step in the secretion of proteins.[14] This study emphasized the advantage of oocytes as a surrogate system for studying the late events in gene expression.

An additional advantage of the oocyte translation system is that a biologically active form of the protein is usually synthesized. The biosynthesis and secretion of catalytically active acetylcholinesterase,[16] β-glucuronidase,[18] and plasminogen activator[17] by oocytes has been demonstrated. The acetylcholinesterase and β-glucuronidase mRNAs are of low abundance, and measurement of biological activity of the translated and secreted products is more sensitive than radiolabeling of the proteins.[18] Biologically active interferons have also been obtained from *Xenopus* oocytes.[19–22] In one case, Soreq *et al.*[22] were able to show that mRNAs lacking 3′-terminal RNA sequences for fibroblast β_1 and β_2 interferons still produced a functional and stable human fibroblast interferon. This work emphasized the usefulness of the oocyte translation system for studying the effect of mRNA structural modifications on translation and on posttranslational processes.

Sumikawa *et al.*[23] demonstrated that oocytes injected with mRNA from the electric organ of *Torpedo marmorata* had the acetylcholine receptor (AchR) localized in the oocyte membrane fraction. The AchR is a pentameric membrane protein composed of four subunits assembled with the stoichiometry $\alpha_2\beta\delta\gamma$. Mishna *et al.*[24] demonstrated that oocytes synthesize and assemble the four subunits of the AchR into the oocyte membrane and maintain biological activity of the receptor. The genes for each subunit of AchR have been independently cloned and individually transfected into monkey COS cells. By injecting the mRNAs from the COS cells Mishna *et al.*[24] were able to evaluate the contribution of each subunit to the ligand binding activity (binding of ^{125}I-α-bungarotoxin) and to the formation of ligand-dependent ion channel. They found that when mRNA for all four subunits is injected into oocytes, functional AchRs appear in the surface membrane. These receptors have appropriate electrophysiological properties and bind the snake toxin used to identify AchRs (α-bungarotoxin). Data obtained with oocytes injected with various combinations of three of the AchR subunit-specific mRNAs suggested that all four subunits were required to elicit a normal nicotinic response to acetylcholine, whereas only the α subunit is indispensable for α-bungarotoxin binding activity.

Oocytes appear to be generally useful for the study of membrane receptors mediating ion fluxes. Recently, Gundersen *et al.*[25] found that mRNA from fetal brain injected into *Xenopus* oocytes directed the translation and membrane insertion of functional serotonin and kainate receptors. These receptors, measured by the appearance of sodium-specific channels in the oocyte plasma membrane, were drug- and voltage-regulated. Houamed *et al.*[26] showed the expression of functional γ-amino butyric acid (GABA), glycine, and glutamate receptors in *Xenopus* oocytes injected with rat brain mRNA. These results show that neurotransmitter receptors can be inserted into the oocyte plasma membrane and furnish another system in which to study receptor–ionophore function. This can now be done for the peripheral nicotinic AchR, the chick brain GABA receptor, and the rat brain serotonin receptor. The GABA, glycine, glutamate, and related acidic amino acid receptors of mammalian brain have been studied in oocytes and shown to exhibit pharmacologically separate identities when their mRNAs are processed in oocytes.

Studies in our laboratory are aimed at understanding the expression of Fc receptors for immunoglobulin molecules. These receptors represent a family of plasma membrane receptors that are encoded by low-abundance mRNA species. We have recently reported that Fc receptor mRNA translated in oocytes leads to the expression of Fc receptors on the oocyte cell surface, which can be detected by the binding of radiolabeled ligands or monoclonal anti-receptor antibodies.[27] This assay may provide a general method for the sensitive and rapid detection of products of rare mRNA species that encode plasma membrane receptors and will facilitate the detailed study of the processes involved in the synthesis and compartmentalization of membrane-associated proteins.

2. Methods

2.1. Maintenance of *Xenopus laevis* and Surgical Removal of Oocytes

Sexually mature female *Xenopus laevis* are obtained from the African Xenopus Facility (P.O. Box 2263, Clarinch 7740, South Africa) and maintained in aerated water tanks containing methylene blue (5 mg/20 gallon tank). For removal of oocytes, the animals are anesthetized on ice for 20 min before surgery and maintained at 4°C throughout the procedure. A unilateral incision is made on the posterior ventral surface through the skin and abdominal muscle to expose the ovary sacs. The ovary sacs are removed by gently pulling with forceps, cut, and immediately placed in Ca^{2+}-free OR-2 saline solution (82 mM NaCl, 2.5 mM KCl, 1.5 mM Na_2HPO_4, 1 mM $CaCl_2$, 1 mM $MgCl_2$, 10 μg/ml gentamycin, 50 mM HEPES, pH 7.2). The abdominal muscles and skin are sutured separately (5-0 chromic gut sutures with an FS-2 cutting needle: Ethicon, Somerville, New Jersey) and the animal is allowed to recover in shallow water containing antibiotics at room temperature.

2.2. Preparation and Injection of Oocytes

The ovary sac is ruptured by gently pulling cords of oocytes with fine forceps. The oocytes are then incubated in Ca^{2+}-free OR-2 saline containing 2 mg/ml collagenase (Type IA, Sigma Chemical Co., St. Louis, Missouri) at room temperature with gentle agitation. After 1 hr the oocytes are transferred to a fresh collagenase solution for an additional 1 hr and are then rinsed in half-strength Leibowitz (L-15) medium (GIBCO Laboratories, Grand Island, New York) supplemented with 100 U/ml of penicillin, 5 μg/ml of gentamycin and 10 mM HEPES, pH 7.4. The oocytes are maintained in this medium at room temperature until injected (up to 48 hr later).

Injection of mRNA can be performed on an air- or oil-driven microinjection apparatus, which consists of a dissecting microscope and a needle drawn from a 25-μl microcap disposable pipette (Drummond Scientific Co.). Our apparatus is oil-driven, and the micrometer drives a plunger on a 100-μl gas-tight Hamilton syringe. Needles with an outer diameter about 150 μm are satisfactory. For injection, large oocytes with uniform vegetal pole pigmentation are selected using micropipettes with disposable plastic tips cut to an inner diameter of about 1.5 mm. The oocytes, in half-strength L-15 medium, are placed in a 60-mm Petri dish that has a polyester monofilament screen (HC7-710, Tetko, Elmsford, New York) adhered to the surface with a few drops of chloroform. The screen prevents the oocytes from rolling when injected. The mRNA (0.5–1 mg/ml in water) is drawn into the needle and approximately 60 nl injected into each oocyte. The oocytes are transferred to 24-well cluster dishes and incubated for 1–3 days at room temperature in half-strength L-15. The needle must be cleaned every few samples by drawing chromerge into the needle followed by extensive rinses with water.

2.3. Preparation of Oocyte Lysates for Radioimmune Assay

Injected oocytes (10–20 per sample) are incubated for 2–3 days, harvested, washed, and lysed in 0.2 ml of 1% NP-40 in the presence of protease inhibitors (0.25 U/ml Aprotonin, 1 mM phenylmethylsulfonyl fluoride). The lysate is subjected to centrifugation (14,000 × g, 4°C) and the supernatant adjusted to 0.2% sodium dodecyl sulfate (SDS). The radioimmune assay, which is based on the immunoprecipitation of ^{125}I-Fab–antigen complexes by polyvalent rabbit IgG bound to fixed *Staphylococcus aureus*, is performed as previously described.[28]

2.4. Oocyte Cell Surface Binding Assay

For binding assays, the oocytes are harvested (10–20 per sample), rinsed in medium, and then incubated for 1 hr at room temperature in medium containing ^{125}I-labeled ligand or monoclonal antibody (1 μg/ml, 0.5 × 10^4 cpm/

ng protein) and [^{14}C]sucrose (0.67 mM sucrose, 3.7 mCi/mmole; New England Nuclear, Boston, Massachusetts) as an impermeant tracer. After washing, oocytes showing intact animal/vegetal pole morphology are individually assayed for ^{125}I in a gamma counter and then prepared for scintillation counting by the addition of 0.1 ml of 0.5 M NH_4OH and 2 ml of Hydrofluor (New England Nuclear). The high end of the ^{14}C spectrum is counted and the counts corrected for spillover of ^{125}I into the ^{14}C channel. Oocytes that take up [^{14}C]sucrose in excess of the mean plus three standard deviations (SD) incorporated by control oocytes are considered nonviable and disregarded. Ligand binding is scored positive if the quantity of ^{125}I-ligand bound is >3 SD above the mean bound by control oocytes. The stimulation index is calculated as average of experimental (cpm bound)/average of controls (cpm bound).

3. Results and Discussion

3.1. Translation of Murine $Fc_{\gamma 2b/\gamma 1}R$ by Oocytes

The J774 mouse macrophage-like cell line and the S49.1 T-cell line express a receptor that binds mouse IgG2b and IgG1 aggregates ($Fc_{\gamma 2b/\gamma 1}R$),[29] while the T-cell line L5178Y does not. mRNA was isolated from J774, S49.1, and L5178Y cell lines by guanidinium isothiocyanate extraction followed by centrifugation on a cesium chloride gradient.[30] Poly A^+ mRNA was isolated by oligo-dT affinity chromatography. The poly A^+ mRNA was injected into *Xenopus* oocytes. In our initial studies, the translated murine $Fc_{\gamma 2b/\gamma 1}R$ was detected by radioimmune assay[28] of oocyte lysates. Briefly, aliquots of cell or oocyte lysates are incubated with radiolabeled Fab fragments of a monoclonal anti-$Fc_{\gamma 2b/\gamma 1}R$ antibody and then the antigen–antibody complexes are immunoprecipitated with rabbit anti-mouse $Fc_{\gamma 2b/\gamma 1}R$ antiserum adsorbed to *Staphylococcus aureus*. Typical results of such an experiment are shown in Table I. Although this approach was feasible for murine $Fc_{\gamma 2b/\gamma 1}R$, it was not for other Fc receptors, for which we lack polyclonal and monoclonal antibodies. In light of previous reports that secreted proteins were synthesized and exported by oocytes, we developed an assay based on the assumption that the oocytes would translate and properly express plasma membrane receptors on their cell surface. In comparison to the radioimmune assay, the single oocyte surface binding assay was less labor-intensive, required fewer oocytes, and gave a higher signal/noise ratio. This could be attributed to the fact that in the radioimmune assay both successfully and unsuccessfully injected oocytes were pooled and assayed.

For cell surface binding assays of *Xenopus* oocytes, mRNA was injected and the oocytes were assayed for the binding of ^{125}I-2.4G2 Fab, a monoclonal antibody that is specific for $Fc_{\gamma 2b/\gamma 1}R$.[27,29] To control for nonviable oocytes, which trap ligand nonspecifically [^{14}C]sucrose, an impermeant tracer, was added to the incubation mixture with the ^{125}I-ligand. Only oocytes that were injected with mRNA from the $Fc_{\gamma 2b/\gamma 1}R$-positive cell lines bound ^{125}I-2.4G2 Fab specifically (Fig. 1). Those oocytes injected with mRNA from L5178Y (an FcR-

Table I. Radioimmune Assay of *Xenopus* Oocyte Lysates

	^{125}I-2.4G2 Fab precipitated, cpm
Oocytes injected with[a]	
ddH$_2$O	115
L5178Y mRNA	160
S49.1 mRNA	2000
J774 mRNA	1800
Control S49.1 cell lysates[b]	
None	115
6 × 10^3 cell equivalents	700
18 × 10^3 cell equivalents	1950

[a] One and one-half microliters of poly A$^+$ mRNA (500 μg/ml) was injected into 20 *Xenopus* oocytes. After 48 hr the oocytes were lysed by sonication and assayed for $Fc_{\gamma 2b/\gamma 1}$ by monoclonal sandwich radioimmune assay.
[b] S49.1 cells grown in spinner culture were concentrated to 5 × 10^6 cells/ml, lysed in 1% NP 40 and 0.2% SDS, and assayed for $Fc_{\gamma 2b/\gamma 1}$ by RIA; 1950 cpm is equivalent to 2 fmoles $Fc_{\gamma 2b/\gamma 1}$.

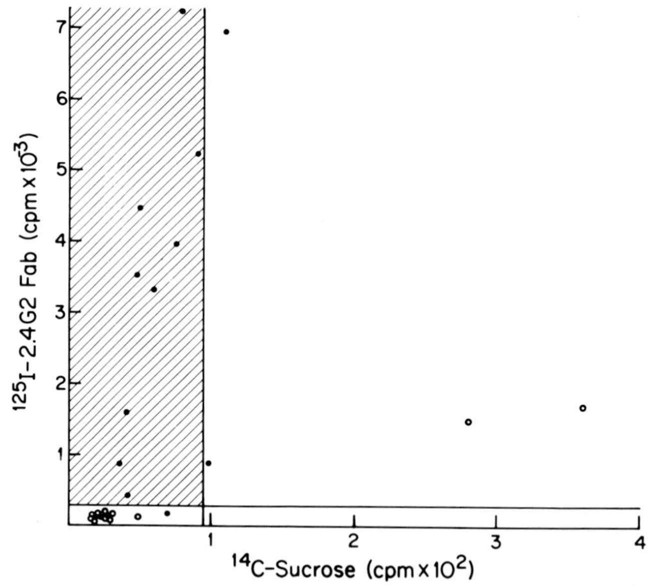

Figure 1. Expression of $Fc_{\gamma 2b/\gamma 1}$ by oocytes injected with J774 mRNA. The oocytes were injected with 60 nl of poly A$^+$ mRNA (1 mg/ml, dissolved in water) isolated from (●) J774 or (○) L5178Y cells, incubated for 2 days, and assayed as described. (From Ref. 27.)

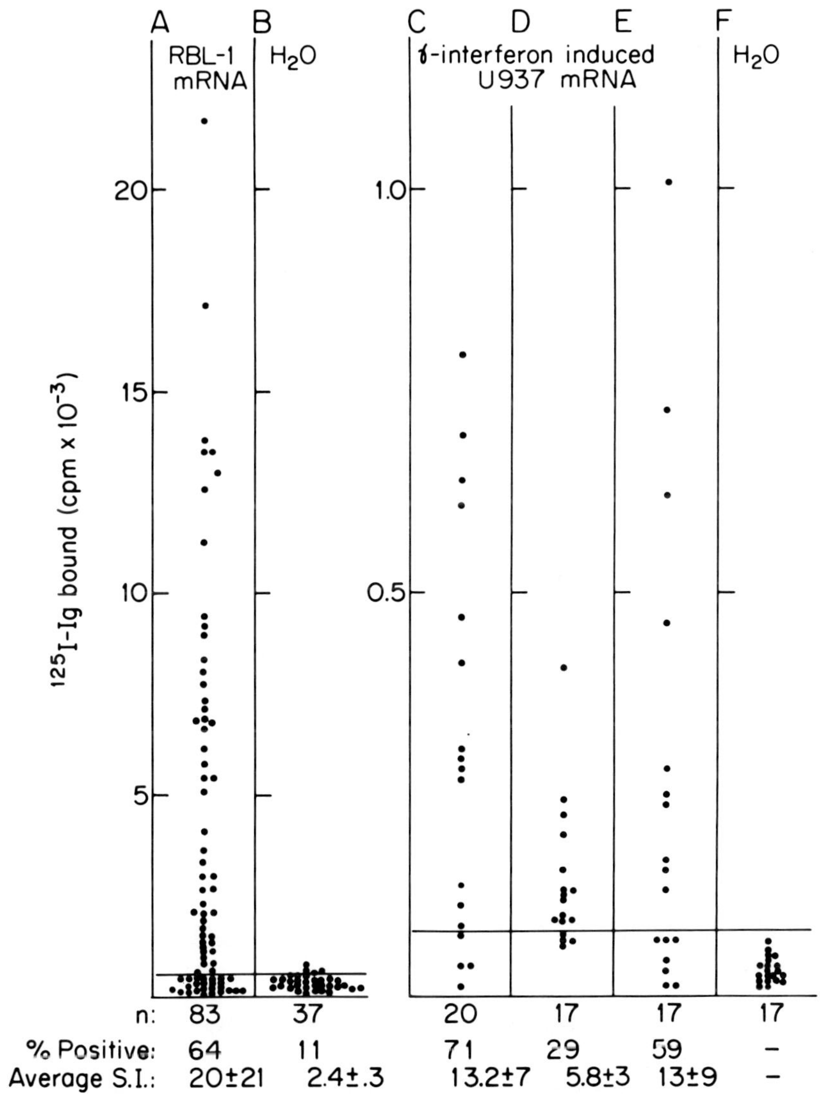

Figure 2. Binding of ^{125}I-ligands by oocytes injected with mRNA from RBL-1 and U937 cells. Oocytes injected with (A) RBL-1 mRNA or (B) water were assayed with ^{125}I-IR-162 IgE myeloma protein (1 μg/ml, 5 × 10^3 cpm/ng). Oocytes injected with (C–E) U937 mRNA or (F) water were assayed with ^{125}I-LPC-1 plus (D) 2 μg/ml of unlabeled LPC-1 or (E) 2 μg/ml of LPC-1 (Fab′)$_2$ fragment. SI, Stimulation index. (From Ref. 27.)

negative T-cell line) that bound ^{125}I-2.4G2 Fab also took up [^{14}C]sucrose, demonstrating that these oocytes were nonviable and that uptake of ligand was thus nonspecific. Binding of ^{125}I-2.4G2 Fab was detected after the injection of as little as 120 pg of mRNA per oocyte and was dependent on the amount of mRNA injected. The percentage of oocytes binding ^{125}I-2.4G2 Fab over background levels reached a plateau at 70% with 6 ng of injected mRNA, and the amount of receptor per oocyte generally began to plateau at 30–60 ng mRNA. Receptor expression was detected 24 hr after injection and increased until day 3.

We have investigated whether radiolabeled monoclonal antibodies specific for J774 cell surface proteins other than FcR were bound by oocytes injected with J774 mRNA. ^{125}I-2E2A, a monoclonal antibody directed against a major 82,000-dalton plasma membrane protein[31] found on J774 cells (6×10^5 sites per cell), binds to oocytes injected with J774 mRNA. The percentage of oocytes binding ^{125}I-2.4G2 Fab and ^{125}I-2E2A over background levels was 80 and 65% respectively. The average stimulation index was 5.4 ± 3.2 for ^{125}I-2E2A Fab and 20 ± 11 for ^{125}I-2.4G2 Fab. These data suggest that binding of monoclonal antibodies to the oocytes plasma membrane is likely to be a general method for the study of cell surface components.

3.2. Expression of Functional Rat $Fc_\epsilon R$ on Oocytes

We investigated the applicability of the oocyte system to translation of other Fc receptors for which we had no monoclonal antibody. The RBL-1 rat basophilic leukemia line (2H3 subline) expresses a high-avidity Fc receptor for IgE ($Fc_\epsilon R$).[32] Individual oocytes injected with RBL-1 mRNA bound as much as 22,000 cpm of ^{125}I-IR-162 rat IgE, compared to an average of 215 ± 36 cpm bound to water-injected oocytes (Figs. 2A and 2B). Comparable data were obtained with a monoclonal mouse IgE,[33] indicating that the IgE bound the oocyte by its Fc domain and not the antigen-combining site. It is apparent that the $Fc_\epsilon R$ on the oocyte plasma membrane was in a conformation that fulfilled the requirements for ligand binding.

3.3. Expression of Functional Human $Fc_\gamma R_{hi}$ on Oocytes

The human histiocyte-like cell line U937 has a high-affinity receptor for IgG ($Fc_\gamma R_{hi}$), the expression of which is amplified by treatment with interferon gamma (IFN-γ)[27,34] (Table II). mRNA isolated from control and IFN-γ-treated U937 cells was injected into oocytes. The oocytes expressed functional human $Fc_\gamma R_{hi}$, as demonstrated by binding of ^{125}I-murine IgG2a (Table II and Fig. 2C). The binding of 1 μg/ml of ^{125}I-IgG2a was inhibited 60% by 2 μg/ml of unlabeled IgG2a, but not by the $F(ab')_2$ fragment (Figs. 2D and 2E). However, tenfold increased binding of ^{125}I-IgG2a was observed on oocytes injected with mRNA from IFN-γ-treated U937 cells compared with untreated U937 cells (Table II),

Table II. Effect of Interferon Gamma on the Expression of $Fc_{\gamma}R_{hi}$[a]

	U937 cells		Oocytes injected with mRNA from U937 cells	
	Untreated	IFN-γ treated	Untreated	IFN-γ treated
FcR per cell[b]	8×10^3	7×10^4	5×10^7	6×10^8
FcR per μm^2 cell surface[c]	8	69	9.7	113

[a] From Ref. 27. U937 cells grown in spinner [(3–4) × 10^5 cells/ml] were treated with 100 U/ml of recombinant IFN-γ. Cells were assayed or mRNA prepared after 18 hr. Binding studies on U937 were performed at 25°C as described,[27] using iodinated IgG2a mouse myeloma protein LPC-1 (1 μg/ml, 8 × 10^3 cpm/ng). Oocytes injected with mRNA were also assayed for binding of ^{125}I-LPC-1. In reticulocyte lysates, both mRNA preparations catalyzed the synthesis of high-molecular-weight proteins, indicating that the mRNA preparations were of good quality.

[b] Data were corrected by subtraction of binding to the FcR-negative cell line MOLT-4 or L5178Y and uninjected oocytes.

[c] The approximate surface areas of the cells were calculated from their diameters.

which suggests that the treatment of the U937 cells with IFN-γ results in induction of mRNA coding for $Fc_{\gamma}R_{hi}$. Interestingly, oocytes express the same number of receptors per μm^3 as U937 cells.[27]

4. Concluding Remarks

We have used three approaches to detect Fc receptors translated in *Xenopus* oocytes. The oocyte translation system enables detection of relatively rare cellular proteins by sensitive radioimmune assay. This approach, in which the oocyte is lysed by detergent, obviously does not depend on cell surface expression of the translated proteins. One disadvantage of the system is that, of necessity, pools of oocytes must go into the lysates. There is considerable variation in the amount of FcR translated by individual oocytes, due to the vagaries of oocyte viability and quality of injection. From the single oocyte binding assays approximately 70% of "injected" oocytes express FcR. The single oocyte binding assay has the twin virtues of requiring less mRNA and having a greater signal/noise ratio. Given the control of an impermeant tracer to assess viability and ligand trapping, the oocyte surface binding assay is quite reliable. Unlike the RIA, however, it depends on the membrane insertion and transport of the newly synthesized protein. We have utilized both monoclonal anti-$Fc_{\gamma2b/\gamma1}R$ antibodies and Ig as ligand to probe the translation of FcRs. In the latter case, not only are FcRs expressed in oocytes, they are localized on the plasma membrane in a functional configuration. Clearly, *Xenopus* oocytes possess all the processing apparatus for posttranslational processing of membrane proteins.

We are interested in cloning the gene(s) for $Fc_{\gamma2b/\gamma1}R$. We have utilized the RIA and ligand binding assay to detect FcR sequences in fractionated mRNA. Fractions containing FcR sequences were then used to construct cDNA libraries. We intend to characterize the cDNA clones by hybrid selection of mRNA and translation in oocytes. This may be problematic because in some cases several polypeptides are required for surface expression of membrane antigens (e.g., for class I and II major histocompatibility antigens). If this is the case for FcR, hybrid selection of mRNA from a single cDNA clone would not result in expression.

The results presented here demonstrate that oocytes efficiently synthesize heterologous plasma membrane proteins and are capable of expressing them in a functional conformation on the plasma membrane. Many monoclonal antibodies (including 2.4G2 IgG) do not immunoprecipitate a detectable reticulocyte lysate translation product. This may be due to the loss of conformational determinants when proteins are not properly modified. In addition, $Fc_{\gamma 2b/\gamma 1}R$ message is of low abundance, making it difficult to immunoprecipitate $Fc_{\gamma 2b/\gamma 1}R$ from [^{35}S]methionine-labeled oocyte lysates. The method of ligand or monoclonal antibody binding to the oocyte surface offers a rapid and sensitive assay for minor mRNA species.

In the future, this technique should be of great utility in the molecular analysis of membrane receptors. In combination with recombinant DNA techniques this may facilitate the cloning and characterization of the genes for membrane proteins.

ACKNOWLEDGMENTS. This work was supported by grants AI-141603, AI-2131501, and CA-30198 from the U. S. Public Health Service. J. C. U. is an American Cancer Society Research Scholar. E. P. and D. A. P. are supported by Damon Runyon–Walter Winchell Cancer Fund Fellowships DRG-565 and DRG-652.

References

1. Gurdon, J. B., Lane, C. D., Woodland, H. R., and Marbaix, G., 1971, Use of frog eggs and oocytes for the study of messenger RNA and its translation in living cells, *Nature* **233**:177–182.
2. Gurdon, J. B., Lingril, J. D. and Marbaix, G., 1973, Message stability in injected frog oocytes: Long life of mammalian α and β globin messages, *J. Mol. Biol.* **80**:539.
3. Mous, J., Peeters, B., Rombauts, W., and Heynes, W., 1982, Assembly, glycosylation and secretion of the oligomeric rat prostatic binding protein in *Xenopus* oocytes, *J. Biol. Chem.* **257**:11822–11828.
4. Mertens, B., and Verhoeven, G., 1981, Synthesis and processing of pre-alpha-2μ-globulin in different translation systems, *FEBS Lett.* **133**:209–212.
5. Bock, S. C., Tiemeier, D. C., Mester, K., Wu, M., and Goldsmith, M. R., 1982, Hybridization-selected translation of *Bombix mori* high-cysteine chorion proteins in *Xenopus laevis* oocytes. *Proc. Natl. Acad. Sci. USA* **79**:1032–1036.
6. Jilka, R. L., Familletti, P., and Pestka, S., 1979, Synthesis and processing of the mouse MOPC-321 k chain in *Xenopus laevis* oocytes, *Arch. Biochem. Biophys.* **192**:290–295.
7. Berridge, M. V., and Lane, C. D., 1976, Translation of *Xenopus* liver messenger RNA in *Xenopus* oocytes: Vitellogin synthesis and conversion to yolk platelet proteins, *Cell* **8**:283–297.
8. Gedami, L., Dixon, G. H., and Gurdon, J. B., 1978, Studies of the injection of poly(A)$^+$ protamine mRNA into *Xenopus laevis* oocytes, *Exp. Cell Res.* **117**:325–334.
9. Matthews, J. A., Brown, J. W. S., and Hall, T. C., 1981, Phaseolin mRNA is translated to yield glycosylated polypeptides in *Xenopus* oocytes, *Nature* **294**:175–176.
10. Richter, J. D., Evers, D. C., and Smith, L. D., 1983, The recruitment of membrane-bound mRNAs for translation in microinjected oocytes, *J. Biol. Chem.* **258**:2614–2620.

11. Valle, G., Besley, J., and Coleman, A., 1981, Synthesis and secretion of mouse immunoglobulin chains from *Xenopus laevis* oocytes, *Nature* **291**:5913.
12. Mous, J., Peeters, B., and Rombauts, W., 1980, Synthesis and core glycosylation of the alpha subunit of human chorionic gonadotropin in *Xenopus* oocytes, *FEBS Lett.* **122**:105–108.
13. DeHerdt, E., Marbaix, G., Tencer, R., and Slegers, H., 1983, Subcellular distribution in *Xenopus laevis* oocytes of a microinjected poly(A)-binding protein from *Artemia salina* gastrulae, *Eur. J. Biochem.* **132**:623–627.
14. Colman, A., Lane, C. D., Craig, R., Boulton, A., Mohun, T., and Morser, J., 1981, The influence of topology and glycosylation on the fate of heterologous secretory proteins made in *Xenopus* oocytes, *Eur. J. Biochem.* **113**:339–342.
15. Colman, A., and Morser, J., 1979, Export of proteins from oocytes of *Xenopus laevis*, *Cell* **17**:517–526.
16. Soreq, H., Parvari, R., and Silman, I., 1982, Biosynthesis and secretion of catalytically active acetylcholinesterase in *Xenopus* oocytes microinjected with mRNA from rat brain and *Torpedo* electric organ, *Proc. Natl. Acad. Sci. USA* **79**:830–834.
17. Mishkin, A., and Soreq, H., 1981, Microinjected *Xenopus* oocytes synthesize active plasminogen activator, *Nucleic Acids Res.* **9**:3355.
18. Labaraca, C., and Paigen, K., 1977, mRNA-directed synthesis of catalytically active mouse β-glucuronidase in *Xenopus* oocytes, *Proc. Natl. Acad. Sci. USA* **74**:4462–4465.
19. Reynolds, F. H., Jr., Premkumar, E., and Petha, P. M., 1975, Interferon activity produced by translation of human interferon messenger RNA in cell free ribosomal systems and in *Xenopus* oocytes, *Proc. Natl. Acad. Sci. USA* **72**:4881–4885.
20. Lebleu, B., Hubert, E., Content, J., DeWit, L., Brande, I. A., and DeClercq, E., 1978, Translation of mouse interferon mRNA in *Xenopus* sequences, *Proc. Natl. Acad. Sci. USA* **78**:1741–1745.
21. Cavalieri, R. L., Havel, E. A., Vilcek, J., and Pestka, S., 1977, Synthesis of human interferon by *Xenopus laevis* oocytes: Two structural genes for interferons in human cells, *Proc. Natl. Acad. Sci. USA* **74**:3287–3291.
22. Soreq, H., Sagar, A. D., and Sehgal, P. B., 1981, Translational activity and functional stability of human fibroblast β_1 and β_2 interferon mRNAs lacking 3′-terminal RNA sequences, *Proc. Natl. Acad. Sci. USA* **78**:1741–1745.
23. Sumikawa, K., Houghton, M., Emtage, J. S., Richards, B. M., and Barnard, E. A., 1981, Active multi-subunit Ach receptor assembled by translation of heterologous mRNA in *Xenopus* oocytes, *Nature* **292**:862–864.
24. Mishna, M., Kurosaki, T., Tobimatsu, T., Morimoto, Y., Noda, M., Yamamoto, T., Terao, M., Lindstrom, J., Takahashi, T., Kuno, M., and Numa, S., 1984, Expression of functional acetylcholine receptor from cloned cDNAs, *Nature* **307**:604–608.
25. Gunderson, C. B., Miledi, R., and Parker, I., 1984, Messenger RNA from human brain induces drug- and voltage-operated channels in *Xenopus* oocytes, *Nature* **308**:421–424.
26. Houamed, K. M., Bilbe, G., Smart, T. G., Constanti, A., Brown, D. A., Barnard, E. A., and Richards, B. M., 1984, Expression of functional GABA, glycine and glutamate receptors in *Xenopus* oocytes injected with rat brain mRNA, *Nature* **310**:318–321.
27. Pure, E., Luster, A. D., and Unkeless, J. C., 1984, Cell surface expression of murine, rat, and human Fc receptors by *Xenopus* oocytes, *J. Exp. Med.* **160**:606–611.
28. Unkeless, J. C., and Healy, G. A., 1983, Quantitation of proteins and internal antigen pools by a monoclonal sandwich radioimmune assay, *J. Immunol. Meth.* **56**:1–12.
29. Unkeless, J. C., 1979, Characterization of a monoclonal antibody directed against mouse macrophage and lymphocyte Fc receptors, *J. Exp. Med.* **150**:580–596.
30. Chirgwin, J. M., Przybyla, A. E., MacDonald, R. J., and Rutter, W. J., 1979, Isolation of biologically active ribonucleic acid from sources enriched in ribonucleases, *Biochemistry* **18**:5294.
31. Mellman, I. S., Steinman, R. M., Unkeless, J. C., and Cohn, Z. A., 1980, Selective iodination and polypeptide composition of pinocytic vesicles, *J. Cell. Biol.* **86**:712–720.
32. Kulczycki, A., Jr., and Metzger, H., 1974, The interaction of IgE with rat basophilic leukemia cells. II. Quantitative aspects of the binding reaction, *J. Exp. Med.* **140**:1676–1684.

33. Liu, F.-T., Bohn, J. W., Ferry, E. L., Yamamoto, H., Molinaro, C. A., Sherman, L. A., Klinman, N. R., and Katz, D. H., 1980, Monoclonal dinitrophenyl-specific murine IgE antibody: Preparation, isolation and characterization, *J. Immunol.* **124**:2728–2732.
34. Guyre, P. M., Morganelli, P. M., and Miller, R., 1983, Recombinant immune interferon increases IgG Fc receptors on cultured mononuclear phagocytes, *J. Clin. Invest.* **72**:393–397.

Part IV

Monoclonal Antibodies in Diagnosis and Therapy

Chapter 28

Antibodies *in Vivo*

EDGAR HABER

1. Introduction

Of all classes of compounds, antibodies provide the greatest range of specificities and affinities. The number of interatomic interactions between an antibody combining site and a large ligand such as a receptor far exceeds those between the common small ligand or drug and its corresponding binding site.[1] As a result, there is increased selectivity and affinity. The very large number of potential antibody specificities provides an opportunity to create a finer degree of selectivity than is possible with simpler compounds. Modern studies in the molecular genetics of antibody synthesis indicate that potentially there are at least ten billion different antibody specificities.[2,3] This should permit the selective recognition of any structure within the human body.

We are in the midst of a period of explosive growth in our ability to make and utilize antibodies. Antibodies have been recognized as serum components since the early 1900s, but their only source was an immunized animal; therefore, supplies were always limited. Even when purified from serum, antibodies were heterogeneous mixtures that varied in their properties from animal to animal. Now antibodies may be produced *in vitro* in a mammalian cell culture by amplifying a single antibody-producing clone.[4] Clones of antibody-producing cells secrete a single antibody that may be considered a pure chemical. Recently, methods have been devised that allow large-scale production of antibodies in this manner in industrial fermenters.[5] It is already possible to transfect lymphoid cells with immunoglobulin genes, which results in the secretion of new proteins.[6,7] Soon mammalian cells will be replaced by yeast or bacteria, through the application of recombinant DNA methods, so that antibodies will be produced as readily as penicillin.

Today, limitations in the use of antibodies as *in vivo* diagnostic and therapeutic agents in clinical medicine relate to their immunogenicity as foreign proteins, their rather long persistence in the circulation, and the formation of

---

EDGAR HABER • Cardiac Unit and Cellular and Molecular Research Laboratory, Massachusetts General Hospital, and Department of Medicine, Harvard Medical School, Boston, Massachusetts 02114.

damaging immune complexes. A partial solution is already at hand and the longer term remedy is in sight.

Two clinical studies have already employed Fab, a smaller fragment of the immunoglobulin molecule.[8,9] Immunoglobulin molecules that bind 2 moles of antigen can be cleaved into fragments by the enzyme papain. The resultant antigen-binding fragment, Fab, binds 1 mole of antigen; the remainder, Fc, contains the complement-binding site. Fab has a number of desirable properties compared with the intact molecule IgG[10]: equilibrium distribution in extracellular fluid is achieved more rapidly; the volume of distribution is greater; and the fragment is eliminated with a far shorter half-life. In addition, when injected intravenously, Fab is less immunogenic than IgG. Complement cannot be fixed because the relevant binding sites on the Fc have been lost, and the immune complexes that may be formed, comprising simply a single antigen molecule with several Fabs attached, are smaller than those that cause nephrotoxicity.

While smaller antibody fragments reduce the risk of immunogenicity, they are not likely to eliminate it entirely. Human immunoglobulins can now be produced by cell fusion techniques *in vitro*.[11,12] An even more promising potential development is the application of molecular genetics techniques. Immunoglobulin genes are now routinely cloned for study.[2,3,13] It is quite reasonable to envision their manipulation and expression as antibody fragments carrying the minimal structure necessary to effect antigen binding. Recombinant DNA methods permit the introduction of human immunoglobulin framework sequences, so that tolerance to intrinsic proteins can prevent the mounting of an immune response.

Applications of antibodies that I would like to discuss include adrenergic receptor blockade, a definition of the role of renin in essential hypertension, the treatment of digitalis intoxication, the evaluation of myocardial infarct size, and the visualization of thrombi *in vivo*. Two of these approaches have reached the point of clinical investigation.

2. Antibodies to the β-Adrenergic Receptor

Pharmacological agonists are often either peptides of modest size or organic compounds, both readily synthesized. For some receptors, a variety of antagonists have been created in the organic chemist's laboratory. Could an antibody for the receptor be obtained by utilizing the ligand (agonist or antagonist) as a template? The vast diversity of antibody combining sites, as suggested above, provides the potential for creating a complementary fit to almost any shape. If a figurative plaster mold could be cast upon the surface of the ligand that bound to the receptor, then a second mold made from the first one should have a perfect fit to the receptor. The well-known immunologic principle of raising antibodies specific for another antibody's combining site (anti-idiotypic antibodies) may be utilized as the vehicle for molding the desired shape.

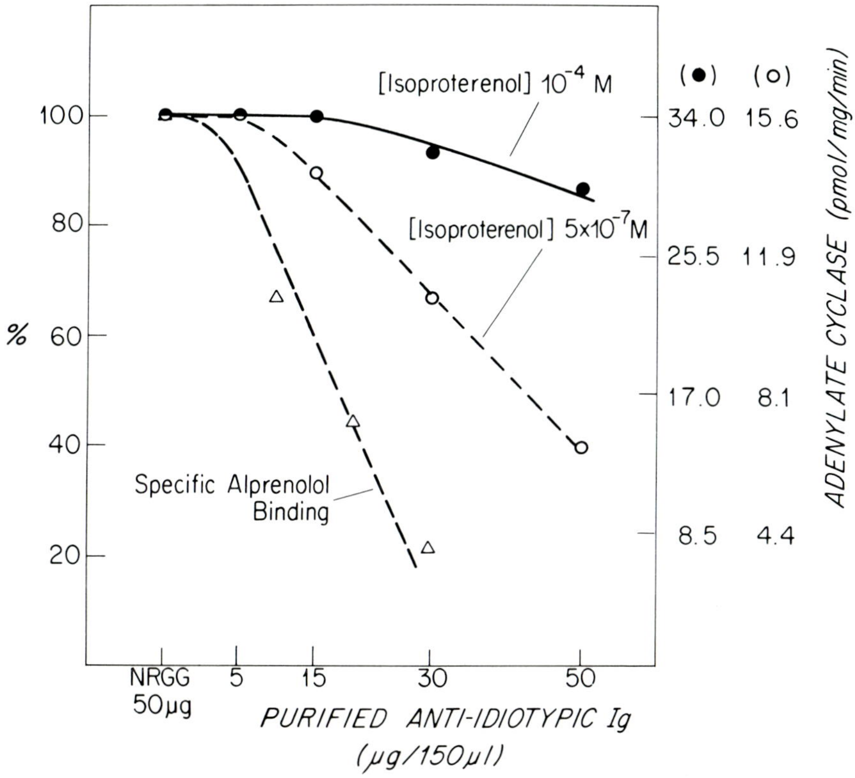

Figure 1. The effects of DEAE-purified Ig fraction on percent [^{3}H]alpronolol (2 nM) binding to turkey erythrocyte membranes and on isoproterenol-mediated adenylate cyclase stimulation. The ability of the anti-idiotypic Ig fraction to inhibit adenylate cyclase stimulation in the turkey erythrocyte membrane was tested at isoproterenol concentrations of 0.5 μM and 0.1 mM in the presence of 0.1 mM GTP. In contrast to the effects seen at the nonsaturating isoproterenol concentration of 0.5 μM, only a slight amount of inhibition is seen at the highest Ig concentrations in the presence of 0.1 mM isoproterenol. NRGG, Normal rabbit gamma globulin. (From Ref. 14 by permission.)

This principle was effected by selecting antibodies that recognized common structures on all β-adrenergic agonists and antagonists. These antibodies were nearly perfect mimics of the receptor, in that they bound all the compounds that would interact with the β-adrenergic receptor, bud did not interact with similar compounds that were neither β-specific agonists nor antagonists. A second generation of antibodies (anti-idiotypic antibodies) was then raised utilizing the first antibodies as immunogens. The anti-idiotypic antibodies were selective β-receptor blockers, shown by their abilities to compete with β-blocking drugs for the receptor and to inhibit the generation of adenylate cyclase when stimulated by isoproterenol[14] (Fig. 1). Potential uses of such receptor-specific antibodies are: the recognition of structural differences among subsets of β-adrenergic receptors; a more rigorous examination of their respective physiological roles utilizing reagents of greater resolution; the isolation of receptors with antibody affinity chromatography; and the ultimate application of antibody fragments as highly selective drugs.

3. Renin-Specific Antibodies

Although renin has been known to play a role in circulatory control since the classic work of Goldblatt in the 1930s,[15] its precise importance in a number of specific circumstances has been in doubt. Much has been learned from the application of inhibitors directed at several of the steps in the sequence leading to angiotensin II, the final product of renin. Most of the inhibitors used, however, lack specificity. The competitive inhibitors of the action of angiotensin II on receptors, such as saralysin, are partial agonists.[16] The angiotensin-converting enzyme is identical to the enzyme that deactivates bradykinin; thus, its inhibitors also affect the kinin system.[17] In addition, compounds such as captopril have been shown to stimulate prostaglandin synthesis.[18] Since both the kinin and the prostaglandin systems affect vasoregulation, it is difficult to define renin's specific role when interpreting experiments in which these inhibitors are used.

A specific antibody for renin should be a highly selective antagonist. Indeed, polyclonal renin-specific antibodies and their Fabs were effective renin-blocking agents in experimental hypertension[19,20] (Fig. 2). Salt-depleted animals showed a marked drop in blood pressure when the antibodies were infused intravenously and in renovascular hypertensive animals, blood pressure was normalized. Monoclonal antibodies to human renin are now available and may provide the potential for utilizing a highly selective renin blocker[21] in examining the role of renin in human essential hypertension, a question that is still largely unsettled.

4. Digoxin-Specific Antibody in the Clinical Reversal of Toxicity

Digitalis intoxication is one of the most frequent adverse drug reactions reported. There is no specific antidote, and the cardiac arrhythmias that are a feature of digitalis intoxication are commonly fatal. We reasoned that if an antibody specific to the digitalis glycosides had a higher affinity for the drug than the physiological receptor, it should be possible simply to transfer the ligand from the receptor to the antibody. If Fab rather than intact antibody was used, the antibody–drug complex would be rapidly excreted in the urine.

After demonstrating safety and effectiveness in animal studies, clinical studies were initiated. Results in 26 patients with life-threatening digitalis intoxication have been reported as the results of a multicenter national trial.[8] Twenty geographically dispersed, university-based centers participated, and patients were chosen for the trial if they presented a life-threatening rhythm

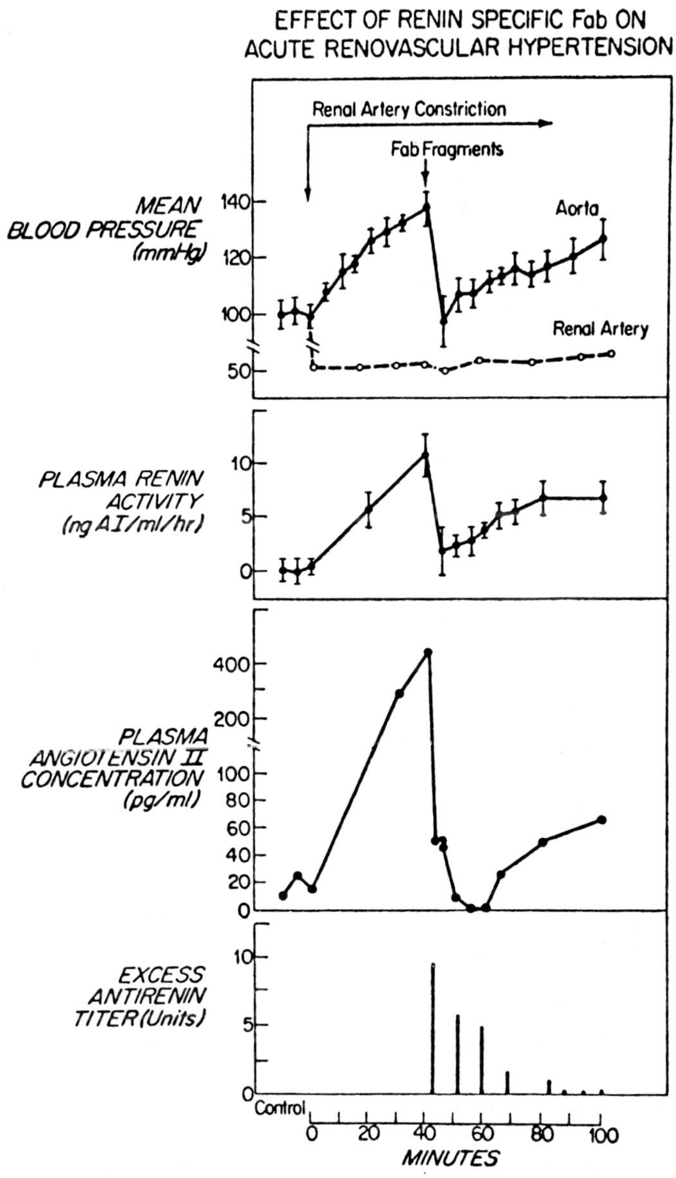

Figure 2. Immediate reduction by renin-specific Fab of systemic blood pressure, plasma renin activity, and angiotensin II levels to normal in acute renovascular hypertension. Duration of action was short-lived (30–60 min). (From Ref. 20 by permission.)

Table I. Results of Digoxin-Specific Fab Treatment (26 patients)[a]

	Number of cases
Manifestation of toxicity	
Refractory ventricular arrythmias	20
Ventricular fibrillation	9
High-grade atrioventricular block	19
Hyperkalemia	10
Result of Fab treatment	
Arrythmia corrected	26
Fully recovered	21
Died	5
Inadequate antibody available	1
Irreversible brain or cardiac damage	4

[a] From Ref. 26 by permission.

disturbance or hyperkalemia and were resistant to conventional therapeutic approaches. The patients ranged in age from 19 months to 35 years, and the overdoses occurred either during the course of therapy or as a result of accidental or suicidal overdose. In each case a dramatic reversal of intoxication symptoms occurred. Five patients died, one because inadequate quantities of Fab were available, and the remaining four because irreversible brain or cardiac damage had occurred by the time the drug was administered. The rest survived without any sequelae. Manifestations of hypersensitivity to the antibody Fab were not observed (Table I).

The history of a recently reported case is typical of the group.[22] The patient was a 34-year-old woman who took 20 mg of digitoxin, a massive overdose, with suicidal intent. She appeared to be well on admission to the hospital, except for nausea, but soon lapsed into a series of life-threatening arrhythmias that included multiple ventricular fibrillations (treated with countershock), as well as asystole (treated with ventricular pacing). At the time the antibody Fab became available to the physicians treating her, she was in shock, aneuric, and exhibited dilated pupils. Her serum potassium was elevated, a grave prognostic sign in digitalis intoxication.[23] Within 1 hr after the intravenous administration of antibody Fab, her atrioventricular conduction returned, and she was soon in normal sinus rhythm. No further dysrhythmias occurred. The patient was discharged from the hospital without sequelae several days later. Figure 3 demonstrates the initial marked increase of serum digitoxin concentration in this patient as tissue-bound drug equilibrated with the antibody (antibody-bound drug is pharmacologically inactive), followed by rapid clearance of both drug and Fab. It should be noted that the half-life of digitoxin in man is normally 7 days, with hepatic metabolism of the drug being the major source of removal. It is apparent that excretion has been markedly accelerated by the antibody Fab, and the half-life seemingly reduced to about 12 hr. Figure 4 shows

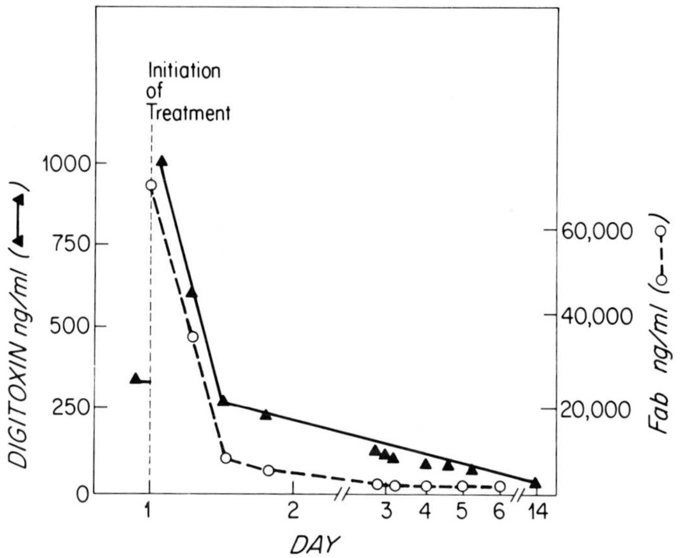

Figure 3. Blood levels of digitoxin and Fab fragments after intravenous administration of antibody Fab to a 34-year-old woman suffering a series of life-threatening arrythmias as a result of a massive overdose (20 mg) of digitoxin. Within 1 hr of intravenous administration of antibody Fab, atrioventricular conduction had returned. (From Ref. 22 by permission.)

that both antibody and Fab appear in the urine largely within the first day after Fab administration.

It should be apparent that this approach could be applied to many other drugs or toxins. Of particular interest is the acceleration of excretion of a substance that is normally metabolized slowly. Digitoxin has half-life of 7 days

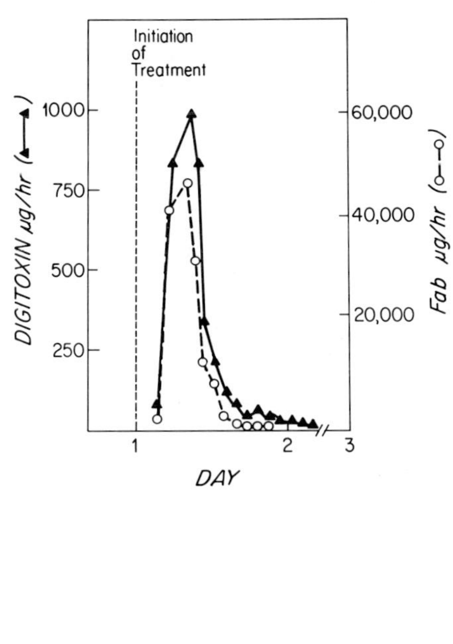

Figure 4. Urinary excretion of digitoxin and Fab fragments following intravenous administration of antibody Fab to a 34-year-woman suffering from digitalis intoxication (20 mg). (From Ref. 22 by permission.)

and is metabolized by the liver. When bound to Fab, it has a biological half-life of less than 1 day (Fig. 3) and is excreted by the kidney (Fig. 4).

5. Imaging of Myocardial Infarcts

The diagnosis of myocardial infarction often does not present a significant challenge to the clinician. Symptoms may be pathognomonic and the so-called objective findings unequivocal. Quite often, however, when it is most important to identify, associated injury or disease masks symptoms and distorts the results of laboratory tests, none of which are entirely specific. Beyond the question of diagnosis is quantification. There have been many attempts at investigating methods for arresting the progress of infarction and salvaging as much tissue as possible. It is very difficult to evaluate the efficacy of these interventions without an objective measure *in vivo* of the extent of cardiac tissue necrosis. Up to the present time, quantification of infarct size has only been possible in retrospect.

The hallmark of cell death is loss of the membrane integrity; when there is no longer a physical separation between inside and outside, the cell ceases to exist. This principle is commonly employed in clinical practice in diagnosing tissue infarction. Intracellular enzymes are lost to extracellular fluid, and their increased concentration in the blood may be used as a measure of tissue necrosis. An alternative approach is measuring the inward diffusion of a marker that is normally excluded from cells. We have selected myocardial infarction as a model and radioactively labeled myosin-specific antibody as a marker.[24] Myosin is the principal protein of the cardiac cell. Its covalent structure is unique to the heart, allowing the development of antibodies that differentiate cardiac myosin from skeletal and smooth muscle myosins. In the intact organism, cardiac myosin is protected from extracellular fluid by the cell's plasma membrane. When cell death occurs and the membrane breaks down, myosin is exposed to extracellular fluid. It is then available to react with labeled antibodies or antibody fragments.

In the first clinical study, Fab fragments of antimyosin antibodies labeled with technetium-99m via a bifunctional chelating agent, diethylene triamine pentaacetic acid, were used in the scintigraphic examination of 32 patients with myocardial infarction and unstable angina pectoris.[9] The results were compared with regional wall motion studies by ventriculography or gated blood pool scanning at 10–14 days following the onset of symptoms. Figure 5 shows a typical antimyosin scintogram of an anterior infarct and a tracing of the late ventriculogram. Concordance in the apparent region of injury defined by these different methods is excellent. Initial clinical studies in over 50 patients show substantial promise that a highly selective method may be developed for imaging and sizing myocardial infarcts. This approach will be of particular value in assessing methods for evaluating reperfusion therapy following coronary thrombosis.

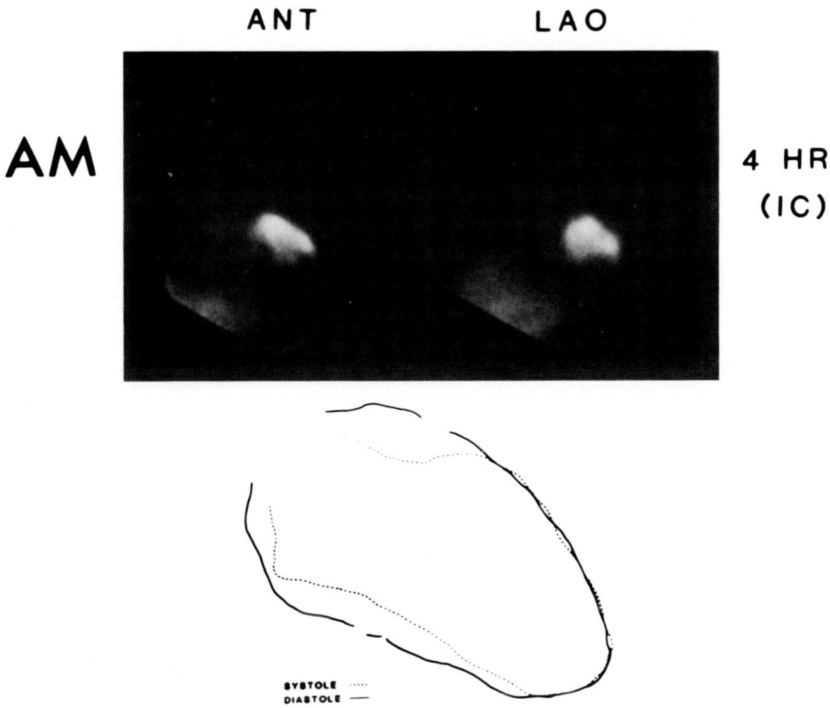

Figure 5. Antimyosin images in the anterior position (top left panel) and left anterior oblique position (top right panel) of a patient with acute anterior infarction. Bottom panel shows end-diastolic (solid lines) and end-systolic (dotted lines) outlines of the contrast ventriculogram performed at 10 days. Akinesis of the anterolateral wall of the left ventricle corresponds to the zone of antimyosin uptake. (From Ref. 26 by permission.)

6. Detecting Thrombi *in Vivo*

It would be highly desirable to have an antibody specific for fibrin that did not react with fibrinogen. Prior attempts to immunize with fibrin have only resulted in antibodies that recognized both fibrin and its precursor. Such antibodies would be unsuitable for detecting the deposition of fibrin *in vivo* since they react with circulating fibrinogen. Most recently a highly specific monoclonal antibody that reacted with fibrin exclusively was described.[25] This was accomplished by immunizing mice, not with fibrin, but with a synthetic peptide that contained the amino acid sequence of the β chain of fibrin at the point of thrombin cleavage. Thrombin, which cleaves both the β and α chains of fibrinogen, reveals two new amino-terminal ends and thus two new antigenic sites. Because these sites represent such a small part of the total fibrin molecule,

Table II. Detection of Human Fibrin: Chicken *ex Vivo* Circulatory Model[a]

Experiment	Paper disk	Circulation *ex vivo*, min	Counts per minute[b]
Ex vivo detection of fibrin disks by intravenous antibody 64C5[c]	Fibrin-coated	0	1,935 ± 250
	Fibrin-coated	10	13,116 ± 450
	Fibrin-coated	60	15,396 ± 600
	Uncoated	60	442 ± 60

[a] From Ref. 25 by permission.
[b] Mean radioactivity associated with ^{125}I-labeled antibody to mouse Fab, used to detect monoclonal antibody 64C5 bound to human fibrin-coated disks. Data are means ± standard deviations, for two separate determinations.
[c] Two disks containing 30–35 μg of human fibrin were placed in a cylindrical plastic chamber and exposed to intravenously administered 64C5 (50 μg) for the indicated time before *in vitro* treatment with the second antibody.

they do not seem to give rise to specific antibodies when immunization with the entire fibrin molecule is undertaken. Emphasizing a single antigenic site by peptide synthesis, however, permits the entire immune response to be directed at the difference between fibrin and fibrinogen.

These monoclonal antibodies have now been shown to localize specifically in thrombi *in vivo* in experimental animals (Table II). In a preliminary study, a thrombus in a coronary artery has been visualized by gamma scintigraphy. The exciting promise of this work is in not only the delineation of thrombi in both arteries and veins, but also the potential for detecting ulcerated atherosclerotic plaques that characteristically have superficial fibrin deposits. It may one day be possible to map potentially troublesome arterial lesions before occlusive thrombosis occurs.

7. How Will Antibodies Be Established as Practical Diagnostic and Therapeutic Agents?

The future of antibodies as therapeutic agents must lie in applying genetic engineering techniques to their modification and manufacture. A minimal antigen-binding site will be created by splicing the appropriate cDNA fragments. A better understanding of structure–function relationships in the antibody combining site will permit refinement of antibody specificity beyond what random selection by the immune system provides. Here site-directed mutagenesis techniques will be applied to change the amino acid sequences of antibodies in order to increase either their affinity or specificity. Appropriate structural changes may also alter antigenicity and gastrointestinal absorptive properties. Finally, the optimally engineered molecules will be expressed by microorganisms in industrial fermenters, so that their ultimate cost may not exceed that of penicillin today.

8. Concluding Comment

I have only scratched the surface of what I believe to be a vast potential for tapping the specificity and selectivity of antibodies as both diagnostic and therapeutic agents in medicine. Wherever there is a unique structure, be it tissue determinant or circulating hormone or drug, an antibody should be able to recognize it. Once recognized, it can be located, blocked, or deactivated. I believe that we are on the brink of a new pharmacology based on the unique resolution of the antibody combining site.

References

1. Poljak, R. J., Amzel, L. M., Avey, H. P., Becka, L. N., and Nisonoff, A. 1972, Structure of Fab' NEW at 6 Å resolution, *Nature New Biol.* **235**:137–140.
2. Sakano, H., Kurosawa, Y., Weigert, M., and Tonegawa, S., 1981, Identification and nucleotide sequence of a diversity DNA segment (D) of immunoglobulin heavy-chain genes, *Nature* **290**:562–565.
3. Early, P., Huang, H., Davis, M., Calame, K., and Hood, L., 1980, An immunoglobulin heavy chain variable region gene is generated from three segments of DNA: V_H, D, and J_H, *Cell* **19**:981–992.
4. Köhler, G., and Milstein, C., 1975, Continuous cultures of fused cells producing antibody of predefined specificity, *Nature* **256**:495–497.
5. Fazekas de St. Groth, S., 1983, Automated production of fused cells secreting antibody of predefined specificity, *J. Immunol. Meth.* **57**:121–136.
6. Rice, D., and Baltimore, D., 1982, Regulated expression of an immoglobulin kappa gene introduced into a mouse lymphoid cell line, *Proc. Natl. Acad. Sci. USA* **79**:7862–7865.
7. Oi, V. T., Morrison, S. L., Herzenberg, L. A., and Berg, P., 1983, Immunoglobulin gene expression in transformed lymphoid cells, *Proc. Natl. Acad. Sci. USA* **80**:825–829.
8. Smith, T. W., Butler, V. P., Jr., Haber, E., Fozzard, H., Marcus, F. I., Bremner, W. F., Schulman, I. C., and Phillips, A., 1982, Treatment of life-threatening digitalis intoxication with digoxin-specific Fab antibody fragments: Experience in 26 cases, *N. Engl. J. Med.* **307**:1357–1362.
9. Khaw, B. A., Gold, H. K., Yasuda, T., Leinbach, R. C., Strauss, H. W., Fallon, J. T., Cahill, S. L., and Haber, E., 1982, Acute myocardial infarct imaging with technetium-99m-DPTA-anti-myosin Fab, *Circulation* **66**:272 (abstract).
10. Smith, T. W., Lloyd, B. L., Spicer, N., and Haber, E., 1979, Immunogenicity and kinetics of distribution and elimination of sheep digoxin-specific IgG and Fab fragments in the rabbit and baboon, *Clin. Exp. Immunol.* **36**:384–396.
11. Olsson, L., and Kaplan, H. S., 1980, Human–human hybridomas producing monoclonal antibodies of predefined antigenic specificity, *Proc. Natl. Acad. Sci. USA* **77**:5429–5431.
12. Croce, C. M., Linnenbach, A., Hall, W., Steplewski, Z., and Koprowski, H., 1980, Production of human hybridomas secreting antibodies to measles virus, *Nature* **288**:488–489.
13. Seidman, J. G., Leder, A., Nau, M., Norman, B., and Leder, P., 1978, A kappa-immunoglobulin gene is formed by site-specific recombination without further somatic mutation, *Science* **202**:11–17.
14. Homcy, C. J., Rockson, S. G., and Haber, E., 1982, An antiidiotypic antibody that recognizes the β-adrenergic receptor, *J. Clin. Invest.* **69**:1147–1154.
15. Goldblatt, H., Lynch, J., Hanzal, R. F., Ramon, F., and Summerville, W. W., 1934, Studies on experimental hypertension. 1. The production of persistent elevation of systolic blood pressure by means of renal ischemia, *J. Exp. Med.* **59**:347–379.

16. Hollenberg, N. K., Williams, G. H., Burger, B., Ishikawa, I., and Adams, D. F., 1979, Blockade and stimulation of renal 1-Sar, 8-Ala angiotensin II in normal man, *J. Clin. Invest.* **57**:39–46.
17. Swartz, S. L., Williams, G. H., Hollenberg, N. K., Moore, T. J., and Dluhy, R. G., 1979, Converting enzyme inhibition in essential hypertension: The hypotensive response does not reflect only reduced angiotensin II formation, *Hypertension* **1**:106–111.
18. Goldstone, R., Martin, K., Zipser, R., and Horton, R., 1981, Evidence for a dual action of converting enzyme inhibitor on blood pressure in normal man, *Prostaglandins* **22**:587–598.
19. Dzau, V. J., Kopelman, R. I., Barger, A. C., and Haber, E., 1980, Renin-specific antibody for study of cardiovascular homeostasis, *Science* **207**:1091–1093.
20. Dzau, V. J., Kopelman, R. I., Barger, A. C., and Haber, E., 1984, Comparison of renin-specific IgG and antibody fragments in studies of blood pressure regulation, *Am. J. Physiol.* **246**:H404–H409.
21. Dzau, V. J., Devine, D., Mudgett-Hunter, M., Kopelman, R. I., Barger, A. C., and Haber, E., 1983, Antibodies as specific renin inhibitors: Studies with polyclonal and monoclonal antibodies and Fab fragments. *Clin. Exper. Hypertension* **A5**(7&8):1207–1220.
22. Aeberhard, P., Bulter, V. P., Smith, T. W., Haber, E., Tse Eng, D., Brau, J., Chalom, A., Glatt, B., Thébaut, J. F., Delangenhagen, B., and Morin, B., 1980, Le traitement d'une intoxication digitalique massive (20 mg de digitoxine) par les anticorps anti-digoxine fractionés (Fab), *Arch. Mal. Coeur* **73**:1471–1478.
23. Bismuth, C., Gaulthier, M., Conso, F., and Efthymiou, M. L., 1973, Hyperkalemia in acute digitalis poisoning: Prognostic significance and therapeutic implications, *Clin. Toxicol.* **6**:153–162.
24. Khaw, B. A., Beller, G. A., Haber, E., and Smith, T. W., 1976, Localization of cardiac myosin-specific antibody in experimental myocardial infarction, *J. Clin. Invest.* **58**:439–446.
25. Hui, K. Y., Matsueda, G. R., and Haber, E., 1983, Monoclonal antibodies to a synthetic fibrin-like peptide bind to human fibrin but not fibrinogen, *Science* **222**:1129–1131.
26. Haber, E., 1984, Monoclonal antibodies: Their potential as *in vivo* diagnostic and therapeutic agents, in: *Monoclonal Antibodies and New Trends in Immunoassays* (C. A. Bizollon, ed.), Elsevier, Amsterdam, pp. 81–90.

Chapter 29

Human Complement-Fixing Antibodies in Transplantation

G. HALE and H. WALDMANN

1. Introduction

It is widely expected that monoclonal antibodies will find many applications in transplantation. They certainly offer significant advantages of exquisite (even if not always predictable) specificity and continuous availability compared with polyclonal antisera. Four major categories of use will be considered here.

1. *In vitro* removal of T cells from allogeneic bone marrow grafts to prevent graft-versus-host disease.
2. *In vitro* removal of residual tumor cells from autologous bone marrow grafts.
3. *In vivo* immunosuppression of recipients of allogeneic bone marrow or organ grafts.
4. *In vivo* serotherapy of neoplasias as an adjunct to cytoreduction prior to an autologous bone marrow graft.

Despite early hopes that tumor-specific antibodies could be obtained, there are few examples, and most studies have been carried out with antibodies specific for differentiation markers on cells of the immune system. Thus, prevention of graft-versus-host disease and treatment of graft rejection are major application areas at present. There is also considerable interest in the use of monoclonal antibodies in autologous marrow grafts, because absolute specificity for tumor cells is not required, only a lack of reactivity with normal hematopoietic stem cells.

Many artificial mechanisms have been proposed for elimination of unwanted cells with monoclonal antibodies. These mostly involve chemical coupling to various drugs, plant or bacterial toxins, radiochemicals, or insoluble polymers and have met with some success. However, our laboratory has concentrated its efforts on exploiting physiological effector mechanisms, such as complement-mediated lysis, antibody-dependent, cell-mediated lysis, and op-

G. HALE and H. WALDMANN • Department of Pathology, Division of Immunology, New Addenbrookes Hospital, University of Cambridge, Cambridge CB2 2QQ, England.

sonization. For various technical reasons, such as ease of large-scale production and clonal stability with respect to loss of Ig secretion, we have chosen to study rat monoclonal antibodies,[1] but the same principles should also apply to mouse antibodies, if differences in the corresponding isotypes are taken into account.

Complement-mediated lysis is a simple and quick method of purging unwanted cells from bone marrow; it can be easily controlled and the effects are easily monitored. Virtually all of the published studies have employed rabbit serum as the source of complement.[2–4] This suffers from some drawbacks; in particular, many batches of rabbit serum must be tested to obtain both efficient antibody-dependent lysis and low nonspecific toxicity.[5] Unwanted "natural" antibodies in the serum that react with human cells could be removed by absorption, or serum from neonates could be used, but it is still possible that sublytic amounts of natural antibodies would remain to give confusing synergistic effects with some monoclonal antibodies.

The advantage of human complement is that large amounts of fresh serum are always freely available and it can be used at high concentrations without risk of nonspecific toxicity. There is little variation among individuals in the lytic effect of human complement when used with autologous cells (Ref. 6, and G. Hale and H. Waldmann, unpublished work). Furthermore, if complement-mediated lysis is contemplated as a possible mechanism for clearance of cells *in vivo*, obviously only human complement can be considered, because infusion of large quantities of animal serum would be unacceptable.

Despite these attractions, human complement has not received much attention in this context, because, unlike polyclonal antisera, only few monoclonal antibodies are good at promoting complement-mediated lysis.

2. Possible Reasons for Poor Lytic Ability of Monoclonal Antibodies

First, only certain Ig isotypes may be able to bind productively to C1q, the first component of the classical complement cascade. The C1q component has six globular heads, at least two of which must bind to the Fc portion of Ig in order to activate subsequent components. Therefore, IgM antibodies, with their five Fc portions, are expected to be much more efficient because a single molecule can fix C1q on a cell surface, whereas at least two molecules of IgG must be adjacent, and on average there must be several thousand per cell to make it probable that two will be sufficiently close.[7,8] The ability of IgG antibodies to activate complement varies among different subclasses and may depend on the source of the complement. For mouse antibodies, ability to fix complement by the classical pathway and lyse cells is in the order IgG2b $\simeq$ IgG2a $>$ IgG3 $>$ IgG1.[9–11] Comparable studies with rat antibodies give the order IgG2b $>$ IgG2a $>$ IgG2c $>$ IgG1.[12,13]

Second, the amount of many individual surface antigens is relatively small. This can be a serious problem because although a single lesion may be adequate to cause lysis of a red cell,[14] many lesions are necessary to lyse a nucleated cell.[15] Furthermore, some types of cell are more resistant to the effects of complement than others, possibly because of differences in the activity of membrane repair mechanisms.[16,17]

Third, cells can evade lysis by a poorly understood process termed "antigenic modulation."[18] This is related to the process of patching and capping induced by the lattice-like interaction between multivalent antibody and multivalent antigen.[19–21] Ultimately this process can result in internalization or shedding of the antigen and antibody,[22] but even partial patching of antibody on the cell surface can inhibit complement lysis.[23,24] This seems paradoxical, because the increased proximity of Fc portions should result in more efficient fixation of C1q. Possibly the antigen–antibody complexes become too closely aggregated to allow insertion of the terminal components of complement that form the lytic lesions. Monoclonal antibodies are assumed to react only with a single antigenic epitope and so should only cause antigenic modulation if the antigen itself is in some way multimeric (e.g., membrane Ig) or is anchored to the cytoskeleton in such a way that antibody binding triggers an active process of aggregation.

Fourth, there is convincing evidence that complement from the same species as the cells is generally less effective than complement from other sources for cell lysis[25] and this is at least partly because of the presence on cell membranes of one or more species-specific, membrane-bound inactivators of key components in the complement cascade.[26,27]

3. Monoclonal Antibodies with Good Lytic Ability

Despite these potential limitations, some mouse monoclonal antibodies have been described, mostly IgM, that do lyse cells with human complement[6,28] and we have identified rat monoclonal antibodies, both IgM and IgG, that also give substantial lysis with human complement.[1] Their isotypes were determined by conventional methods and confirmed by agglutination of red cells coupled with mouse monoclonal antibodies specific for the different rat isotypes.[29,30] IgG subclasses in the rat are IgG1, IgG2a, IgG2b, and IgG2c.[31] Although IgG1 comprises 25–30% of the total Ig in normal rat serum,[31] we have not detected any in our fusions, although others have obtained them,[13,32] particularly after immunizing with protein antigens.[33] We frequently obtained IgM, IgG2a, and IgG2b antibodies and rarely IgG2c. Studies using aggregated myeloma proteins in solution had indicated that the ability of rat immunoglobulins to fix human complement was in the order IgG2b > IgG2a > IgG1 > IgG2c.[12] However, the lytic capacity of our monoclonal antibodies depended more strongly on which antigens they recognized (Table I). When comparing different antibodies of the same specificity, the order deduced with myeloma proteins appears to hold true.

Table I. Lysis of Human Cells by Rat Monoclonal Antibodies with Human Complement

Antibody	Isotype	Specificity[a]	Representative cells	Lysis[b]
YTH 62.7	IgM	CAMPATH-1	T and B cells	+ + +
YTH 66.9	IgM	CAMPATH-1	T and B cells	+ + +
YTH 34.5	IgG2a	CAMPATH-1	T and B cells	+ +
YTH 86.1	IgG2c	CAMPATH-1	T and B cells	+
YAML 8.13	IgM	HLA class 2	B cells	+ + +
YCL 6.8	IgG2a	HLA class 2	B cells	+ + +
YAML 555.6	IgG2a	HLA class 2	B cells	+ + +
YHB 6.14	IgG2b	HLA class 2	B cells	+ + +
YTH 76.3	IgG2a	HLA class 1	T and B cells	+ +
YHB 66.25	IgM	LCA	T and B cells	—
YAML 501.4	IgG2a	LCA	T and B cells	—
YAML 568.4	IgG2a	LCA	T and B cells	—
YTH 5.3	IgG2b	LCA	T and B cells	—
YTH 24.5	IgG2b	LCA	T and B cells	—
YTH 54.12	IgG2b	LCA	T and B cells	—
YTH 75.6	IgG2b	LCA	T and B cells	—
YHB 143.6	IgG2c	LCA	T and B cells	—
YTH 36.11	IgG2a	CAMPATH-4	T cells	—
YTH 67.1	IgG2a	CAMPATH-4	T cells	—
YTH 26.5	IgG2b	CAMPATH-4	T cells	—
YTH 27.7	IgG2a	CAMPATH-5	Subset of T and B cells	—
YTH 56.8	IgG2a	CAMPATH-5	Subset of T and B cells	—
YTH 80.101	IgG2b	CAMPATH-5	Subset of T and B cells	—

[a] Antigenic specificities were defined by cell distribution, immunoprecipitation, and inhibition assays.[40,41,75,85] CAMPATH-1, -4, and -5 refer to specificities defined by these antibodies not yet related to other lymphocyte antigens. LCA, Leukocyte-common antigen.
[b] Lysis of ^{51}Cr-labeled cells was measured by the release of radioactivity when incubated with antibodies and human complement,[40] and scored as follows: (—) 0–10%, (+) 11–50%, (+ +) 51–90%, (+ + +) 91–100%.

4. Therapeutic Applications

4.1. Elimination of T Cells from Marrow Grafts

It is well established in animal models that graft-versus-host disease can be abrogated by purging the donor marrow of mature T cells,[34–36] and after some unsuccessful attempts, it has now been shown that T-cell depletion prevents graft-versus-host disease in humans.[4,37,38] In one study[4] 14 patients received HLA-matched marrow transplants treated *in vitro* with rabbit complement and a mixture of mouse monoclonal antibodies against different T-cell antigens. This gave >99% depletion of T cells after two cycles of treatment. However, because of the variability in potency and stem cell toxicity between different batches, it is difficult to obtain large quantities of suitable rabbit serum, so the marrow first had to be fractionated to obtain a concentrated suspension of mononuclear cells. After *in vitro* lysis, it also needed to be thoroughly washed to remove the foreign proteins.[39] Such extensive manipulation can lead to loss and clumping of cells.

All of these problems are avoided by using human complement, which is readily available from the marrow donor. Alternatively, an even simpler technique would be merely to coat the unseparated marrow cells with antibody and to rely on the recipient's complement system. This would eliminate the need for incubation with serum and the consequent washing of the cells to remove potentially anaphylatoxic fragments of activated complement components.

Among the rat monoclonal antibodies described above, one group was particularly efficient at lysis with human complement; the prototype antibody in this group is the IgM CAMPATH-1,[40,41] which has a specificity not yet reported among mouse monoclonal antibodies. It recognizes human T and B lymphocytes at most stages of differentiation, as well as monocytes, but is unreactive with other types of blood cells, including granulocytes, erythroid cells, platelets, and colony-forming cells. Binding of CAMPATH-1 to lymphocytes did not induce any patching or capping, and treatment with CAMPATH-1 and human complement abolished >99% of T-cell activity in proliferation assays. Therefore it appeared ideal for removal of T cells from bone marrow grafts in order to prevent graft-versus-host disease. Serum from well over 150 donors has been tested with CAMPATH-1 and invariably supports lysis of lymphocytes.

A small series of 11 allogeneic marrow transplants from matched siblings has been carried out using one cycle of treatment with CAMPATH-1 and donor complement *in vitro*.[42] Preparation of mononuclear cells from the marrow aspirate was unnecessary, and a simple buffy coat fraction made with hydroxyethyl starch was used. Depletion of E rosette-positive cells was greater than 99%, which compares well with small-scale incubations with CAMPATH-1[40] and the alternative procedure using rabbit complement in two cycles.[4] Rapid engraftment was documented in all patients, and so far none have developed graft-versus-host disease, though five have died of leukemic relapse, infection, or other complications (follow up 3–12 months). Similar studies are being carried out in several other centers in Germany and England and the incidence of graft-versus-host disease so far is very low (follow up 3–15 months, Table II). Although complement has been added *in vitro* so that T-cell depletion could be measured, CAMPATH-1 might be equally effective by just coating the cells *in vitro* and exploiting the recipient's complement system.

It could be questioned whether removal of B cells from the marrow graft by CAMPATH-1, while not necessary for elimination of graft-versus-host disease, might be disadvantageous to the immune reconstitution of the recipient. It is well known that conventional bone marrow transplantation causes long-term immunologic abnormalities,[43] and so far the long-term effects of lymphocyte depletion have not been reported. However, we do know that at least one patient with severe combined immunodeficiency, transplanted with CAMPATH-1-treated marrow from a haploidentical parent following ablative conditioning, has recovered good T-cell and B-cell function by 6 months post-transplant.[44] This indicates that CAMPATH-1 does spare the stem cells that give rise to T and B lymphocytes. A more serious problem, which will probably

Table II. Matched Bone Marrow Transplants Depleted of T Cells with CAMPATH-1[a]

Center	Clinician	Number of patients	Diseases	Other immunosuppression	GVHD >Grade 2	Graft failure
Jerusalem	S. Slavin	15	Leukemia, SAA, thalassemia, osteopetrosis	none	0	3 (1SAA)
Ulm	W. Heit	17	Leukemia	none	0	2
Hammersmith	E. C. Gordon-Smith J. Goldman	29	SAA, Fanconi anaemia, leukemia	CyA	3	4 (3SAA)
Westminster	J. Barrett	14	Leukemia	CyA	0	1
Munich	H. Kolb	9	Leukemia	CyA	0	2

[a] Abbreviations: GVHD, graft-versus-host disease; SAA, severe aplastic anaemia; CyA, cyclosporin A.

apply to any technique of T-cell depletion, is the increased risk of graft rejection once the immunosuppressive effect of graft-versus-host disease has been eliminated[45] and we noted cases of late graft failure in the patients who received HLA-matched, CAMPATH-1-treated marrow[42] (Table II). This problem may be overcome by increased conditioning, although another possibility could be to remove antigen-presenting cells from the marrow if they provoke the strongest immune response, as seems to be the case for a least some organ transplants.[46,47]

4.2 Autologous Bone Marrow Transplantation

The majority of patients with disseminated malignant disease who might be eligible for bone marrow transplantation do not have a suitable matched donor. Autologous bone marrow transplantation would be the treatment of choice if we could be confident that residual tumor cells in the marrow would not contribute to a subsequent relapse.[48] The main difficulty is to ensure complete elimination of all tumor cells, because even a 0.1% contamination of the treated marrow represents about 10^7 cells. It is unlikely that a single antibody will be able to give complete elimination, because expression of membrane antigens is usually heterogenous, and so there will always be some cells that bind very few molecules of a particular antibody. Therefore it is logical to use a cocktail of antibodies with different specificities.[49] Such a cocktail would advantageously include antibodies that activate a variety of physiological effector mechanisms, and then in principle the marrow could be coated with the mixture and infused without need for further manipulations. The choice of an ideal combination may be a lengthy process because appropriate clinical trials will take several years. Therefore we believe that there will be advantages in choosing reagents with a rather broad reactivity with different types of tumor cells, which can be standardized for use in many different situations. CAMPATH-1 may be useful in autologous transplants for lymphoid malignancies because it has already been tested in allogeneic transplants and it recognizes cells from virtually all cases of lymphoid leukemia[50] and non-Hodgkin lymphoma[51] (also G. Hale and H. Waldmann, unpublished work).

4.3. Serotherapy

Consideration of the problem of relapse after marrow transplantation brings to mind that present regimes of intensive chemotherapy and radiotherapy for conditioning are still not adequate to remove all residual disease.[45,52–54] It would be difficult to further escalate present treatment without unacceptable toxicity to other organs, but monoclonal antibodies might offer a useful extra modality of therapy. Many different antibodies have been tested in humans with varied success, and several potential problems, such as antigenic modulation, provocation of an immune response, and presence of free antigen in the serum, have been identified.[55] The optimum effector mechanisms have not yet been defined and the role of human complement has not been studied in detail. First it was essential to establish whether complement-fixing antibodies can be administered safely.

Previous experience with polyclonal antisera has shown that intravenous infusion of antibodies can be associated with reactions such as chills, fever, and rashes and occasionally serum sickness, probably associated with the formation of immune complexes and activation of complement.[56,57] Monoclonal antibodies are highly specific and much more active; therefore smaller doses are likely to be administered. Nevertheless, it was thought necessary to check the safety of intravenous infusion of an IgM complement-fixing antibody. CAMPATH-1 recognizes lymphocytes from cynomolgus monkeys[41] and it was tested by injection into two animals. To the first, weekly injections were given to provoke a strong antibody response to the rat Ig, and to the other, daily injections were given to simulate the proposed therapeutic dose regime.[51] Neither monkey developed any signs of toxicity. The level of circulating lymphocytes and hemolytic complement fell rapidly after each antibody injection to recover partially during 24 hr. After 7 days, anti-rat Ig could be detected in the serum, and from this time antibody injections had progressively smaller effects on the lymphocyte count, but the drop in complement level was even more marked, presumably due to the formation of immune complexes. Other monkeys were injected with IgG antibodies of the same specificity as CAMPATH-1 that fix complement only weakly, but in these animals there was no significant effect on lymphocyte counts or on complement levels until after day 7.[51]

Two patients with advanced lymphoid malignancies (non-Hodgkin lymphoma and B-cell chronic lymphocytic leukemia) were treated with CAMPATH-1 (90 mg/day) for 4 and 9 days respectively. Both had very high white cell counts (24×10^9 and 70×10^9) at the start of treatment, and the cells were sensitive to CAMPATH-1 plus complement *in vitro*. After each injection there was a sharp decrease in the number of circulating leukemic cells, accompanied by an equally sharp fall in the level of hemolytic complement (Fig.

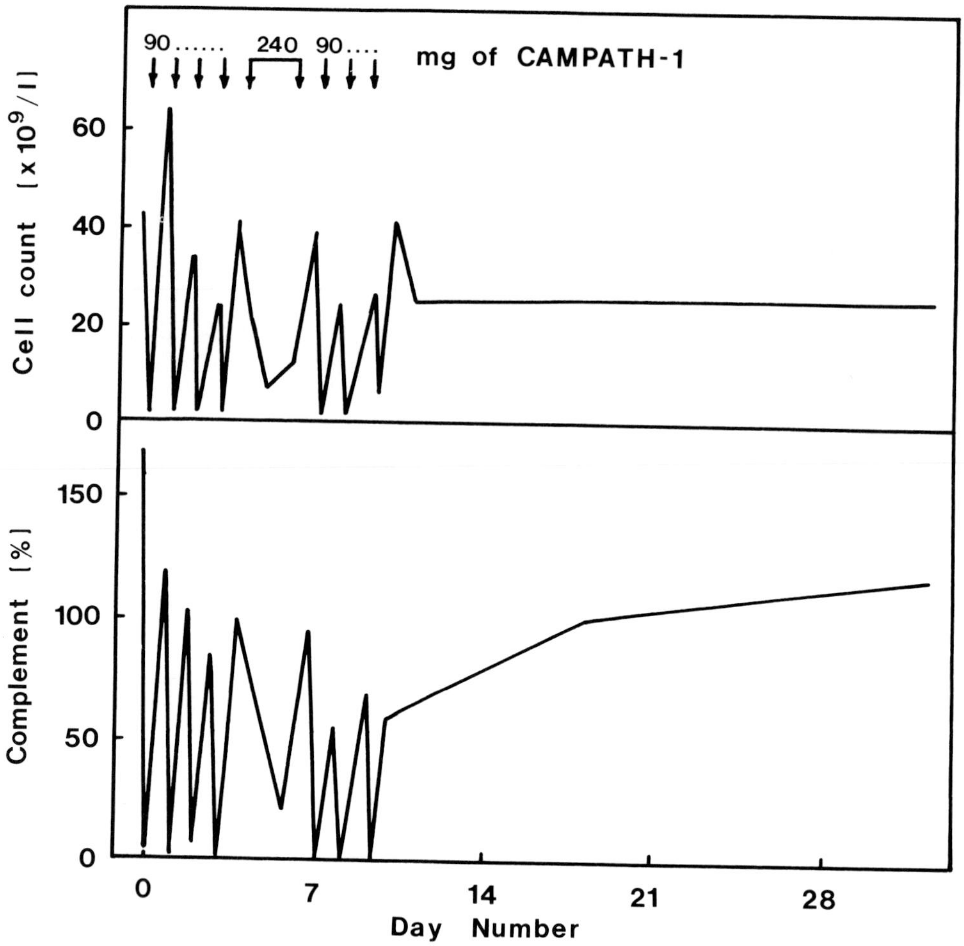

Figure 1. Serotherapy of B-cell chronic lymphocytic leukemia with CAMPATH-1. Daily injections of 90 mg of CAMPATH-1 were given for 10 days except that on days 5–6 a continuous infusion of 240 mg was given at 10 mg/hr. The levels of white cells (>95% lymphocytes) and hemolytic complement were monitored.

1). After 24 hr, the cell counts had returned to the starting level, but the level of complement, particularly the C4 component, had not completely recovered. Although there was little or no clinical improvement, the antibody injections were well tolerated, with no untoward side effects. In these two patients with very high cell burdens, the availability of complement appeared to limit the rate at which cells could be lysed.[51] Since then 43 recipients of organ grafts (who have low to normal lymphocyte counts) have been treated prophylactically with CAMPATH-1 at 25–50 mg/day for 10 days immediately posttransplant to assess its potential use as an immunosuppressant (R. Calne, G. Hale, and H. Waldmann, unpublished work). Reduction in the lymphocyte count was accompanied by only a modest decrease (about 10%) in complement levels. The 23 patients who received liver transplants were also treated with conventional steroid immunosuppressants (prednisolone plus imuran) and none of them had any adverse reactions to the antibody injections. The remaining 20 patients had kidney or kidney plus pancreas grafts and received cyclosporin A as the standard immunosuppressant.[58,59] Of these, 13 had no reactions, but seven had various acute reactions to the first injection (two patients) or subsequent ones. These reactions included chills (three), nausea (two), urticaria (two), hypotension (one; antibody had been diluted in the wrong diluent and contained aggregates when injected), and bronchospasm (one; the only patient given antibody while under anaesthetic). All responded rapidly to appropriate treatment. In most cases antibody therapy was discontinued after any adverse reaction, however mild, but more recently symptoms can be avoided by giving 100 mg of hydrocortisone just before the antibody injection if necessary.

These observations are similar to the clinical experience with other monoclonal antibodies, most of which are IgG and do not fix human complement.[55,60,61] In fact, several authors have suggested that the clinical reactions are mainly a consequence of intravascular cell lysis[62–64] and monoclonal antibodies that do not react with circulating cells may fail to provoke any such reactions.[65]

There seems to be no *a priori* reason why complement-fixing or IgM antibodies should not be used for serotherapy, but their value remains to be proven. There has not yet been sufficient followup on the transplant recipients to enable us to draw conclusions about the prophylactic value of CAMPATH-1, and firm results will await the performance of a properly controlled trial.

5. Techniques for Enhancing Complement-Mediated Lysis

Many monoclonal antibodies are poorly lytic with human complement, and this appears to be at least partly related to the nature of the antigen. Antibodies such as CAMPATH-1 give potent lysis, but there are potentially useful reagents that are less effective. However, there are several ways in which the lytic ability of an antibody can be enhanced.

5.1. Development with Antiglobulins

One way of enhancing lysis is to add an appropriate antiglobulin that fixes complement more efficiently. Such antiglobulins have regularly been used to enhance the hemolytic efficiency of monoclonal IgG antibodies in plaquing assays for B cells[66] and more recently to enable hematopoietic progenitor cells to be tested for their expression of histocompatibility antigens.[67] There has also been much interest in the complement-fixing ability of so-called "rheumatoid factor." This is a form of antibody found in the sera of patients with rheumatoid arthritis and predominantly consists of IgM, which recognizes aggregated or antigen-bound human IgG. Early studies suggested that it fixed complement poorly, if at all, but subsequent reports showed that under appropriate conditions polyclonal IgM anti-IgG could give enhanced lysis.[68] Recently a mixture of five mouse IgM monoclonal antibodies specific for mouse IgG1 was shown to improve lysis of human T cells coated with either of two monoclonal IgG1 anti-T-cell antibodies.[69] Unlike xenogeneic antiglobulin reagents, rheumatoid factors have only low affinity for free IgG in solution. This is a distinct advantage because it means that cells need not be washed free of the first antibody before adding the developing reagent.

Complement fixation in the presence of a developing antibody may be brought about by several possible mechanisms, involving the Fc of either or both antibodies. Out of a range of mouse monoclonal anti-rat Ig antibodies, only certain ones gave enhanced lysis with rat monoclonal antibodies, and even then, not all of the rat antibodies were developed as expected (T. St. J. Alderson, M. R. Clark, and G. Hale, unpublished work). For example, MAR 18.5, a mouse antibody against rat κ light chains,[70] was found to develop only IgG2b antibodies against the leukocyte common antigen and not IgG2a antibodies with identical specificity. This suggests that in some instances aggregation of the first antibody may be a more significant effect of the anti-Ig than contribution of a new Fc. Aggregation of IgG molecules to produce enchanced lytic ability has also been achieved by using protein A or concanavalin A as specific cross-linking agents.[71,72]

5.2. Synergy

Initiation of the complement cascade requires C1q attachment by more than one globular head and there must be an adequate density of antibody molecules on the cell surface to bring this about.[7,8] Clearly, improved lysis might be expected by using a mixture of two or more antibodies binding to different determinants. In the special case of two antibodies binding to different epitopes on the same antigen molecule there is the potential for much greater than additive lysis, since the effective concentration of adjacent Fc regions is substantially increased, first because each antigen molecule can bear two antibody molecules, and second, because groups of antigen molecules can become linked in catenary chains.[13] This phenomenon is termed synergistic lysis. It was first clearly demonstrated by Elliot *et al.*[73] using polyclonal antibodies against different surface antigens on guinea pig L_2C leukemic lymphocytes. These observations were extended by Howard *et al.*[74] using human complement and rat monoclonal antibodies against rat major histocompatibility antigens. They showed that at least one of the synergistic pair must be an IgG2b antibody, which is the optimum subclass for fixing human C1q.[13]

To test the generality of these findings in a system that might be directly applicable to human therapy, we have carried out similar experiments using

Table III. Synergistic Lysis with Pairs of Monoclonal Antibodies against the Leukocyte Common Antigen

			Percent lysis with human complement					
			Second antibody					
First antibody	Isotype	Inhibition group	YAML 501.4	YAML 568.4	YTH 5.3	YTH 24.5	YTH 54.12	YTH 75.6
YAML 501.4	IgG2a	Q	0					
YAML 568.4	IgG2a	P	0	0				
YTH 5.3	IgG2b	P	0	0	0			
YTH 24.5	IgG2b	P	0	0	0	7		
YTH 54.12	IgG2b	Q	0	4	51	64	6	
YTH 75.6	IgG2b	P	1	3	0	8	66	10

rat monoclonal antibodies against the human leukocyte common antigen.[75] This is a family of related glycoproteins with apparent molecular weights of 170,000–220,000 present on all leukocytes but not found on other tissues.[76] We anticipate that antibodies against the leukocyte common antigen will be useful *in vivo* for immunosuppression and eradication of residual leukemic cells prior to marrow transplantion or for purging organ grafts of passenger leukocytes to reduce their immunogenicity.

Monoclonal antibodies against the human leukocyte common antigen are poorly lytic with complement (Table I), but because of its large size it should be a good target for synergistic antibodies. We isolated a series of rat monoclonal antibodies of different isotypes and by means of competitive binding assays with purified antigen defined two distinct groups that recognize different epitopes (or different sets of overlapping epitopes). All possible pairs were tested for synergistic lysis with human complement and we found that only IgG2b antibodies from different groups could cooperate significantly (Table III). The maximum lysis corresponded to about 75% of that obtained with CAMPATH-1, which was a considerable improvement on the effect of the individual antibodies alone. It remains to be seen whether further improvement can be achieved by adding more antibodies against yet other epitopes on this molecule. An optimum combination of synergistic antibodies could be better than a polyclonal antiserum, because inhibitory nonlytic antibodies could be excluded.

5.3. Monovalent Antibodies

As described earlier, one of the ways by which cells can evade complement-mediated lysis is brought about by rapid redistribution of antibody–antigen complexes on the cell surface (antigenic modulation). This process generally depends on bivalent antibody binding, and for it to occur with monoclonal antibodies it presumably requires the antigen molecules to also be at least bivalent (with respect to the relevant epitope). A good example of such

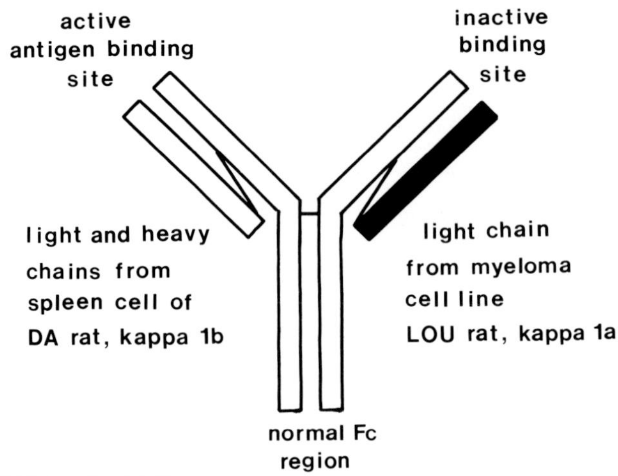

Figure 2. Diagram of monovalent antibody. The hybrid molecules were separated from bivalently active molecules by affinity chromatography using Sepharose-bound MRC OX12, which selectively binds the κ 1a allotype.[86]

an antigen is cell surface IgM present on all B cells and it has been shown that bivalent antibody is essential for antigenic modulation in this case.[23] Rabbit antibodies against surface Ig on guinea pig L_2C tumor cells were partially digested with papain. Because of the unusual asymmetric glycosylation of rabbit IgG, a single Fab fragment was removed to leave Fab/c derivatives with a single binding site and an intact Fc region. These monovalent antibodies showed no tendency to induce patching or capping and gave enhanced cell killing both *in vitro* and *in vivo*.[77]

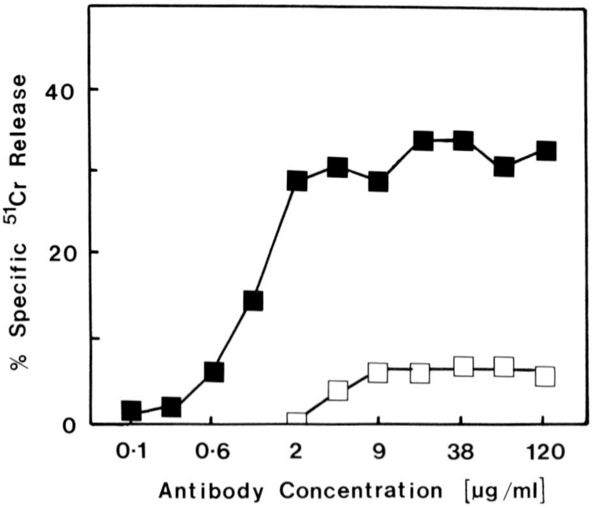

Figure 3. Improved lytic effect of monovalent antibody compared with unfractionated antibody. Human lymphocytes were labeled with ^{51}Cr and incubated with (■) monovalent YTH 12.5 or (□) unfractionated YTH 12.5, in the presence of human complement.[78] Released radioactivity was counted as a measure of cell lysis and expressed relative to that released by CAMPATH-1, which kills all lymphocytes.

Unfortunately, most monoclonal antibodies cannot be digested in the same way. In the mouse, only IgG2b yields Fab/c (Parham, this volume, Chapter 8). However, other properties of hybrid myelomas can be exploited to produce functionally monovalent antibodies in good yield.[78] Hybrids between Ig-producing cells show codominant expression of all the parental immunoglobulin chains, which can recombine more or less at random.[33,79] Many myeloma lines used for cell fusion have been selected for lack of production of Ig chains, but we have made rat–rat hybrid myelomas using the Y3. Ag1.2.3 myeloma line (LOU strain), which produces a κ light chain with the 1a allotype.[80] When fused with spleen cells from a DA rat (κ 1b allotype) all of the hybrids were found to secrete antibodies containing both types of light chains. By means of an affinity column of mouse monoclonal antibody specific for the κ 1a allotype, we were able to separate monovalent antibodies with mixed light chains from the bivalent antibodies (Fig. 2). Two IgG2b antibodies against human T cells were separated in this way and it was shown that the fraction containing monovalent antibody was unable to cause patching or capping, but did give significantly enhanced lysis compared with the unfractionated antibody (Fig. 3).

5.4. Agents That Modify the Ability of Cells to Resist Complement Lysis

So far we have focused on established ways of manipulating antibodies to increase their lytic potential, but it may also be possible to modify the cells to make them more sensitive to lysis. For example, erythrocytes from patients with paroxysmal nocturnal hemoglobinuria (PNH) are abnormally sensitive to complement lysis and this has been ascribed to a lack of the membrane protein decay-accelerating factor (DAF), the normal function of which is to accelerate the dissociation of cell-bound C3-convertase and thus inhibit the complement cascade, presumably as a protective measure against accidental complement attack. Treatment of normal erythrocytes with specific antibodies against DAF rendered them as sensitive to complement as the PNH cells.[26]

Nucleated cells also possess enzyme systems that are able to repair membrane lesions by *de novo* synthesis of lipids, and this accounts for the necessity for multiple hits by complement to obtain cell lysis.[15] Various metabolic inhibitors that interfere with lipid synthesis have been shown to enhance complement-mediated lysis,[81–84] including chemotherapeutic drugs such as adriamycin, vincristine, and azacytidine.[83] Some of these might have a role in conjunction with monoclonal antibodies for increased conditioning of patients with leukemia prior to transplantation.

6. Conclusion

During the past ninety years there have been many attempts to use antibodies for treatment of cancer and immunosuppression, but they have met with only partial success. The major problem has been the difficulty in obtaining reproducible results, because it was impossible to produce sufficiently well-defined reagents. This has been overcome since the advent of monoclonal antibody technology, but now we are faced with a new problem, that of testing and choosing among many antibody specificities. In addition, there are many ancillary technologies (conjugation of drugs, toxins, radioisotopes, etc.) whose safety and effectiveness also need to be evaluated. We choose to exploit human complement-mediated cell lysis because it offers little if any additional hazard, is easily tested *in vitro*, and involves the minimum technical difficulty. The reason it had previously been neglected is that very few monoclonal antibodies have been reported that are lytic with human complement. Perhaps it should not be surprising to find that cells have mechanisms to protect themselves against lysis. Presumably, the major role of the humoral immune system is the rapid destruction of invading microorganisms. Self cells need to be protected from the potentially damaging effects of bystander lysis and low levels of antibodies that recognize self determinants. Nevertheless, monoclonal antibodies can be found that are the optimum isotype for complement fixation and recognize suitable antigens, which do lyse cells efficiently with human complement. We have described in some detail one such antibody, CAMPATH-1, in order to show its potential application in several areas of clinical transplantation. The lytic ability of less efficient antibodies could be enhanced by several strategems.

Lysis with monoclonal antibodies and human complement appears to be an excellent method of removing unwanted cells from bone marrow for transplantation. The use *in vivo* of antibodies that fix human complement does not appear to involve any additional risk compared with non-complement-fixing antibodies, and they may be very potent for eliminating cells. It seems logical that the optimum cocktail of monoclonal antibodies for serotherapy will include reagents that interact with the whole range of physiological effector mechanisms.

Acknowledgments. We thank the Medical Research Council (U.K.) for financial support. Many colleagues contributed to the work described here, particularly T. St. J. Alderson, C. Bindon, Dr. M. R. Clark, Dr. S. P. Cobbold, J. Free, P. Lovat, and Dr. D. Swirsky, as well as the clinical teams referred to in the text.

References

1. Clark, M., Cobbold, S., Hale, G., and Waldmann, H., 1983, Advantages of rat monoclonal antibodies, *Immunol. Today* **4**:100–101.
2. Ritz, J., Sallan, S. E., Bast, R. C., Lipton, J. M., Clavell, L. A., Feeney, M., Hercend, T., Nathan, D. G., and Schlossman, S. F., 1983, Autologous bone marrow transplantation in cALLa positive acute lymphoblastic leukemia after *in vitro* treatment with J5 monoclonal antibody and complement, *Lancet* **2**:60–63.

3. Sharp, T. G., Sachs, D. H., Fauci, A. S., Messerschmidt, G. L., and Rosenberg, S. A., 1983, T cell depletion of human bone marrow using monoclonal antibody and complement mediated lysis, *Transplantation* **35:**112–120.
4. Prentice, H. G., Blacklock, H. A., Janossy, G., Gilmore, M. J. M. L., Price-Jones, L., Tidman, N., Trejdosiewicz, L. K., and Skeggs, D. B. L., Panjwani, D., Ball, S., Graphakos, S., Patterson, J., and Hoffbrand, A. V., 1984, Depletion of T lymphocytes in donor marrow prevents significant graft versus host disease in matched allogeneic leukemic marrow transplant recipients, *Lancet* **1:**472–476.
5. Jansen, J., Falkenburg, J. H. F., Stepan, D. E., and LeBien, T. W., 1984, Removal of neoplastic cells from autologous bone marrow grafts with monoclonal antibodies, *Sem. Haematol.* **21:**164–181.
6. Stepan, D. E., Bartholomew, R. M., and LeBien, T. W., 1984, *In vitro* cytodestruction of human leukemic cells using murine monoclonal antibodies and human complement, *Blood* **63:**1120–1125.
7. Borsos, T., and Rapp, H. J., 1965, Complement fixation on cell surfaces by 19S and 7S antibodies, *Science* **150:**505–506.
8. Hughes-Jones, N. C., and Ghosh, S., 1981, Anti-D-coated Rh positive red cells will bind the first component of the complement pathway, C1q, *FEBS Lett.* **128:**318–320.
9. Klaus, G. G. B., Pepys, M. B., Kitajima, K., and Askonas, B. A., 1979, Activation of mouse complement by different classes of mouse antibody, *Immunology* **38:**687–695.
10. Neuberger, M. S., and Rajewsky, K., 1981, Activation of mouse complement by monoclonal mouse antibodies, *Eur. J. Immunol.* **11:**1012–1016.
11. Oi, V. T., Vuong, T. M., Hardy, R., Reidler, J., Dangl, J., Herzenberg, L. A., and Stryer, L., 1984, Correlation between segmental flexibility and effector function of antibodies, *Nature* **307:**136–140.
12. Fust, G., Medgyesi, G. A., Bazin, H., and Gergely, J., 1980, Differences in the ability of rat IgG subclasses to consume complement in homologous and heterologous serum, *Immunol. Lett.* **1:**249–253.
13. Hughes-Jones, N. C., Gorick, B. D., and Howard, J. C., 1983, The mechanism of synergistic complement-mediated lysis of rat red cells by monoclonal IgG antibodies, *Eur. J. Immunol.* **13:**635–640.
14. Borsos, T., Rapp, H. J., and Mayer, M. M., 1961, Studies on the second component of complement. I. The reaction between EAC'1,4 and C'2: Evidence on the single site mechanism of immune hemolysis and determination of C'2 on a molecular basis, *J. Immunol.* **87:**310–325.
15. Koski, C. L., Ramm, L. E., Hammer, C. H., Mayer, M. M., and Shin, M. L., 1983, Cytolysis of nucleated cells by complement: Cell death displays multi hit characteristics, *Proc. Natl. Acad. Sci. USA* **80:**3816–3820.
16. Lerner, R. A., Oldstone, M. B., and Cooper, N. R., 1971, Cell-cycle dependent immune lysis of Moloney virus transformed lymphocytes: Presence of viral antigens, accessibility to antibody and complement activation, *Proc. Nat. Acad. Sci. USA* **68:**2584–2588.
17. Ohanian, S. H., Borsos, T., and Rapp, H. J., 1973, Lysis of tumour cells by antibody and complement 1. Lack of correlation between antigen content and lytic susceptibility, *J. Natl. Cancer Inst.* **50:**1313–1320.
18. Boyse, E. A., and Old, L. J., 1969, Some aspects of normal and abnormal cell surface genetics, *Annu. Rev. Genet.* **3:**269–291.
19. Gordon, J., Daniele, S., Robinson, F., and Stevenson, G. T., 1981, Antigenic modulation of lymphocyte surface immunoglobulin yielding resistance to complement-mediated lysis I. Characterization with syngeneic and xenogeneic complements, *Immunology* **42:**7–12.
20. Stackpole, C. W., Jacobson, J. B., and Lardis, M. P., 1974, Antigenic modulation *in vivo* I. Fate of thymus leukemia (TL) antigen–antibody complexes following modulation of TL antigenicity from the surfaces of mouse leukemia cells and thymocytes, *J. Exp. Med.* **140:**939–953.
21. Taylor, R. B., Duffus, W. P. H., Raff, M. C., and de Petris, S., 1971, Redistribution and pinocytosis of lymphocyte surface immunoglobulin molecules induced by anti-immunoglobulin antibody, *Nature* **233:**225–229.

22. Schreiner, G. F. and Unanue, E. R., 1976, Membrane and cytoplasmic changes in B lymphocytes induced by ligand–surface immunoglobulin interaction, *Adv. Immunol.* **24**:37–165.
23. Gordon, J., and Stevenson, G. T., 1981, Antigenic modulation of lymphocyte surface immunoglobulin yielding resistance to complement-mediated lysis. II. Relationship to redistribution of the antigen, *Immunology* **42**:13–17.
24. Gordon, J., Anderson, V. A., and Stevenson, G. T., 1982, Loss of surface-bound antibody accompanying the anti-complementary modulation of leukemic B cell immunoglobulin: Contrasting effects of antibodies directed against idiotypic and constant regions, *J. Immunol.* **128**:2763–2769.
25. Hansch, G. M., Hammer, C. H., Vanguri, P., and Shin, M. L., 1981, Homologous species restriction in lysis of erythrocytes by terminal complement proteins, *Proc. Natl. Acad. Sci. USA* **78**:5118–5121.
26. Pangburn, M. K., Schreiber, R. D., and Muller-Eberhard, H. J., 1983, Deficiency of an erythrocyte membrane protein with complement regulatory activity in paroxysmal nocturnal hemoglobinuria, *Proc. Natl. Acad. Sci. USA* **80**:5430–5434.
27. Okada, H., Tanaka, H., and Okada, N., 1983, Prevention of complement activation on the homologous cell membrane of nucleated cells as well as erythrocytes, *Eur. J. Immunol.* **13**:340–344.
28. Kasubowski, P. A., Terasaki, P. I., Chia, D. S., Kukes, G. D., Hardiwidjaja, S. I., and Cicciarelli, J. C., 1984, A cytotoxic monoclonal antibody to colon adenocarcinoma, *Cancer Res.* **44**:1194–1199.
29. Springer, T. A., Bhattacharya, A., Cardoza, J. T., and Sanchez-Madrid, F., 1982, Monoclonal antibodies specific for rat IgG1, IgG2a and IgG2b subclasses and kappa chain monotypic and allotypic determinants: Reagents for use with rat monoclonal antibodies, *Hybridoma* **1**:257–273.
30. Aqel, N. M., Clark, M., Cobbold, S. P., and Waldmann, H., 1984, Immunohistological screening in the selection of monoclonal antibodies: The use of isotype-specific antiglobulins, *J. Immunol. Meth.* **69**:207–214.
31. Bazin, H., Beckers, A., and Querinjean, P., 1974, Three classes and four subclasses of rat immunoglobulins: IgM, IgA, IgE, and IgG1, IgG2a, IgG2b, IgG2c, *Eur. J. Immunol.* **4**:44–48.
32. Springer, T. A., 1980, Cell surface differentiation in the mouse: Characterization of jumping and lineage specific antigens using xenogeneic rat monoclonal antibodies, in: *Monoclonal Antibodies* (R. Kennett, T. McKearn, and K. Bechtol, eds.), Plenum Press, New York, pp. 185–217.
33. Milstein, C. and Cuello, C., 1983, Hybrid myelomas and their use in immunohistochemistry, *Nature* **305**:537–540.
34. Rodt, H., Kolb, H. J., Netzel, B., Rieder, I., Janka, G., Belohradsky, B., Haas, R. J., and Thierfelder, S., 1979, GVHD suppression by incubation of bone marrow grafts with anti-T cell globulin: Effect in the canine model and application to clinical bone marrow transplantation, *Transplant. Proc.* **11**:962–966.
35. Vallera, D. A., Soderling, C. C. R., Carlson, G. J., and Kersey, J. H., 1981, Bone marrow transplantation across major histocompatibility barriers in mice. Effect of elimination of T cells from donor grafts by pretreatment with monoclonal anti-Thy-1 plus complement or antibody alone, *Transplantation* **31**:218–222.
36. Wagemaker, G., Vriesendorp, H. M., and van Bekkum, D. W., 1981, Successful bone marrow transplantation across major histocompatibility barriers in rhesus monkeys, *Transplant. Proc.* **13**:875–830.
37. Reisner, Y., Kapoor, N., Kirkpatrick, D., Pollack, M. S., Cunningham-Rundles, S., Dupont, B., Hodes, M. Z., and Good, R. A., O'Reilly, R. J., 1983, Transplantation for severe combined immunodeficiency with HLA-A,B,C,D,DR incompatible parental marrow cells fractionated by soybean agglutinin and sheep red blood cells, *Blood* **61**:341–348.
38. Filipovich, A. H., Vallera, D. A., Youle, R. J., Quinones, R. A., Neville, D. M., and Kersey, J. H., 1984, *Ex vivo* treatment of donor bone marrow with anti-T cell immunotoxins for the prevention of graft versus host disease, *Lancet* **1**:469–472.

39. Gilmore, M. J. M. L., Prentice, H. G., Price Jones, E., Blacklock, H. A., Tidman, N., Schey, S., Goldstein, G., Janossy, G., and Hoffbrand, A. V., 1983, Allogeneic bone marrow transplantation: The monitoring of granulocyte macrophage colonies following the collection of bone marrow mononuclear cells and after the subsequent *in vitro* cytolysis of OKT3 positive lymphocytes, *Br. J. Haematol.* **55:**587–593.
40. Hale, G., Bright, S., Chumbley, G., Hoang, T., Metcalf, D., Munro, A. J., and Waldmann, H., 1983, Removal of T cells from bone marrow for transplantation: A monoclonal antilymphocyte antibody that fixes human complement, *Blood* **62:**873–882.
41. Hale, G., Hoang, T., Prospero, T., Watt, S. M., and Waldmann, H., 1983, Removal of T cells from bone marrow for transplantation: Comparison of rat monoclonal anti-lymphocyte antibodies of different isotypes, *Mol. Biol. Med.* **1:**305–319.
42. Waldmann, H., Or, R., Hale, G., Weiss, L., Cividalli, G., Samuel, S., Manor, D., Brautbar, C., Polliack, A., Rachmilewitz, E. A., and Slavin, S., 1984, Elimination of graft versus host disease by *in vitro* depletion of alloreactive lymphocytes using a monoclonal rat anti-human lymphocyte antibody (CAMPATH-1), *Lancet* **2:**483–486.
43. Witherspoon, R. P., Lum, L. G., and Storb, R., 1984, Immunologic reconstitution after human marrow grafting, *Sem. Haematol.* **21:**2–10.
44. Morgan, G., Linch, D. C., Davies, E. G., Sieff, C., Chessells, J. M. C., Hale, G., Waldmann, H., and Levinsky, R. J., 1985, Successful haploidentical mismatched bone marrow transplantation in severe combined immunodeficiency: T Cell removal using CAMPATH-1 monoclonal antibody plus E rosetting, *Br. J. Haematol.*, In press.
45. Van Bekkum, D. W., 1984, Conditioning regimes for marrow grafting, *Sem. Haematol.* **21:**81–90.
46. Lafferty, K. J., Prowse, S. J., Simeonovic, C. J., and Warren, H. S., 1983, Immunobiology of tissue transplantation: A return to the passenger leucocyte concept, *Annu. Rev. Immunol.* **1:**143–174.
47. Silvers, W. K., Bartlett, S. T., Chen, H.-D., Fleming, H. L., Naji, A., and Barker, C. F., 1984, Major histocompatibility complex restriction and transplantation immunity. A possible solution to the allograft problem, *Transplantation* **37:**28–32.
48. Dicke, K. A., Jagannath, S., Spitzer, G., Poynton, C., Zander, A., Vellekoop, L., Reading, C. L., Jehn, U. W., and Tindle, S., 1984, The role of autologous bone marrow transplantation in various malignancies, *Sem. Haematol.* **21:**109–122.
49. Treleavan, J. G., Gibson, F. M., Ugelstad, J., Rembaum, A., Philip, T., Caine, G. D., and Kemshead, J. T., 1984, Removal of neuroblastoma cells from bone marrow with monoclonal antibodies conjugated to magnetic microspheres, *Lancet* **1:**70–73.
50. Hale, G., Swirsky, D., Waldmann, H., and Chan, L. C., 1984, Reactivity of rat monoclonal antibody CAMPATH-1 with human leukaemia cells and its possible application for autologous bone marrow transplantation, *Br. J. Haematol.* **60:**41–48.
51. Hale, G., Swirsky, D. M., Hayhoe, F. G. J., and Waldmann, H., 1983, Effects of monoclonal antilymphocyte antibodies *in vivo* in monkeys and humans, *Mol. Biol. Med.* **1:**321–334.
52. Zwaan, F. E., and Jansen, J., 1984, Bone marrow transplantation in acute nonlymphoblastic leukemia, *Sem. Haematol.* **21:**36–42.
53. Buckner, C. D., and Clift, R. A., 1984, Marrow transplantation for acute lymphoblastic leukemia, *Sem. Haematol.* **21:**43–47.
54. Speck, B., Gratwohl, A., Osterwalder, B., and Nissen, C., 1984, Bone marrow transplantation for chronic myeloid leukemia, *Sem. Haematol.* **21:**48–52.
55. Ritz, J., and Schlossman, S. F., 1982, Utilization of monoclonal antibodies in the treatment of leukemia and lymphoma, *Blood* **59:**1–11.
56. Cosimi, A. B., 1981, The clinical value of anti-lymphocyte globulin, *Transplant. Proc.* **13:**462–468.
57. Harkiss, G. D., Brown, D. L., Cory-Pearce, R., and English, T. A. H., 1983, Serial analysis of circulating immune complexes, complement and anti-thymocyte globulin antibodies in heart transplant patients, *J. Clin. Immunol.* **3:**117–126.
58. Calne, R. Y., 1980, Transplant surgery: Current status, *Br. J. Surg.* **67:**765–771.

59. Calne, R. Y., 1984, Paratopic segmental pancreas grafting: A technique with portal venous drainage, *Lancet* **1**:595–597.
60. Oldham, R. K., 1983, Monoclonal antibodies in cancer therapy, *J. Clin. Oncol.* **1**:582–590.
61. Levy, R., and Miller, R. A., 1983, Biological and clinical implications of lymphocyte hybridomas: Tumor therapy with monoclonal antibodies, *Annu. Rev. Med.* **34**:107–116.
62. Shield, C. F., Cosimi, A. B., Tolkoff-Rubin, N., Rubin, R. N., Herrin, J., and Russell, P. S., 1979, Use of antithymocyte globulin for reversal of acute allograft rejection, *Transplantation* **28**:461–464.
63. Cosimi, A. B., Burton, R. C., Colvin, R. B., Goldstein, G., Delmonico, F. L., LaQuaglia, M. P., Tolkoff-Rubin, N., Rubin, R. H., Herrin, J. T., and Russell, P. S., 1981, Treatment of acute renal allograft rejection with OKT3 monoclonal antibody, *Transplantation* **32**:535–539.
64. Nelson, P. W., Cosimi, A. B., Delmonico, F. L., Rubin, R. H., Tolkoff-Rubin, N. E., Fang, L., and Russell, P. S., 1983, Antithymocyte globulin as the primary treament for renal allograft rejection, *Transplantation* **36**:587–589.
65. Takahashi, H., Okazaki, H., Terasaki, P. I., Iwaki, Y., Kinukawa, T., Taguchi, Y., Chia, D., Hardiwidjaja, S., Miura, K., Ishizaki, M., and Billing, R., 1983, Reversal of transplant rejection by monoclonal antiblast antibody, *Lancet* **2**:1155–1157.
66. Dresser, D. W. and Wortis, H. H., 1965, Use of an antiglobulin serum to detect cells producing antibody with low haemolytic efficiency, *Nature* **208**:859–860.
67. Fitchen, J. H., Ruisso, C., and Ferrone, S., 1984, Complement-dependent killing of human hematopoietic progenitor cells with non complement-fixing monoclonal antibodies in an antiglobulin assay, *Blood* **63**:873–877.
68. Tanimoto, K., Cooper, N. R., Johnson, J. S., and Vaughan, J. H., 1975, Complement fixation by rheumatoid factor, *J. Clin. Invest.* **55**:437–445.
69. Carson, D. A., 1984, Increase in the complement-fixing ability of murine IgG anti-lymphocyte antibodies by addition of monoclonal IgM rheumatoid factors, *J. Immunol. Meth.* **68**:103–108.
70. Lanier, L. L., Gutman, G. A., Lewis, D. E., Griswold, S. T., and Warner, N. L., 1982, Monoclonal antibodies against rat immunoglobulin kappa chains, *Hybridoma* **1**:125–131.
71. Langone, J. J., 1982, Enhancing effect of concanavalin A on the hemolytic effect of anti-Forssman IgG: The role of C1, *J. Immunol.* **129**:1159–1164.
72. Langone, J. J., Boyle, M. D. P., and Borsos, T., 1984, Studies on the interaction between protein A and immunoglobulin G. 1. Effect of protein A on the functional activity of IgG, *J. Immunol.* **131**:327–332.
73. Elliot, E. V., Pinder, A., Stevenson, F. K., and Stevenson, G. T., 1978, Synergistic cytotoxic effects of antibodies directed against different cell surface determinants, *Immunology* **34**:405–409.
74. Howard, J. C., Butcher, J. W., Galfre, G., Milstein, C., and Milstein, C. P., 1979, Monoclonal antibodies as tools to analyse the serological and genetic complexities of major transplantation antigens, *Immunol. Rev.* **47**:139–175.
75. Bindon, C. I., Hale, G., Clark, M., and Waldmann, H., 1985, Therapeutic potential of monoclonal antibodies to the leucocyte common antigen: Synergy and interference in complement-mediated lysis, *J. Immunol.,* In press.
76. Dalchau, R., Kirkley, J., and Fabre, J. W., 1980, Monoclonal antibody to a human leukocyte specific membrane glycoprotein probably homologous to the leukocyte common antigen of the rat, *Eur. J. Immunol.* **10**:737–744.
77. Glennie, M. J., and Stevenson, G. T., 1982, Univalent antibodies kill tumour cells *in vitro* and *in vivo, Nature* **295**:712–714.
78. Cobbold, S. P., and Waldmann, H., 1984, Therapeutic potential of monovalent monoclonal antibodies, *Nature* **308**:460–462.
79. Cotton, R. G. H., and Milstein, C., 1973, Fusion of two immunoglobulin-producing myeloma cells, *Nature* **244**:42–43.
80. Galfre, G., Milstein, C., and Wright, B., 1979, Rat × rat hybrid myelomas and a monoclonal anti-Fd portion of mouse IgG, *Nature* **277**:131–133.

81. Schlager, S. I., Ohanian, S. H., and Borsos, T., 1978, Correlation between the ability of tumor cells to resist humoral immune attack and their ability to synthesize lipid, *J. Immunol.* **120:**463–471.
82. Schlager, S. I., 1982, Relationship between cell-mediated and humoural immune attack on tumour cells II. The role of cellular lipid metabolism and cell surface charge in the outcome of immune attack, *Cell. Immunol.* **66:**300–316.
83. Segerling, M., Ohanian, S. H., and Borsos, T., 1975, Chemotherapeutic drugs increase killing of tumor cells by antibody and complement, *Science* **188:**55–56.
84. Hansch, G. M., Betz, M., and Shin, M., 1984, Cytolysis of nucleated cells by complement. Inhibition of membrane transmethylation enhances cell death by C5b-9, *J. Immunol.* **132:**1440–1444.
85. Waldmann, H., Cobbold, S., Wilson, A., Clark, M., Watt, S., Hale, G., and Tighe, H., 1985, Rat monoclonal antibodies for bone marrow transplantation—The CAMPATH series, in: *Microenvironments in the Lymphoid System,* (G. G. B. Klaus, ed.), Plenum Press, New York, pp. 869–878.
86. Hunt, S. V., and Fowler, M. H., 1981, A repopulation assay for B and T lymphocyte stem cells employing radiation chimaeras, *Cell Tiss. Kinet.* **14:**445–464.

Chapter 30

Manipulation of T-Cell Populations to Abrogate Allograft Rejection

CHARLES B. CARPENTER

1. Introduction

Selective intervention in the afferent or efferent arcs of the immune response *in vivo* has become a possibility because specific subsets of interacting cells can be identified by monoclonal antibodies directed to surface molecules that relate to specific functions. A subset of cells thus identified can be targeted for destruction, either by opsonization and/or complement-mediated lysis, or by internalization of toxins that have been conjugated to the antibody molecules. Other possibilities relate to the inhibition by specific monoclonal antibodies of cell surface receptors or interaction sites without actually destroying the cell, or to the neutralization of secreted molecules [e.g., interleukin 2 (IL-2) or interferon gamma (IFN-γ)].

Before embarking upon selective immune intervention in humans, however, it has been necessary to evaluate some of the fundamental properties of xenogeneic monoclonal immunoglobulin molecules in clinical situations, using those that offer some benefit to patients. The organ transplant recipient is often in need of increased immunosuppressive therapy in order to overcome a cell-mediated rejection reaction that threatens survival of the organ. These rejection episodes in patients receiving baseline therapy with azathioprine plus prednisone, or cyclosporine plus prednisone, are generally treated with short courses of glucocorticoid hormones in high doses or by the globulin fractions of xenogeneic antilymphocyte sera. Monoclonal versions of the latter, in the form of anti-T-cell monoclonals reactive with all T lymphocytes, have been subjected to *in vivo* trial in the setting of an acute rejection episode, and are the principal subject of this chapter. Before discussing therapeutic trials, major features of the human allotransplant rejection response need review.

2. The Nature of Allograft Rejection

Since the kidney has been transplanted and studied most extensively, most data on the nature of the rejection process derive from renal transplantations,

CHARLES B. CARPENTER • Brigham and Women's Hospital, Harvard Medical School, Boston, Massachusetts 02115.

although in experimental animal models the lesions in rejecting cardiac grafts are similar. The patterns of rejection found in human renal allografts are varied, but all are similar to those produced in various animal models. Differences between humans and the inbred rat model of renal transplantation, for example, are more in the time or sequence of appearance of various lesions than in their character. Differences are due to the influence of various modifying factors, especially those of immunosuppressive therapy and of chronic uremia, itself an immunodepressant. Also, virtually all recipients have been primed allogeneically by blood transfusions.

Various pathological and clinical patterns characterize the rejected allograft. The classic form of rejection is called cellular rejection—microscopically showing cellular infiltration of the renal parenchyma.[1,2] Within a few hours after transplantation, a few small lymphocytes are found in contact with the endothelial cells lining the peritubular capillaries and venules in the cortex and outer medulla. Between 2 and 3 days later larger cells with abundant basophilic cytoplasm begin to appear. These are predominantly activated T (thymic-dependent) lymphocytes, while a few of the host cells entering the kidneys are macrophages. The infiltrating cells lie close to the endothelial cells lining the small intertubular capillaries and venules, and there is evidence of reactive changes in the endothelial cells and focal injury to the vessels. At first, the cellular infiltration is focal, but later the cells are distributed diffusely in the interstitium. Another group of cells entering the kidney are part of the plasma cell series and originate from B (bone marrow-derived) lymphocytes. The progressive disruption of peritubular capillaries and venules, together with the accumulation of large quantities of fluid and cells in the interstitium, produces a fall in total renal blood flow.

Allografts transplanted into presensitized recipients may be rejected quickly. Such an immediate failure is commonly termed *hyperacute rejection*. About 80% of patients who have preformed cytotoxic antibodies in their sera to the donor's lymphocytes reject allografts immediately after transplantation. Early biopsies of hyperacutely rejecting allogeneic kidneys show a linear localization of IgG and C3 on the glomerular and peritubular capillary walls,[3,4] and ultrastructurally there are platelet aggregates in many of the capillary lumena. Soon polymorphonuclear leukocytes line the capillary walls and most of the intrarenal capillaries and arterioles are blocked by microthrombi, with ensuing cortical necrosis.

Months or years after human transplantation, function may gradually deteriorate without there being any clear-cut rejection episode. Kidneys undergoing *chronic rejection* show severe narrowing of arteries and thickening of the glomerular capillary basement membrane. The arterial narrowing is most common in the interlobular and arcuate vessels (with a thickened intima and ruptured internal elastic lamina), but the endothelial lining remains intact. Serial biopsies of chronically rejecting kidneys have shown derivation of these lesions from continual or intermittent formation of platelet and fibrin aggregates on the vessel wall.[4,5] The mural deposits become covered by endothelium and

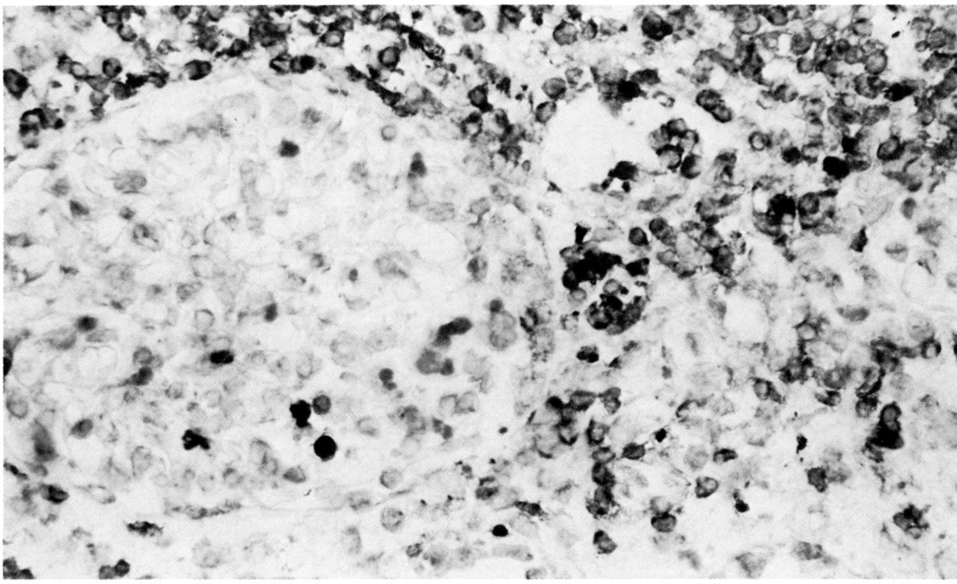

Figure 1. Renal allograft biopsy showing cellular infiltration. The immunoperoxidase technique has been employed to identify cells bearing the T11 pan-T-cell marker. Positive cells, stained darkly on their surfaces, constitute the majority of infiltrating cells in the interstitial areas. The glomerulus on the left has only a few darkly stained neutrophils. The latter are nonspecifically positive because of endogenous peroxidase, and these can be discerned in the controls incubated without anti-T11. (Photograph courtesy of Gwen Mazoujian, by permission from Ref. 26.)

incorporated into the intima, which often contains IgM and complement, emphasizing the role of the humoral system in this form of rejection.

2.1. Acute Cellular Rejection

Tritiated-thymidine labeling studies have suggested that the large lymphoid cells with pyroninophilic cytoplasm that appear in the lymphoid tissues probably give rise to clones of immunologically committed cells, which migrate into the circulation and reach the graft. Even after reaching the peritubular capillaries, some of the lymphoid cells undergo division. An average of 4% of the infiltrating cells lying in a renal allograft 4 days after transplantation incorporate tritiated thymidine within 30 min of the injection of the isotope into the renal artery, indicating that these cells are actively synthesizing DNA and presumably can and will divide.[6] Although a variety of mononuclear cell types are present in the rejection lesion,[7,8] there is some evidence that rejection of solid tissue allografts is, in fact, initiated by T lymphocytes.[9,10] Labeled T lymphocytes have been shown to accumulate in graft infiltrates and have been shown to be present in such tissue sections when stained with anti-T cell antibodies[11,12] (Fig. 1).

2.2. Cytotoxic Cells

Since T cells sensitized *in vitro* or *in vivo* produce target cell injury when confronted with cells bearing the antigens of the immunizing donor,[13] it has been assumed that this is the primary mode of graft injury. Indeed, cytolytically active cells (CTLs) have been recovered from graft infiltrates[14,15] and in a model system in which infiltrating cells are extracted from sponges implanted in allogeneic hosts.[16] Although "killer" cell activity can be attributed to T cells in the early-rejecting rat allograft infiltrate, they are not the only cell type with cytolytic activity. The cell types known to have cytotoxic potential are listed in Table I. Although the classic CTL is a T lymphocyte directed to class I antigens on donor target cells, some cytotoxic T lymphocytes (T_C) are directed to class II antigens. T-Cell-mediated cytotoxicity is clonally determined, i.e., each T cell has receptors for a single antigenic determinant and is therefore exquisitely specific in the same way that each antibody molecule is precisely targeted to its antigenic determinant. Antibodies may result in graft injury by fixation of Clq and activation of the complement cascade, or may induce the second major type of cell-mediated cytotoxicity, called antibody-dependent, cell-mediated cytotoxicity (ADCC). This reaction is mediated by a variety of cell types, all of which must have surface receptors for the Fc portion of IgG. These cells, having no specificity themselves for the antigen, effect injury to target cells by mechanisms similar to that of the T_C when lymphocytes are involved, or by lysosomal enzymes and other toxins in the case of polymorphs and activated macrophages. Evidence of a common mode of cell-mediated injury by T cells comes from the fact that activated T cells, while bearing clonally determined antigen receptors, also express F_C receptors and can be cytotoxic via the ADCC mechanism to a totally different target cell, as long as the latter is coated with IgG. The role of natural killer (NK) cells in graft rejection is unclear, but they are present in the inflammatory response found in rejection.[17] They have no specificity to donor target histocompatibility antigens, but react with determinants present on immature and neoplastic cells. Since cell surface expression of donor histocompatibility antigens (and possibly other molecules) is increased by host release of IFN-γ[18] during rejection activity, NK cells might injure donor endothelium via a target molecule not expressed on normal cells. There is new evidence that noncytotoxic T helper cells, the type that mediate delayed-type hypersensitivity (DTH) to antigens such as tuberculin, can, under some circumstances, provide the principal effector mechanism for graft rejection.[19,20] In such cases, the mediators of injury may include secreted lymphokines and recruitment and activation of macrophages. Experimental studies illustrate, therefore, a variety of potential mechanisms at play in the rejection process.

2.3. Human Studies

The infiltrating cells from rejecting human renal allografts have been studied in a limited number of cases. Donor-specific CTLs are demonstrable in the

Table I. Varieties of Cytotoxic Killer Cells[a]

	Cytotoxic T lymphocytes (CTL)		Antibody-dependent, cell-mediated cytotoxic cells (ADCC)	Natural killers (NK)
Cell type	Lymphocytes	Lymphocytes	B and "null" lymphocytes, large granular lymphocytes, polymorphs, macrophages, activated T cells	Large granular lymphocytes
Phenotype	T4	T8	F_C Receptor	F_C Receptor
Clonal	Yes	Yes	No	No
Specificity	Fine, usually to class II HLA	Fine, usually to class I HLA	Via IgG	Neoplasms, thymocytes, fetal fibroblasts, bone marrow
Restricted by HLA	Yes	Yes	No	No

[a] From Ref. 26 by permission.

population of monodisperse lymphoid cells prepared from rejecting renal tissue. The degree of this activity correlates with the intensity of cellular rejection as scored by the pathologist.[14] These grafts differ from those in the animal model because they represent clinical failures in drug-modified recipients who have undergone one or more rejection episodes prior to the decision to remove the nonfunctioning graft. In all cases, the degree of lysis produced by graft cells exceeds that produced by peripheral blood cells. In states of chronic allostimulation, cellular effector mechanisms of a non-T cell type exist; perhaps they are examples of NK-like activity.

Detailed studies by Busch and co-workers[8,21] on the cytological profiles of the interstitial infiltrates present in 24 rejected and excised human renal allografts have been correlated with the surface marker and functional studies performed in parallel. Four patterns of human rejection have emerged from these studies employing tissue sections and surface markers on monodisperse cell suspensions. In all of these the density of cellular infiltration was the same.

Type 1: Marked *humoral rejection* with arteritis having deposits of IgG and/or IgM. Cellular infiltrate is mostly with Ig-positive lymphocytes. Donor-specific CTL activity is low. The possibility of a secondary cellular mechanism (ADCC) exists.

Type 2B: Mixed B- and T-cell proportions with variable degrees of arteritis. CTL activity is highest in this group.

Type 3: Highest proportion of plasma cells and T cells, low CTL reactivity, and chronic obliterative vasculitis.

Type 2A: Low numbers of plasma cells and Ig-positive cells, moderate numbers of T cells and macrophages, leaving 15–35% "null" cells.

These subdivisions reflect, of course, only the spectrum of cellular patterns seen, but they show clearly that there is no single cell type that predominates in all rejections. None of these findings could be directly related to known histocompatibility factors nor to doses of immunosuppressive therapy used. It should be emphasized that these grafts were all unsuccessful; namely, they were removed because of function too poor to sustain life. The patterns seen, therefore, represent the host's successful circumvention of clinical immunosuppression. Monoclonal antibodies derived from mice immunized to human lymphocytes are useful for the immunohistologic identification of various functional subsets of cells in biopsies of allografts.[17,22] The techniques are generally those of indirect immunofluorescence, or of localization of peroxidase bound to second or third antibodies in sandwich techniques. The varieties of specific monoclonal antibodies available are reviewed in a subsequent section. Figure 1 shows an example of immunoperoxidase staining of infiltrating T cells in a rejecting renal allograft. Careful quantitation of T-cell and B-cell subsets is possible, although the overall anatomic pattern of infiltration discerned is the most consistent finding in studies so far. The typical rejecting lesion shows predominance of T helper (T_H) cells in discrete clusters of infiltrating cells, while T cytotoxic/suppressor cells predominate in peritubular areas when infiltrates are diffuse.[22] NK cells, marked by a specific monoclonal antibody, are also present. As monoclonal antibodies specific for precise functional programs of T helper and T cytotoxic/suppressor subsets become available, more useful data on a variety of cellular rejecting lesions will be forthcoming.

3. Monoclonal Anti-T-Cell Antibodies

A number of epitopes on molecules characteristic of some or all T lymphocytes can be defined by monoclonal antibodies. Phenotypically stable functional T-cell subsets exist, and states of differentiation from immature thymocyte to mature peripheral T cell can be defined. During maturation in the thymus, T cells diverge into two major subsets, generally having helper/inducer or suppressor functions, respectively.[23–25] Table II shows the major T-cell structures so far defined and their expression at various states of differentiation. The T4 and T5/T8 are not coexpressed on mature cells, and are the major markers distinguishing the two major subsets. The paradigm of the immune response begins with helper (inducer) T4-positive cells interacting in a clonally determined manner with nominal antigen presented concurrently with self class II molecule on macrophages and dendritic cells. Allogeneic class II (HLA-D/DR in man) is perceived as modified self and provides the basis for the mixed lymphocyte reaction (MLR).[26] Lymphocytes bearing the T8 (T5) antigen recognize nominal antigen presented concurrently with self class I molecules (HLA-A, B, C) and, following delivery of interleukin-2 (IL-2) and other helper signals secreted from T4-positive cells, proliferate and differentiate into T8-positive cytotoxic cells. Allogeneic class I molecules provide antigenic stimuli directly, since they are perceived as modified self. The dichotomy of the preference of T4-positive cells for class II and of T8-positive cells for class I targets has been confirmed by the fact that when cytotoxic cells are found against class II antigens, they are of the T4-positive phenotype, although a few clones have been described that do not fit this functional dichotomy. It is postulated that T4 and T8 represent nonpolymorphic receptors for HLA molecules of class II and class I, respectively.[27] Suppressor T cells are of the T8 phenotype, even though they behave as if primed to class II-related antigens; hence, T8-positive cells include both cytotoxic and suppressor subsets. The T4-positive population is also heterogeneous, containing separate inducer subsets for suppression and help. Sera of patients with active juvenile rheumatoid arthritis (JRA) contain anti-T-cell antibodies reactive with 40% of the T4-positive inducer population. The T4-positive, JRA-positive subset provides the help necessary for activation of T8-positive cells to become suppressor effector cells, while the T4-positive, JRA-negative cell subset is the major population responding to soluble antigens.[28]

Several "second generation" monoclonal antibodies are now being defined. In general, these antibodies cut across several cell types, but overlap in differing patterns. For example, TQ1 is present on 70–85% of T4-positive and 50% of T8-positive lymphocytes. It is absent on macrophages, but is present on a fraction of normal B and null cells, and on non-T-lymphoblastoid cell lines.[29] The T4-positive, JRA-positive cells are included within the T4-positive,

Table II. Monoclonal Antibodies to Human T-Cell Surface Antigens[a]

Monoclonal antibody	Specificity	Approximate molecular weight of antigen (reduced), kD	Cell surface expression (reactivity with antibodies)		
			Thymocytes[b]	Peripheral T cells	Non-T cells
Anti-T1	Total peripheral T	69	M	All	0
Anti-T3	Total peripheral T	19	M	All	0
Anti-T4	Helper/inducer	62	C, M	60%	0
Anti-T5	Suppressor	30 + 32	C, M	25%	0
Anti-T8	Suppressor	30 + 32	C, M	30%	0
Anti-T6[c]	Thymic antigen, TL-like	49	C	None	0
Anti-T9[d]	Transferrin receptor	94	I	None	0
Anti-T10[d]	Thymic antigen	45	I, C, M	5%	10%
Anti-T11	E Rosette receptor	50	I, C, M	All	≤10%
Anti-T12	Mature intravascular T	120	M	All	0
Anti-TQ1	(70–85%: T4; 50%: T8)	80	M (<2%)	60%	<10%
Anti-9.3	(100%: T4; 50%: T8)	44	C, M	60–80%	0
Anti-3A.1	(70%: T4; 100%: T8)	40	I, C, M	85%	0

[a] From Ref. 26 by permission.
[b] Ten percent of thymocytes are immature (I); 80% are intermediate or common (C); 10% are mature (M), i.e., similar to peripheral cells.
[c] T6 is β_2-microglobulin-associated.
[d] T9 and T10 antigens are not T-lineage-specific and are found on normal and malignant populations of non-T cells. In addition, both antigens are expressed on a fraction of peripheral T cells following mitogen stimulation.

TQ1-positive subset, while the major portion of helper activity for immunoglobulin production is found in the 15–30% of T4-positive, TQ1-negative cells. Another monoclonal of recent interest is called 9.3,[25] and this reacts with nearly all T4-positive cells and approximately 50% of T8-positive cells. Within the T8-positive population 9.3 marks the cytotoxic, but not the suppressor cell precursors.[30] After expansion and differentiation of cytotoxic clones in MLR, cytotoxic effector cells are much less susceptible to lysis by 9.3 antibody and complement; hence, this monoclonal antibody may not prove useful in distinguishing mature cytotoxic and suppressor cells.

Additional monoclonal antibodies to T-cell surface structures that represent states of activation (e.g., class II, IL-2 receptors, Ta-1, and others)[31–36] are of increasing interest, not only as markers to dissect the kinetics of the immune response, but also as potential therapeutic agents in the selective elimination of activated clones.

3.1. Selection of a Monoclonal Antibody as Therapy for Acute Rejection

Given the heterogeneity of human rejection patterns and the current uncertainty of how best to approach selective immune alteration in individual patients,[26] initial clinical trials with monoclonal antibodies have involved use of pan-T-cell antibodies in the setting of acute cellular rejection episodes. The end point of reversal is generally clear-cut, and although the target cells may include suppressor as well as effector T cells, reversal of the acute episode can be accomplished by monoclonal antibodies directed to sites on mature functional T cells. The results, as reviewed below, indicate that T cells are the important effectors in most cases of acute renal allograft rejection.

Since each monoclonal antibody is a unique molecule, molecular size, binding site affinity, and complement-fixing ability all may be important factors in *in vivo* efficacy. For example, IgM is more than five times larger than IgG and around 80% of a dose is restricted to the intravascular space after intravenous administration. In contrast, more than half of infused IgG equilibrates into extravascular spaces.[37] Also, five times as much IgM by weight is needed to provide a molar equivalent to IgG. The IgM molecules are almost always effective complement-fixers and promote opsonization into phagocytic cells and the reticuloendothelial system very efficiently. IgG subclasses vary in their complement-fixing and opsonizing ability, with IgG1 antibodies sometimes being poor complement-fixers. If they have not been aggregated in the process of preparation, xenogeneic plasma proteins generally behave physiologically. Once a host makes an immune response to the foreign protein, however, rapid immune elimination occurs. During this phase, the possibility of a serum sickness-like reaction exists. Since studies on immunoglobulin distribution and catabolism have been conducted with labeled polyclonal mixtures, it is possible that a few individual monoclonals could show aberrant behavior because of the nature of their Fab or Fc portions.

In interrupting the process of T-cell-mediated graft rejection it has been assumed that the target cells need to be cleared from the graft and eliminated. Antibodies that fix complement and promote phagocytosis have therefore been employed. On the other hand, if one plans to block a specific cell receptor or to neutralize a secreted product (e.g., IL-2), it might be optimal to avoid complement activation. In any case, high affinity is of importance, particularly if one wants to use as low a dose as possible and attain maximum specificity. To some extent, *in vivo* effects can be anticipated by *in vitro* study of the interaction between a given monoclonal antibody and a cell type. The most important phenomenon in this regard is termed modulation; that is, the removal of antibody-complexed antigen from the cell surface. The T-cell antigens T1 and T3 behave similarly, with rapid independent capping *in vitro* of these molecules upon several minutes of incubation at 37°C with the respective antibodies. Reexpression of T1 and T3 commences promptly when the antibodies are removed and synthesis of new molecules continues.[38,39] In contrast, modulation of T4, T8, T11, and T12 occurs to a limited degree or not at all. The significance of modulation lies in its potential to circumvent cell clearance and destruction. The next question to ask is whether modulation is related to any further effects upon the function of the targeted cells. In the case of T3, it is. Incubation of mature T cells with anti-T3 produces a vigorous polyclonal mitogenic response *in vitro*, an effect related to the close association of the invariant T3 molecule to the polymorphic 49K, 43K heterodimer that is the T-cell receptor for antigen.[38,40] Hence, anti-T3 has the potential, not only of blockading antigen receptors, but of nonspecifically activating all mature T cells, with an intense outpouring of helper factors, suppressor factors, interleukins, and interferons. In contrast, the other T-cell monoclonals are not mitogenic. If the object is to eliminate cell types by complement-mediated lysis, or by opsonization through the reticuloendothelial system, a stable nonmodulating molecule, such as T12, offers a better target than T3.

When monoclonal antibodies are infused into the vascular space they will, of course, bind to antigens and antigen-bearing cells of the blood. Depending upon the degree to which an antibody molecule equilibrates into extravascular spaces, other cells and tissues will be exposed to the antibody. In the case of the lymphocyte, 95% of total body cells are extravascular at any one moment, yet the considerable volume of recirculation of lymphocytes from lymphatic channels (e.g., thoracic duct) to blood brings large numbers of lymphocytes to the intravascular compartment, where they can be intercepted by antibody. Hence, the accessibility to the targeted cells depends both upon the extravascular penetration of a given monoclonal antibody and the degree of influx of cells into the blood compartment. Additional considerations in a rejecting kidney include the extent to which inflammation permits greater extravascular diffusion and the counterbalancing effect of reduced blood flow to the organ. At present these factors are mostly deduced from experience in clinical trials, since methods for direct sampling and study of lymphocyte pool sizes in man are limited. In general, successful protocols have employed both IgG and IgM antibodies, providing daily intravenous doses, which maintain continuous levels of monoclonal antibodies in blood.

Finally, the distribution of the target antigen on tissues other than peripheral lymphoid populations is of potential concern. For example, antibodies such as anti-T11 would have potential for destruction of immature thymic stem cells and could in theory establish a long-lasting immunologic defect. Similarly, antibodies such as CBL1,[41] directed to activated T cells and B cells, but also to normal monocytes and bone marrow stem cells, have potential for producing bone marrow suppression.

3.2. Testing in Primates

Mouse monoclonal antibodies to human lymphocyte subsets cross-react extensively with subhuman primate lymphocytes. Cosimi *et al.*[42] first reported that OKT4 (anti-T4) given to cynomolgus monkeys could prolong kidney graft survival. In ten recipients given sufficient antibody (0.5–1.0 mg/kg per day) intravenously, T4 cells were cleared from the circulation and free circulating levels of OKT4 could be obtained. Allograft survival was extended to as long as 7 weeks after a 1- to 2-week course of therapy. Jonker *et al.*[43] used a rhesus monkey skin graft model to assess the immunosuppressive effects of OKT4 and OKT4A given daily in doses of 4–5 mg to animals weighing 2–4 kg. These antibodies administered separately or together prolonged skin graft survival beyond the 8.5- to 13-day control range, up to 19 days. When OKT4 and OKT4A were administered separately, T4 cells were not at all eliminated from the circulation; rather, the antibody-coated cells continued to circulate. When both monoclonals were given to the same recipient there was rapid disappearance of circulating T4 cells; however, skin graft survival was not further improved. These authors showed that OKT4 and OKT4A had the same titers against rhesus cells as human cells, as measured by fluorescence intensity of stained cells; hence, difficulty in clearance of rhesus cells *in vivo* would not appear to be related to weak cross-reactivity. OKT8A cross-reacts rather weakly with rhesus lymphocytes, yet when 5 mg of OKT8A was given intravenously to two monkeys on a daily basis there was slow elimination of T8 cells from the blood over a 4- to 5-day period. Skin graft rejection times were not altered, however.[43]

OKT11A, directed to the E rosette receptor on all T cells, demonstrated apparent *in vivo* modulation of T11 from circulating cells during the first week of administration in the rhesus skin graft model.[43] This was surmised because the percentages of T4 and T8 cells did not change. However, there were up to 30% mouse globulin-coated cells in the circulation, and in the cynomolgous monkey model, Giorgi *et al.*[44] found that the initial disappearance of T11 cells with maintenance of T4 and T8 positivity could be accounted for by coating of sites by the OKT11A monoclonal antibody. As noted above, anti-T11 does not modulate human cells *in vitro*. In neither monkey study was there a demonstration of prolonged allograft survival with administration of OKT11A. Bieber *et al.*[45] have reported some effect of two E-rosette blocking monoclonal antibodies in the rhesus skin graft model. Further comparison with OKT11A cannot be made at this time.

It is likely that careful study in subhuman primate models will continue to provide valuable information on monoclonals of potential interest for human trials, although some caution is needed in interpretation of cellular clearance patterns, since subtle differences in complement fixation or interaction with phagocytic cells may exist among primate species.

4. Pan-T-Cell Monoclonal Antibodies in Renal Transplantation

4.1. OKT3

Cosimi *et al.*[46,47] provided the initial evaluation of OKT3 (anti-T3) therapy in eight cadaver graft recipients receiving baseline treatment with azathioprine and prednisone. All of these patients received cadaver allografts and had biopsy-proven evidence for an acute rejection episode 6–16 days after transplantation. After some initial variation in dose, the protocol evolved to administration of 5 mg of OKT3 intravenously daily for 14 to 29 days with concomitant reduction in both azathioprine and prednisone doses to 0.4 mg/kg during monoclonal therapy. There was rapid and complete clearance of all detectable OKT3 cells within minutes of infusion, and this persisted for the duration of therapy. All patients developed chills and spiking fevers within an hour of the first infusion, sometimes accompanied by dyspnea and wheezes. In all eight patients there was reversal of rejection activity, even in the first four patients receiving a 1–2 mg/day dose of OKT3, an amount that barely produced free plasma antibody levels. The higher dose (5 mg) was adopted in the second group to see if the recurrent rejection episodes occurring after cessation of OKT3 could be prevented. In this initial trial, the four patients with the higher dose did indeed show more stable courses, and three of them were not subjected to the need for additional rejection therapy. During an overall followup period of 12–18 months seven of the eight patients experienced further rejection episodes, and three of these were irreversible with conventional therapy.

Analysis of T-cell-subset alterations in the peripheral blood of the OKT3-treated patients[48] showed that the initial lymphopenia was maintained with virtually no T3 cells in the blood until 2–3 days after therapy was discontinued; however T4, T8, and T11A cells were present at around one-third of the normal concentrations after 3–4 days, and this number rose further after 5–7 days. When these cells were cultured *in vitro*, reactivity with OKT3 was restored, indicating that modulation of T3 by the antibody occurs *in vivo*.

A multicenter randomized trial of OKT3 therapy in reversing acute rejection episodes is in progress. Virtually all rejections are reversed by OKT3, but a large percentage of patients will experience subsequent rejections; hence, the combined effect of this monoclonal antibody, which activates T cells in a polyclonal fashion while blocking and modulating T-cell antigen receptors, is to stop all immediate injury to the graft, but it does not establish a state of sustained unresponsiveness. Another trial of OKT3 as the sole daily therapy for 31 days, starting on the day of transplantation,[49] has confirmed the *in vivo* modulating effects of this monoclonal antibody, as well as a high incidence of severe rejection activity after therapy was stopped.

4.2. Anti-T12

From a series of monoclonal anti-T-cell antibodies prepared and characterized by Reinherz, Schlossman, and co-workers,[23,38] an IgM antibody directed to the 120-kD T12 molecule was selected for trial. T12 is limited in expression to mature, immunologically active T lymphocytes, and interaction with anti-T12 does not result in rapid modulation of the antigen-bearing molecule;[38] hence, interaction with IgM anti-T12 should result in a stable target for complement-mediated lysis or opsonization of the cells. Further, since interaction with anti-T12 does not result in mitogenic stimulation of T cells *in vitro*, anti-T12 *in vivo* would not be expected to produce nonspecific immune effects, because of generalized activation of T cells. The initial trial involved either cadaver or living related donor renal allografts. They had clinical and biopsy evidence of an acute rejection episode occurring within 3 months of transplantation. Clinical signs included fever, graft enlargement, and/or tenderness and decreased renal function.[50,51] Percutaneous needle biopsies were quickly processed to confirm the presence of significant degrees of cellular rejection, marked by infiltration of mononuclear cells. In all cases, patients would otherwise have received a steroid pulse consisting of methylprednisolone, 1 g intravenously daily for 3 days. Baseline immunosuppression with oral prednisone and either azathioprine or cyclosporine was decreased slightly or not altered during anti-T12 treatment. Patients received an antibody dose of 200 μg/kg daily over a 2- to 4-hour period, with adjustments to maintain a predose free antibody titer of 1:2–1:4, as determined by reaction of the patients' sera with normal reference lymphocytes.

There were no discernible febrile or systemic reactions to the infusions, although seven patients were initially febrile as part of their rejection episodes. One patient developed fever, low back pain, and a transient rash on day 8 of therapy, and was subsequently shown to have developed anti-mouse antibodies at that time.

There were three general patterns of response. Seven patients had prompt and complete resolution of their rejection episodes without additional therapy (Fig. 2). All patients in this group have maintained functioning grafts over a followup period of over 1 year. Only one of these seven patients required treatment for subsequent acute rejections. Four patients had equivocal responses, with no improvement in the serum creatinine after 5 days of therapy, and according to protocol, anti-T12 was discontinued. Following additional antirejection therapies with steroids and/or plasmapheresis, these four patients

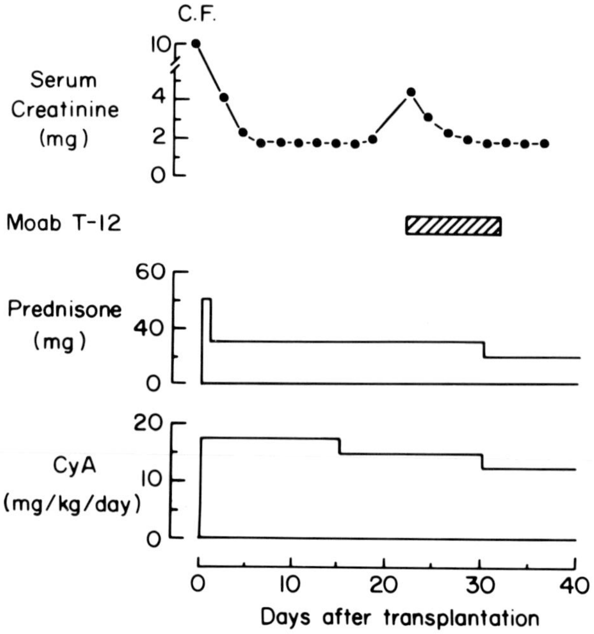

Figure 2. Reversal of acute renal allograft rejection with anti-T12 administered intravenously for 10 days. The initial fall in serum creatinine to a level of 1.9 mg/dl indicated the initial achievement of normal renal function in this patient treated with cyclosporine and prednisone. Twenty-two days after transplantation, graft tenderness and a reduced urine output heralded an acute rejection episode, which was confirmed by biopsy and a rise in serum creatinine. The addition of anti-T12 effected complete reversal. (From Ref. 51 by permission.)

attained functioning kidneys. It is difficult to assess the relative roles of acute tubular necrosis and nephrotoxicity from cyclosporine in this group, and interpretation of the effects of anti-T12 is uncertain. It is noteworthy that complete clearing of the cellular infiltration in one anuric kidney occurred without concomitant diuresis and return of renal function until 2 weeks later. Eight patients failed to respond to treatment with anti-T12. Five of these are considered true failures. Of the other three, the first patient treated was given only 100 μg/kg doses and did not attain free serum antibody levels. Another withdrew from the protocol after four doses, and a third patient had already been subjected to severe unremitting rejection, and was unresponsive to steroid pulses, antithymocyte globulin, and plasmapheresis. Four of the five anti-T12 failures had, in addition to cellular infiltration on biopsy, moderate to severe signs of humoral vasculitis, and subsequently lost their grafts. Rapid clearance of T lymphocytes occurred following the first anti-T12 infusion. Thereafter, a steady rise occurred over a 2- to 4-day period in T3-positive, T12-negative cells and T lymphopenia no longer existed. The distribution between T4 helper/inducer and T8 suppressor cells was generally reestablished to pretreatment levels. Figure 3 illustrates this phenomenon for a patient showing normal percentages of T3-, T4-, and T8-positive cells but no T12-positive cells, a pattern that persisted as long as anti-T12 was continued, with prompt reemergence of T12-positive cells thereafter. Since the T12-negative T cells were shown to be negative for mouse globulin as well, the possibility that T12 had been modulated *in vivo* by interaction with antibody was considered, even though modulation cannot be induced *in vitro*. When cells from anti-T12-treated patients are cul-

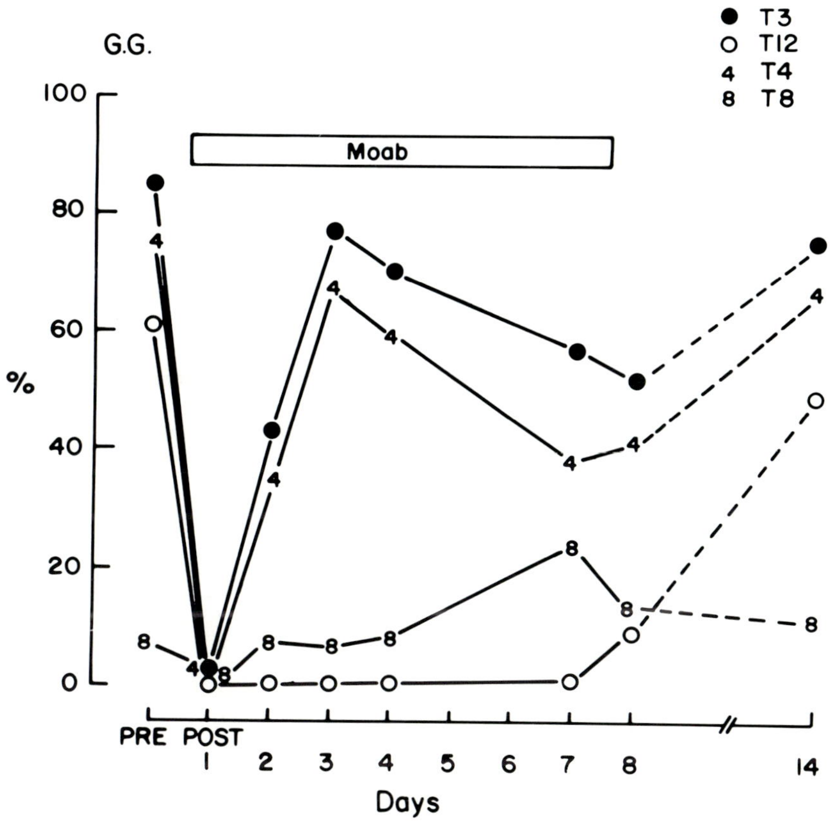

Figure 3. Phenotypes of peripheral T lymphocytes in a patient given daily intravenous infusions of anti-T12 for treatment of acute renal allograft rejection. Immediately after the first infusion all T cells were cleared from the circulation, and T12-positive cells did not reappear until therapy was discontinued. In contrast, T3-, T4-, and T8-positive cells returned to their original levels within 2 days. In some cases, this repopulation takes a day or two longer, but the overall pattern is seen in all patients whether rejection activity is reversed or not. (From Ref. 51 by permission.)

tured *in vitro* for several days, T12 positivity appears in some cases, suggesting that some type of modulation occurs *in vivo*. Preliminary functional experiments on the T12-negative, T3-positive cells show them to have reduced capability in MLR. The alternative explanation that anti-T12 selects for a minor subpopulation of cells is being explored. Analysis of T-cell clones shows that such T3-positive, T12-negative cells can exist.[52] When one considers the prodigious rate at which the thoracic duct alone returns circulating lymphocytes to the intravascular compartment,[53] it is conceivable that such T12-negative cells are normally present in lymph, and accumulate as the T12-positive cells are eliminated. The reverse process occurs as anti-T12 therapy is withdrawn.

Among the 12 patients with equivocal or no response to anti-T12, several failures appear to be related to persistent cellular infiltration with T12-negative cells, so it appears that some cases escape from anti-T12 by modulation, or by expansion of T12-negative functional populations. There seems to be no difficulty with penetration of the IgM antibody into tissue, since cellular infiltration can be cleared from a kidney in the anuric stage of acute tubular necrosis.[50] Alternatively, there may be a greater degree of cellular traffic in and out of a rejecting graft than had been assumed, and the monoclonal antibody may act principally within the vascular compartment. Acute febrile or other reactions to anti-T12 have not occurred, and while immunity developed in more than half of the patients to mouse globulin, mild anaphylaxis occurred in only one recipient, and all serum antibody responses were IgM.

4.3. Monoclonal Antibodies to Activated Cells

An antiblast/monocyte monoclonal antibody (CBLI) that prolonged skin grafts in rhesus monkeys[54] was administered to 19 Japanese patients with acute renal allograft rejection.[55] None of the recipients developed fever or other side effects, and lymphopenia did not occur, nor was there a depression in platelet, granulocyte, or monocyte counts during or after the 9-day course of intravenous therapy. This was somewhat unexpected, since CBLI reacts *in vitro* with bone marrow cells and peripheral blood monocytes. Most of the patients were judged to be resistant to a steroid pulse given shortly before the initiation of CBLI therapy, and 17 of the 19 had their rejections reversed. Five patients experienced subsequent rejections during a 1- to 12-month followup period. Further study of this antibody is showing it to be less effective than in the original study. Nevertheless, it represents a different approach to selective targeting of activated clones. There are several new candidate antibodies to activation antigens on T cells, and also on B cells.

5. Immunogenicity of Mouse Immunoglobulins

Antibody responses to the foreign mouse globulins are common, and at present are a major barrier to repeated courses of therapy. Antilymphocyte globulins have been known to elicit similar responses, although the large protein doses used clinically may paralyze the response. Small doses of rabbit antithymocyte IgG are known to be more immunogenic in rats than normal IgG, however.[56] The doses of monoclonal antibodies now being used are in a reasonable range for eliciting immunity, and since all of the antibodies reviewed above induce immunity in man and/or monkeys, it is clear that they are not immunosuppressive to themselves as antigens. Prior sensitization to mice is unlikely to play a role, since all patients treated are first shown to have negative immediate type skin reactions to mouse monoclonals, and baseline serum antibody titers are usually negative.

The anti-mouse response occurred in 13 of 17 patients receiving OKT3.[49,57] It is predominantly IgG, and there is further evidence for increased specificity to OKT3 itself. Jaffers *et al.*[57] describe two patients whose sera reacted with OKT3 only, indicating a possible specificity to idiotype. In the CBLI study, 14 of 19 patients rapidly developed antibodies to mouse within 2 weeks, and in some cases during the course of therapy.[55] No clinical reactions were noted in the latter cases, however, and their rejections continued to respond. In the anti-T12 study 8 of 14 patients studied developed an anti-mouse response, but this was entirely of the IgM class; furthermore, these sera were as reactive with the anti-T6 (IgG) control, having a different idiotype and isotype, as with the anti-T12 (IgM). Three patients developed the anti-mouse response during therapy on the 7th to 9th days. All of these showed a concomitant return of T12-positive lymphocytes, but only one developed mild anaphylactoid symptoms.[50,51] There have been no reports of serum sickness reactions from any of the trials.

The impact of anti-mouse immunity is that it limits the treatment course should antibodies develop before the full therapeutic effect is obtained, and it would be unlikely that subsequent courses of mouse monoclonal antibodies could be given to immunized patients, especially if a strong IgG response was made initially. In this regard, the relatively weaker immunogenicity of anti-T12, inducing as it does a predominant IgM response, may allow more leeway in its repeated use. It is also possible that tolerance to mouse immunoglobulins can be induced in advance by intravenous administration of deaggregated normal IgG or by other maneuvers.

6. Conclusion

The relative safety and efficacy of the intravenous administration of mouse monoclonal antibodies in humans seem established. The contrasting immediate and long-term effects of two pan-T-cell antibodies, anti-T3 (OKT3) and anti-T12, provide a clear illustration that the fine specificity of an antibody can be more important than the cellular target. Both of these antibodies react with the same major population of mature T cells, and both fix complement. Anti-T3 produces very complicated effects because it activates T cells via the associated T-cell antigen receptor, but also can lose efficacy as the target molecule is rapidly modulated. Anti-T3 therapy induces severe toxic reactions during the first infusion, but is highly effective in reversing acute rejections. In followup, recurrent rejections are common. Anti-T12 is completely nontoxic and appears to act principally by clearing T12-positive cells from the graft and blood. Not all rejections respond, yet those that do are not subject to recurrent rejection. Therapeutic trials such as these are providing important material for functional studies. More precise intervention in rejection will be possible by targeting activated cells, specific receptors, or secreted mediators. If study of biopsy material with monoclonal antibodies leads to evidence that some cases of rejection are primarily effected by NK cells or other non-T cells, then selective use of a relevant monoclonal antibody could be employed. More important, however, will be the selective induction of unresponsiveness by targeting components of the effector response while sparing those of the suppressor system to prevent the generation of rejection episodes in the first place. It is already known that examples of success in renal transplantation are associated with the presence of donor-specific suppressor T cells.[58] It should be possible to induce the appropriate systems selectively, to the advantage of all graft recipients.

ACKNOWLEDGMENT. Supported in part by NIH grant AI-19414.

References

1. Carpenter, C. B., 1981, The cellular basis of allograft rejection, *Immunol. Today* **2:**50.
2. Strom, T. B., Tilney, N. L., Paradysz, J. M., Bancewicz, J., and Carpenter, C. B., 1977, Cellular components of allograft rejection: Identity, specificity, and cytotoxic function of cells infiltrating acutely rejecting allografts, *J. Immunol.* **118:**2020.
3. Williams, G. M., Hume, D. M., Hudson, R. P., Morris, P. J., Kano, K., and Milgrom, F., 1968, "Hyperacute" renal homograft rejection in man, *N. Engl. J. Med.* **279:**611.
4. Busch, G. J., Reynolds, E. S., Galvanek, E. G., Braun, W. E., and Dammin, G. J., 1971, Human renal allografts: The role of vascular injury in early graft failure, *Medicine* **50:**29.
5. Porter, K. A., The effects of antibodies on human renal allografts, 1976, *Transplant. Proc.* **8:**189.
6. Porter, K. A., Joseph, N. H., Rendall, J. M., Stolinski, C., Hoehn, R. J., and Calne, R. Y., 1964, The role of lymphocytes in the rejection of canine renal homotransplants, *Lab. Invest.* **13:**1080.
7. Tilney, N. L., Strom, T. B., MacPherson, S. G., and Carpenter, C. B., 1976, Studies on infiltrating host cells harvested from acutely rejecting rat cardiac allografts, *Surgery* **79:**209.
8. Busch, G. J., Schamberg, J. F., Moretz, R. C., Strom, T. B., Tilney, N. L., and Carpenter, C. B., 1976, T and B cell patterns in irreversibly rejected human renal allografts: Correlation of morphology with surface markers and cytotoxic capacity of the isolated lymphoid infiltrate, *Lab. Invest* **35:**272.
9. Berke, G., and Amos, D. B., 1973, Mechanism of lymphocyte-mediated cytolysis; The LMC cycle and its role in transplantation immunity, *Transplant. Rev.* **17:**71.
10. Tilney, N. L., and Ford, W. L., 1974, The migration of rat lymphoid cells into skin grafts, *Transplantation,* **17:**12.
11. Bhan, A. K., Reinisch, C. L., Levey, R. H., McCluskey, R. T., and Schlossman, S. E., 1975, T-cell migration into allografts, *J. Exp. Med.* **141:**1210.
12. Balch, C. M., Wilson, C. B., Lee, S., and Feldman, J. D., 1973, Thymus-dependent lymphocytes in tissue sections of rejecting rat renal allografts, *J. Exp. Med.* **138:**1584.
13. Cerottini, J. C., and Brunner, K. T., 1974, Cell-mediated cytotoxicity, allograft rejection, and tumor immunity, *Adv. Immunol.* **18:**67.
14. Strom, R. B., Tilney, T. B., Carpenter, C. B., and Busch, G. J., 1975, Identity and cytotoxic capacity of cells infiltrating renal allografts, *N. Engl. J. Med.* **292:**1257.
15. Tilney, N. L., Strom, T. B., MacPherson, S. G., and Carpenter, C. B., 1975, Surface properties and functional characteristics of infiltrating cells harvested from acutely rejecting cardiac allografts in inbred rats, *Transplantation* **20:**323.
16. Roberts, P. J., and Hayry, P., 1976, Sponge matrix allografts. A model for analysis of killer cells infiltrating mouse allografts, *Transplantation* **21:**437.
17. Hancock, W. W., 1984, Analysis of intragraft effector mechanisms associated with human renal allograft rejection: Immunohistological studies with monoclonal antibodies, *Immunol. Rev.* **77:**61.
18. Pober, J. S., Gimbrone, M. A., Jr., Cotran, R. S., Reiss, C. S., Burakoff, S. J., Fiers, W., and Ault, K. A., 1983, Ia expression by vascular endothelium is inducible by activated T cells and by human γ-interferon, *J. Exp. Med.* **157:**1339.
19. Loveland, B. E., and McKenzie, I. F. C., 1982, Which T cells cause graft rejection? *Transplantation* **33:**217.

20. Dallman, M. J., and Mason, D. W., 1982, Role of thymus derived and thymus-independent cells in murine skin allograft rejection, *Transplantation* **33:**221.
21. Busch, G. J., Schamberg, J. F., Moretz, R. C., Strom, T. B., Tilney, N. L., and Carpenter, C. B., 1977, Four patterns of human renal allograft rejection: A cytologic and *in vitro* analysis of the infiltrate in 24 irreversibly rejected kidneys, *Transplant. Proc.* **9:**37.
22. Hall, B. M., Bishop, G. A., Farnsworth, A., Duggin, G. G., Horvath, J. S., Sheil, A. G. R., and Tiller, D. J., 1984, Identification of the cellular subpopulation infiltrating rejecting cadaver renal allografts, *Transplantation* **37:**564.
23. Reinherz, E. L., and Schlossman, S. F., 1980, The differentiation and function of human T lymphocytes, *Cell* **19:**821.
24. Reinherz, E. L., Kung, P. C., Goldstein, G., and Schlossman, S. F., 1979, A monoclonal antibody with selective reactivity with functionally mature thymocytes and all peripheral human T cells, *J. Immunol.* **123:**1312.
25. Hansen, J. A., Martin, P. J., and Nowinski, R. C., 1980, Monoclonal antibodies identifying a novel T-cell antigen and Ia antigens of human lymphocytes, *Immunogenetics* **10:**247.
26. Carpenter, C. B., and Milford, E. L., 1985, Renal transplantation: Immunobiology, in: *The Kidney* (B. M. Brenner and F. C. Rector, eds.), 3rd ed., W. B. Saunders, Philadelphia, in press.
27. Reinherz, E. L., Meuer, S. C., and Schlossman, S. F., 1983, The delineation of antigen receptors on human T lymphocytes, *Immunol. Today* **4:**5.
28. Morimoto, C., Reinherz, E. L., Borel, Y., and Schlossman, S. F., 1983, Direct demonstration of the human suppresor inducer subset by anti-T cell antibodies, *J. Immunol.* **130:**157.
29. Reinherz, E. L., Morimoto, C., Fitzgerald, K. A., Hussey, R. E., Daley, J. F., and Schlossman, S. F., 1982, Heterogeneity of human $T4^+$ inducer T cells defined by a monoclonal antibody that delineates two functional subpopulations, *J. Immunol.* **128:**463.
30. Damle, N. K., Mohagheghpour, N., Hansen, J. A., and Engleman, E. G., 1983, Alloantigen-specific cytotoxic and suppressor T lymphocytes are derived from phenotypically distinct precursors, *J. Immunol.* **131:**2296.
31. Evans, R. L., Faldetta, T. J., Humphreys, R. E., Pratt, D. M., Yunis, E. J., and Schlossman, S. F., 1978, Peripheral human T cells sensitized in mixed leukocyte culture synthesize and express Ia-like antigens, *J. Exp. Med.* **148:**1440.
32. Reinherz, E. L., Kung, P. C., Pesando, J. M., Ritz, J., Goldstein, G., and Schlossman, S. F., 1979, Ia determinants on human T cell subsets defined by monoclonal antibody: Activation stimuli required for expression, *J. Exp. Med.* **150:**1472.
33. Uchiyama, T., Nelson, D. L., Fletcher, T. A., and Waldmann, T. A., 1981, A monoclonal antibody (antitac) reactive with activated and functionally mature human T cells II. Expression of tac antigen on activated cytotoxic killer T cells, suppressor cells, and on one of two types of helper cells, *J. Immunol.* **126:**1398.
34. Leonard, W. J., Depper, J. M., Uchiyama, T., Smith, K. A., Waldmann, T. A., and Greene, W. C., 1982, A monoclonal antibody that appears to recognize the receptor for human T-cell growth factor; partial characterization of the receptor, *Nature* **300:**267.
35. Meuer, S. C., Hussey, R. E., Fabbi, M., Fox, D., Acuto, O., Fitzgerald, K. A., Hodgdon, J. C., Protentis, J. P., Schlossman, S. F., and Reinherz, E. L., 1984, An alternative pathway of T-cell activation: A functional role for the 50 kD T11 sheep erythrocyte receptor protoin, *Cell* **36:**897.
36. Fox, D. A., Hussey, R. E., Fitzgerald, K. A., Acuto, O., Poole, C., Palley, L., Daley, J. F., Schlossman, S. F., and Reinherz, E. L., 1984, Ta_1, a novel 105 kD human T cell activation antigen defined by a monoclonal antibody, *J. Immunol.* **133:**1250.
37. Schultze, H. E., and Heremans, J. F., 1966, Nature and metabolism of extracellular proteins, in: *Molecular Biology of Human Proteins*, Volume 1, Elsevier, Amsterdam, pp. 473–477.
38. Reinherz, E. L., Meuer, S., Fitzgerald, K. A., Hussey, R. E., Levine, H., and Schlossman, S. F., 1982, Antigen recognition of human T lymphocytes is linked to surface expression of the T3 molecular complex, *Cell* **30:**735.
39. Estabrook, A., Berger, C. I., Mittler, R., LoGerfo, P., Hardy, M., and Edelson, R. L., 1983, Antigenic modulation of human T-lymphocytes by monoclonal antibodies, *Transplant. Proc.* **15:**651.

40. Van Wauwe, F. P., DeMay, J. R., and Goossener, J. G., 1980, OKT3: A Monoclonal anti-human T lymphocyte antibody with potent mitogenic properties, *J. Immunol.* **124**:2708.
41. Billing, R., Wells, J., Zettel, D., and Terasaki, P. I., 1982, Monoclonal and heteroantibody reacting with different antigens common to human blast cells and monocytes, *Hybridoma* **1**:303.
42. Cosimi, A. B., Burton, R. C., Kung, P. C., Colvin, R., Goldstein, G., Lifter, J., Rhodes, W., and Russell, P. S., 1981, Evaluation in primate renal allograft recipients of monoclonal antibody to human T-cell sub-classes, *Transplant. Proc.* **13**:499.
43. Jonker, M., Malissen, B., van Vreeswijk, W., Mawas, C., Goldstein, G., Tax, W., and Balner, H., 1983, *In vivo* application of monoclonal antibodies specific for human T cell subsets permits the modification of immune responsiveness in rhesus monkeys, *Transplant. Proc.* **15**:635.
44. Giorgi, J. V., Burton, R. C., Barrett, L. V., Delmonico, F. L., Goldstein, G., and Cosimi, A. B., 1983, Immunosuppressive effect and immunogenicity of OKT11A monoclonal antibody in monkey allograft recipients, *Transplant. Proc.* **15**:639.
45. Bieber, C. P., Howard, F. D., Pennock, J., Wong, J., Shorthouse, R., and Stinson, E. B., 1981, Preparation, characterization and primate testing of monoclonal antithymocyte globulin, *Transplantation* **31**:283.
46. Cosimi, A. B., Colvin, R. B., Burton, R. C., Rubin, R. H., Goldstein, G., Kung, P., Hansen, W. P., Delmonico, F. L., and Russell, P. S., 1981, Use of monoclonal antibodies to T cell subsets for immunologic monitoring and treatment in recipients of renal allografts, *N. Engl. J. Med.* **305**:308.
47. Cosimi, A. B., Burton, R. C., Colvin, R. B., Goldstein, G., Delmonico, F. L., LaQuaglia, M. P., Tolkoff-Rubin, N., Rubin, R. H., Herrin, J. T., and Russell, P. S., 1981, Treatment of acute renal allograft rejection with OKT3 monoclonal antibody, *Transplantation* **32**:535.
48. Cosimi, A. B., 1983, The clinical usefulness of antilymphocyte antibodies, *Transplant. Proc.* **15**:583.
49. Chatenoud, L., Baudrihaye, M. F., Chkoff, N., Kreis, H., and Bach, J. F., 1983, Immunologic followup of renal allograft recipients treated prophylactically by OKT3 alone, *Transplant. Proc.* **15**:643.
50. Kirkman, R. L., Araujo, J. L., Busch, G. J., Carpenter, C. B., Milford, E. L., Reinherz, E. L., Schlossman, S. F., Strom, T. B., and Tilney, N. L., 1983, Treatment of acute renal allograft rejection with monoclonal anti-T12 antibody, *Transplantation* **36**:620.
51. Carpenter, C. B., Milford, E. L., Reinherz, E. L., Schlossman, S. F., Tilney, N. L., Strom, T. B., Kirkman, R. L., Busch, G. J., and Araujo, J. L., 1983, Monoclonal anti-T12 antibody as therapy for renal allograft rejection, *Trans. Assoc. Am. Physicians* **96**:84.
52. Hercend, T., Reinherz, E. L., Meuer, S., Schlossman, S. F., and Ritz, J., 1983, Phenotypic and functional heterogeneity of human cloned natural killer cell lines, *Nature* **301**:158.
53. Tilney, N. L., and Murray, J. E., 1967, The thoracic duct fistula as an adjunct to immunosuppression in human renal transplantation, *Transplantation* **5**:1204.
54. Billing, R., and Chatterjee, S., 1983, Prolongation of skin allograft survival in monkeys treated with anti-Ia and anti-blast/monocyte monoclonal antibodies, *Transplant. Proc.* **15**:649.
55. Takahashi, H., Okazaki, H., Terasaki, P. I., Iwaki, Y., Kinukawa, T., Chia, D., Miura, K., Ishizaka, M., Taguchi, Y., and Billing, R., 1983, Reversal of transplant rejection by monoclonal antiblast antibody, *Lancet* **2**:1155.
56. Guttmann, R. D., Carpenter, C. B., Lindquist, R. R., and Merrill, J. P., 1967, Renal transplantation in the inbred rat. III. A study of heterologous antithymocyte sera, *J. Exp. Med.* **126**:1099.
57. Jaffers, G. J., Colvin, R. B., Cosimi, A. B., Giorgi, J. V., Goldstein, G., Fuller, T. C., Kurnick, J. T., Lillehei, C., and Russell, P. S., 1983, The human immune response to murine OKT3 monoclonal antibody, *Transplant. Proc.* **15**:646.
58. Charpentier, B. M., Lang, P. P., Martin, B., and Freis, D., 1982, Specific recipient–donor unresponsiveness mediated by a suppressor cell system in human kidney allograft tolerance, *Transplantation* **33**:470.

Chapter 31

Serotherapy and Bone Marrow Transplantation

JEROME RITZ, STEPHEN E. SALLAN, ROBERT C. BAST, Jr., TAK TAKVORIAN, and STUART F. SCHLOSSMAN

1. Introduction

Within the human hematopoietic system, monoclonal antibodies have been used to identify a large number of surface antigens expressed by both normal and malignant cells, and in many instances it has now been possible to ascribe specific functions to individual cell surface molecules. Since monoclonal antibodies can be produced in large quantities and can be easily purified, it has also been possible to explore the potential therapeutic applications of these unique reagents. As a result, several different antibodies have been used in serotherapy trials in patients with refractory leukemia or lymphoma[1–5] and in several solid tumors.[6] In each of these studies, antibodies have been infused, with the hopes that antibody-bound tumor cells would subsequently be eliminated by natural effector mechanisms. In addition, monoclonal antibodies have also been utilized under more controlled circumstances *in vitro* in order to deplete specific target cells from bone marrow prior to either autologous[7] or allogeneic marrow transplantation.[8] In order to demonstrate the potential utility of these reagents, this chapter will focus on the specific clinical applications of monoclonal antibodies in patients with acute lymphoblastic leukemia (ALL). Although other clinical situations and other monoclonal antibodies with different specificity will undoubtedly present unique problems, much of the information gained in patients with ALL will be applicable to other leukemias and lymphomas and, to a lesser extent, to solid tumors as well.

JEROME RITZ, ROBERT C. BAST, Jr., and STUART F. SCHLOSSMAN • Division of Tumor Immunology, Dana–Farber Cancer Institute and Department of Medicine, Harvard Medical School, Boston, Massachusetts 02115. TAK TAKVORIAN • Division of Medical Oncology, Dana–Farber Cancer Institute and Department of Medicine, Harvard Medical School, Boston, Massachusetts 02115. STEPHEN E. SALLAN • Division of Pediatric Oncology, Dana–Farber Cancer Institute and Department of Pediatrics, Harvard Medical School, Boston, Massachusetts 02115.

Table I. Expression of CALLA in Leukemia

	Number tested	Number reactive	Percent positive
ALL			
Non-T-cell	214	173[a]	81
T-cell	40	5	12.5
AML	278	0	0
CLL			
B-cell	28	0	0
T-cell	6	0	0
CML			
Stable phase	26	0	0
Blast crisis	27	12	44
Total	619		

[a] Determined by indirect immunofluorescence reactivity with J5 monoclonal antibody.

2. Acute Lymphoblastic Leukemic Antigens: Targets for Immunotherapy

2.1. Common ALL Antigen (CALLA)

CALLA is a 100-kD cell surface glycoprotein that can be identified by specific murine monoclonal antibodies such as J5 (IgG2a)[9] and J13 (IgM). As summarized in Table I, CALLA is expressed on leukemic cells from approximately 80% of patients with non-T-cell ALL and 40% of patients with chronic myelocytic leukemia (CML) in blast crisis. Leukemic cells from patients with AML or CML in stable phase do not express CALLA.[10] In addition, CALLA is expressed by tumor cells from most patients with nodular, poorly differentiated lymphocytic lymphoma and Burkitt lymphoma, and approximately 40% of T-cell lymphoblastic lymphomas.[11] In normal bone marrow, approximately 1% of mononuclear cells express CALLA. Regenerating marrow and fetal hematopoietic tissues contain a larger fraction of CALLA-positive cells (2–5%). Although it had been postulated that these normal CALLA-positive cells could have been early marrow stem cells, treatment of bone marrow with J5 antibody and rabbit C did not selectively deplete committed myeloid stem cells (BFU-E, CFU-E, CFU-C) or mixed granuloerythropoietic colonies (CFU-G/E).[12] Hokland *et al.*[13] purified normal CALLA-positive cells from fetal tissues and showed that the phenotype of these cells is similar to that of non-T ALL cells. However, the majority of TdT-positive cells were found in the CALLA-negative fraction, as were all myeloid stem cells (CFU-C). CALLA is also expressed by other tissues, including terminally differentiated granulocytes,[14,15] renal glomerulus,[16] and proximal renal tubule and cultured fibroblasts.[15] Although CALLA present in these various tissues may have slightly different molecular weights, and may therefore be biochemically distinct from CALLA on ALL cells, each of these tissues is reactive with CALLA-specific antibodies and could potentially limit the effectiveness of anti-CALLA antibody *in vivo*. This type

Table II. gp26 Expression in Lymphocytic Leukemias

	Number tested	Number positive	Percent positive
Non-T-cell ALL			
CALLA-positive	30	25[a]	83
CALLA-negative	16	11	68
T-cell ALL	17	4	24
CLL			
B-cell	17	6	25
T-cell	2	1	50

[a] Determined by indirect immunofluorescence reactivity with J2 monoclonal antibody.

of reactivity is not, however, a major obstacle to selective treatment of bone marrow *in vitro*.

2.2. Twenty-six thousand-Dalton ALL-Associated Antigen

In addition to CALLA, ALL cells have been found to express other leukemia-associated antigens that are not found on normal circulating lymphocytes. One of these antigens is a 24- to 26-kD protein that has been identified by a series of monoclonal antibodies, including J2 (IgM),[17] J30 (IgG2), J47 (IgG1), BA-2,[18] Du-ALL-1,[19] and SJ-9A4.[20] In the majority of cases of non-T-cell ALL, leukemic cells express both CALLA and gp26 antigen. However, as shown in Table II, these two antigens are not always coexpressed and there are instances where only one of these antigens is present. Thus, in over 90% of cases of non-T-cell ALL, leukemic cells will express at least one of these antigens, which independently might serve as a target for monoclonal antibody directed therapy.

Although ALL cells most frequently express both CALLA and gp26 and undifferentiated lymphoid cells in fetal marrow and fetal liver also coexpress these antigens, it is also evident that the expression of these antigens on other hematopoietic cells is widely divergent. As shown in Table III, gp26 is ex-

Table III. Expression of gp26 Antigen in Normal Hematopoietic Tissues

	Percent positive cells
Normal or regenerating bone marrow	2–5
Fetal liver or fetal bone marrow	5–10
Thymus	30
Activated peripheral blood T cells	30–40 after 3–4 days
Mature platelets	100%
Myeloid precursor cells	
CFU-G/M, BFU-E, CFU-E, CFU-Mega	Negative
CFU-G/E/M mixed colonies	Negative

pressed on various hematopoietic and lymphoid cell populations of different lineages that are not CALLA-positive. Within nonhematopoietic tissues, gp26 is also expressed by various tissues, including smooth muscle and distal renal tubules.

3. Results of Clinical Studies

3.1. Serotherapy with Anti-CALLA Monoclonal Antibodies

Previous reports have presented the results of serotherapy in four patients with CALLA-positive ALL who received multiple infusions of J5 monoclonal antibody.[2] Each patient had relapsed multiple times before serotherapy and their tumor cells had become resistant to standard chemotherapy. Three of the patients had circulating lymphoblasts, which were cleared rapidly after the initial infusion of J5 antibody. Analysis of leukemic cells in these patients indicated that J5 antibody was binding to the cell surface after antibody infusion and that human complement (C3) was being deposited on the surface, after which they were cleared rapidly from the circulation. J5 antibody also rapidly bound to bone marrow lymphoblasts, but there was no decrease in the percentage of these cells during serotherapy in any patient. In two patients treated with J13, an IgM monoclonal antibody specific for CALLA, similar clinical results were obtained, suggesting that reticuloendothelial clearance rather than complement-mediated lysis was the primary mechanism by which circulating lymphoblasts were cleared during serotherapy.

Although there were rapid decreases in numbers of circulating leukemic cells after J5 antibody infusion, not all circulating blasts could be eliminated by serotherapy. Phenotypic analysis of leukemic cells during the course of serotherapy suggested that this resistance was due in part to a profound change in expression of CALLA on the cell surface. Whereas before serotherapy it appeared that all leukemic cells expressed CALLA and were reactive with J5 antibody, during therapy persistent leukemic cells expressed much less CALLA and were unreactive with J5 antibody. This change in phenotype was not due to selection of CALLA-negative lymphoblasts present before serotherapy, but to a loss of CALLA from the surface of CALLA-positive leukemic cells. Furthermore, this loss occurred in bone marrow cells as well as in circulating lymphoblasts. This antigenic modulation appeared to be induced directly by the presence of J5 antibody and it was shown that leukemic cells *in vivo* reexpressed CALLA when J5 antibody was no longer detectable in patients' serum. *In vitro* studies with leukemic cells and CALLA-positive cell lines confirmed the finding that antigenic modulation occurs in response to the binding of J5 antibody to cell surface antigen.[21] Although antigenic modulation is a known mechanism whereby murine leukemia cells can evade host immune defenses, this phenomenon had not been demonstrated previously for human leukemia cells. Additionally, there was no evidence in the patients of circulating blocking factors that could have inhibited the binding of J5 antibody to the leukemic

Table IV. Potential Limitations of Serotherapy with Monoclonal Antibody

1.	Circulating blocking factor
2.	Antigenic modulation
3.	Inability to eliminate antibody-coated cells
4.	Heterogeneous expression of target antigen by tumor cells
5.	Cross-reactivity with normal cellular antigens
6.	Immunogenicity of murine antibody
7.	Toxicity of monoclonal antibody infusion

cells. The toxicity of antibody infusion was minimal and consisted only of asymptomatic fevers in two of the four patients treated with J5 antibody and both patients treated with J13 antibody. Renal toxicity was not observed.

Although the analysis of patients receiving anti-CALLA antibodies suggested that antigenic modulation was a major mechanism whereby cells might become resistant to antibody infusion *in vivo*, other studies utilizing other reagents in patients with leukemia and lymphoma have identified several other factors that can significantly limit the effectiveness of monoclonal antibody infusion. These factors are summarized in Table IV and reviewed in Ref. 22. It should be noted that although not all factors become evident in every patient, at least one of these factors was shown to limit the effective elimination of tumor cells in almost every patient. In fact, in only one patient thus far has there been a sustained clinical response to antibody infusion[5] and resistance has developed in all other patients.

3.2. *In Vitro* Depletion of Tumor Cells with Monoclonal Antibody prior to Autologous Marrow Transplantation

Many of the limitations associated with *in vivo* serotherapy can be circumvented by the use of monoclonal antibodies *in vitro*: the therapeutic environment can be carefully controlled; circulating blocking factors can be removed completely; rabbit complement can be used to lyse leukemic cells before antigenic modulation can occur; and multiple treatments with antibody and complement can be used to ensure lysis of all antibody-coated cells. Furthermore, any potential toxicity produced by reactivity of monoclonal antibody with nonhematopoietic tissues can be avoided.

One disadvantage of this approach is that it can only be used in clinical situations when tumor cells remaining *in vivo* can be eradicated by high dose chemotherapy and/or total body irradiation (TBI). Although these ablative regimens may not be useful in patients with many solid tumors, numerous studies have demonstrated that bone marrow transplantation in conjunction with ablative therapy can be an effective treatment for patients with acute leukemia and lymphoma. Unfortunately, only 40% of patients have normal histocompatible

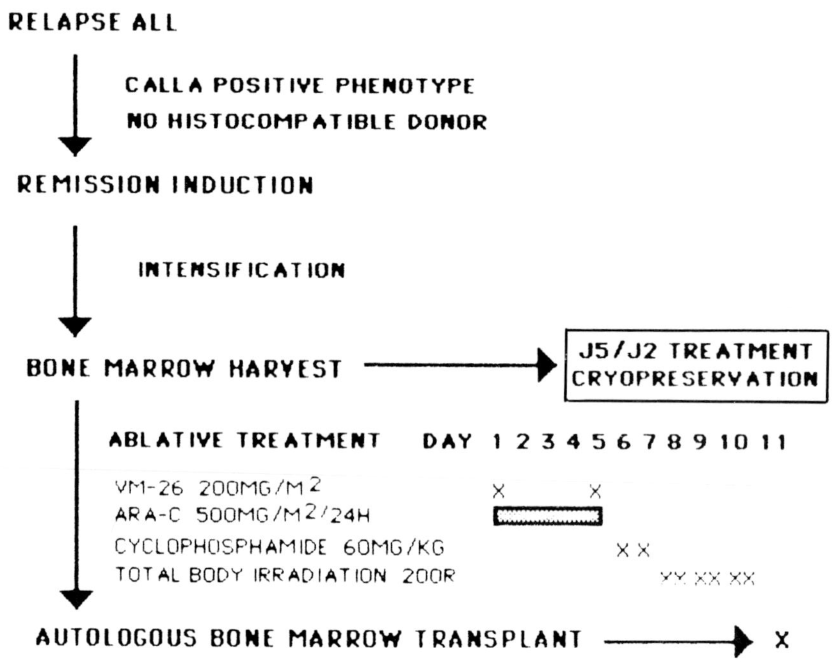

Figure 1. Schematic protocol for autologous bone marrow transplantation in patients with relapsed CALLA-positive acute lymphoblastic leukemia.

donors, and autologous transplantation is limited by the presence of residual leukemic cells in remission bone marrow.

We therefore began a clinical study in which J5 monoclonal antibody was used to eliminate residual CALLA-positive leukemic cells from remission bone marrow prior to autologous transplantation.[7] The clinical protocol for this study is presented schematically in Fig. 1. Patients with ALL who had relapsed with CALLA-positive leukemic cells following standard chemotherapy were considered eligible for this protocol, but those having normal identical twins or histocompatible siblings were excluded from study. Patients who failed to achieve complete remission with chemotherapy alone were also excluded.

After reinduction of remission in our first three patients, bone marrow was harvested under general anesthesia and mononuclear cells were purified by Ficoll-Hypaque density sedimentation and cryopreserved without *in vitro* antibody treatment. This constituted a "backup marrow," which could be used in the event that *in vitro* antibody and complement-treated bone marrow failed to engraft. Patients then received intensification chemotherapy with VM-26, cytosine arabinoside (Ara-C), and L-asparaginase, and central nervous system prophylaxis with intrathecal Ara-C and hydrocortisone.

After recovery from intensification chemotherapy, the first three patients underwent a second bone marrow harvest from which mononuclear cells were isolated and treated with J5 antibody and rabbit complement prior to cryopreservation. Our method for *in vitro* treatment of bone marrow, which included three separate incubations with monoclonal antibody and complement, was based on previous studies that determined the optimal conditions for lysis of small numbers of CALLA-positive tumor cells in the presence of a large excess of normal marrow.[23] After J5-antibody-treated marrow was shown to engraft in the first three patients, the separate backup marrow was eliminated from the clinical protocol and patients currently undergo only one marrow harvest under general anesthesia after recovery from intensification chemotherapy. One day after marrow harvest and *in vitro* antibody treatment, patients began receiving ablative treatment with VM-26, Ara-C, cyclophosphamide, and total body irradiation (TBI) as shown in Fig. 1. Approximately 12 hr following TBI, cryopreserved marrow that had been treated *in vitro* was thawed rapidly and reinfused through a central venous catheter. Patients did not receive additional chemotherapy or immune suppression following autologous transplantation.

Fourteen patients have met these criteria and have received autologous J5-treated marrow. Within this group, five patients relapsed and four patients expired in remission within 3 months of transplantation. All relapses occurred in bone marrow with CALLA-positive lymphoblasts. The remaining five patients continue in unmaintained remission and two of these patients have now been followed for greater than 3 years posttransplant. We have recently compared the status of these 14 patients receiving autologous J5-treated marrow with a comparable group of pediatric patients with ALL in second or third remission who were referred to one of three transplant centers where they received normal allogeneic marrow from histocompatible siblings. The results of this comparison, which are shown in Fig. 2, indicate that there is no significant difference in outcome between the two groups of patients. In both groups, >50% of patients failed within 1 year of transplant and there was no significant difference with respect to incidence of relapse or failure from other causes. These results are also similar to other published studies of allogeneic histocompatible marrow transplantation in patients with ALL in second or subsequent remission.[24]

Although results of J5 autologous marrow transplantation were comparable to results of standard allogeneic marrow transplantation, we have also attempted to improve upon the results of this study. As expected, the primary cause of failure in over one-third of patients was relapse leukemia. In our autologous transplants, it is evident that relapse can occur from either inadequate elimination of leukemic cells from the marrow or from inadequate "ablative" therapy in the patient. For this reason, studies were undertaken to improve the *in vitro* treatment of bone marrow and these experiments indicated that addition of J2 antibody to J5 antibody consistently enhanced the elimination of tumor cell targets *in vitro*.[25] As noted previously, J2 antibody also reacted with ALL cells in the majority of patients with non-T-cell ALL and was not present on normal bone marrow progenitors. The ability of J2-antibody-treated marrow to engraft has now been confirmed *in vivo* and we have therefore modified the *in vitro* treatment of all patients on this study to include both J5 and J2 antibodies.

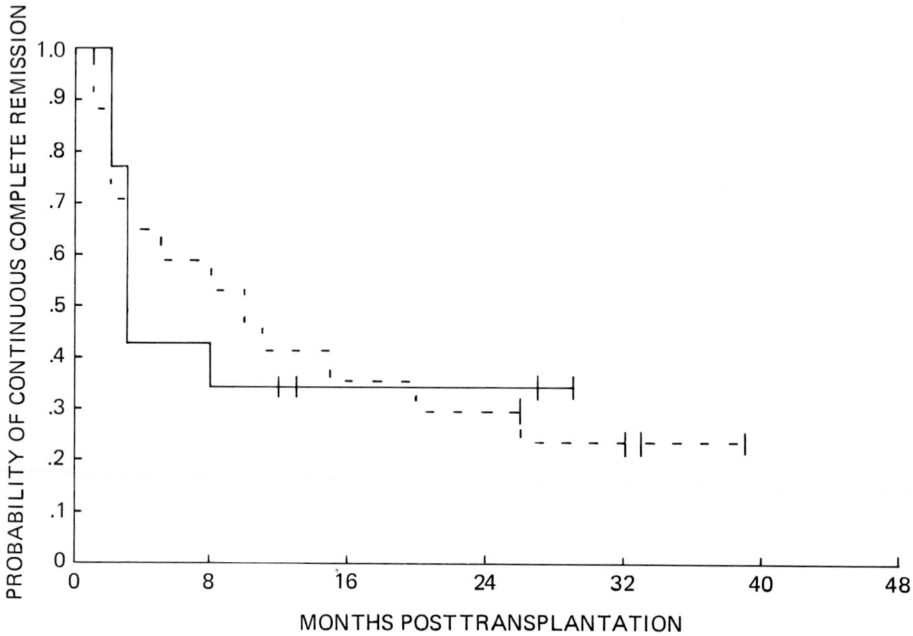

Figure 2. Comparison of results of (—) autologous (14 patients) vs. (- - -) allogeneic (17 patients) marrow transplantation for patients with ALL in second or third remission.

In addition to autologous marrow transplantation in ALL, *in vitro* treatment with monoclonal antibodies has been utilized to facilitate treatment of other hematopoietic malignancies that often involve bone marrow. In particular, Nadler *et al.*[26] have recently reported the results of autologous bone marrow transplantation in eight patients with relapsed non-Hodgkin lymphoma. Patients received ablative therapy consisting of cyclophosphamide (60 mg/kg iv ×2) and TBI (200 rad ×6). All patients had B-cell lymphoma, and marrow was harvested before initiation of this ablative regimen and treated *in vitro* with anti-B1 antibody and rabbit complement to remove residual tumor cells. Despite the fact that these were generally older patients (median age 44), all patients tolerated the chemotherapy/TBI regimen and all patients were reconstituted with anti-B1-treated marrow. Although six of the eight patients had relapsed more than once previously, only three of the eight patients have relapsed following autologous transplantation. Of the five surviving patients, four are alive more than 1 year posttransplant in unmaintained complete remission.

4. Discussion

Although the development of monoclonal antibodies reactive with human tumor cells has circumvented many of the limitations that previously have been associated with antibody-directed therapy, it should be emphasized that the therapeutic use of monoclonal antibodies is still in an early phase of clinical evaluation. Major limitations still exist[22] and only a relatively small number of patients have been treated under various protocols. Nevertheless, considerable information has been obtained from these early trials that has been used in a constructive way to direct current (and future) studies with monoclonal antibodies.

In vivo serotherapy with J5 monoclonal antibody in patients with CALLA-positive ALL did not produce a consistent clinical response in our patients. However, there was evidence of antibody binding and activation of complement on the surface of leukemic cells in peripheral blood and bone marrow as well as clearance of some circulating tumor cells. Furthermore, this was accomplished without significant toxicity to normal hematopoietic cells or to non-hematopoietic tissues.

The use of monoclonal antibodies *in vitro* eliminates some of the problems associated with *in vivo* administration. Unfortunately, the application of *in vitro* therapy is limited to clinical situations where the bulk of tumor cells *in vivo* can be treated with conventional drugs and irradiation. In our study, *in vitro* treatment with J5 antibody was used specifically to eradicate residual leukemia cells from patients with CALLA-positive ALL in second or subsequent remission. Previous experience in several centers had indicated that conventional chemotherapy in this situation results in very few long-term responses.[24] However, supralethal chemotherapy and TBI in conjunction with syngeneic or allogeneic histocompatible bone marrow transplantation has resulted in a substantial percentage of long-term survivors.[24] Unfortunately, 60% of patients do not have normal histocompatible donor marrow, and autologous bone marrow transplantation in patients with leukemia is limited by the presence of residual tumor cells, even during complete remission. In this clinical setting, the results in our first 14 patients suggest that *in vitro* treatment of marrow with J5 monoclonal antibody is capable of selectively eradicating residual leukemia cells without affecting hematopoietic progenitor cells, which are necessary for autologous engraftment.

Although our current regimen of "ablative" therapy in conjunction with J5 treatment *in vitro* appears to be effective in over one-third of our patients, significant numbers of patients relapse following either autologous or allogeneic marrow transplantation and this clearly indicates a need for improvement of both the patients' "ablative" therapy as well as the *in vitro* bone marrow treatment. For this reason, we have recently modified the *in vitro* treatment to include both J2 and J5 antibodies.[25] Improvements are also needed in the chemotherapy and TBI that patients receive prior to marrow infusion, since, given the high relapse rate following transplantation of normal allogeneic marrow, it is likely that inadequate patient treatment is the primary cause of relapse. Hopefully, these modifications will continue to improve the efficacy of autologous marrow transplantation for patients with relapsed leukemia.

In addition to the use of monoclonal antibodies to remove residual ALL cells, it is also evident that similar techniques can be used to remove other types of residual tumor cells prior to autologous marrow transplantation. In particular, the same techniques have recently been applied in patients with relapsed non-Hodgkin lymphoma.[26] Although lymphoma cells are not always histologically evident in marrow at the time of presentation, bone marrow is a frequent site of lymphoma relapse and tumor cells can sometimes be detected in marrow that is histologically normal.[27] Moreover, as in the case of acute leukemia, B-cell lymphomas are amenable to treatment with intensive chemotherapy and TBI, which can result in long-term remission in some patients, even though standard dose chemotherapy is not effective.[28] Thus, the ability to remove residual tumor cells prior to autologous transplantation through the use of monoclonal antibodies will hopefully allow additional patients to receive more effective treatment of their disease. As antibodies selectively reactive with various other tumor cells become available and as techniques for *in vitro* depletion become more effective, additional therapeutic benefits are likely to be obtained.

ACKNOWLEDGMENTS. This work was supported in part by NIH grant CA 34183. J.R. is a Scholar of the Leukemia Society of America.

References

1. Nadler, L. M., Stashenko, P., Hardy, R., Kaplan, W. D., Button, L. N., Kufe, D. W., Antman, K. H., and Schlossman, S. F., 1980, Serotherapy of a patient with a monoclonal antibody directed against a human lymphoma associated antigen, *Cancer Res.* **40:**3147–3154.
2. Ritz, J., Pesando, J. M., Sallan, S. E., Clavell, L. A., Notis-McConarty, J., Rosenthal, P., and Schlossman, S. F., 1981, Serotherapy of acute lymphoblastic leukemia with monoclonal antibody, *Blood* **58:**141–152.
3. Miller, R. A., Oseroff, A. R., Stratte, P. T., and Levy, R., 1983, Monoclonal antibody therapeutic trials in seven patients with T cell lymphoma, *Blood* **62:**988–995.
4. Dillman, R. O., Shawler, D. L., Sobol, R. E., Collins, H. A., Beuregard, J. C., Wormsley, S. B., and Royston, I., 1982, Murine monoclonal antibody therapy in two patients with chronic lymphocytic leukemia, *Blood* **59:**1036–1045.
5. Miller, R. A., Maloney, D. A., Warnke, R., and Levy, R., 1982, Treatment of B cell lymphoma with monoclonal anti-idiotype antibody, *N. Engl. J. Med.* **306:**517–522.
6. Sears, H. F., Herlyn, D., Steplewski, Z., and Koprowski, H., 1984, Effects of monoclonal antibody immunotherapy on patients with gastrointestinal adenocarcinoma, *J. Biol. Resp. Modif.* **3:**138–150.
7. Ritz, J., Sallan, S. E., Bast, R. C., Lipton, J. M., Clavell, L. A., Feeney, M., Hercend, T., Nathan, D. G., and Schlossman, S. F., 1982, Autologous bone marrow transplantation in CALLA positive acute lymphoblastic leukemias after *in vitro* treatment with J5 monoclonal antibody and complement, *Lancet* **ii:**60–63.
8. Reinherz, E. L., Geha, G., Rappeport, J. M., Wilson, M., Penta, A. C., Hussey, R. E., Fitzgerald, K. A., Daley, J., Levine, H., Rosen, F. S., and Schlossman, S. F., 1982, Immune reconstitution in severe combined immunodeficiency following transplantation with T lymphocyte depleted HLA haplotype mismatched bone marrow, *Proc. Natl. Acad. Sci. USA* **79:**6047–6051.
9. Ritz, J., Pesando, J. M., Notis-McConarty, J., Lazarus, H., and Schlossman, S. F., 1980, A monoclonal antibody to human acute lymphoblastic leukemia antigen, *Nature* **283:**583–585.

10. Greaves, M. F., Hariri, G., Newman, R. A., Sutherland, D. R., Ritter, M. A., and Ritz, J., 1983, Selective expression of the common acute lymphoblastic leukemia (gp100) antigen on immature lymphoid cells and their malignant counterparts, *Blood* **61:**628–639.
11. Ritz, J., Nadler, L. M., Bhan, A. K., Notis-McConarty, J., Pesando, J. M., and Schlossman, S. F., 1981, Expression of common acute lymphoblastic leukemia antigen (CALLA) by lymphomas of B cell and T cell lineage, *Blood* **58:**648–652.
12. Clavell, L. A., Lipton, J. M., Bast, R. C., Kudisch, M., Pesando, J. M., Schlossman, S. F., and Ritz, J., 1981, Absence of common ALL antigen on bi-potent myeloid, erythroid and granulocyte progenitors, *Blood* **58:**333–336.
13. Hokland, P., Rosenthal, P., Griffin, J. D., Nadler, L. M., Daley, J. F., Hokland, M., Schlossman, S. F., and Ritz, J., 1983, Purification and characterization of fetal hematopoietic cells which express the common acute lymphoblastic leukemia antigen (CALLA), *J. Exp. Med.* **157:**114–129.
14. Cossman, J., Neckers, L. M., Leonard, W. J., and Greene, W. C., 1983, Polymorphonuclear neutrophils express the common acute lymphoblastic leukemia antigen, *J. Exp. Med.* **157:**1064–1069.
15. Braun, M. P., Martin, P. J., Ledbetter, J. A., and Hansen, J. A., 1983, Granulocytes and cultured human fibroblasts express common acute lymphoblastic leukemia associated antigens, *Blood* **61:**718–725.
16. Metzgar, R. S., Borowitz, M. F., Jones, N. H., and Dowell, B. L., 1981, Distribution of common acute lymphoblastic leukemia antigen in nonhematopoietic tissues, *J. Exp. Med.* **154:**1249–1254.
17. Hercend, T., Nadler, L. M., Pesando, J. M., Reinherz, E. L., Schlossman, S. F., and Ritz, J., 1981, Expression of a 26,000 dalton glycoprotein on activated human T cells, *Cell. Immunol.* **64:**192–199.
18. LeBien, T., Kersey, J., Nakazawa, S., Minato, K., and Minowada, J., 1982, Analysis of human leukemia/lymphoma cell lines with monoclonal antibodies BA-1, BA-2 and BA-3, *Leukemia Res.* **6:**299–305.
19. Jones, N. H., Borowitz, M. J., and Metzgar, R. S., 1982, Characterization and distribution of a 24,000 molecular weight antigen defined by a monoclonal antibody (DU-ALL-1) elicited to common acute lymphoblastic leukemia (cALL) cells, *Leukemia Res.* **6:**449–464.
20. Komada, Y., Peiper, S. C., Melvin, S. L., Metzgar, D. W., Tarnowski, B. H., and Green, A. A., 1983, A monoclonal antibody (SJ-9A4) to p24 present on common ALLs, neuroblastomas and platelets. I. Characterization and development of a unique radioimmunometric assay, *Leukemia Res.* **7:**487–498.
21. Ritz, J., Pesando, J. M., Notis-McConarty, J., and Schlossman, S. F., 1980, Modulation of human acute lymphoblastic leukemia antigen induced by monoclonal antibody *in vitro*, *J. Immunol.* **125:**1506–1514.
22. Ritz, J., and Schlossman, S. F., 1982, Utilization of monoclonal antibodies in the treatment of leukemia and lymphoma, *Blood* **59:**1–11.
23. Bast, R. C., Ritz, J., Lipton, J. M., Feeney, M., Sallan, S. E., Nathan, D. G., and Schlossman, S. F., 1983, Elimination of leukemic cells from human bone marrow using monoclonal antibody and complement, *Cancer Res.* **43:**1389–1394.
24. Johnson, F. L., Thomas, E. D., Clark, B. S., Chard, R. L., Harmann, J. R., and Storb, R., 1981, A comparison of marrow transplantation with chemotherapy for children with acute lymphoblastic leukemia in second or subsequent remission, *N. Engl. J. Med.* **305:**846–851.
25. Bast, R. C., DeFabritiis, P., Lipton, J. M., Gelber, R., Maver, C., Nadler, L. M., Sallan, S. E., and Ritz, J., 1985, Elimination of malignant clonogenic cells from human bone marrow using multiple monoclonal antibodies and complement, *Cancer Res.* **45:**499–503.
26. Nadler, L. M., Takvorian, T., Botnick, L., Bast, R. C., Finberg, R., Hellman, S., Canellos, G. P., and Schlossman, S. F., 1984, Anti-B1 monoclonal antibody and complement treated autologous bone marrow transplantation for relapsed B cell non-Hodgkin's lymphoma, *Lancet* **ii:**427–434.

27. Benjamin, D., Magrath, I. T., Douglass, E. C., and Corash, L. M., 1983, Derivation of lymphoma cell lines from microscopically normal bone marrow in patients with undifferentiated lymphomas: Evidence of occult bone marrow involvement, *Blood* **61:**1017–1019.
28. Philips, G. L., Herzig, R. H., Lazarus, H. M., Fay, J. W., Wolff, S. N., Mill, W. B., Lin, H., Thomas, P. R. M., Glasgow, G. P., Shina, D. C., and Herzig, G. P., 1984, Treatment of resistant malignant lymphoma with cyclophosphamide, total body irradiation, and transplantation of cryopreserved autologous marrow, *N. Engl. J. Med.* **310:**1557–1561.

Part V

T-Cell Clones and Their Products

Chapter 32

The Murine T-Cell Antigen:Ia Receptor: Functional and Structural Analysis with a Monoclonal Antireceptor Antibody

JONATHAN KAYE

1. Introduction

Antigen specificity is intrinsic to the T-cell as well as the B-cell compartment of an immune response. However, the term T cell applies to a heterogeneous population of lymphocytes. T cells were originally divided into subsets based on apparent function, subsequently classified by surface phenotype, and more recently classified by their antigen recognition properties. As a population, T cells are capable of recognizing a large number of diverse antigens. Like B-cell antigen recognition, mediated by membrane immunoglobulin, T-cell antigen recognition is a clonally distributed property such that any given T cell and its progeny are, allowing for an expected degree of cross-reactivity, monospecific. Unlike B cells, however, helper T lymphocytes, which induce B-cell growth and antibody secretion, and cytolytic T cells, which are capable of destroying virally infected cells, only recognize foreign antigen in conjunction with self major histocompatibility complex (MHC) glycoproteins on the surface of another cell. In immunologic slang, the dual specificity of these T-cell subsets for foreign antigen and self MHC molecules has been termed "MHC restriction," since the ability of the T cell to recognize foreign antigen in this case is restricted by MHC molecules. In general, helper T cells recognize antigen in conjunction with class II MHC molecules (Ia antigens), and cytolytic T cells recognize foreign antigen in conjunction with class I MHC molecules.

The specificity of MHC-restricted T-cell antigen recognition is the result of a T-cell integral membrane receptor for antigen and MHC molecules. Although countless experiments have demonstrated the existence of such a receptor functionally, only recently has the receptor protein actually been iden-

JONATHAN KAYE • Department of Biology, University of California, San Diego, La Jolla, California 92093.

tified. The difficulty in identifying the T-cell antigen receptor was twofold. First, the heterogeneity of the immune response to a particular antigen made homogeneous receptor material difficult to obtain. Second, the ligand for the receptor, an integral membrane MHC glycoprotein apparently complexed with foreign antigen on a cell surface, made isolation of the T-cell receptor by binding to its ligand technically unachievable. The former problem has been overcome by the identification of growth factors necessary for the *in vitro* propagation and cloning of functional antigen-specific T-cell lines, and by the development of somatic cell fusion techniques. The complexity of the ligand for the receptor, however, remains a major stumbling block to performing direct antigen-binding studies. Nevertheless, several laboratories have been able to isolate T-cell antigen : MHC receptors by producing monoclonal antibodies reactive with cloned T-cell lines or T-cell hybrids. The following sections detail the production of such a monoclonal antibody, reactive with antigen:Ia receptors on a cloned murine helper T-cell line, and the structural and functional information gained from its use. This chapter particularly emphasizes the power of a monoclonal antireceptor antibody with agonist activity in revealing the details of cell activation. Although this discussion specifically addresses the issues of helper T-cell function and the structure of the T-cell antigen:Ia receptor, the approaches used are of general applicability in receptor systems.

2. Approaches to Isolating the T-Cell Antigen : MHC Receptor

As with the production of any monoclonal antibody of a desired specificity, a good selection procedure is of utmost importance. Two approaches for screening for antireceptor monoclonal antibodies have proved successful. The first takes advantage of the clonally distributed nature of T-cell antigen recognition. Thus, T cells with different antigen and/or MHC specificities will have different receptor structures that can be differentiated serologically. In practice, monoclonal antibodies can be produced against a homogeneous population of T cells and screened for the ability to bind to the T cells used for immunization but not to T cells with similar functional properties but with a different antigen specificity.[1–4] This procedure should select for antibodies that bind variable portions of the antigen : MHC receptor. Such monoclonal antibodies have been termed "clonotypic," analogous to anti-idiotypic antibodies, which bind immunoglobulin variable region determinants. The alternative approach, described in detail below, is to screen for monoclonal antireceptor antibodies by the ability to inhibit or mimic T-cell activation induced by antigen.[5,6] The functional method of screening for monoclonal antibodies against cell surface components is of general applicability in any system with an appropriate *in vitro* assay for cell activation. This "shotgun" approach has the potential of uncovering any cell surface component involved in the function studied, but as a consequence requires other criteria to determine the specificity of the antibody. For example, the production of monoclonal antibodies that inhibit T-cell function originally resulted in the identification of T-cell surface proteins other than the antigen receptor, but nevertheless important for T-cell interactions.[7] Interestingly, with one exception,[4] all of the reported antireceptor monoclonal antibodies obtained by immunization with whole cells bind exclusively to the cells used for immunization.[1–6,8,9] The inability to obtain anti-constant-region antibodies by this protocol may be due to the highly conserved nature of the T-cell antigen receptor constant region and/or the orientation of the receptor in the cell membrane. Thus far, antibodies against antigen receptor determinants shared between T cells have generally been produced by immunization with purified receptor.[10–12]

Antibodies produced against cell surface receptors can have antagonist[13,14] or agonist activity.[14–17] What determines the ability of an antireceptor antibody to block or transduce a signal to the cell is unclear. In some cases, the determinant recognized by the antibody apparently determines its biological properties.[14] In other cases, of which the T-cell antigen receptor is probably one, some intrinsic property of the receptor-bearing cell may be the deciding factor. However, in either situation, monoclonal antireceptor antibodies can potentially be used as specific probes to study cell activation as well as for affinity purification of cell surface receptors. In the case of T-cell activation, where the antigen receptor interacts with a ligand on the surface of an accessory cell, antibodies with agonist activity allow one to determine the requirements and pathways of T-cell growth and differentiation in the absence of other cell types. This has obvious advantages for biochemical analysis of the process of cell activation.

3. The Production of Antireceptor Antibodies against Murine Helper T-Cell Lines

T-Cell hybrids,[5,8] T-cell tumors,[1,3,4] and cloned T-cell lines[2,6,9] have been used successfully to produce antireceptor antibodies and to characterize biochemically the T-cell antigen receptor. The advantage of using transformed T-cell tumor or hybrid lines as immunogens and for biochemical analysis is the ease in obtaining large numbers of cells and the ability to propagate such cells in the absence of other cell types. However, the phenotypic stability of T-cell hybrids can vary and they have obvious limitations for the study of normal T-cell growth and differentiation. For these reasons, our laboratory has relied exclusively on cloned T-cell lines to analyze T-cell antigen recognition. Methods for the production and cloning of T-cell lines have been described in detail elsewhere (Refs. 6 and 18, and Krensky *et al.*, this volume, Chapter 35). Briefly, antigen-primed lymph node T cells are expanded *in vitro* in the presence of antigen and a source of syngeneic antigen-presenting cells and then cloned in agar. Colonies of cells are plucked from the agar and expanded in the presence of antigen, syngeneic antigen-presenting cells, and a source of growth factors. Cell lines established from these colonies can undergo multiple rounds of recloning by the method of limiting dilution. The demonstration of the monoclonality of these lines is often a problem when cloning frequencies are poor.

However, the importance of establishing monoclonality depends on the problem being addressed. As will be discussed later, monoclonality can be demonstrated with a clonotypic antireceptor monoclonal antibody.

In general, we have found that cloned T-cell lines established by this protocol are of the helper T-cell phenotype, that is, Ig^-, Thy-1^+, L3T4^+, and Lyt-2^-. The expression of Lyt-1 on these cells is variable. As expected for helper T cells, these cells are antigen-specific and self-Ia restricted when either the initiation of DNA synthesis or secretion of the T-cell growth factor interleukin 2 (IL-2) is used as a measure of cell activation. A relatively high frequency of antigen-specific T-cell clones are also activated by a particular allogeneic Ia glycoprotein in the absence of antigen.[18,19] This alloreactivity reflects a cross-reaction of self Ia recognition, a point we will discuss in detail below. Helper T cells take their name from their ability to stimulate B cells. Cloned helper T cells activate B cells *in vitro* in an antigen-specific and self-Ia restricted manner, as measured by the induction of B-cell proliferation[20] and by the induction of polyclonal or antigen-specific immunoglobulin secretion.[21]

Two cloned helper T-cell lines, D10.G4.1 and D8, have been analyzed in detail.[6] These T cells were derived from the pooled lymph node T cells of two AKR/J mice immunized with a mixture of egg white proteins. The line D10.G4.1, twice recloned by limiting dilution, is specific for conalbumin and I-A^k (the superscript refers to the strain of origin of the Ia glycoprotein), while T-cell line D8 is specific for ovalbumin and I-A^k. The specificity of the activation of these T cells is shown in Table I, as measured by the induction of thymidine incorporation into DNA. The D10.G4.1 cells are also alloreactive, and are activated by I-A^b glycoproteins in the absence of conalbumin (Table I), whereas D8 cells have no known alloreactivity. Although phenotypically and functionally indistinguishable, helper T-cell clones D10.G4.1 and D8 were predicted to possess different antigen receptor variable regions based on their distinct antigen and Ia activation requirements.

In an attempt to identify cell surface molecules involved in helper T-cell antigen recognition, antisera were initially raised against D10.G4.1 and D8 cells in BALB.K mice.[6] The characterization of these antisera established the method of screening for a monoclonal antireceptor antibody. The choice of BALB.K mice as recipients for these immunizations eliminated the potential production of anti-MHC antibodies (AKR and BALB.K mice are both H-2^k) that might have influenced screening assays while favoring the production of antibodies directed against other alloantigens. We have also produced an anti-D10.G4.1 antiserum with similar properties to those described below, although of lower titer, in (AKR $\times$ C57BL6) (H-2^k $\times$ H-2^b) F_1 mice, but have been unsuccessful in limited attempts to produce a similar anti-D10.G4.1 antiserum in AKR mice. These results are consistent with the idea that other cell surface alloantigens may act as helper determinants for the production of antireceptor antibodies.

Anti-D10.G4.1 antisera were initially screened for the ability to inhibit cloned T-cell proliferation induced by conalbumin and syngeneic antigen-presenting cells. However, these antisera were instead found to be potent stimulators of D10.G4.1 proliferation in the absence of antigen. This response did

Table I. Specificity of Cloned Helper T-Cell Lines D10.G4.1 and D8

Experiment	T Clone[a]	MHC haplotype of antigen-presenting Cells[b]	Antigen[c]	Response[d]
I	D8	H-2^k	—	45
	D8	H-2^k	CA	64
	D8	H-2^k	OVA	10,925
	D10.G4.1	H-2^k	—	236
	D10.G4.1	H-2^k	CA	14,237
	D10.G4.1	H-2^k	OVA	338
II	D8	H-2^k	—	45
	D8	H-2^k	OVA	10,920
	D8	H-2^d	—	85
	D8	H-2^d	OVA	154
III	D10.G4.1	H-2^k	—	330
	D10.G4.1	H-2^k	CA	10,993
	D10.G4.1	H-2^d	—	558
	D10.G4.1	H-2^d	CA	659
IV	D10.G4.1	H-2^k	—	136
	D10.G4.1	H-2^k	CA	45,395
	D10.G4.1	H-2^b	—	57,433

[a] 2×10^4 cloned T cells/200 μl culture.
[b] 2×10^5 H-2^k, H-2^d or H-2^b mitomycin C-treated spleen cells/culture.
[c] OVA (ovalbumin) or CA (conalbumin) at 200 μg/ml.
[d] Mean [^{3}H]-thymidine incorporation of triplicate cultures pulsed for the final 16 hr of a 65-hr culture period.

require the presence of accessory cells, as will be discussed below, as a source of a growth factor. Six out of six mice tested after two to four weekly immunizations of D10.G4.1 cells in saline had positive sera. Subsequently, an antiserum against D8 cells that induced D8 cell proliferation in the absence of antigen and the presence of accessory cells was produced in one of two mice given seven weekly immunizations of cloned T cells. The reason for the greater immunogenicity of D10.G4.1 cells is unknown. Our laboratory has made many immunizations of mice with cloned T-cell lines. Of these, responses to D10.G4.1 cells have been uniquely potent. Thus, in raising antireceptor antibodies, it is well to try many different immunogens in a variety of recipient strains or species. The ability of anti-D10 and anti-D8 antisera to induce T-cell clone proliferation was specific for the immunizing cells.[6] In addition, normal or mitogen-activated AKR T cells did not absorb out the mitogenic activity of anti-D10 antiserum. These results suggested that these antisera might be reacting with a variable portion of the T-cell antigen receptor on the appropriate T-cell clone.

Subsequent experiments demonstrated that anti-D10 and anti-D8 antisera would induce T-cell clone proliferation in the absence of accessory cells if the monokine interleukin 1 (IL-1) was added to the culture.[6] This proved to be the basis for a simple screening procedure for a monoclonal antibody possessing the same biological properties as anti-D10 antiserum. An initial attempt to produce a monoclonal anti-D10 antibody using hyperimmunized and rested

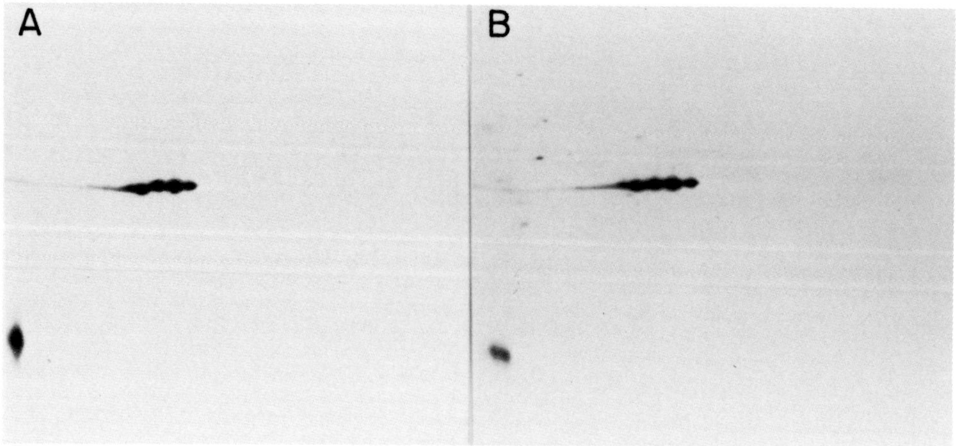

Figure 1. Two-dimensional gel analysis of monoclonal antibody 3D3. (A) 2.5×10^6 3D3 hybridoma cells or (B) a twice recloned subclone, 3D3.D4.C5, were incubated at 37°C with [^{35}S]methionine in 1 ml of medium. After 5 hr, culture supernatant was collected, saturated ammonium sulfate added to 50%, and the precipitate analyzed by nonequilibrium pH gradient electrophoresis (horizontal direction, acid to the left) followed by SDS–PAGE on a 10% polyacrylamide slab gel (vertical direction), both under reducing conditions.

mice was unsuccessful. A second successful fusion used BALB.K mice primed with D10.G4.1 cells in saline and boosted 3 weeks later with the same. Three days later, the immune spleen cells from these mice were fused to P3X63-Ag8.653 cells in polyethylene glycol by standard procedures.[22] The resulting hybridoma cells were screened for the ability of their antibodies to induce D10.G4.1 proliferation in the presence of IL-1 in a 2-day assay. Out of 120 hybridomas obtained from this fusion, one, designated 3D3, was positive in this assay.[6] This hybridoma was subsequently cloned in agar and by the method of limiting dilution with no loss in biological activity. The monoclonality of this hybridoma was verified by two-dimensional gel analysis of biosynthetically labeled culture supernatants as shown in Fig. 1. The single light chain spot and the clonotype of heavy chain spots due to glycosylation is a typical pattern for a monoclonal antibody. Monoclonal antibody 3D3 has been typed as an IgG1κ on the basis of its binding characteristics to protein A[23] and its reaction with isotype-specific antisera.

The binding of monoclonal antibody 3D3 to D10.G4.1 cells can be detected by immunofluorescence as shown in Fig. 2. However, 3D3 does not bind the AKR helper T-cell clone D8,[24] nor AKR lymph node T cells (Fig. 2). The lack of binding of this monoclonal antibody to other T cells is correlated with the inability of the antibody to activate T cells other than the T-cell clone D10.G4.1. The clonotypic nature of this antibody and its ability to mimic antigen and Ia in D10.G4.1 activation strongly suggested that this monoclonal antibody bound a variable portion of the T-cell antigen receptor. The cumulative evidence,

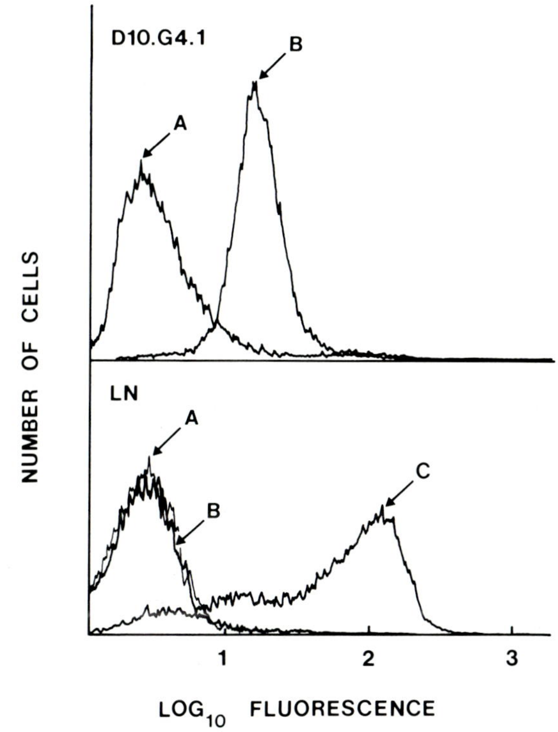

Figure 2. Monoclonal antibody 3D3 binds D10.G4.1 cells but not AKR lymph node cells. (Top) D10.G4.1 cloned T cells or (bottom) AKR lymph node cells were (A) stained with fluorescein-avidin alone (B) or stained with 3D3–biotin followed by fluorescein–avidin. (C) Lymph node cells stained with a monoclonal anti-Thy-1 antibody. Stained cells were analyzed by FACS.

described below, demonstrates that this is indeed the case. Note that antireceptor antibody 3D3 binds essentially all of the cells of the D10.G4.1 T-cell line (Fig. 2), direct evidence for the monoclonality of this cell line.

4. The Biological Activity of a Monoclonal Antireceptor Antibody

4.1. The Role of Growth Factors in Helper T-Cell Activation

The interaction of a helper T lymphocyte with antigen and Ia molecules on the surface of a specialized antigen-presenting cell or a B cell initiates a cascade of events that affects both cell types. Although the initiation of this interaction is a highly specific cell-to-cell interaction, a series of soluble mediators amplify and control subsequent events. The activation of the helper T cell is initially mediated by an autocrine pathway involving the secretion and reception of IL-2.[25] Interleukin 1, produced by macrophages and possibly B cells,[26] is involved in the amplification of these early events.[27] The interaction of IL-2 and its receptor results in a secondary release of lymphokines by the T cell, such as B-cell growth factors[28,29] and interferon gamma,[30] which operate on cells in the local environment. The IL-2:IL-2 receptor interaction also induces expression of transferrin receptors on the T cell,[31] a necessary prerequisite for the subsequent initiation of DNA synthesis and T-cell growth. The study of these complex pathways has been hampered by the necessity for an accessory cell, that is, an Ia-bearing antigen-presenting cell, to activate the T cell via its antigen receptor. Many investigators have circumvented this problem by using mitogenic plant lectins to study T-cell activation. However, while T-cell activation by mitogen and antigen:Ia share many properties, the ability of lectins to bind many different cell surface proteins may not accurately reflect activation via a receptor–ligand interaction. This is not a problem with a monoclonal antibody against the T-cell antigen receptor, in essence a specific, soluble, high-affinity artificial ligand for the receptor. The agonist activity of monoclonal antibody 3D3 has been used to detail the events surrounding the activation of D10.G4.1 helper T cells, as will be described in the following sections.

Anti-D10.G4.1 hybridoma supernatants were initially screened at a concentration of 5% for the ability to induce T-cell clone proliferation. A subsequent titration of 3D3 culture supernatants revealed that this concentration was in great excess; culture supernatants at a dilution of $1:10^5$ had potent activity.[6] Figure 3 shows a titration of purified antibody, demonstrating that the peak induction of D10.G4.1 DNA synthesis is achieved at 1–10 ng/ml of monoclonal antibody. This same concentration of monoclonal antibody also induces D10.G4.1-dependent B-cell proliferation (Fig. 3) and B-cell immunoglobulin secretion.[32] Thus, monoclonal antibody 3D3, by binding to the antigen:Ia receptor, elicits the complete repertoire of helper T-cell functions from cloned D10.G4.1 cells. Also, this antibody does not inhibit activation of D10.G4.1 over a range of concentrations greater than 10^4.

As noted previously, the entry of helper T cells into S phase can be separated into two events: the secretion of the growth factor IL-2 and the expression of surface receptors for IL-2. *In vivo* these events presumably happen in tandem as a result of the interaction of the T cell and an antigen-bearing accessory cell. *In vitro*, however, these events are separable. Monoclonal antibody 3D3 induces IL-2 secretion from D10.G4.1 cells in the absence of any other cell type or exogenous factor (Fig. 4). This finding suggests that the interaction of the T-cell receptor with its natural ligand, antigen and Ia, is also likely to be sufficient to initiate IL-2 secretion. In contrast, some,[33–36] but by no means all,[34,37,38] studies of mitogen activation have suggested that a second signal, IL-1, is required for secretion of IL-2. There are no detectable effects of IL-1 on IL-2 synthesis by D10.G4.1 (Fig. 4). Rather, as described below, the results demonstrate that the primary role of IL-1 in the growth of these helper T cells is to promote the expression of IL-2 receptors.

Although D10.G4.1 cells will secrete IL-2 in the presence of 3D3, they will proliferate only minimally unless accessory cells or IL-1 is added to the culture (Fig. 4). Although homogeneous preparations of IL-1 have not been used, we have verified that the active component of crude preparations is indeed IL-1, by inhibition with specific anti-IL-1 antisera.[39] In the absence of 3D3, D10.G4.1 cells do not respond to IL-1 or the accessory cells. All our evidence suggests

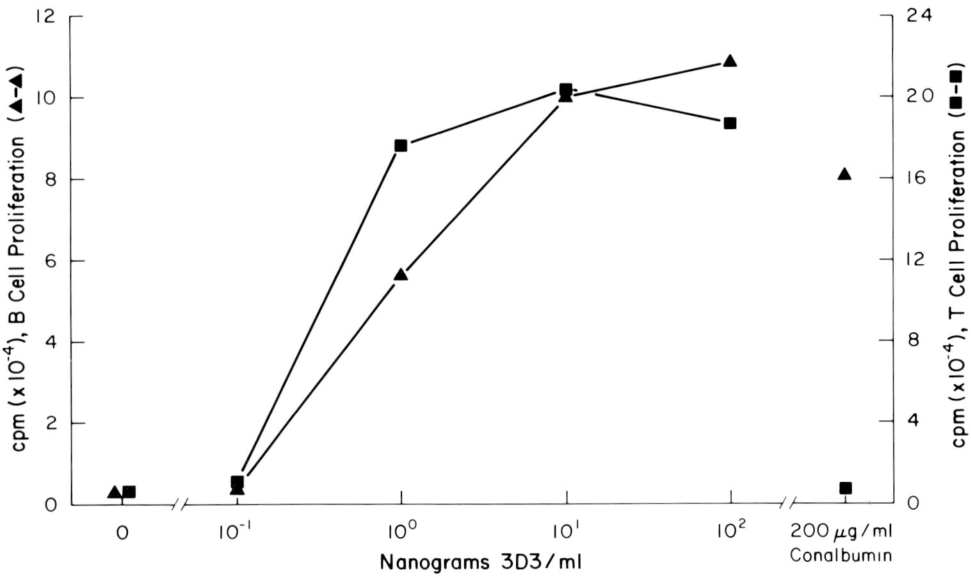

Figure 3. Induction by monoclonal antireceptor antibody 3D3 of D10.G4.1 proliferation and D10.G4.1-dependent B-cell proliferation. (■) D10.G4.1 proliferation measured in a 65-hr assay containing 2×10^4 cloned T cells, 1% of a partially purified IL-1-rich P388D1 supernatant, and various concentrations of 3D3, or 200 μg/ml conalbumin. (▲) B-cell proliferation measured in a 48-hr assay containing 2×10^4 mitomycin C-treated D10.G4.1 cells, 2×10^5 BALB.K B cells (anti-Thy-1 plus complement-treated spleen), and various concentrations of 3D3. Data are expressed as the mean cpm [^{3}H]thymidine incorporation of triplicate cultures. (From Ref. 24 by permission.)

that the accessory cells function solely as a source of IL-1. In our hands, cultured splenic cells produce significant amounts of IL-1. Whether activated D10.G4.1 cells can also induce IL-1 secretion is currently under examination.

Since D10.G4.1 cells activated by 3D3 released significant amounts of IL-2 but did not proliferate in the absence of IL-1, the effects of IL-1 on IL-2 receptor expression were examined. D10.G4.1 cells cultured overnight with 3D3 or IL-1 and stained with a monoclonal anti-IL-2 receptor antibody show no increase in IL-2 receptor expression. However, cells incubated with 3D3 *and* IL-1 exhibit an eightfold increase in the intensity of fluorescent staining with an anti-IL-2 receptor antibody.[39]

Because the IL-1 receptor has not been characterized, it is not known whether 3D3 induces the expression of IL-1 receptors on D10.G4.1 cells, or alternatively, whether IL-1 receptors are constituitively expressed and the effects of IL-1 require perturbation of the antigen receptor as well. In this regard, this system is ideally suited for the attempted isolation of IL-1 receptors, once again by screening for antireceptor monoclonal antibodies in a functional assay. It should also be noted that the IL-1 dependence of D10.G4.1 proliferation in response to 3D3 can be used as a simple and sensitive assay for IL-1.[40] The

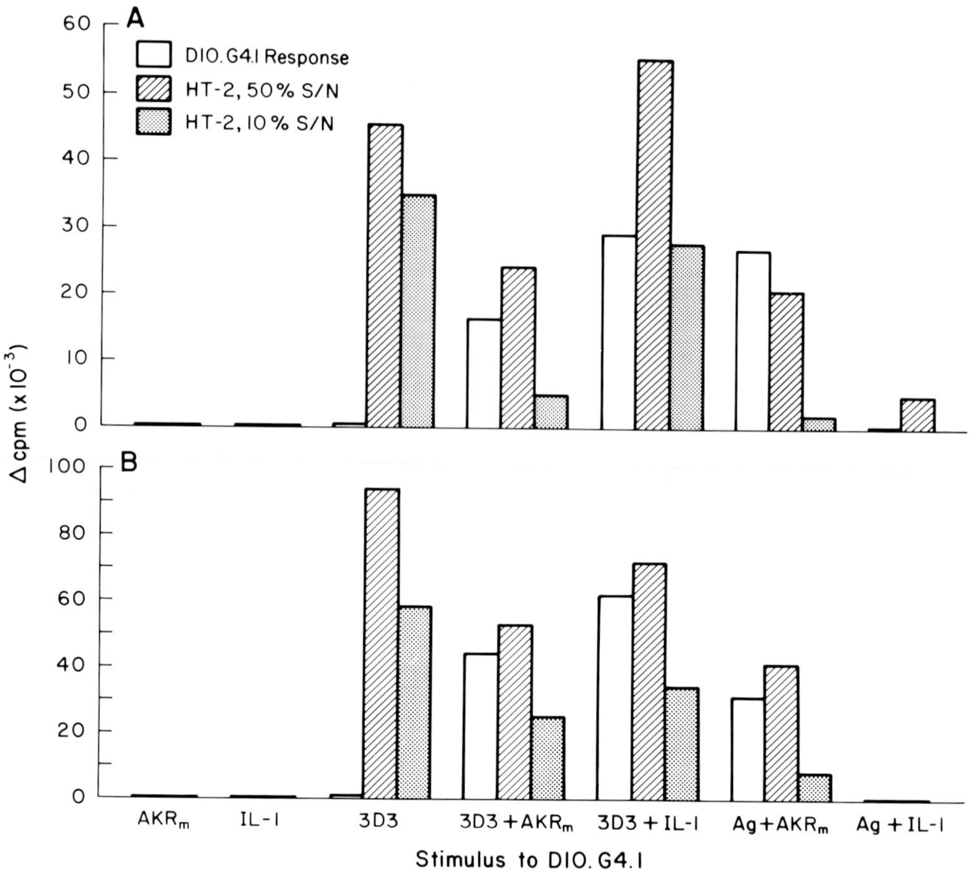

Figure 4. (A, B) Independent experiments showing 3D3 induction of IL-2 production from D10.G4.1 cells, but not their proliferation unless IL-1 or accessory cells are present. D10.G4.1 proliferation (open bars) was measured in a 65-hr assay containing 2×10^4 cloned T cells and various additions (2×10^5 mitomycin C-treated AKR/J spleen cells; 1% IL-1-containing supernatant; 10 ng/ml 3D3; 200 μg/ml conalbumin as antigen, Ag) per 0.2 ml culture. At 48 hr, 100 μl of supernatant per D10.G4.1 culture was removed and assayed for IL-2 by the ability to stimulate HT-2 cell proliferation (1×10^4 HT-2 cells/100 μl culture) in a 24-hr assay at a concentration of 50% (striped bars) or 10% (stipled bars). The cultures were replenished with 100 μl fresh medium and the incubation continued overnight to measure D10.G4.1 proliferation. Data are expressed as mean Δcpm [^{3}H]thymidine incorporation of triplicate cultures. (From Ref. 39 by permission.)

ability to utilize the T-cell mitogens concanavalin A or phytohemagglutinin in place of 3D3 has made this assay generally applicable.

In summary, the interaction of 3D3 and the D10.G4.1 antigen receptor results in the secretion of IL-2 from the T cell. In the presence of IL-1, there is also a significant increase in the surface expression of IL-2 receptors, which correlates with the initiation of DNA synthesis. However, recent results in our laboratory suggest that the regulation of T-cell growth may have further complexities. Although 3D3 induces IL-2 secretion from, but not growth of, D10.G4.1 cells, exogenously supplied IL-2, including recombinant human-derived IL-2, can induce D10.G4.1 cell proliferation, presumably by interaction with a basal level of IL-2 receptors. This paradox appears to be the result of an inhibitory activity in D10.G4.1 culture supernatants that prevents D10.G4.1 growth in the presence of endogenously produced IL-2, but interestingly enough has little or no inhibitory effect on the response of the IL-2 indicator T-cell line HT-2 to IL-2. It is possible that the increased expression of IL-2 receptors on D10.G4.1 cells in the presence of 3D3 and IL-1 is secondary to an alteration in this inhibitory activity. The identification of the molecule responsible for this activity, its mode of action, and the effect of 3D3 and IL-1 on its production are currently under investigation.

4.2. Receptor Aggregation as the Signal for T-Cell Activation

The ability to alter the valency of antibody molecules without altering their specificity allows one to distinguish receptor occupancy from receptor cross-linking as the initiating signal for cell activation. For example, monovalent Fab fragments of anti-thyrotropin receptor antibodies have been reported to mimic hormone action.[41] In contrast, the cross-linking of B-cell antigen receptors with anti-immunoglobulin antibody triggers the B cell, causing a physical association between membrane immunoglobulin and cytoskeletal elements,[42] patching and capping of the membrane immunoglobulin, and B-cell proliferation.[43] Similarly, bivalent but not monovalent antibodies to the C3b receptor on human polymorphonuclear leukocytes induce internalization of that receptor.[44] Downmodulation of receptors following ligand binding has also been reported for the insulin receptor,[45] the epidermal growth factor receptor,[46] and the macrophage Fc receptor,[47] apparently as a result of the enhanced degradation of internalized ligand–receptor complexes.

Overnight activation of D10.G4.1 cells with biotinylated 3D3 also causes a decrease in the expression of antigen:Ia receptors as detected by subsequent staining with 3D3–biotin and fluorescein–avidin.[48] This downmodulation of receptors is not merely secondary to cell activation, since mitogen stimulation of D10.G4.1 cells has no effect on the 3D3 determinant. Similarly, downmodulation of the antigen receptor-associated T3 molecule on human T-cell clones has been reported as a result of the binding of anti-T3 or anti-antigen receptor monoclonal antibodies.[2]

In order to determine the role of receptor cross-linking in the activation of D10.G4.1 cells, a monovalent Fab fragment was prepared from monoclonal antibody 3D3 by papain digestion.[24] Papain coupled to carboxymethylcellulose beads was used to facilitate removal of the enzyme. Monovalent Fab fragments of 3D3 were separated from undigested intact antibody by protein A–Sepharose affinity chromatography. Although concentrations of 3D3 as low as 1 ng/ml can induce proliferation of D10.G4.1 cells in the presence of IL-1, an Fab frag-

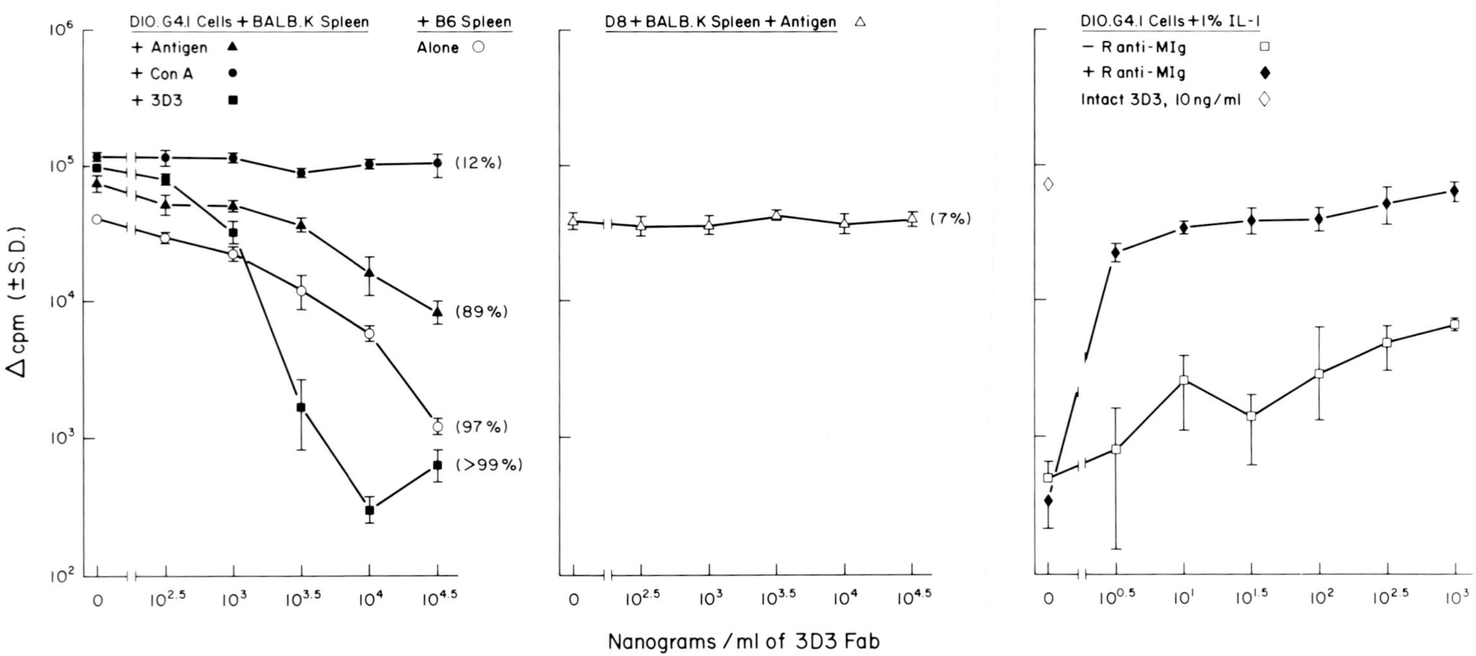

Figure 5. An Fab fragment of monoclonal antibody 3D3 blocks antigen/Ia- but not mitogen-induced activation of D10.G4.1 cells. (Right) D10.G4.1 proliferation measured in a 65-hr assay containing 2×10^4 cloned T cells, 1% of a partially purified IL-1-rich supernatant, and various concentrations of a 3D3 Fab fragment (◆) in the presence or (□) absence of 10 μg/ml affinity-purified rabbit anti-mouse Ig antibody, and for comparison, (◇) in the presence of 10 ng/ml intact 3D3 and 1% IL-1. (Left) D10.G4.1 proliferation measured in an assay containing 2×10^4 cloned T cells 2×10^5 mitomycin C-treated BALB.K (H-2^k) spleen cells, various concentrations of a 3D3 Fab fragment, and (▲) 200 μg/ml conalbumin, (●) 2.5 μg/ml concanavalin A, or (■) 10 ng/ml intact 3D3. (○) D10.G4.1 proliferation assayed in the presence of 2×10^5 mitomycin C-treated C57BL6 (H-2^b) spleen cells and various concentrations of a 3D3 Fab fragment. (Middle) (△) D8 proliferation assayed in a 65-hr assay containing 2×10^4 cloned T cells, 2×10^5 mitomycin C-treated BALB.K spleen cells, 200 μg/ml ovalbumin, and various concentrations of a 3D3 Fab fragment. Parentheses give the percent inhibition of the response for cultures containing 30 μg/ml ($10^{4.5}$ μg/ml) Fab fragment. All data are expressed as the mean Δcpm [^{3}H]thymidine incorporation of triplicate cultures ± SD. (From Ref. 24 by permission.)

ment of 3D3 has no effect even at 1000 times higher concentration (Fig. 5, right panel). A change in the valency of an IgG can radically alter its avidity.[49] However, two observations suggest that the inactivity of the monovalent 3D3 Fab fragment is due to the valency change and not to an inability to bind D10.G4.1 cells: (1) rabbit anti-mouse immunoglobulin antibody can restore the activity of the Fab fragment (Fig. 5, right panel), and (2) at concentrations of Fab fragment that can inhibit responses (see below) and thus bind the T cell, the Fab fragment does not stimulate. Thus, cross-linking of receptors appears to be necessary for 3D3-induced activation of D10.G4.1 cells. Because Ia, and presumably antigen, are expressed in multiple copies on an antigen-presenting cell surface, it is likely that they, too, are capable of aggregating T-cell receptors. It is not expected that a high percentage of the Ia molecules will be complexed with an appropriate fragment of the protein antigen at any given time, and thus it is unlikely that a high percentage of T-cell receptors can be engaged by the antigen-presenting cell. This "spare receptor hypothesis" has precedent with peptide hormones; it has been reported that maximal stimulation can occur at hormone concentrations that result in occupancy of only 1% of the total hormone binding sites.[50]

Other clonotypic monoclonal antireceptor antibodies have been reported to stimulate T-cell activation only when coupled to Sepharose beads, in effect increasing their valency and cross-linking ability.[51,52] Similarly, antagonist anti-hormone receptor antibodies can be converted to agonists in the presence of a second layer anti-immunoglobulin.[14] The unique ability of soluble 3D3 to activate D10.G4.1 cells appears to be an intrinsic property of the cloned T cells and not the monoclonal antibody, since a monoclonal antibody produced by Haskins *et al.*[11] and reactive with a shared T-cell receptor determinant blocks the activation of some T-cell clones but activates D10.G4.1 cells.

Although 3D3 could mimic the action of antigen and Ia, it remained to be demonstrated that the molecule bearing the 3D3 determinant was actually involved in antigen and Ia recognition. Because 3D3 Fab fragments were unable to trigger D10.G4.1 cells but maintained the binding specificity of the intact antibody, they could be used to address this issue. As expected, the Fab fragment of 3D3 completely inhibits D10.G4.1 proliferation induced by the intact monoclonal antibody in the presence of IL-1 or accessory cells (Fig. 5, left panel). Fifty percent inhibition is observed at approximately a 100-fold excess concentration of Fab fragment to the intact antibody. More importantly, an Fab fragment of 3D3 also inhibits, by 90% at 30 μg/ml, D10.G4.1 proliferation in response to antigen and syngeneic antigen-presenting cells (Fig. 5, left panel). In contrast, D10.G4.1 proliferation induced by the mitogenic lectin concanavalin A (Fig. 5, left panel), or by rabbit anti-mouse brain serum[24] (mitogenic by virtue of its interaction with the Thy-1 glycoprotein on D10.G4.1 cells[53]), is not inhibited by 3D3 Fab. An Fab fragment of 3D3 also does not inhibit D8 cell proliferation induced by antigen (Fig. 5, middle panel), consistent with the lack of binding of the monoclonal antibody to D8 helper T cells.[24]

4.3. Interaction of the Antigen Receptor with Allogeneic Ia Molecules: Use of Monovalent Fab Fragments of Antireceptor Monoclonal Antibodies as Probes of Receptor Affinity

The identification and subsequent characterization of the major histocompatibility complex was a consequence of the study of two nonphysiological T-cell-mediated phenomena: graft rejection and the *in vitro* mixed lymphocyte reaction. These phenomena are the result of recognition of allogeneic MHC antigens by T cells. When compared to the frequency of T cells that respond to a given foreign protein antigen, the frequency of T cells that will respond to a particular allogeneic MHC difference is extremely high.[54–56] The analysis of cloned T-cell lines has demonstrated that the high frequency of alloreactive T cells in mixed populations is the result of a relatively frequent cross-reaction of antigen-specific, self MHC-restricted T cells with allogeneic MHC antigens.[18,19] D10.G4.1 cells display this property and can be activated by conalbumin in conjunction with I-A^k glycoproteins or by I-A^b glycoproteins in the absence of conalbumin (Table I). An Fab fragment of monoclonal antibody 3D3 blocks the proliferation D10.G4.1 cells in response to I-A^b-bearing cells as well as to conalbumin and I-A^k (Fig. 5, left panel). This is the first direct demonstration that the receptor that mediates recognition of antigen and self Ia also mediates recognition of allogeneic Ia antigens. Approximately a twofold higher concentration of 3D3 Fab fragment is necessary to cause 50% inhibition of the response of D10.G4.1 cells to conalbumin and I-A^k as compared to the concentration necessary to inhibit by 50% the D10.G4.1 activation induced by I-A^b. These results suggest that the D10.G4.1 receptor has a lower affinity for I-A^b than for conalbumin and I-A^k. As mentioned above, one would not expect a high percentage of the Ia molecules on an antigen-presenting cell to be complexed with the appropriate fragment of antigen at any given moment. However, all of the Ia molecules on an allogeneic antigen-presenting cell may be capable of acting as a ligand for the T-cell receptor on an alloreactive T cell. Given that receptor aggregation appears to be the primary signal for T-cell activation, we have proposed[24] that alloreactivity is a low-affinity cross-reaction of the antigen:Ia receptor with a ligand in high multiplicity, while the physiological interaction of the T cell with antigen and self Ia is the result of a higher affinity interaction of the receptor with a ligand at low multiplicity.

These results also illustrate the potential application of blocking studies using Fab antireceptor antibody fragments in determining the relative affinity of the receptor for diverse ligands. This is especially valuable when ligands are complex or not available in pure form, as in this case.

5. Structural Analysis of the T-Cell Antigen:MHC Receptor

The specificity of monoclonal antibodies has made them of widespread use for affinity purification. However, despite their antigen specificity, "nonspecific" protein–protein interactions or the presence of immunoglobulin binding proteins, such as Fc receptors, can thwart attempts to use antibodies as a means for one-step purification. Nevertheless, immunoprecipitation analysis has become a standard, relatively simple means for the identification and characterization of cell proteins. In my hands, antibodies coupled to Sepharose beads have yielded more specific immunoprecipitations than two-step procedures, such as the isolation of antibody–antigen complexes with insoluble forms of protein A. Extensive preclearing of cell lysates with inappropriate antibodies on Sepharose also enhances immunoprecipitation specificity. Finally, I have found it extremely useful, especially for immunoprecipitation from biosynthetically labeled cells, to block nonspecific interactions with an unlabeled lysate of an inappropriate cell type. For example, immunoprecipitation of the T-cell antigen receptor in the presence of an unlabeled B-cell tumor lysate greatly enhances specificity. This technique is generally applicable in any system in which a cell type exists that does not express the relevant protein. However, one must be cautious that the protein in question is not expressed cytoplasmically as well as lacking on the cell surface. In addition, there is the danger that one may fail to detect associated proteins that may be shared between cell types although the protein under initial study is not. These potential problems can be easily overcome by performing immunoprecipitations in the presence and absence of the blocking lysate, in combination with careful comparisons with control immunoprecipitates.

The T-cell antigen:MHC receptor has now been identified on various cytolytic or helper, human or murine, T-cell clones, hybrids, or tumors by immunoprecipitation with monoclonal antireceptor antibodies. There is universal agreement that the receptor is a disulfide-linked heterodimer of 80–90 kD, composed of an acidic (or α) chain and a basic (or β) chain.[1–5,8,9] I have characterized the antigen:Ia receptor on D10.G4.1 helper T cells using monoclonal antibody 3D3.[24] Immunoprecipitations with monoclonal antibody 3D3 from detergent lysates of surface iodinated D10.G4.1 cells followed by two-dimensional gel analysis have demonstrated that the receptor on these cells is a disulfide-linked heterodimer comprised of a 42-kD α chain and a 42-kD β chain. Charge microheterogeneity has been observed for both cell surface receptor chains.

The two-dimensional gel pattern obtained from 3D3 immunoprecipitates of D10.G4.1 cells biosynthetically labeled with [^{35}S]methionine (Fig. 6) or [^{35}S]cysteine is more complex. The major internal form of the receptor α chain is 38 kD, a precursor of the 42-kD surface α chain as demonstrated by pulse-chase experiments. Other minor internal forms of the α chain can be detected with molecular weights as low as 35,000. Given that these minor forms are more acidic than the major internal pool of α chains, it is likely that they are directly converted to higher molecular weight surface chains. The β chain also exists in several forms distinguishable by charge and apparent molecular weight (Fig. 6), although precursor–product relationships between these forms could not be determined by pulse-chase experiments. No internal monomeric pools of α or β chains have been detected.

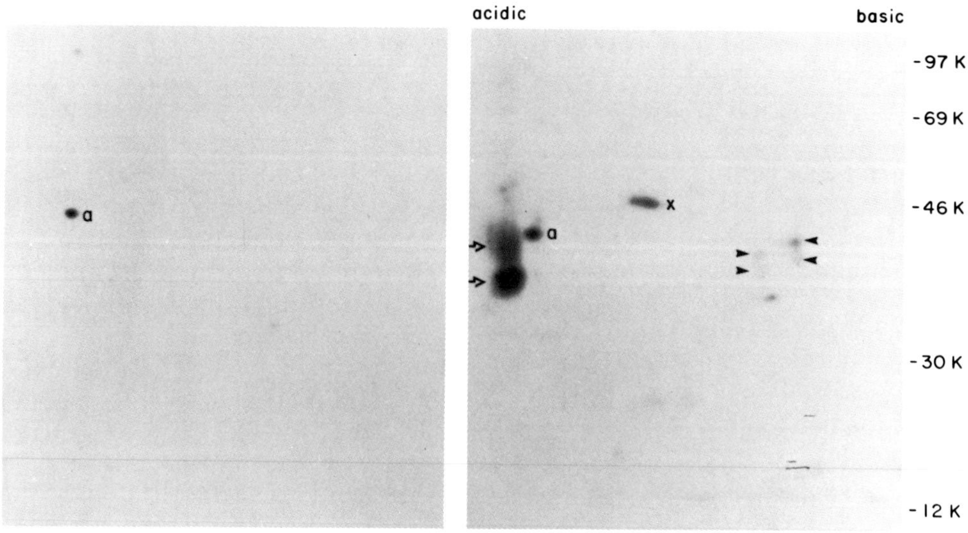

Figure 6. Identification of internal and surface forms of the D10.G4.1 antigen: Ia receptor. D10.G4.1 cells were labeled with [^{35}S]methionine for 4 hr, lysed in NP40, and immunoprecipitated with (left) a control monoclonal antibody (Y3P, anti-Ia) or (right) 3D3. Immunoprecipitates were analyzed under reducing conditions as in Fig. 1. Acidic (open arrows) and basic components (closed arrows) of the heterodimer are indicated. Actin (a) has been identified based on electrophoretic mobility in both dimensions, and X denotes material believed to be nonspecifically precipitated in this experiment. (From Ref. 24 by permission.)

The microheterogeneity of the D10.G4.1 α and β chains is almost entirely due to N-linked glycosylation. Two-dimensional gel analysis of 3D3 immunoprecipitates of cells labeled in the presence of tunicamycin, an inhibitor of asparagine-linked carbohydrate, reveals a single 31-kD β-chain spot and two 31-kD α-chain spots that differ only slightly in charge.[57]

Other investigators have compared the receptor on different cloned T-cell lines or T-cell hybrids and directly demonstrated the presence of variable and constant peptides.[3,58,59] The β chain of the human or murine T-cell antigen: MHC receptor has recently been demonstrated to be encoded by V, D, J, and C region genes, analogous to those of immunoglobulin heavy chain genes.[60,61] Isolated β-chain cDNAs encode a mature protein of approximately 32 kD,[62,63] in close agreement with the size of the D10.G4.1 receptor β-chain immunoprecipitated in the presence of tunicamycin. Recently, a putative α-chain gene has been identified from a cloned murine cytolytic T-cell line.[63] Surprisingly, there are no potential N-linked glycosylation sites, whereas the D10.G4.1 α chain is clearly N-glycosylated.[57] More recently, a different gene has been isolated. It is a better candidate for the α subunit gene, because it contains potential N-glycosylation sites.[64,65]

6. Conclusions

T-Cell antigen recognition is a cell-to-cell interaction involving a number of cell surface proteins on the T cell as well as on the antigen-bearing cell. The production of antireceptor monoclonal antibodies in a situation where the receptor ligand is in essence another cell was central to the identification and biochemical characterization of the specific T-cell antigen:MHC receptor protein. The recent advances in knowledge of the protein structure as well as the gene structure of this receptor have now set the stage for detailed analysis of structure–function relationships of T-cell antigen recognition and for analysis of the development of the self restricted T-cell repertoire.

Just as important, however, is the ability of some antireceptor antibodies to mimic the action of the natural ligand and thus serve as specific probes of cell activation. The regulation of the autocrine pathway of T-cell activation is of particular interest, since such pathways may be particularly susceptible to disruption leading to the self-sustaining growth of the transformed cell. The finding that cellular homologues of viral oncogenes in two instances encode growth factors[66] or their receptors[67] has further emphasized the importance of understanding the molecular events of normal cellular growth and differentiation. Monoclonal antibodies hold great potential in this regard.

ACKNOWLEDGMENTS. The author would like to thank Dr. C. A. Janeway, Jr. for his support and input into this work, and Laurie Hauer for typing the manuscript. The author was initially supported by NIH grant T32-AI-07019 and subsequently by NIH grant CA-29606.

References

1. Allison, J. P., McIntyre, B. W., and Bloch, D., 1982, Tumor-specific antigen of murine T-lymphoma defined with monoclonal antibody, *J. Immunol.* **129:**2293–2300.
2. Meuer, S. C., Fitzgerald, K. A., Hussey, R. E., Hodgdon, J. C., Schlossman, S. F., and Reinherz, E. L., 1983, Clonotypic structures involved in antigen-specific human T cell function, *J. Exp. Med.* **157:**705–719.
3. Acuto, O., Hussey, R. E., Fitzgerald, K. A., Protentis, J. P., Meuer, S. C., Schlossman, S. F., and Reinherz, E. L., 1983, The human T cell receptor: Appearance in ontogeny and biochemical relationship of alpha and beta subunits on IL-2 dependent clones and T cell tumors, *Cell* **34:**717–726.
4. Bigler, R. D., Fisher, D. E., Wang, C. Y., Rinnooy Kan, E. A., and Kunkel, H. G., 1983, Idiotype-like molecules on cells of a human T cell leukemia, *J. Exp. Med.* **158:**1000–1005.
5. Haskins, K., Kubo, R., White, J., Pigeon, M., Kapler, J., and Marrack, P., 1983, The major histocompatibility complex-restricted antigen receptor on T cells. I. Isolation with a monoclonal antibody, *J. Exp. Med.* **157:**1149–1169.
6. Kaye, J., Porcelli, S., Tite, J., Jones, B., and Janeway, C. A., Jr., 1983, Both a monoclonal antibody and antisera specific for determinants unique to individual cloned helper T cell lines can substitute for antigen and antigen-presenting cells in the activation of T cells, *J. Exp. Med.* **158:**836–856.

7. Sanchez-Madrid, F., Krensky, A. M., Ware, C. F., Robbins, E., Strominger, J. L., Burakoff, S. J., and Springer, T. A., 1982, Three distinct antigens associated with human T-lymphocyte mediated cytolysis: LFA-1, LFA-2, and LFA-3, *Proc. Natl. Acad. Sci. USA* **79:**7489–7493.
8. Samelson, L. E., Germain, R. N., and Schwartz, R. H., 1983, Monoclonal antibodies against the antigen receptor on a cloned T cell hybrid, *Proc. Natl. Acad. Sci. USA* **80:**6972–6976.
9. Staerz, U. D., Pasternack, M. S., Klein, J. R., Benedetto, J. D., and Bevan, M. J., 1984, Monoclonal antibodies specific for a murine cytotoxic T lymphocyte clone, *Proc. Natl. Acad. Sci. USA* **81:**1799–1803.
10. McIntyre, B. W., and Allison, J. P., 1983, The mouse T cell receptor: Structural heterogeneity of molecules of normal T cells defined by xenoantiserum, *Cell* **34:**739–746.
11. Haskins, K., Hannum, C., White, J., Roehm, N., Kubo, R., Kappler, J., and Marrack, P., 1984, The antigen-specific, major histocompatibility complex-restricted receptor on T cells. VI. An antibody to a receptor allotype, *J. Exp. Med.* **160:**452–471.
12. Brenner, M. B., Trowbridge, I. S., McLean, J., and Strominger, J. L., 1984, Identification of shared antigenic determinants of the putative human T lymphocyte antigen receptor, *J. Exp. Med.* **160:**541–551.
13. Leonard, W. J., Depper, J. M., Uchiyama, T., Smith, K. A., Waldmann, T. A., and Greene, W. C., 1982, A monoclonal antibody that appears to recognize the receptor for human T cell growth factor; partial characterization of the receptor, *Nature* **300:**267–269.
14. Podesta, E. J., Solano, A. R., Attar, R., Sanchez, M. L., and Molina Y Vedia, L., 1983, Receptor aggregation induced by antilutropin receptor antibody and biological response in rat testis Leydig cells, *Proc. Natl. Acad. Sci. USA* **80:**3986–3990.
15. Jacobs, S., Chang, K.-J., and Cuatrecasas, P., 1978, Antibodies to purified insulin receptor have insulin-like activity, *Science* **200:**1283–1284.
16. Leiber, D., Harbon, S., Guillet, J.-G., Andre, C., and Strosberg, A. D., 1984, Monoclonal antibodies to purified muscarinic receptor display agonist-like activity, *Proc. Natl. Acad. Sci. USA* **81:**4331–4334.
17. Schreiber, A. B., Lax, I., Yarden, Y., Eshhar, Z., and Schlessinger, J., 1981, Monoclonal antibodies against receptors for epidermal growth factor induce early and delayed effects of epidermal growth factor, *Proc. Natl. Acad. Sci. USA* **12:**7535–7539.
18. Sredni, B., and Schwartz, R. H., 1981, Antigen specific proliferating T lymphocyte clones. Methodology, specificity, MHC restriction and alloreactivity, *Immunol. Rev.* **54:**187–223.
19. Janeway, C. A., Jr., Lerner, E. A., Conrad, P. J., and Jones, B., 1982, The precision of self and non-self major histocompatibility complex encoded antigen recognition by cloned T cells, *Behring Inst. Mitt.* **70:**200–209.
20. Jones, B., and Janeway, C. A., Jr., 1981, Cooperative interaction of B lymphocytes with antigen-specific helper T lymphocytes is MHC restricted, *Nature* **292:**547–549.
21. Bottomly, K., Jones, B., Kaye, J., and Jones, F., III, 1983, Subpopulations of B cells distinguished by cell surface expression of Ia antigens. Correlation of Ia and idiotype during activation by cloned Ia-restricted T cells, *J. Exp. Med.* **158:**265–279.
22. Lerner, E. A., 1981, How to make a hybridoma, *Yale J. Biol. Med.* **54:**387–402.
23. Ey, P. L., Prowse, S. J., and Jenkin, C. R., 1978, Isolation of pure IgG1, IgG2a and IgG2b immunoglobulins from mouse serum using protein A Sepharose, *Immunochemistry* **15:**429–436.
24. Kaye, J., and Janeway, C. A., Jr., 1984, The Fab fragment of a directly activating monoclonal antibody that precipitates a disulfide-linked heterodimer from a helper T cell clone blocks activation by either allogeneic Ia or antigen and self-Ia, *J. Exp. Med.* **159:**1397–1412.
25. Cantrell, D. A., and Smith, K. A., 1983, Transient expression of interleukin 2 receptors: Consequences for T cell growth, *J. Exp. Med.* **158:**1895–1911.
26. Scala, G., Kuang, Y. D., Hall, R. E., Muchmore, A. V., and Oppenheim, J. J., 1984, Accessory cell function of human B cells. I. Production of both interleukin 1-like activity and an interleukin 1 inhibitory factor by an EBV-transformed human B cell line, *J. Exp. Med.* **159:**1637–1652.
27. Mizel, S. B., and Ben-Zvi, Amos, 1980, Studies on the role of lymphocyte-activating factor (interleukin 1) in antigen-induced lymph node lymphocyte proliferation, *Cell. Immunol.* **54:**382–389.

28. Howard, M., Matis, L., Malek, T. R., Shevach, E., Kell, W., Cohen, D., Nakanishi, K., and Paul, W. E., 1983, Interleukin 2 induces antigen-reactive T cell lines to secrete BCGF-I, *J. Exp. Med.* **158:**2024–2039.
29. Inaba, K., Granelli-Piperno, A., and Steinman, R. M., 1983, Dendritic cells induce T lymphocytes to release B cell-stimulating factors by an interleukin 2-dependent mechanism, *J. Exp. Med.* **158:**2040–2057.
30. Kasahara, T., Hooks, J. J., Dougherty, S. F., and Oppenheim, J. J., 1983, Interleukin 2-mediated immune interferon (IFN-γ) production by human T cells and T cell subsets, *J. Immunol.* **130:**1784–1789.
31. Neckers, L. M., and Cossman, J., 1983, Transferrin receptor induction in mitogen-stimulated human T lymphocytes is required for DNA synthesis and cell division and is regulated by interleukin 2, *Proc. Natl. Acad. Sci. USA* **80:**3494–3498.
32. Tite, J. P., Kaye, J., and Jones, B., 1984, The role of B cell surface Ia antigen recognition by T cells in B cell triggering. Analysis of the interaction of cloned helper T cells with normal B cells in differing states of activation and with B cells expressing the *xid* defect, *Eur. J. Immunol.* **14:**553–561.
33. Smith, K. A., Lachman, L. B., Oppenheim, J. J., and Favata, M. F., 1980, The functional relationship of the interleukins, *J. Exp. Med.* **151:**1551–1556.
34. Gillis, S., and Mizel, S. B., 1981, T-cell lymphoma model for the analysis of interleukin 1-mediated T-cell activation, *Proc. Natl. Acad. Sci. USA* **78:**1133–1137.
35. Rock, K. R., 1982, The role of Ia molecules in the activation of T lymphocytes. I. The activation of an IL 1-dependent IL 2-producing T cell hybridoma by con A requires an interaction, which is not H-2 restricted, with an Ia-bearing accessory cell, *J. Immunol.* **129:**1360–1366.
36. Smith, K. A., 1984, Lymphokine regulation of T cell and B cell function, in: *Fundamental Immunology* (W. E. Paul, ed.), Raven Press, New York, pp. 559–576.
37. Harwell, L., Skidmore, B., Marrack, P., and Kappler, J., 1980, Concanavalin A-inducible, interleukin-2-producing T cell hybridoma, *J. Exp. Med.* **152:**893–904.
38. Gillis, S., and Watson, J., 1980, Biochemical and biological characterization of lymphocyte regulatory molecules. V. Identification of an interleukin 2-producing human leukemia T cell line. *J. Exp. Med.* **152:**1709–1719.
39. Kaye, J., Gillis, S., Mizel, S. B., Shevach, E. M., Malek, T. R., Dinarello, C. A., Lachman, L. B., and Janeway, C. A., Jr., 1984, Growth of a cloned helper T cell line induced by a monoclonal antibody specific for the antigen receptor: Interleukin 1 is required for the expression of receptors for interleukin 2, *J. Immunol.* **133:**1339–1345.
40. Kaye, J., and Janeway, C. A., Jr., 1984, Induction of receptors for interleukin 2 requires T cell Ag:Ia receptor crosslinking and interleukin 1, *Lymphokine Res.* **3:**175–182.
41. Rees Smith, B., Pyle, G. A., Petersen, V. B., Hall, R., 1977, Interaction of thyroid-stimulating antibodies with the human thyrotropin receptor, *J. Endocrinol.* **75:**401–407.
42. Braun, J., Hochman, P. S., and Unanue, E. R., 1982, Ligand-induced association of surface immunoglobulin and detergent-insoluble cytoskeletal matrix of the B lymphocyte, *J. Immunol.* **128:**1198–1204.
43. Sieckmann, D. G., Asofsky, R., Mosier, D. E., Zitron, I. M., and Paul, W. E., 1978, Activation of mouse lymphocytes by anti-immunoglobulin. I. Parameters of the proliferative response, *J. Exp. Med.* **147:**814–829.
44. Fearon, D. T., Kaneko, I., and Thomson, G. G., 1981, Membrane distribution and adsorptive endocytosis by C3b receptors on human polymorphonuclear leukocytes, *J. Exp. Med.* **153:**1615–1628.
45. Kasuga, M., Kahn, C. R., Hedo, J. A., Obberghen, E. V., and Yamada, K. M., 1981, Insulin-induced receptor loss in cultured human lymphocytes is due to accelerated receptor degradation, *Proc. Natl. Acad. Sci. USA* **78:**6917–6921.
46. Carpenter, G., and Cohen, S., 1976, ^{125}I-Labelled human epidermal growth factor. Binding, internalization, and degradation in human fibroblasts, *J. Cell. Biol.* **71:**159–171.
47. Mellman, I. S., Unkeless, J., Steinman, R. M., and Cohn, Z. A., 1983, Selective internalization and degradation of macrophage Fc receptors during receptor mediated phagocytosis, *J. Cell. Biol.* **96:**887–895.

48. Kaye, J., Jones, B., and Janeway, C. A., Jr., 1984, The structure and function of T cell receptor complexes, *Immunol. Rev.* **81:**40–63.
49. Ways, J. P., and Parham, P., 1983, The binding of monoclonal antibodies to cell surface molecules. A quantitative analysis with immunoglobulin G against two alloantigenic determinants of the human transplantation antigen HLA-A2, *Biochem. J.* **216:**423–432.
50. Medelson, C., Dufau, M., and Catt, K., 1975, Gonadotropin binding and stimulation of cyclic adenosine 3′:5′ monophosphate and testosterone production in isolated Leydig cells, *J. Biol. chem.* **250:**8818–8823.
51. Meuer, S. C., Hodgdon, J. C., Hussey, R. E., Protentis, J. P., Schlossman, S. F., and Reinherz, E. L., 1983, Antigen-like effects of monoclonal antibodies directed at receptors on human T cell clones, *J. Exp. Med.* **158:**988–993.
52. Kappler, J., Kubo, R., Haskins, K., White, J., and Marrack, P., 1983, The mouse T cell receptor: Comparison of MHC-restricted receptors on two T cell hybridomas, *Cell* **34:**727–737.
53. Jones, B., 1983, Evidence that the Thy-1 molecule is the target for T cell mitogenic antibody against brain-associated antigens, *Eur. J. Immunol.* **13:**678–684.
54. Simonsen, M., 1968, The clonal selection hypothesis evaluated by grafted cells reacting against their hosts, *Cold Spring Harbor Symp. Quant. Biol.* **32:**517–523.
55. Lindahl, K. F., and Wilson, D. B., 1977, Histocompatibility antigen-activated cytotoxic T lymphocytes. II. Estimates of the frequency and specificity of precursors, *J. Exp. Med.* **145:**508–522.
56. Kronke, M., Scheurich, P., Pfizenmaier, K., Rollinghoff, M., and Wagner, H., 1982, T–T Cell interactions during *in vitro* cytotoxic T lymphocyte responses. V. Precursor frequencies and specificity of alloreactive helper T cells, *J. Exp. Med.* **156:**41–54.
57. Kaye, J., and Janeway, C. A., Jr., 1984, The α and β subunits of a murine T cell antigen/Ia receptor have a molecular weight of 31,000 in the absence of N-linked glycosylation, *J. Immunol.* **135:**1–3.
58. Kappler, J., Kubo, R., Haskins, K., Hannum, C., Marrack, P., Pigeon, M., McIntyre, B., Allison, J., and Trowbridge, I., 1983, The major histocompatibility complex-restricted antigen receptor on T cells in mouse and man: Identification of constant and variable peptides, *Cell* **35:**295–302.
59. Reinherz, E. L., Meuer, S. C., Fitzgerald, A., Hussey, R. E., Hodgdon, J. C., Acuto, O., and Schlossman, S. F., 1983, Comparison of T3-associated 49- and 43-kilodalton cell surface molecules on individual human T-cell clones: Evidence for peptide variability in T cell receptor structures, *Proc. Natl. Acad. Sci. USA* **80:**4104–4108.
60. Chien, Y.-H., Gascogne, N. R. J., Kavaler, J., Lee, N. E., and Davis, M. M., 1984, Somatic recombination in a murine T cell receptor gene, *Nature* **309:**322–326.
61. Siu, G., Clark, S. P., Yoshikai, Y., Malissen, M., Yanagi, Y., Strauss, E., Mak, T. W., and Hood, L., 1984, The human T cell antigen receptor is encoded by variable, diversity, and joining gene segments that rearrange to generate a complete V gene, *Cell* **37:**393–401.
62. Hedrick, S. M., Nielsen, E. A., Kavaler, J., Cohen, D. I., and Davis, M. M., 1984, Sequence relationships between putative T cell receptor polypeptides and immunoglobulins, *Nature* **308:**153–158.
63. Saito, H., Kranz, D. M., Takagaki, Y., Hayday, A. C., Eisen, H. N., and Tonegawa, S., 1984, Complete primary structure of a heterodimer T cell receptor deduced from cDNA sequences, *Nature* **309:**757–762.
64. Chien, Y., Becker, D. M., Lindsten, T., Okamura, M., Cohen, D. I., and Davis, M. M., 1984, A third type of murine T-cell receptor gene, *Nature* **312:**31–35.
65. Saito, H., Kranz, D. M., Takagaki, Y., Hayday, A. C., Eisen, H. N., and Tonegawa, S., 1984, A third rearranged and expressed gene in a clone of cytotoxic T lymphocytes, *Nature* **312:**36–40.
66. Deuel, T. F., Huang, J. S., Huang, S. S., Stroobant, P., and Waterfield, M. D., 1983, Expression of a platelet-derived growth factor-like protein in simian sarcoma virus transformed cells, *Science* **221:**1348–1350.
67. Downward, J., Yarden, Y., Mayes, E., Scrace, G., Totty, N., Stockwell, P., Ullrich, A., Schlessinger, J., and Waterfield, M. D., 1984, Close similarity of epidermal growth factor receptor and v-*erb*-B oncogene protein sequences, *Nature* **307:**521–527.

Chapter 33

Functional T-Cell Hybridomas

KENNETH L. ROCK

1. Introduction

A significant technical advance in the field of immunology is the ability to isolate homogeneous and monospecific populations of lymphocytes. Among the several methodologies that have been employed, somatic cell hybridization is proving to be a powerful tool in the isolation and characterization of T-lymphocyte clones. The technique of cell fusion is similar to that used to generate monoclonal antibodies. However, the initial lymphocyte selection as well as the identification and characterization of hybridomas differ considerably. Once derived, the T-cell hybridomas are useful, sometimes uniquely so, for a wide range of applications.

This chapter provides an overview of both the methods and applications of T-cell hybridoma technology. The methods reviewed include the initial selection and fusion of T cells as well as the subsequent screening, passage, cloning, and storage of hybrids. Where possible, general strategies are covered.

The potential applications of T-cell hybrids are illustrated with examples from a variety of experimental systems. The various distinct types of T cells that have been immortalized are reviewed. Their use in the generation of T-cell products is discussed, as is their application to basic immunologic problems. Other examples cover the analysis of the lymphocyte membrane and the use of mutant or variant hybrid clones.

2. Methodology

2.1. A Comparison of Normal Clones versus Hybrid Clones

Two strategies have been employed to generate clonal populations of T lymphocytes. The first is to propagate normal T cells via the physiological signals that stimulate and maintain proliferation.[1–4] The second is to immortalize T lymphocytes by malignant transformation. This has been accomplished

KENNETH L. ROCK • Department of Pathology, Harvard Medical School, Boston, Massachusetts 02115.

by direct transformation in a few cases[5] and more generally through somatic cell hybridization to malignant T-cell tumors. This latter approach is the subject of the current chapter. However, at the outset it should be emphasized that both strategies have their advantages and disadvantages. These general properties should be considered by the investigator in choosing the optimal technology for a particular experimental system.

A comparison of several general properties of T-cell hybridomas vs. normal T-cell clones is outlined below. Both types of T-cell lines have variable stability, although the nature of the instability is different for each. T-Cell hybridomas are karyotypically unstable.[6] These cells will continue to grow, but may lose immunologic activity, presumably due to chromosomal loss. Strategies to overcome this problem are outlined below. On the other hand, T-cell clones are karyotypically stable but may undergo "crisis" periods where they grow poorly or die. Aside from these periods, function is usually maintained, especially when functional activity is selected during passage, i.e., via serial restimulation. Clones that are maintained solely in growth factor may also lose activity with time.

T-Cell hybridomas have a number of favorable growth characteristics relative to normal clones.[7] First, these cells easily grow in standard tissue culture media supplemented solely with fetal calf serum. In contrast, normal clones are highly fastidious and require growth factors (e.g., interleukin 2) and/or restimulation with antigen and filler cells. Additional manipulation of the normal clones may be required, e.g., isolation on density gradients. Second, T-cell hybridomas grow to a density of $(1-1.5) \times 10^6$ cells/ml, while normal clones may only achieve maximum densities of tenfold less and growth may be erratic. Therefore, to generate comparable cell yields, considerably more media and constituents (e.g., antigen and growth factors) are required. Cell numbers of over 10^8 may be difficult to achieve with normal clones. Third, T-cell hybrids can be available daily. Normal clones may only be usable at a particular point in the restimulation cycle, e.g., 14 days poststimulation.[1] In this case, cells would only be available for experimentation once every 2 weeks or multiple passes must be maintained. Fourth, hybridomas are easily frozen and recovered. Some laboratories have had success with recovering normal clones from frozen storage, but in general, this has been difficult. Finally, "normal" clones may in fact have abnormalities.[8]

Taken together, the requirements of hybridomas relative to clones for culture conditions, passage, cell numbers, and storage, are highly favorable. However, the hybridomas are not well suited for all experimental systems. They cannot be used in direct proliferative assays, since they are autonomously growing. This eliminates a very direct and simple measure of T-cell activation that may be more sensitive and measure additional activation events than lymphokine assays. There is the potential for contributions of two genomes to a particular activity or phenotype, and in general T-cell hybridomas may be a poor model for resting T cells.[7] Additionally, their malignant nature as well as histocompatibility constraints will limit their usefullness for *in vivo* experiments. Finally, optimal tumor parents are not available in all species (see

Section 2.3). Normal clones would appear to circumvent several of these limitations, although any cultured clonal population may have *in vivo* limitations (e.g., lack appropriate receptors[9]).

2.2. Normal T Cell for Fusion

Before reviewing the methodology for T-cell hybridization, it is essential to consider the diversity of T lymphocytes. The T-cell compartment is considerably more heterogeneous than that of B lymphocytes. This heterogeneity encompasses differences in function, surface phenotype, specificity, and physiology. These differences must be considered in devising an optimal strategy for the fusion and identification of any particular cell type. Therefore, a brief overview of the various T-cell subsets will be presented.

The T lymphocytes can be roughly divided into three compartments. The first is T inducer (helper) cells. This class of cells mediates a variety of activities that tend to activate or help responses of other cells. Included in these activities is "help" for both B cells and T cells, lymphokine production, proliferation, macrophage activation, and delayed-type sensitivity. Several of these activities may be mediated by the same cell, although there is some evidence to suggest cases of functional segregation. These cells corecognize foreign antigens (protein or haptens) in association with major histocompatibility complex (MHC) class II gene products (Ia molecules) on the surface of Ia-bearing cells (macrophages, dendritic cells, and B lymphocytes). Alternatively, T inducer cells can respond to foreign (allogeneic) Ia molecules. In addition to the triggering of their antigen/MHC receptor, these cells may also require additional hormonal-like factors for activation. These factors include interleukin 1 (IL-1; monocyte-derived) and IL-2 (which the inducer cell both produces and consumes). The activated or effector state of these cells is transient. In addition to pan-T-cell markers, these cells are distinguished by the expression of L3T4 (mouse) or T4 (human).

The second subset of T cells are cytotoxic T lymphocytes (CTL). These cells bind to and lyse their target cells. Their specificity is for viral or hapten antigens in association with class I MHC molecules. Alternatively, CTLs can respond to allogeneic class I molecules on a cell surface. A specialized antigen-presenting cell has not been defined. In addition to the triggering of the antigen/MHC receptor on these cells, they require soluble factors (IL-2 and possibly cytotoxic differentiation factor, both T-inducer cell-derived) for activation. Once activated, the duration of the effector state is not well defined, but in some cases lytic activity may be sustained. Classically, these cells bear the Lyt-2 (mouse) or T8 (human) antigens on their surface. There are rare exceptions to these phenotypes, for example, L3T4/T4 bearing CTLs with specificity for class II MHC molecules as well as helper-cell-independent, lymphokine-producing CTL.

The third set of T lymphocytes are the suppressor T cells (Ts). These cells function to down regulate immune responses of B cells or other T lymphocytes. In the most intensively studied systems, there appear to be at least three Ts cells (Ts_1, Ts_2, and Ts_3) interacting in a cascadelike pathway. Their specificity is incompletely understood. They appear capable of binding free antigen. It has been suggested that at least some Ts cells have additional specificity for MHC controlled determinants (I-J) whose expression is on suppressor cells. Once activated, the effector function of these cells may be sustained. The cell surface phenotype is distinct for each member of the suppressor pathways.

2.2.2. T-Cell Selection for Fusion

The potential for the successful isolation of hybrid clones will depend on both the ease of hybrid detection and the frequency of the desired cell type in the population being fused. The screening of hybridomas is the most laborious step and its complexity will determine the limits on the number of clones that can be analyzed. For *in vitro* lymphokine assays several hundred clones can be assayed. On the other hand, for *in vivo* assays, e.g., for DTH or Ts factor, many fewer clones can be analyzed. Considering these limitations, the frequency of the desired cell type in the initial population must be high enough to be detected in the sample size being screened. The following sections will consider the general strategies that have been adopted to isolate successfully various types of T-cell hybrids.

2.2.2a. Immunization. In some cases where a frequent cell function (e.g., IL-2 production) is sought and there is a means of bypassing receptor specificity (e.g., with mitogens), freshly dissected T cells may be fused.[10,11] When the cell of interest is of low frequency, as is the case for T cells of a defined specificity, then this cell type must be clonally expanded by immunization to antigen. In most cases, priming is done *in vivo*, since primary responses are difficult to achieve *in vitro* (an exception is allogeneic MHC stimulation). The nature of the *in vivo* immunization will depend on the cell type of interest. Inducer cells are optimally primed by a midrange of antigen (e.g., 25–200 μg), usually with adjuvant and given subcutaneously or intraperitoneally. CTLs may be most optimally primed by live infection (for viral-specific cells) or subcutaneous injection of haptenating compounds or hapten coupled to cell surfaces. The T suppressor cells tend to be activated by either very low or high antigen doses in the absence of adjuvant. Intravenous injection of antigen coupled to the surface of splenocytes is a potent immunogen for Ts_1 and Ts_2. Certain suppressor cells are activated by Ts factor alone (Ts_2) or together with subcutaneous immunization (Ts_3). A more detailed consideration of immunization protocols for these various cell types is beyond the scope of this chapter, but is no different from priming for heterogeneous T-cell responses. In any new system optimal conditions must be determined empirically.

2.2.2b. Further Cell Selection. In most cases, simple immunization is not sufficient for specific cell isolation. This can be appreciated if one considers the frequencies involved. For example, the frequency of a hapten-specific CTL in a naive animal may be on the order of 1:25,000. After a single immunization, its frequency may be 1:8000. During hybridization there appears to be preferential fusion of activated cells, which will increase the frequency of specific hybrids by an unknown factor, possibly tenfold. In this case, approximately 800 clones would need to be sampled to obtain a single positive hybrid. Since not all hybrid clones are sufficiently stable or active to warrant further study, a much larger screen would be required. Therefore, additional initial selection is necessary.

Two strategies have been employed to enrich for antigen-specific T lymphocytes. The first is to supply the requisite signals for continued clonal expansion *in vitro*. The specific cells increase in number and the irrelevant cells are diluted and/or die out. After a single restimulation, frequencies of greater than 1:100 can be achieved. Therefore, with the preferential fusion of activated T cells, specific hybrid clones may be as frequent as one in five.

The requisite signals for continued cell growth will depend on the cell type of interest. As outlined in Section 2.2.1, T inducer cells will require both antigen and Ia-bearing accessory cells. If T-cell purification depletes the latter or if T cells are harvested from *in vitro* culture for restimulation, accessory cell addition will be required. Some investigators have added exogenous sources of lymphokines, e.g., IL-2.[12] However, additional factors are not generally necessary, since inducer cells can induce or produce them.[13,14] CTLs will require antigen/MHC stimulation as well as helper factors. The latter will be generated in cultures from T-inducer cell-accessory cell stimulation. If these cells have been depleted, they must be reconstituted or a source of helper factor added. Supernatant from mitogen-stimulated T cells (from which mitogen has been removed or inactivated) or from secondary mixed lymphocyte cultures are convenient bulk sources of helper factor.[4]

Optimal cell densities for restimulation are 2.5–7.5 million responder cells per milliliter for the *in vitro* culture. Subsequent restimulations utilize 10- to 100-fold lower density. Five million irradiated, erythrocyte-free spleenoytes per milliliter are usually sufficient for accessory and/or stimulation function. Culture vessel geometry will affect optimal densities, with the surface area for growth being the most important variable. As a rule of thumb, the better the responses being generated *in vitro*, e.g., levels of antigen-specific proliferation, the greater the likelihood of successful hybrid isolation. Precise determination of specific cell frequency is usually not necessary. It is our impression that little additional improvement is obtained by more than two *in vitro* restimulations, and in fact, that long-term T-cell lines do not serve as good fusion partners.

The second approach is to isolate directly the cell type of interest. This strategy is necessary when the conditions required for *in vitro* clonal expansion are unknown. For example, this approach has been employed in the isolation of antigen-specific Ts cell hybrids.[15] Specific Ts cells can be affinity-purified by binding to and elution from antigen coupled to an insoluble matrix, resulting in at least 100-fold enrichment.

Table I. Representative Tumor Parents

Species	Tumor	Origin	Ref.
Mouse	BW5147	Spontaneous AKR lymphoma	16, 17
	EL4	Benzopyrine C57BL/6 lymphoma	16, 18
	FS6.14.13.AZ	B6D2F$_1$ × BW5147 hybridoma	10
Rat	W/FUC58N.T.	Gross MLV WISTAR/FURTH	19
Human	CEM	T-Cell lymphoma	20, 21
	DIRII	Clone of KE37	22
	J3R7	Clone of JURKAT	20
	SH9	Clone of HUT102-82	23

2.3. Tumor Parent

The tumor lines most commonly used for somatic hybridization are listed in Table I. All of these are *in vitro*-adapted and have a selectable marker, most often hypoxanthine-guanosine phosphoribosyltransferase (HGPRT) deficiency. In murine systems, the most commonly employed parent is a spontaneous AKR T-cell lymphoma, BW5147.[16,17] In the rat and human there is much less consensus as to the best tumor parent. Mouse–rat fusions have been successfully generated, with apparent stability.[19] Individual sublines of a tumor may vary considerably in their fusion frequencies. If drug-resistant revertants arise, they should be selected against prior to fusion (e.g., passage in 8-azaguanine).

It is not always known precisely what effect the tumor parent confers on the phenotype of a somatic hybrid apart from immortality. It is clear that BW5147 is compatible with many if not all T-cell subsets. Thus, functional T-inducer, T-suppressor, and CTL hybrids have been successfully generated. It has been reported that the tumor parent may affect the activation state of its hybrid progeny. For example, it has been reported that the tumor parent will determine the requirement of a CTL hybridoma for factors.[19] It is probable that the tumor parent will donate its complement of activities and receptors. In addition, the tumor parent may be induced to express previously silent gene products in the hybrid state.[24,25] For BW5147, there is no known immune function or specificity. It possesses a rearranged gene for the β chain of the T-cell receptor.[26] An example where BW5147 has contributed to the specificity of a T helper factor has been reported, although this case may be exceptional.[27] Several of the tumor parents produce lymphokines upon mitogen stimulation (e.g., FS6.14.13.AZ, EL4, JURKAT). This may facilitate the construction of antigen-specific, lymphokine-producing hybrids, but may be disadvantageous if hybridomas making only a single or a limited spectrum of lymphokines are desired.

Some tumor parents have additional limitations. One problem can be long doubling times (e.g., several days). Where possible, faster growing variants should be sought.[20] Additionally, it has been reported that several human T-cell tumors are adversely sensitive to exogenous thymidine.[20] In these cases, selection with HAT media slows their growth rate and/or results in poor hybrid yields. A strategy to circumvent this problem is to substitute azaserine for aminopterin during hybrid selection, which eliminates the need for thymidine.[20] Where examined, this has increased the apparent fusion frequency by fourfold with a marked increase in active clones. Finally, several *in vitro* passaged tumors may carry infections that will be inherited by their hybrid progeny. Of particular importance is infection with a variety of mycoplasma species. This can affect cell growth as well as having a variety of independent biological effects. Mycoplasma infection can be difficult to eradicate. Cell lines can also carry chronic viral infections. In particular, human T-cell tumors may carry human T-cell leukemia virus, which is expressed by the hybrid progeny.[23]

2.4. Cell Fusion

The mechanics of cell hybridization are similar to that used for B-cell fusions. The following is the protocol employed in our laboratory (modified from what was originally provided to us by J. Kappler and P. Marrack) with the most critical variables noted:

1. Harvest tumor parent (BW5147). It is important that it be in log phase growth, which for this tumor parent occurs at a density $<10^6$ cells/ml.
2. Mix normal T-cell source with the tumor parent in a ratio of 4:1.
3. Wash cells three times with room-temperature, serum-free, phosphate-buffered saline (PBS), pH 7.4, at room temperature.
4. Decant supernatant and respin pellet.
5. Warm tube to 37°C, aspirate all supernatant, and loosen pellet by vigorously tapping.
6. Add 1 ml of 40% polyethylene glycol (PEG)/PBS at 37°C continuously over 45 sec with mixing. Continue incubation for an additional 45 sec without mixing. Different lots of PEG will significantly affect fusion frequencies. This must be determined empirically and optimal length of incubation in PEG may have to be adjusted. Pretested PEG can be obtained from the American Type Culture Collection.
7. Dilute PEG with 37°C PBS. It is important that this dilution be gradual. We start by adding 1 ml of PBS over 30 sec, and subsequently add an identical volume plus 1 ml every 30 sec (e.g. 1 ml → 2 ml → 3 ml) to a total volume of 50 ml.
8. Incubate for 5 min at 37°C.
9. Centrifuge, decant supernatant, and replace with 50 ml PBS. Do not triturate the pellet. Invert the tube several times and centrifuge.
10. Resuspend the pellet gently with a large-bore pipette in complete media, 37°C (e.g., Dulbecco's modified Eagle's medium, DMEM). We use DMEM with 4.5 g/liter glucose, 10% FCS, and antibiotics. This

medium requires a 10% CO_2 environment. The FCS should be screened to give good cloning efficiency of the tumor parent. Cells should be plated so that a single clone arises per well. The requisite dilution will depend on the fusion frequencies. In our hands, we distribute 2.5×10^4 BW5147 in 100 μl per well in 96-well flat-bottom microtiter plates and expect growth in approximately one in three wells. Filler cells are not necessary with BW5147.

11. After 24 hr at 37°C, the medium is replaced with 100 μl HAT[28]-containing medium at 37°C.
12. Cultures are fed every 5 days with 50–100 μl HAT medium.
13. With BW5147, hybrids will appear between days 7–21. When they achieve ½–¾'s confluence they are transferred to 1- to 2-ml macrowells in HAT medium. Transfer of low-density wells or over dilution will result in poor yields.
14. Subsequently, the macrowells are passaged at least two times in HT medium before changing to regular medium.

2.5. Hybridoma Screening

As noted earlier, screening and initial maintenance of the hybridomas is the most labor-intensive phase of the procedure. Prior to this stage, the screening assays should be optimized and streamlined. Details on specific immunologic assays are beyond the scope of this chapter. This section will focus on the general approach, potential pitfalls, and limitations of this process.

Three forms of screening assays may be considered. The first measures an activity directly in the hybridoma culture supernatant. Obviously, this requires a hybrid that will constitutively make a soluble product. This has been successfully applied to the identification of Ts hybridomas (see Section 3.2) and several lymphokine-producing hybrids.[20,23,29,40] This approach will not identify the majority of lymphokine-producing clones, since, except for Ts cells, stimulation is required for factor production (see Section 2.2.1). The second screening assay stimulates a T-cell hybrid response. This is necessary for an activity that requires triggering or a cell–cell interaction. Most inducer and CTL hybridomas would be screened in this manner. This approach requires expansion of the hybridoma to at least a 1-ml culture to achieve sufficient cell numbers. Finally, a two-stage screening procedure may be employed. The first stage identifies cells of potential interest, which are then assayed for a specific immunologic function. This approach may be considered when a screening assay is not amenable to large numbers of samples. For example, the specific immunologic assay for the identification of antigen-specific Ts cells for DTH is performed *in vivo*.[15] This requires one to several mice per hybrid clone. The identification of a specific Ts marker, I-J, in a rapid first-stage screen markedly reduces the number of cells assayed *in vivo*. This approach has also been employed for T inducer cells using an anticlonotypic antibody.[30]

Several pitfalls and limitations should be considered. First, the effect of the constituents of the medium on screening assays should be tested. The presence of HAT may interfere with certain assays. For example, the exogenous thymidine will compete for the incorporation of labeled thymidine. Additionally, T-cell hybrids removed directly from HAT medium will die if cultured in the absence of HT. This will not influence lymphokine production over 18–24 hr, but may affect longer term cultures. Other constituents to be considered are FCS (some lots are highly mitogenic) and mycoplasma if present. Second, it is possible to get false-positive results. The unfused normal T cells are HGPRT-positive and not eliminated by HAT selection. Ordinarily, they will be diluted and/or die out, but under some circumstances may undergo limited expansion. These cells may contribute to observed activity. Also, some T-cell products, e.g., suppressor factors, may be released from dead cells. Finally, irradiated "filler" cells may be immunologically competent (e.g., they can produce lymphokines). If every hybrid initially tests positive and quickly loses activity, these possibilities should be considered. Third, in those cases where many true-positive hybridomas are expected, it is best to design the screening assay to distinguish levels of activity, not simply positive and negative clones.

Once hybridomas of interest have been identified, the first priority is to freeze several aliquots (see Section 2.6). This will conserve the features of the original isolate and provide insurance in the case of laboratory accidents (e.g., contamination). Additionally, cells should be weaned off aminopterin and subsequently passaged in regular medium (see Section 2.4). In general, newly derived hybridomas tolerate the extremes of cell density poorly. It is safest to split cultures conservatively at 1:10 when densities are $(5–8) \times 10^5$/ml. They may not tolerate densities of $>8 \times 10^5$/ml or very high dilution. Established hybridomas will grow to densities of $\geq 1.5 \times 10^6$ and can be routinely passed at 1:100.

The stability of T-cell hybrids is highly variable and initially is difficult to predict. Two rough indicators that predict stability are high levels of reactivity/activity and a high frequency of active subclones. If possible, it is best to monitor activity over several months of passage to identify stable lines. Activity frequently can be stabilized through multiple subclonings (see Section 2.6). Established clones should periodically be restarted from frozen stock (see Section 2.6).

2.6. Cloning and Storage

Hybridomas of interest should be cloned. Inactive but proliferating variants will arise with passage, especially early after fusion. Cloning assures a single cell of origin, aids in stabilization, and may recover cells with higher activity.

We recommend cloning by limiting dilution for murine hybridomas. Alternatively, cells can be cloned by dispersion in soft agar, micromanipulation, or flow cytometry. However, the necessary experience or equipment for these techniques is less generally available. Limiting dilution relies on statistical probability of clonal origin.[31] Hybrid cells grow in single-cell suspension and should not bind other cells that could prejudice clonality by this technique. For BW5147-derived hybrids, cells in log-phase growth are diluted to 2–3 cells/ml and distributed in 100-μl aliquots to 96-well flat-bottomed microtiter wells. Cloning frequencies are usually improved by the addition of filler cells, e.g., 5×10^5 erythrocyte-depleted, irradiated spleenocytes per well. The hybridoma should be nonreactive to the filler cell employed (i.e., not alloreactive or antigen-stimulated). The medium employed is that routinely used for hybrid passage. Some laboratories add sources of conditioned medium (e.g., medium from B-lymhoblastoid cell cultures) to aid cloning efficiency. Once plated, cultures should be fed with medium every 5 days. Depending on doubling times, clones will be visible after 7–14 days. They would then be assayed as described in Section 2.5. We routinely screen 25 clones per hybrid. In those cases where hybrids are unstable or of low activity, one may need to screen 100 or more clones. It is best to clone from cells that have not been in extended passage, so as to have a higher frequency of active cells in the initial population.

Most T-cell hybridomas can be easily frozen and recovered. The methods follow standard protocols as described for B-cell hybridomas (Eshhar, this volume, Chapter 1).

3. Applications

The following sections will overview the types of T-cell hybridomas that have been constructed and their various uses. Examples have been picked to highlight various applications. These examples and the corresponding references are not exhaustive, but should serve as an introduction to the literature.

3.1. Types of T-Cell Hybridomas

Lymphocytes from the various T-cell subsets have been successfully hybridized. There has been considerable success in the immortalization of T-inducer cells. Large panels of lymphokine-producing hybrids have been constructed (see Section 3.2). In some cases, both a specific function (e.g., lymphokine production) and a known specific receptor have been introduced and selected (see Section 3.2). These cells are the equivalent of antigen-specific, MHC-restricted, and/or alloreactive proliferating cells. Among this set of cells are clones that mediate help for B-cell antibody responses.[32] Hybrids that mediate delayed-type hypersensitivity have also been described.[33] Numerous laboratories have successfully constructed T-suppressor hybridomas from various members of the suppressor cascade, including Ts_1, Ts_2, and Ts_3 (see Sections 2.2.1 and 3.2). CTL hybridomas have been derived, although there is less experience with this cell type.[19,34] In all categories both constitutive and stimulation-dependent phenotypes have been observed. Among the latter, both lym-

Table II. Lymphokines Produced by T-Cell Hybridomas

Lymphokine	Example	Species	Ref.
IL-2	FS6.14.13, FS7.20	Mouse	10, 37
IL-2	L-18	Human	38
IL-3	123	Mouse	39
GMCSF	123	Mouse	39
TRF	B151K12, 14G3	Mouse	40, 41
BCDF	90E	Human	42
ILX	FS7.20	Mouse	37
IaIF	FS7.20	Mouse	37
MAF	FS7.20, 24/G1	Mouse	37, 43
γ-Interferon	FS7.20	Mouse	37
γ-Interferon	L23, L-265	Human	23, 38
CDF	AOFS21.10.9	Mouse	44
BCGF	FS6.14.13, T91	Mouse	10, 45
BCGF	77A, 2B11	Human	42, 46
AEF	Hyb 34	Mouse	29

phokine-dependent and -independent forms have been described.[13,19] Finally, both specific and nonspecific thymocyte hybridomas have been identified.[35,36]

3.2. Use for T-Cell Products

Hybridomas producing both antigen-specific and -nonspecific factors have been constructed. Table II lists lymphokines (antigen-nonspecific factors) produced by representative T-cell hybrids. It is important to note that many of these eponyms specify a biological activity identified in a particular assay system. Some factors may have pleiotropic effects and may therefore have several names associated with them. For example, current evidence suggests that macrophage-activating factor, IL-X, and Ia-inducing factor are identical with interferon gamma.[37] Furthermore, the potential exists for indirect effects. For example, IL-2 may stimulate T cells in culture to secrete other factors (e.g., B-cell stimulatory factors).

The hybridomas listed in Table II produce their factors either constitutively or after stimulation with polyclonal mitogens, which bypass receptor specificity. The latter may require subsequent removal or inactivation, which is easily accomplished for some mitogens (e.g., Con A). To be activated by mitogen, an occasional hybrid may require additional activation signals (e.g., accessory cells or IL-1.[13] Those that are directly triggered allow for a unicellular origin of factor to be assured.

Antigen-specific hybridomas that secrete lymphokines in response to stimulation with specific antigen are listed in Table III. They can also be activated by mitogen, and would be expected to make a range of factors similar to those listed in Table II.

Table III. Antigen-Specific T-Cell Hybridomas That Produce Lymphokines

Class of antigen	Specificity: Antigen	Specificity: MHC	Ref.
Protein	KLH	IA^d	12
	HGG	IA^d	12
	OVA	IA^d	53
	KLH	IA^b	6
	Cytochrome c	IA^d	54
	Insulin	IA^d	55
Amino acid copolymer	GAT	IA^d	14
	GAT	IA^d	14
	GLØ	IE^d	56
	TGAL	IA^d	58
Hapten	TNP	IA^d	58
Allo or auto MHC		IA^d	59
		IE^d	59
		IA^k	36
		IE^k	36
		D^d	60

T-cell hybridomas are of obvious use as defined sources of T-cell products for characterization. Hybridomas can vary considerably in the amount of factor produced. High-level factor-producing hybrids should be screened for during isolation and subsequent cloning. If factors are being induced with mitogen, maximum levels of activity are obtained usually within 18 hr of culture. Factor production can be accomplished under serum-free conditions, which aids in biochemical characterization.

It is important to realize that while hybridoma products will be monoclonal in origin, the production of multiple, molecularly distinct factors from a single clone is frequently observed (see Table II). In fact, analysis of multiple independent T-cell hybridoma clones as well as karyotypically distinct variants may help to elucidate which activities are mediated by separate factors.[37] Those activities that segregate can be inferred to have a molecularly distinct origin. Furthermore, the existence of variation among hybrid clones is potentially useful in dissecting lymphokine requirements for immune responses, e.g., in the analysis of B-cell activation.[11] In this case, T-helper hybridomas that fail to activate B-cell responses can be used to identify the requisite signals that they lack but that can be found in the supernatant of other hybrid clones.[32] From such an analysis, the requirement for several lymphokines for successful T–B cell collaboration could be defined.

Examples of T-cell hybridomas that produce antigen-specific factors are listed in Table IV. The largest experience is with T-suppressor hybridomas. A majority of these produce their factors constitutively.

Table IV. Antigen-Specific T-Cell Hybridomas That Produce Antigen-Specific Factors

Activity	Specificity	Species	Ref.
TsF	GAT	Mouse	47
TsF	KLH	Mouse	48
TsF_1	ABA	Mouse	49
TsF_1	NP	Mouse	15
TsF_2	NP	Mouse	15
TsF_3	NP	Mouse	15
TsF	LDH	Mouse	50
TsF	IgE	Mouse	51
TsF	Ig	Human	22
THF	CGG	Mouse	27
THF	KLH	Mouse	52

3.3. Analytical Uses

A second major use of hybridoma technology is in the analysis of the properties of individual T cells as well as the underlying cellular and molecular events important for their activation. Selected examples will be cited to illustrate this application. First, hybrid clones are well suited to analyze individual T-lymphocyte specificities. Hybridomas were among the first examples of autoreactive, MHC-specific T-cell clones.[14,55] Further, cells with unexpected specificities have been documented, e.g., with specificity both for Ia molecules alone and for the same Ia molecule plus antigen[14] and with specificity for antigen alone.[61] Also, using this approach, it has been possible to probe and define the specificity of thymocyte clones.[36] One advantage of hybrid clonal analysis is that subsequent to fusion, T-cell specificity will not bias growth rates as might occur with T-cell lines requiring receptor stimulation. Another potential advantage of hybridomas is that they are not passaged with filler cells or specific antigen that could carry over into test cultures. This was of importance in defining the antigen-specific yet autoreactive phenotype described above. It also has allowed the activity of T-suppressor factors to be assessed in the complete absence of antigen (to which they may normally be complexed). A potential limitation to consider is the possibility that multiple fusion events could in theory occur and influence clonal specificity.

Hybridomas have been used to explore the molecular events underlying T-cell activation. It has been possible to identify precisely the determinants on antigens that are critical to T-inducer cell activation. This has been accomplished using species variants of proteins with limited amino acid substitutions, peptides isolated after proteolytic fragmentation, and, ultimately, synthetic peptides.[53,54] Since most of the inducer hybrids appear to lack requirements for second signals (lymphokines), it has been possible to use metabolically inactivated presenting cells to define what modifications of an antigen are required for successful presentation.[54] Hybridomas have also been important in dissecting the role of Ia molecules in antigen presentation. It has been shown that distinct Ia molecules influence the fine antigenic specificity of single hybrid clones, suggesting a close physical association between the two ligands.[54] Using chemically related but nonactivating antigens as structural analogues, it has been possible to define a specific, competitive site of antigen association with an antigen-presenting cell.[56,58] Furthermore, using alloreactive T-cell hybrids to probe Ia molecular determinants, it was possible to detect alterations of Ia-associated determinants.[59] These findings suggest an underlying specific antigen–Ia molecule association. Finally, the receptor basis for dual specificity was analyzed by fusing two T cells with distinct specificities for both antigen and Ia, thus introducing receptors of distinct specificity into the same membrane.[12] The resultant hybrid progeny were then tested to see if mixing of antigen and Ia specificities occurred; it did not.

3.4. Cell Surface Analysis

The availability of large numbers of homogeneous T cells has been useful for the study of the structure and function of plasma membrane-associated proteins. This is well illustrated in the case of the antigen/MHC receptor of T lymphocytes. Individual lymphocytes differ in their receptor specificity, and therefore the frequency of any particular receptor is quite low. To characterize this receptor, homogeneous, monospecific T-cell hybrids were used as immunogens to develop clone-specific, monoclonal antibodies.[57,62] The availability of functional T-cell clones allowed the identification of specific antibodies. Thus, antibodies could be screened for their ability to inhibit both antigen-specific activation and binding as well as to stimulate clone-specific activation.[57,62] Both normal clones and T-cell hybrids have been instrumental in this analysis. Hybrid sources, however, provide greater amounts of material for biochemical characterization. Also, the ability to generate large numbers of hybrid clones has allowed the identification of independent isolates reactive with the same antibody.[30] An analysis of their fine specificity for both antigen and MHC has suggested the existance of a single receptor. The availability of well-defined functional clones has also aided the characterization of nonpolymorphic cell surface determinants.[63]

Hybridomas have been useful as homogeneous sources of T lymphocytes for which the conditions necessary for normal clonal growth ar unknown. For example, thymocyte hybridomas corresponding to immature T-cell forms have been constructed. These have been useful to identify the pattern of expression of various cell surface determinants.[35]

3.5. A Tool for Mutation and Variants

Hybridomas are well suited for the generation of cellular variants for the study of structure–function relationships. Hybridoma growth is not dependent on immunologic function, and therefore cells with altered expression of immunologically relevant structures can be selected. Such variants can be generated spontaneously (e.g., by karyotypic instability) or with mutagens. As noted in Section 3.2, cellular variants have been used to dissect independent lymphokines and to analyze lymphokine action. The correlation between karyotype and function has been used to try to identify the chromosomal localization of genes.[6] Finally, hybrids have been selected to lack expression of a particular cell surface determinant. Using hybrids that are negative for L3T4 (the murine equivalent of the human T4 antigen), it has been shown that this molecule is not absolutely required for immunologic activity.[63] However, when present, it contributes to the activation of T cells. The negative variants have been useful in defining the potential for Ia molecule interaction with L3T4 molecules.[64]

3.6. Analysis of T-Cell Genes

Homogeneous T-cell lines and hybrids are an important source of genetic material for the cloning and characterization of genes expressed in T lymphocytes. They have been employed to probe the configuration of immunoglobulin genes in T cells[65] and to clone and analyze the genes encoding the T-cell antigen/MHC receptor.[26] T-Cell hybrids transfected with cloned antigen/MHC receptor genes may play an important role in future studies on the molecular basis of T-cell antigen recognition and function.

References

1. Fathman, C. G., and Kimoto, M., 1980, Studies utilizing murine T cell clones: Ir genes, Ia antigens and MLR stimulating determinants, *Immunol. Rev.* **54:**57–59.
2. Sredni, B., and Schwartz, R. H., 1980, Alloreactivity of an antigen-specific T cell clone, *Nature* **287:**855–857.
3. Fresno, M., Nabel, G., McVay-Boudreau, L., Furthmeyer, H., and Cantor, H., 1981, Antigen-specific T lymphocyte clones. I. Characterization of a T lymphocyte clone expressing antigen-specific suppressive activity, *J. Exp. Med.* **53:**1246–1259.
4. Nabholz, M., Engers, H. D., Collavo, D., and North, M., 1978, Cloned T-cell lines with specific cytotoxic activity, *Curr. Top. Microbiol. Immunol.* **81:**176–187.
5. Yefenof, E., Azar, Y., Eidelsztein, P., and Ben-Sasson, S. Z., 1982, Immortalization of antigen-specific helper T cells by transformation with the radiation leukemia virus (Rad Lv), *J. Immunol.* **128:**625–628.
6. Marrack, P., and Kappler, J., 1983, Use of somatic cell genetics to study chromosomes contributing to antigen plus I recognition by T cell hybridomas, *J. Exp. Med.* **157:**404–418.
7. Rock, K. L., and Benacerraf, B., 1983, MHC-restricted T cell activation: Analysis with T cell hybridomas. *Immunol. Rev.* **76:**29–57.
8. Johnson, J. P., Cianfriglia, M., Glasebrook, A. L., and Nabholz, M., 1982, Karyotypic evolution of cytolytic T cell lines, in: *Isolation, Characterization and Utilization of T Lymphocyte Clones* (C. G. Fathman and F. W. Fitch eds.), Academic Press, New York, pp. 183–191.
9. Gallatin, W. M., Weissman, J. L., and Butcher, E. C., 1983, A cell-surface molecule involved in organ specific homing of lymphocytes, *Nature* **304:**30–34.

10. Harwell, L., Skidmore, B., Marrack, P., and Kappler, J., 1980, Concanavalin A-inducible, interleukin-2 producing T cell hybridoma, *J. Exp. Med.* **152:**893–904.
11. Leibson, H. J., Marrack, P., and Kappler, J. W., 1981, B Cell helper factors. I. Requirement for both interleukin-2 and another 40,000 mol. wt. factor, *J. Exp. Med.* **154:**1681–1693.
12. Kappler, J. W., Skidmore, B., White, J., and Marrack, P., 1981, Antigen inducible, H-2 restricted, interleukin-2 producing T cell hybridomas. Lack of independent antigen and H-2 recognition, *J. Exp. Med.* **153:**1198–1214.
13. Rock, K. L., 1982, The role of Ia molecules in the activation of T lymphocytes. I. The activation of an IL-1 dependent IL-2 producing T cell hybridoma by Con A requires an interaction, which is not H-2 restricted with an Ia-bearing accessory cell, *J. Immunol.* **129:**1360–1366.
14. Rock, K. L., and Benacerraf, B., 1983, The role of Ia molecules in the activation of T lymphocytes. III. Antigen-specific, Ia restricted interleukin 2-producing T cell hybridomas with detectable affinity for the restricting I-A molecule, *J. Exp. Med.* **157:**359–364.
15. Minami, M., Okuda, K., Furusawa, S., Benacerraf, B., and Dorf, M. E., 1981, Analysis of T cell hybridomas. I. Characterization of H-2 and Igh-restricted monoclonal suppressor factors, *J. Exp. Med.* **154:**1390–1402.
16. Hammerling, G. J., 1977, T Lymphocyte tissue culture lines produced by cell hybridization, *Eur. J. Immunol.* **7:**743–746.
17. Godsby, R. A., Osbourne, B. A., Simpson, E., and Herzenberg, L. A., 1977, Hybrid cell line with T-cell characteristics, *Nature* **267:**707–708.
18. Taniguchi, M., and Miller, J. F. A. P., 1978, Specific suppressive factors produced by hybridomas derived from the fusion of enriched suppressor T cells and a T lymphoma cell line, *J. Exp. Med.* **148:**373–382.
19. Silva, A., MacDonald, H. R., Conzelman, A., Corthesy, P., and Nabholz, M., 1983, Rat and mouse T-cell hybrids with inducible specific cytolytic activity, *Immunol. Rev.* **76:**105–130.
20. Foung, S. K. H., Sasaki, D. T., Grumet, F. C., and Engleman, E. G., 1982, Production of functional human T–T hybridomas in selection media lacking aminopterin and thymidine, *Proc. Natl. Acad. Sci. USA* **79:**7484–7488.
21. Kaplan, J., Shope, T. C., and Peterson, W. D., 1974, Epstein–Barr virus negative human malignant T cell lines, *J. Exp. Med.* **139:**1070–1076.
22. Grillot-Courvalin, C., Dellagi, K., Chevalier, A., and Brouet, J. C., 1982, Characterization of a suppressor factor produced by a human T cell hybridoma, *J. Immunol.* **129:**1008–1016.
23. Le, J., Vilcek, J., Saxinger, C., and Prensky, W., 1982, Human T cell hybridomas secreting immune interferon, *Proc. Natl. Acad. Sci. USA* **79:**7857–7861.
24. Kontaiainen, S., Simpson, E., Bohrer, E., Beverly, P. C. L., Herzenberg, L. A., Fitzpatrick, W. C., Vogt, P., Torano, A., McKenzie, I. F. C., and Feldman, M., 1978, T-cell lines producing antigen-specific suppressor factors, *Nature* **274:**477–480.
25. Kontaiainen, S., Culbert, E. J., Ceka, M., Simpson, E., McKenzie, I. F. C., and Feldman, M., 1981, T Cell hybridomas producing hapten-specific suppressor factors, *Immunology* **43:**747–754.
26. Hedrick, S. M., Cohen, D. I., Nielsen, E. A., and Davis, M. M., 1984, Isolation of cDNA clones encoding T cell-specific membrane-associated proteins, *Nature* **308:**149–153.
27. Lonai, P., Ritton, S., Sarelkoul, H. F. J., Piur, J., and Hammerling, G. J., 1981, Two separate genes regulate self-Ia and carrier recognition. H-2 restricted helper factors secreted by hybridoma cell lines. *J. Exp. Med.* **154:**1910–1921.
28. Littlefield, J. W., 1964, Selection of hybrids from matings of fibroblasts *in vitro* and their presumed recombinants, *Science* **145:**709–719.
29. Katz, D. H., Bechtold, T. E., and Altman, A., 1980, Construction of T cell hybridomas secreting allogenic effect factor, *J. Exp. Med.* **152:**956–968.
30. Marrack, P. C., Shimonkevitz, R., Hannum, C., Haskins, K., and Kappler, J., 1983, The major histocompatibility complex restricted antigen receptor on T cells. IV. An anti-idiotypic antibody predicts both antigen and I-specificity, *J. Exp. Med.* **158:**1635–1646.
31. Lefkovits, J., and Waldman, H., 1979, *Limiting Dilution Analysis of Cells in the Immune System*, Cambridge University Press, Cambridge.

32. Roehm, N. W., Marrack, P., and Kappler, J. W., 1983, Helper signals in the plaque-forming cell response to protein-bound haptens, *J. Exp. Med.* **158:**317–333.
33. Minami, M., Okuda, K., Sunday, M. E., and Dorf, M. E., 1982, H-2K-, H-2I-, and H-2D-restricted hybridoma contact sensitivity effector cells, *Nature* **297:**231–233.
34. Kaufmann, Y., Berke, G., and Eshhar, Z., 1981, Cytotoxic T lymphocyte hybridomas that mediate specific tumor-cell lysis *in vitro, Proc. Natl. Acad. Sci. USA* **78:**2502–2506.
35. Owen, F. L., 1982, Products of the Ig T-C region on chromosome 12 are maturational markers for T cells. Sequence of appearance in immunocompetant T cells parallels ontogenetic appearance of Thy^{d}, $Tind^{d}$, and TSU^{d}, *J. Exp. Med.* **156:**703–718.
36. Yeh, E. T. H., Benacerraf, B., and Rock, K. L., 1984, Analysis of thymocyte MHC-specificity with thymocyte hybridomas, *J. Exp. Med.* **160:**799–813.
37. Zlotnik, A., Roberts, W. K., Vasil, A., Blumenthal, E., Larosa, F., Leibson, H. J., Endres, R. O., Graham, S. D., White, J., Hill, J., Henson, P., Klein, J. R., Bevan, M. J., Marrack, P., and Kappler, J. W., 1983, Coordinate production by a T cell hybridoma of gamma interferon and three other lymphokine activities: Multiple activities of a single lymphokine, *J. Immunol.* **131:**794–800.
38. Le, J., Vilcek, J., Sadlik, J. R., Cheung, M. K., Balazs, J., Sarngadharan, M. G., and Presnky, W., 1983, Lymphokine production by human T cell hybrids, *J. Immunol.* **130:**1231–1235.
39. Schrader, J. W., Clark-Lewis, I., Crapper, R. M., and Wong, G. W., 1983, P-Cell stimulating factor: Characterization, action on multiple lineages of bone marrow derived cells and role in oncogenesis, *Immunol. Rev.* **76:**79–104.
40. Takatsu, K., Tanaka, K., Tominaga, A., Kumahara, Y., and Hamaoka, T., 1980, Antigen-induced T cell replacing factor (TRF). III. Establishment of T cell hybrid clone continuously producing TRF and functional analysis of released TRF, *J. Immunol.* **125:**2646–2653.
41. Elkins, K., and Cambier, J. C., 1983, Constitutive production of a factor supporting B lymphocyte differentiation by a T cell hybridoma, *J. Immunol.* **130:**1247–1251.
42. Okada, M., Sakaguchi, N., Yoshimura, N., Hara, H., Shimizu, K., Yoshida, N., Yoshizaki, K., Kishimoto, S., Yamamura, Y., and Kishimoto, T., 1983, B Cell growth factors and B cell differentiation factor from human T hybridomas. Two distinct kinds of B cell growth factors and their synergism in B cell proliferation, *J. Exp. Med.* **157:**583–590.
43. Schreiber, R. D., Altman, A., and Katz, D. H., 1982, Identification of a T cell hybridoma that produces large quantities of macrophage activating factor, *J. Exp. Med.* **156:**677–689.
44. Raulet, D. H., and Bevan, M. J., 1982, A differentiation factor required for the expression of cytotoxic T-cell function, *Nature* **296:**754–757.
45. Garchon, H.-J., Levi-Strauss, M., Carnaud, C., and Bach, J.-F., 1983, Soluble factors for B cell activation: A T cell hybridoma that secretes a specific B cell growth factor, *J. Immunol.* **131:**777–780.
46. Butler, J. L., Muraguchi, A., Lane, H. C., and Fauci, A. S., 1983, Development of a human T–T cell hybridoma secreting B cell growth factor, *J. Exp. Med.* **157:**60–68.
47. Kapp, J. A., Araneo, B. A., and Clevinger, B. C., 1980, Suppression of antibody and T cell proliferative responses to L-glutamic $acid^{60}$-L-$alanine^{30}$-L-$tyrosine^{10}$ by a specific monoclonal T cell factor, *J. Exp. Med.* **152:**235–240.
48. Tokuhisa, T., and Taniguchi, M., 1982, Two distinct allotype determinants on the antigen-specific suppressor and enhancing T cell factors that are encoded by genes linked to the immunoglobulin heavy chain locus, *J. Exp. Med.* **155:**126–139.
49. Whitaker, R. B., Nepom, J. T., Sy, M.-S., Takaoki, M., Gramm, C. F., Fox, I., Germain, R. N., Nelles, M. J., Greene, M. I., and Benacerraf, B., 1981, Suppressor factor from a T cell hybrid inhibits delayed-type hypersensitivity responses to azobenzenearsonate, *Proc. Natl. Acad. Sci. USA* **78:**6441–6445.
50. Ikezawa, Z., Baxevanis, C. N., Nonaka, M., Abe, R., Tada, T., Nagy, Z. A., and Klein, J., 1983, Monoclonal suppressor factor specific for lactate dehydrogenase B. I. Mechanism of interaction between the factor and its target cells, *J. Exp. Med.* **157:**1855–1866.
51. Suemura, M., Ishizaka, A., Kobatake, S., Sugimura, K., Maeda, K., Nakanishi, K., Kishimoto, S., Yamamura, Y., and Kishimoto, T., 1983, Inhibition of IgE production in B hybridomas by IgE class-specific suppressor factors from T hybridomas, *J. Immunol.* **130:**1056–1065.

52. Hiramatsu, K., Miyatani, S., Kim, M., Yamada, S., Okumura, K., and Tada, T., 1981, Unique T cell Ia antigens expressed on a hybrid cell line producing antigen-specific augmenting T cell factors, *J. Immunol.* **127:**1118–1122.
53. Shimonkevitz, R., Kappler, J., Marrack, P., and Grey, H., 1983, Antigen-recognition by H-2 restricted T cells. I. Cell free antigen processing, *J. Exp. Med.* **158:**303–316.
54. Heber-Katz, E., Schwartz, E. R., Matis, L. A., Hannum, C., Fairwell, T., Appella, E., and Hansburg, D., 1982, Contribution of antigen-presenting cell major histocompatibility complex gene products to the specificity of antigen induced T cell activation, *J. Exp. Med.* **155:**1086–1099.
55. Glimcher, L. H., and Shevach, E. M., 1982, Production of autoreactive I region restricted T cell hybridomas, *J. Exp. Med.* **156:**640–645.
56. Rock, K. L., and Benacerraf, B., 1984, Inhibition of antigen-specific T lymphocyte activation by structurally related Ir gene-controlled polymers. II. Competitive inhibition of I-E restricted antigen-specific responses, *J. Exp. Med.* **160:**1864–1879.
57. White, J., Haskins, K. M., Marrack, P., and Kappler, J. W., 1983, Use of I-region restricted antigen-specific T cell hybridomas to produce idiotypically specific anti-receptor antibodies, *J. Immunol.* **130:**1033–1037.
58. Rock, K. L., and Benacerraf, B., 1983, Inhibition of antigen-specific T lymphocyte activation by structurally related Ir gene controlled polymers. Evidence of specific competition for accessory cell antigen-presentation, *J. Exp. Med.* **157:**1618–1634.
59. Rock, K. L., and Benacerraf, B., 1984, Selective modification of a private Ia allostimulating determinant upon antigen association with antigen presenting cells, *J. Exp. Med.* **159:**1238–1252.
60. Endres, R. O., Marrack, P., and Kappler, J., 1983, An IL-2 secreting T hybridoma that responds to a self-class I histcompatibility antigen in the H-2D region, *J. Immunol.* **131:**1656–1662.
61. Carel, S., Bron, C., and Corradin, G., 1983, T-Cell hybridoma specific for a cytochrome peptide: Specific antigen-binding and interleukin-2 production, *Proc. Natl. Acad. Sci. USA* **80:**4832–4836.
62. Haskins, K., Kubo, R., White, J., Pigeon, M., Kappler, J., and Marrack, P., 1983, The major histocompatibility complex restricted antigen receptor on T cells. I. Isolation with a monoclonal antibody, *J. Exp. Med.* **157:**1149–1169.
63. Marrack, P., Endres, R., Shimonkevitz, R., Zlotnik, A., Dialynas, D., Fitch, F., and Kappler, J., 1983, The major histocompatibility complex-restricted antigen receptor on T cells. II. Role of the L3T4 product, *J. Exp. Med.* **158:**1077–1091.
64. Greenstein, J. L., Kappler, J., Marrack, P., and Burakoff, S. J., 1984, The role of L3T4 in recognition of Ia by a cytotoxic, H-2D^{d}-specific T cell hybridoma, *J. Immunol.* **159:**1213–1224.
65. Kronenberg, M., Kraig, E., Siu, G., Kapp, J. A., Kappler, J., Marrack, P., Pierce, C. W., and Hood, L., 1983, Three T cell hybridomas do not contain detectable heavy chain variable gene transcripts, *J. Exp. Med.* **158:**210–227.

Chapter 34

The Mechanisms That Control the Proliferation and Activity of Cytolytic T Lymphocytes

MARKUS NABHOLZ

1. Introduction

The discovery in 1975 that culture supernatants of mitogen-activated leukocyte populations contained a lymphocyte-specific growth factor [T-cell growth factor (TCGF) = interleukin 2 (IL-2)][1] provided the cornerstone for the development of cellular immunology in the last decade.

The early experiments on the sensitivity of normal lymphocytes to the growth-promoting activity of IL-2 led to a testable hypothesis concerning the proliferative response of T cells to antigenic stimulation.[2,3] Further support for this hypothesis was obtained when IL-2 was purified and specific cell surface receptors for this lymphokine demonstrated by direct binding assays.[4] The isolation of monoclonal antibodies against the receptor has allowed the biochemical characterization and isolation of a cDNA clone coding for the receptor molecule.[5–10]

The discovery of IL-2 has been instrumental for the isolation of cloned cell lines derived from mature functional T lymphocytes (for review see Ref. 11). Such cell lines, in turn, have become important tools for the analysis of the functional role of cell surface molecules such as Lyt-2 (for review see Ref. 12), and have played an essential role in the identification of the molecules responsible for specific antigen recognition by T cells.[13]

These developments have resulted in a significant shift in the nature of the questions that we ask about lymphocyte "activation." The results of the complex experimental systems of classical cellular immunology were interpreted in terms of simple but necessarily highly speculative models. Now these systems have given way to much simpler ones that begin to yield the complex molecular answers characteristic of cellular biology.

MARKUS NABHOLZ • Genetics Unit, Swiss Institute for Experimental Cancer Research (ISREC), Epalinges, Switzerland.

In this chapter I will discuss some of the problems of the cellular biology of T cells, especially cytolytic T lymphocytes (CTL), and outline the experimental approaches that we use to attack them. These include the use of T-cell hybrids. All our work was done with murine cell lines, but there is no indication that any of the conclusions reached do not also apply to human lymphocytes.

2. The Control of Lymphocyte Proliferation

2.1. The Discovery of IL-2 and the Basic Model

Shortly after the discovery of IL-2 it became clear that normal small lymphocytes could not respond to this growth factor, and that responsiveness was induced in T cells by a short exposure of leukocyte populations to mitogenic lectins such as concanavalin A (Con A) or antigenic stimuli.[3,14,15] Absorption experiments showed that T blasts but not small resting T cells removed IL-2 from the surrounding culture fluids.[14] These results led to the hypothesis proposed more or less simultaneously by several groups that resting T cells could not respond to IL-2 because they lacked specific cell surface receptors for the growth factor, and that mitogenic or antigenic stimulation induced the expression of such receptors and thereby IL-2 responsiveness.[3,15] Formally this model is quite analogous to one recently proposed for the growth control of fibroblasts, according to which induction of proliferation in resting cells requires, first, "competence" factors that induce these cells to become responsive to other, so-called "progression" factors.[16]

Strong support for this type of model for T-lymphocytes came when pure radio labeled IL-2 was used to measure IL-2 binding to cells directly.[4] Such measurements revealed a class of specific IL-2 receptors with the expected very high affinity on CTL lines and T blasts, and they confirmed the earlier absorption data.

In 1982 Waldmann's group[5] isolated a monoclonal antibody that reacted with activated human T cells and turned out to be specific for IL-2 receptors.

Using this antibody as well as radiolabeled IL-2, Cantrell and Smith[17] showed that in human leukocytes phytohemagglutinin (PHA) stimulation induced the appearance of IL-2 receptors before the onset of DNA synthesis. After some days of IL-2-promoted proliferation the IL-2 receptor content of the cells and their capacity to respond to IL-2 declined, but both could be reinduced by a short reexposure to PHA. In the meantime similar experiments with T-cell clones rather than mass cultures have been reported (see below). While they supported the model on T-cell activation, they could not provide any answers to a number of questions concerning the molecular mechanisms of this process and about the role of IL-2 in the control of immune responses. Some of these questions are:

1. How does interaction with an antigenic stimulator cell or a lectin trigger the expression of IL-2 receptors and IL-2 responsiveness?

2. Are these two characteristics equivalent, i.e., is the appearance of IL-2 receptors on a lymphocyte plasma membrane sufficient to render this cell capable to respond to IL-2?
3. How does IL-2 work? Does it have other effects on cells apart from the induction of proliferation?
4. Does the growth of all lymphocytes depend on IL-2?

2.2. All Lymphocytes May Be IL-2 Dependent

The observations that led to the discovery and characterization of IL-2 suggested that this factor was specific for T cells, hence its early name, T-cell growth factor (TCGF). For about 9 years, it remained controversial whether IL-2 had any direct effects on B lymphocytes, but recent results prove that mouse B lymphocytes activated with a combination of lipopolysaccharide (LPS) and anti-immunoglobulin antibodies can respond to IL-2. The evidence can be summarized as follows: (1) Highly purified activated B cells proliferate in response to immunoaffinity-purified as well as to recombinant IL-2. (2) Such B cells bind IL-2 with the same affinity as T blasts and their response to IL-2 can be inhibited by a monoclonal antibody raised against a CTL line and specific for the mouse IL-2 receptor. (3) This antibody immunoprecipitates a similar molecule from both surface-labeled T and B blasts (Ref. 18, and J. Lowenthal, unpublished results). Similar experiments show that activated human B cells can also respond to IL-2.[19]

What remains to be determined is whether all T and B lymphocytes can be made IL-2 responsive, and whether there are alternative pathways to promote lymphocyte proliferation. In the case of T cells there is no evidence for a mode of proliferation that is independent of IL-2 (I am, of course, only referring to normal T lymphocytes and not T-cell tumors or cell lines derived from such). There are certainly T-cell clones that can proliferate in the absence of exogenously supplied IL-2, but many of these secrete detectable amounts of IL-2,[20] and for the others this possibility has not been ruled out. Recently we have made some observations that bear on this point. They were made with hybrids derived from a cross between a murine IL-2-dependent CTL line and a rat thymoma. Certain hybrid clones were partially dependent on IL-2: they would grow in its absence, but very much more slowly than in its presence.[21] Subcloning experiments ruled out intrahybrid heterogeneity. We found detectable IL-2 activity in the concentrated culture supernatants of some of such hybrids, but not in those of others with a similar behavior. We then compared the growth rate of such cells in normal stationary conditions to that in cultures maintained on a slowly rocking platform. The results were clear: addition of IL-2 to cells in stationary cultures only had an effect when the cells were seeded at a low density. In presence of added IL-2 the cells in the moving cultures grew as well as those in stationary cultures, whereas in its absence the initial growth rate in the latter condition was virtually zero even at relatively high inoculum densities (A. Silva, unpublished results). The experiments strongly suggest that cells that both produce and consume IL-2 can establish around them an IL-2 gradient so that the local concentration is high enough to maintain their proliferation even if the average IL-2 concentration does not reach easily detectable levels.

My own prejudice is that all mature T cells depend on IL-2 for proliferation.

What about immature thymic T cells? The rate of cell turnover in the thymus is large and at least partly due to rapid cell proliferation. But most thymocytes never leave the thymus and presumably die. The large majority of thymocytes do not express detectable IL-2 receptors[4] and so far have been refractory to any attempts to induce them to respond to IL-2. It may thus be that most thymocyte proliferation *in situ* is IL-2 independent. This is what we assumed in the interpretation of the behavior of hybrids derived from AKR thymomas. There is evidence that these tumors are derived from and therefore representative of cortical thymocytes.[22] They do not produce detectable IL-2 and do not express IL-2 receptors (Refs. 4 and 23, and J. Lowenthal, unpublished results). Their growth cannot be inhibited by anti-IL-2-receptor antibodies. In crosses between AKR thymomas and murine IL-2-dependent CTL lines, IL-2 dependence behaves like a dominant heritable trait and its expression is correlated with that of other characteristics of mature CTLs not found in AKR thymomas.[24,25,51] We proposed that IL-2 dependence is a characteristic of mature T cells and controlled by a gene that is not yet active in immature thymocytes. Its activation during T-cell differentiation would lead to the expression of the mature T-cell phenotype. According to this hypothesis, the proliferation of immature T cells is controlled not by IL-2, but by other signals or factors, and the transformation with murine leukemia virus that makes the thymoma cells independent of these does not the abolish IL-2 dependence of mature T cells. At present these speculations await confirmation or refutation by further experiments.

One recent finding that casts some doubt on the IL-2 independence of immature T cells is the observation that a fraction of thymocytes, namely about one-half of the about 2% of thymocytes that express neither of the mature T-cell marker antigens (Lyt-2 and L3T4 in the mouse) express large numbers of specific receptors for IL-2.[52] These can be detected by measuring specific binding of ^{3}H-IL-2 or with an anti-IL-2-receptor antibody. Such antibodies precipitate from these cells a molecule that is very similar to the IL-2 receptor of mature T cells. There is evidence that suggests that among the Lyt-2^-, $T4^-$ thymocytes are the elusive precursors of both cortical[26] and medullary thymocytes.[27] If the precursors can be shown to be IL-2 responsive, then this would suggest that also the thymic precursors of mature T cells depend on IL-2 for their growth.

2.3. The Mechanism of Induction of IL-2 Responsiveness

Early experiments with mass cultures of more or less purified normal peripheral T cells indicated that a few hours of exposure to a mitogenic lectin was sufficient to induce T cells to become IL-2 responsive.[15] Recently we have reinvestigated this question using a CTL clone that requires periodic restimulation with appropriate antigenic stimulator cells to respond to IL-2. Monoclonal antibodies against the Lyt-2 or the LFA-1 antigens of the responder cells or against the stimulating H-2 antigen can inhibit the induction of IL-2 responsiveness in these cells, but only when they are added before or at the same time as the stimulator cells. After 3 hr of exposure to the antigenic stimulation the antibodies are no longer inhibitory. After such a short antigenic stimulation the cells can be driven through about six to seven divisions (in 4–5 days) by immunoaffinity-purified IL-2 before they again become refractory to the growth factor. This return to IL-2 unresponsiveness takes place even when the cells are maintained in an excess of IL-2, and is preceded by a gradual decline in the number of IL-2 receptors/cell from a maximal level 2 days after antigenic stimulation.[28–31]

While these and similar experiments from other laboratories confirm the basic features of the model described earlier in more precisely defined experimental systems, they do not tell us anything about the mechanism by which antigenic stimuli induce expression of IL-2 receptors. They do not even rule out that the stimulator cells contribute, besides antigenic determinants, other signals or factors required for the induction of IL-2 receptor expression and IL-2 responsiveness. The available information with regard to this latter point is confusing: there are indeed indications that antigen-dependent CTL clones of the type described above require more than antigen and IL-2 to grow. They do not respond to stimulation with mitogenic lectins (J. Lowenthal, unpublished; H. v. Boehmer, personal communication) or with tumor cell lines that express the appropriate antigenic determinants (as shown by the fact that they are specifically lysed by the CTL clones). Certain human cytolytic T-cell clones, on the other hand, can be stimulated to express increased levels of IL-2 receptors with anticlonotypic monoclonal antibodies, apparently in the absence of other cells.[32]

2.4. Normal pCTL Can Be Induced to Proliferate by Lectin and Pure IL-2

Most CTLs are derived from small Lyt-2$^+$ peripheral lymphocytes (pCTL). Ironically, at present the requirements for the induction of the proliferation of normal pCTLs have been determined more clearly than those of antigen-dependent CTL clones, although they have been, until recently, quite controversial. Certain groups have steadfastly maintained that Lyt-2$^+$ T cells could be induced to become IL-2 responsive by mitogenic lectins in the absence of other cell types.[15] However, because these experiments were done with relatively high cell concentrations, it was difficult to prove the point, and others postulated a requirement for an interaction between Lyt-2$^+$ cells with "accessory" cells.[33] Neither side could rule out a requirement for other factors contaminating the crude or "semipurified" IL-2 preparations used, and the need for such additional factors has indeed been postulated by yet others (H. Wagner, personal communication). Recent experiments in our laboratory have clearly shown that about one-third of all splenic Lyt-2^+ cells will proliferate when exposed to an optimal dose of mitogenic lectin and immunoaffinity-purified or recombinant IL-2 from bacteria.[34] Individual cells (isolated by micromanipulation) can respond in the absence of any other cells. In a sufficiently high concentration of IL-2 they will undergo at least eight to nine divisions. When the IL-2 concentration is lowered to about 1 U/ml, the initial rate of proliferation does not change, but thymidine incorporation and cell division cease earlier. This argues against the possibility that pCTLs can only respond to IL-2 and mitogen when the IL-2 concentration is so high as to overcome the requirement for other factors needed in physiological conditions.

To conclude this section, it should perhaps be pointed out that whereas it is obvious that IL-2-dependent cells need to express IL-2 receptors to be able to respond to this growth factor, this does not mean that this is the only change required for a resting lymphocyte to become IL-2 responsive. It is quite conceivable that this requires the activation of other genes whose products play a role in the transmission of the signals that IL-2 produces when it interacts with its receptor.

2.5. The Mechanism of Action of IL-2

We do not know what makes a cell dependent on IL-2 (or, for that matter, on any other growth factor). The finding described earlier that in crosses between IL-2-independent AKR thymomas and CTL lines the IL-2 dependence of the latter is inherited like a dominant genetic trait suggests that IL-2 dependence is imposed by a *trans*-acting gene that blocks progression of the cells through the cell cycle. IL-2 in some way relieves this block.

IL-2 has several of the characteristics of other growth factors: it binds to specific receptors, is internalized, and is degraded.[4] It acts like a "progression" factor in that it allows responsive cells to progress from the G_1 phase of the cell cycle into S phase.[35] However, as for other growth factors and polypeptide hormones, the molecular mechanism(s) by which IL-2 stimulates cells is (are) not known. The response that is usually measured is cell proliferation or DNA synthesis, but from what we know about other polypeptide growth factors and hormones, it would not be surprising if IL-2 induces several other cellular activities. There are indeed already indications that this is so: as I will discuss later, IL-2 seems to play a crucial role in the induction of cytolytic activity in pCTLs. Recently we have found that it can have a rather surprising effect on the expression of its own receptors: certain hybrids between the rat thymoma W/Fu(C58/NT)D and mouse CTLs (PC60) that grow independently of IL-2 do not express detectable high-affinity IL-2 receptors (<200/cell) when they are cultured in normal medium. However, these cells can be induced to express several thousand high-affinity IL-2 receptors/cell by transferring them to medium supplemented with supernatants from Con A-stimulated spleen cells

(CS).[36] The induction is mediated by two synergizing factors, interleukin 1 (IL-1) and IL-2. Treatment with either factor alone does not induce any detectable high-affinity receptors (Ref. 36, and F. Erard, unpublished results). Neither the shift of the cells from normal to CS-supplemented medium or the reverse has any detectable effect on the growth rate of the cells.[37] Thus it is very unlikely that exposure to CS induces the cells to become IL-2 dependent. If we accept that IL-2 acts on cells exclusively through specific receptors, we have to explain the effect of IL-2 on the expression of its own receptors by postulating either that IL-1 by itself induces on PC60 the appearance of low-affinity or an undetectable number of high-affinity IL-2 receptors, or that such receptors are already present on noninduced cells but that IL-1 is required to render the cells capable of responding to IL-2. Evidence for the existence of a class of low-affinity IL-2 receptors on human T cells has recently been reported[38] and activated mouse lymphocytes also express both high- and low-affinity IL-2 binding sites.[53,54] Whatever the role of IL-1, the experiments clearly show that IL-2 can regulate the expression of its own receptors in an unusual way: it induces an increase in their number or affinity rather than the more frequently observed downregulation. The fact that the growth of PC60 cells is not dependent on IL-2 suggests that the pathways by which this factor stimulates CTLs to enter into S phase and induces increased IL-2 receptor expression are not identical.

The finding that IL-2 receptor induction (as well as induction of cytolytic activity; see below) in PC60 cells requires IL-1 seems to contradict the requirements described earlier of normal pCTLs, and one might be tempted to dismiss the behavior of PC60 as the artifactual result of an artificial cell line. On the contrary, I believe that these cells will be very useful for the analysis of the molecular mechanisms by which these factors act, since I do not think that these cells have "invented" new ways of responding to IL-1 and IL-2. One possible explanation for the IL-1 requirement of PC60 may be that the rat thymoma has imposed on them some characteristics of helper T cells, which may have more complex requirements for activation than pCTLs. There is indeed a recent report showing that T-cell clones with the characteristics of T helper cells require IL-1 to express IL-2 receptors and to become IL-2 responsive.[39] Whether IL-2 is also required for the mitogen- or antigen-induced receptor expression by pCTLs is not yet clear, but recently we have found that it does indeed increase receptor expression on antigen-independent CTL lines arrested in G_1 by IL-2 deprival (R. Sekaly, unpublished results).

3. The Control of the Expression of CTL-Effector Function

3.1. The Mechanism of CTL-Mediated Target Cell Lysis

In addition to antigen-specific lysis, recent investigations have shown that most or all CTLs express other effector functions: they secrete IFN-γ and, less frequently, IL-2 and other lymphokines.[40] However, production of lymphokines is not an exclusive property of CTL.[11]

The mechanism(s) by which CTLs destroy target cells is (are) still not clearly established, although recent experiments from several laboratories suggest that an essential component of the lytic machinery is a molecular complex, called polyperforin, which resembles the tubular polymers of complement component C9 in the membrane attack complex.[41–43] It appears that the nonpolymerized precursors of polyperforin are contained in granular organelles characteristic of CTLs. At present the most plausible model of the cytolytic interaction between CTLs and target cells postulates that the binding of a CTL to its target via its antigen-specific receptors induces the CTL to secrete the granules containing the polyperforin precursors into the space between itself and the target cell. The perforin molecules insert into and form lesions or channels in the target cell membrane.

Using the rat thymoma × mouse CTL hybrid PC60, we have obtained a series of results that lend further support to this model.[55] This hybrid has no detectable cytolytic activity when cultured in normal medium, but acquires CTL activity when exposed for more than 1 day to both IL-1 and IL-2. When we compared the membranes of cells of the parental murine CTL line B6.1 cultured under conditions where the cells attack each other (i.e., in the presence of Con A) with those of induced and noninduced PC60 cells, we found on B6.1 as well as on membranes of cytolytically active PC60 the two types of polyperforin complexes observed previously on other CTL lines by Podack and Denner.[41,42] Membranes of noninduced PC60 cells, on the other hand, contained only the smaller (6-nm inner diameter) type of polyperforin (polyperforin 2). When cells of CTL lines are broken by nitrogen cavitation and their contents fractionated on Percoll density gradients one can isolate cytoplasmic granules that contain a distinct set of proteins, most of which are also found in purified assembled polyperforin. Under appropriate conditions the granules display strong cytolytic and hemolytic activity. Induced PC60 cells contain hemolytic granules of a similar density and protein composition as the parental CTL line, whereas no such granules could be isolated from the same cells in their noninduced state, and they lacked at least one of the proteins characteristic of assembled polyperforins.

It is clear that the data still leave open many of the questions concerning the precise molecular mechanisms of the formation of polyperforin. The experimental evidence for the role of polyperforin in CTL activity is still not conclusive, and we have no good ideas concerning how the insertion of polyperforin channels into the target cells leads to the death of the latter. Nevertheless, it is the first time that clearly identifiable molecular structures have been implicated in CTL activity, and an unequivocal answer as to their importance will very likely already have been provided when this book appears in print.

3.2. The Requirements for the Induction of CTL Activity

Induction of cytolytic activity in pCTLs is as yet a poorly understood process (although now that the structural basis for cell-mediated cytolysis begins to appear less nebulous this will, I expect, change rapidly) and the requirements for such induction have been quite controversial (for discussion and references, see Ref. 11). Early *in vitro* work with mass cultures of leukocytes had shown that aquisition of CTL activity was a relatively late consequence of antigenic stimulation of peripheral T cells. Nevertheless, it did not appear to require DNA synthesis. Other studies strongly suggest (but do not prove) that the transition from pCTLs to CTLs is reversible, i.e., that active CTLs can return to a cell physiological state similar or identical to that of virgin inactive pCTLs (for review see Ref. 44).

The discovery of IL-2 raised the question of whether this factor was required for pCTL activation, and in 1982 several reports appeared claiming that the appearance of CTL activity in mitogen- or antigen-stimulated leukocyte cultures depended not only on IL-2 but also required other "differentiation" factors,[45–50] In none of these studies was it clear whether IL-2 was required only to promote the proliferation of activated CTLs to a level where they represented a sufficiently large fraction of the cells to be detectable, or whether it had other functions in CTL maturation. Our own involvment in these problems stems from the discovery that certain hybrids between the rat thymoma W/Fu(C58/NT)D and mouse CTL displayed inducible CTL activity.[21,37] As described earlier, induction of some such hybrids (including PC60) requires both IL-1 and IL-2,[36] but it is not dependent on DNA synthesis or cell division.[21] Since the proliferation of these hybrids neither in their induced nor in their noninduced state appears to depend on IL-2, these results clearly indicate that IL-2 plays a role in the induction of CTL activity that is different from its effects on cell proliferation.

Before we had identified the non-IL-2 factor required for the induction of the PC60 hybrid as IL-1, we considered the possibility that it was identical with the postulated CTL differentiation factors. As a consequence, we attempted to set up experimental systems in which these factors could be measured, but we encountered considerable difficulties to doing so. These eventually led us to carry out the experiments that demonstrated that mitogenic lectin and IL-2 are necessary and sufficient to induce the proliferation of pCTLs. The same experiments failed to reveal any requirements for other factors for the induction of cytolytic activity, and proliferation of pCTLs was invariably associated with the appearance of lectin-dependent CTL activity.[34]

The simplest hypothesis that accounts for all our findings is that pCTLs require the same signals to become cytolytically active as to proliferate, namely lectin or antigenic stimulation and IL-2, but that expression of cytolytic activity is not simply a secondary consequence of the entry of the cells into the cell cycle. The latter conclusion is based not only on the findings with PC60, but also on the observation that most established CTL lines retain their cytolytic activity even when their growth is arrested by IL-2 deprivation.

When we compare the requirements for the appearance of CTL activity with those for the induction of lymphokine secretion we find that they seem quite different: CTL clones, most of which are constitutively cytolytic, require lectin or antigenic stimulation but not IL-2 to secrete IFN-γ, IL-2, or colony-stimulating factor. That lymphokine secretion and the expression of ctyolytic activity are controlled by different mechanisms is also suggested by the behavior of some of the hybrids described earlier between AKR thymomas and murine CTL lines. Among these there is a class that is IL-2 independent and does not express CTL activity, but can still be induced to secrete IFN-γ by exposure to Con A or the appropriate antigenic stimulators (W. Haas, personal communication).

4. Concluding Remarks on the Role of T-Cell Hybrids

I believe that this review illustrates why and how somatic hybrids between cells representing different stages of T-lymphocyte differentiation can be useful for the investigation of the mechanisms controlling T-cell development and activation. They are clearly artificial cells and it would be foolish to expect them to display a phenotype identical to that of a particular normal T-cell type. However, it is precisely their abnormality that makes them useful, because it leads us to new questions or suggests answers to old ones, and sometimes makes these hybrids more amenable to molecular analysis than cell lines with more normal characteristics. The rat thymoma × mouse CTL hybrid PC60 is a case in point: not only does its behavior suggest new ideas about the role of IL-1 and IL-2 in the control of CTL activity and of IL-2 receptor expression—ideas that certainly have to be tested in experiments with normal cells—but, in addition, it provides us with a very reliable quantitative assay for IL-1. Finally, in these cells the regulation of CTL activity and IL-2 receptor expression is uncoupled from that of proliferation, something that is likely to be very handy in studies on the molecular mechanisms controlling these functions.

These considerations point out that hybrids will be most useful in areas of research where the interpretation of their behavior in molecular terms begins to be possible. They clearly assume that however abnormal the behavior of a cell may be, it is still governed by the same molecular interactions that operate in normal cells.

ACKNOWLEDGMENTS. I would like to thank my colleagues Rod Ceredig, François Erard, John Lowenthal, Rob MacDonald, Danièle Masson, Tito Silva, Jürg Tschopp, and Rudolf Zubler for many stimulating discussions and good ideas, and for permission to cite their unpublished results. The work in my laboratory has been supported by the Swiss National Science Foundation and the Swiss Cancer League.

References

1. Morgan, D. A., Ruscetti, F. W., and Gallo, R. C., 1976, Selective *in vitro* growth of T-lymphocytes from normal human bone marrows, *Science* **193**:1007–1008.
2. Coutinho, A., Larsson, E., Grönvik, K., and Andersson, J., 1979, Studies on T-lymphocyte activation. II. The target cells for concanavalin A-induced growth factors, *Eur. J. Immunol.* **9**:587–592.

3. Bonnard, G. D., Yasaka, K., and Jacobson, D., 1979, Ligand-activated T cell growth factor-induced proliferation: Absorption of T-cell growth factor by activated T-cells, *J. Immunol.* **123:**2704–2708.
4. Robb, R. J., Munck, A., and Smith, K. A., 1981, T Cell growth factor receptors. Quantitation, specificity, and biological relevance, *J. Exp. Med.* **154:**1455–1474.
5. Leonard, W. J., Depper, J. M., Uchiyama, T., Smith, K. A., Waldmann, T. A., and Greene, W. C., 1982, A monoclonal antibody that appears to recognize the receptor for human T-cell growth factor; partial characterization of the receptor, *Nature* **300:**267–269.
6. Osawa, H., and Diamantstein, T., 1983, The characteristics of a monoclonal antibody that binds specifically to rat T lymphoblasts and inhibits IL-2 receptor functions, *J. Immunol.* **30:**51–55.
7. Malek, T. R., Robb, R. J., and Shevach, E. M., 1983, Identification and initial characterization of a rat monoclonal antibody reactive with the murine interleukin 2 receptor–ligand complex, *Proc. Natl. Acad. Sci. USA* **80:**5694–5698.
8. Leonard, W. J., Deeper, J. M., Robb, R. J., Waldmann, T. A., and Greene, W. C., 1983, Characterization of the human receptor for T-cell growth factor, *Proc. Natl. Acad. Sci. USA* **80:**6957–6961.
9. Leonard, W. J., Depper, J. M., Crabtree, G. R., Rudikoff, S., Pumphrey, J., Robb, R. J., Krönke, M., Svetlic, P. B., Peffer, N. J., Waldmann, T. A., and Greene, W. C., 1984, Molecular cloning and expression of cDNAs for the human interleukin-2 receptor, *Nature* **311:**626–631.
10. Nikaido, T., Shimizu, A., Ishida, N., Sabe, H., Teshigawara, K., Maeda, M., Uchiyama, T., Yodoi, J., and Honjo, T., 1984, Molecular cloning of cDNA encoding human interleukin-2 receptor, *Nature* **311:**631–635.
11. Nabholz, M., and MacDonald, H. R., 1983, Cytolytic T lymphocytes. *Annu. Rev. Immunol.* **1:**273–306.
12. Möller, G. (ed.), 1982, Effects of anti-membrane antibodies on killer T cells, *Immunol. Rev.* **68:**1–218.
13. Reinherz, E. L., Meuer, S. C., Fitzgerald, K. A., Hussey, R. E., Hodgdon, J. C., Acuto, O., and Schlossmann, S. F., 1983, Comparison of T3 associated 49/43 kD cell surface molecules on individual human T cell clones: Evidence for peptide variability in T cell receptor structure, *Proc. Natl. Acad. Sci. USA* **80:**4104–4108.
14. Smith, K. A., 1980, T-Cell growth factor, *Immunol Rev.* **51:**336–357.
15. Larsson, E.-L., and Coutinho, A., 1979, The role of mitogenic lectins in T-cell triggering, *Nature* **280:**239–241.
16. Pledger, W. J., Stiles, C. D., Antoniades, H. N., and Scher, C. D., 1978, An ordered sequence of events is required before BALB/c–3T3 cells become committed to DNA synthesis, *Proc. Natl. Acad. Sci. USA* **75:**2839–2843.
17. Cantrell, D. A., and Smith, K. A., 1983, Transient expression of interleukin 2 receptors. Consequences for T cell growth, *J. Exp. Med.* **158:**1895–1911.
18. Zubler, R. H., Lowenthal, J. W., Erard, F., Hashimoto, N., Devos, R., and MacDonald, H. R., 1984, Activated B cells express receptors for, and proliferate in response to, pure interleukin 2, *J. Exp. med.* **160:**1170–1183.
19. Tsudo, M., Uchiyama, T., and Uchino, H., 1984, Expression of TAC antigen on activated normal human B cells, *J. Exp. Med.* **160:**612–617.
20. MacDonald, H. R., Ceredig, R., and Cerottini, J.-C., 1984, Heterogeneity of lymphokine production by T lymphocytes: Analysis of established clones and primary limiting dilution microcultures, in: *Progress in Immunology V* (Y. Yanraniura and T. Tada, eds.), Academic Press, New York, pp. 247–258.
21. Silva, A., MacDonald, H. R., Conzelmann, A., Corthésy, P., and Nabholz, M., 1983, Rat × mouse T-cell hybrids with inducible specific cytolytic activity, *Immunol. Rev.* **76:**105–129.
22. Cloyd, M. W., 1983, Characterization of target cells for MCF viruses in AKR mice, *Cell* **32:**217–225.
23. Gillis, S., Scheid, M., and Watson, J., 1980, Biochemical and biologic characterization of lymphocyte regulatory molecules. III. The isolation and phenotypic characterization of interleukin-2 producing T cell lymphomas, *J. Immunol.* **125:**2570–2578.

24. Conzelmann, A., Corthésy, P., and Nabholz, M., 1982, Correlation between cytolytic activity, growth factor dependence and lectin resistance in cytolytic T cell hybrids, in: *Isolation, Characterization and Utilization of T Lymphocyte Clones* (C. G. Fathman and F. W. Fitch, eds.), Academic Press, New York, pp. 205–215.
25. Conzelmann, A., Silva, A., Cianfriglia, M., Tougne, C., Sekaly, R. P., and Nabholz, M., 1982, Correlated expression of TCGF-dependence, sensitivity to *Vicia villosa* lectin and cytolytic activity in hybrids between cytolytic T cells and T lymphomas, *J. Exp. Med.* **156:**1335–1351.
26. Ceredig, R., Sekaly, R. P., and MacDonald, H. R., 1983, Differentiation *in vitro* of lyt-2^{+} thymocytes from embryonic lyt-2^{-} precursors, *Nature* **303:**248–250.
27. Mathieson, B. J., and Fowlkes, B. J., 1984, Cell surface antigen expression on thymocytes: Development and phenotypic differentiation of intrathymic subsets, *Immunol. Rev.* **82:**141–173.
28. Lowenthal, J. P., Tougne, C., MacDonald, H. R., Smith, K. A., and Nabholz, M., 1985, Antigenic stimulation regulates the expression of IL-2 receptors in a cytolytic T lymphocyte clone, *J. Immunol.* **134:**931–939.
29. Andrew, M. E., Braciale, V. L., and Braciale, T. J., 1984, Regulation of interleukin 2 receptor expression of murine cytotoxic T lymphocyte clones, *J. Immunol.* **132:**839–844.
30. Hemler, M. E., Brenner, M. B., McLean, J. M., and Strominger, J. L., Antigenic stimulation regulates the level of expression of interleukin 2 receptor on human T cells, *Proc. Natl. Acad. Sci. USA* **81:**2172–2175.
31. Reske-Kunz, A. B., von Steldern, D., Rüde, E., Osawa, H., and Diamantstein, T., 1984, Interleukin 2 receptors on an insulin-specific T cell line: Dynamics of receptor expression, *J. Immunol.* **133:**1356–1361.
32. Meuer, S. C., Hussey, R. E., Cantrell, D. A., Hodgdon, J. C., Schlossman, S. F., Smith, K. S., and Reinherz, E. L., 1984, Triggering of the T3-Ti antigen–receptor complex results in clonal T-cell proliferation through an interleukin 2-dependent autocrine pathway, *Proc. Natl. Acad. Sci. USA* **81:**1509–1513.
33. Hünig, T., Loos, M., and Schimpl, A., 1983, The role of accessory cells in polyclonal T cell activation. I. Both induction of interleukin-2 production and interleukin-2 responsiveness by concanavalin A are accessory cell dependent, *Eur. J. Immunol.* **13:**1–6.
34. Erard, F., Corthésy, P., Nabholz, M., Lowenthal, J. W., Zaech, P., Plaetinck, G., and MacDonald, H. R., 1985, Interleukin 2 is both necessary and sufficient for the growth and differentiation of lectin-stimulated cytolytic T lymphocyte precursors, *J. Immunol.* **134:**1644–1652.
35. Sekaly, R. P., MacDonald, H. R., Zaech, P., and Nabholz, M., 1982, Cell cycle regulation of cloned cytolytic T cells by T-cell growth factor: Analysis by flow microfluorometry, *J. Immunol.* **129:**1407–1415.
36. Erard, F., Corthésy, P., Smith, K. A., Fiers, W., Conzelmann, A., and Nabholz, M., 1984, Characterization of soluble factors which induce the cytolytic activity and the expression of T cell growth factor receptors of a T cell hybrid, *J. Exp. Med.* **160:**584–599.
37. Conzelmann, A., Corthésy, P., Cianfriglia, M., Silva, A., and Nabholz, M., 1982, Hybrids between rat lymphoma and mouse T cells with inducible cytolytic activity, *Nature* **298:**170–172.
38. Robb, R. J., Greene, W. C., and Rusk, C. M., 1984, Low and high affinity cellular receptors for interleukin 2. Implications for the level of Tac antigen, *J. Exp. Med.* **160:**1126–1146.
39. Kaye, J., Gillis, S., Mizel, S. B., Shevach, E. M., Malek, T. R., Dinarello, C. A., Lachman, L. B., and Janeway, Jr., C. A., 1984, Growth of a cloned helper T cell line induced by a monoclonal antibody specific for the antigen receptor: Interleukin 1 is required for the expression of receptors for interleukin 2, *J. Immunol.* **133:**1339–1345.
40. Kelso, A., and Glasebrook, A. L., 1984, Secretion of interleukin 2, macrophage-activating factor, interferon and colony-stimulation factor by alloreactive T lymphocyte clones, *J. Immunol.* **13:**2924–2931.
41. Dennert, G., and Podack, E. R., 1983, Cytolysis by H-2 specific T killer cells, *J. Exp. Med.* **157:**1483–1495.
42. Podack, E. R., and Königsberg, P. Y., 1984, Cytolytic T-cell granules: Isolation, structural, biochemical and functional characterization, *J. Exp. Med.* **160:**695–710.

43. Henkart, P. A., Millard, P. J., Reynolds, C. W., and Henkart, M. P., 1984, Cytolytic activity of purified cytoplasmic granules from cytotoxic rat large granular lymphocyte tumors, *J. Exp. Med.* **160:**75–93.
44. Engers, H. D., and MacDonald, H. R., 1976, Generation of cytolytic T lymphocytes *in vitro*, in: *Contemporary Topics in Immunobiology* (W. O. Weigle, ed.), Plenum Press, New York, pp. 145–190.
45. Raulet, D. H., and Bevan, M. J., 1982, A differentiation factor required for the expression of cytotoxic T cell function, *Nature* **296:**754–757.
46. Wagner, H., Hardt, C., Rouse, B. T., Röllinghoff, M., Schenrich, P., and Pfizenmaier, K., 1982, Dissection of the proliferative and differentiative signals controlling murine cytotoxic T lymphocyte responses, *J. Exp. Med.* **155:**1876–1881.
47. Kanagawa, O., 1983, Three different signals are required for the induction of cytolytic T lymphocytes from resting precursors, *J. Immunol.* **131:**606–610.
48. Männel, D. N., Falk, W., and Dröge, W., 1983, Induction of cytotoxic T cell function requires sequential action of three lymphokines, *J. Immunol.* **130:**2508–2510.
49. Garman, R. D., and Fan, D. P., 1983, Characterization of helper factors distinct from interleukin-2, necessary for the generation of allospecific cytolytic T lymphocytes, *J. Immunol.* **130:**756–762.
50. Finke, J. H., Scott, J., Gillis, S., and Hilfiker, M. L., 1983, Generation of alloreactive cytotoxic T lymphocytes: Evidence for a differentiation factor distinct from IL-2, *J. Immunol.* **130:**763–767.
51. Nguyen, T., and Nabholz, M., 1985, Glucocorticoid resistance is a dominant trait in hybrids between cytolytic T-lymphocyte lines and AKR-thymomas, manuscript submitted.
52. Ceredig, R., Lowenthal, J. W., Nabholz, M., and MacDonald, H. R., 1985, Expression of Interleukin 2 receptors as a differentiation marker on intrathymic stem cells, *Nature* **314:**98–109.
53. Lowenthal, J. W., Zubler, R. H., Nabholz, M., and MacDonald, H. R., Similarities between Interleukin 2 receptor number and affinity on activated B and T lymphocytes, manuscript submitted.
54. Lowenthal, J. W., Corthesy, P., Tougue, C., Lees, R., MacDonald, H. R., and Nabholz, M., manuscript in preparation.
55. Masson, D., Corthesy, P., Nabholz, M., and Tschopp, J., 1984, Appearance of cytolytic granules upon induction of cytolitic activity in CTL-hybrids, manuscript submitted.

Chapter 35

Human Cytolytic T-Lymphocyte Clones and Their Function-Associated Cell Surface Molecules

ALAN M. KRENSKY, STEVEN J. MENTZER, JULIA L. GREENSTEIN, MARY CRIMMINS, CAROL CLAYBERGER, TIMOTHY A. SPRINGER, and STEVEN J. BURAKOFF

1. Introduction

Cytolytic T lymphocytes (CTLs) are important effectors in the recognition of viruses,[1] allografts,[2] and some tumors.[3] A molecular understanding of the CTL–target cell interaction therefore may be relevant to the etiology and/or treatment of a variety of disease states. Tissue culture techniques, first reported by Gillis and Smith,[4] have allowed the generation of long-term T-cell lines that retain function. A number of human long-term cytolytic T lymphocyte lines have been generated by continued stimulation of peripheral blood lymphocyte lines with "foreign" cells in the presence of the T-cell growth factor interleukin 2 (IL-2).[5,6] We have used CTL lines and clones to define target antigens recognized by human allogeneic lymphocytes, to correlate lymphocyte phenotype with antigen specificity, and to generate monoclonal antibodies that block lymphocyte function. Our findings have provided new insights into the cell surface molecules involved in the CTL–target cell interaction. In this chapter we describe our methodologies for the generation and maintenance of CTL lines and

ALAN M. KRENSKY and CAROL CLAYBERGER • Department of Pediatrics, Stanford University School of Medicine, Stanford, California 94305. STEVEN J. MENTZER • Division of Pediatric Oncology, Dana-Farber Cancer Institute, and Department of Surgery, Harvard Medical School, Boston, Massachusetts 02115. JULIA L. GREENSTEIN • Division of Pediatric Oncology, Dana-Farber Cancer Institute, and Department of Pathology, Harvard Medical School, Boston, Massachusetts 02115. MARY CRIMMINS • Division of Pediatric Oncology, Dana-Farber Cancer Institute, Boston, Massachusetts 02115. TIMOTHY A. SPRINGER • Laboratory of Membrane Immunochemistry, Dana-Farber Cancer Institute, and Department of Pathology, Harvard Medical School, Boston, Massachusetts 02115. STEVEN J. BURAKOFF • Division of Pediatric Oncology, Dana-Farber Cancer Institute, and Department of Pediatrics, Harvard Medical School, Boston, Massachusetts 02115.

clones and the use of these cells in concert with monoclonal antibodies to define and analyze function-associated cell surface molecules.

2. Methods

2.1. Generation of T-Cell Growth Factors (Conditioned Medium)

Although interleukin 2 (IL-2) is requisite for the proliferation and maintenance of human T cells, it may not be sufficient for the long-term maintenance and cloning of CTLs. We have found that IL-2 produced by the T-cell tumor Jurkat or by recombinant techniques support short-term CTL growth and proliferation but poorly maintains long-term growth or the cloning of human CTLs. These findings suggest that other, as yet undefined factors may also be required for optimal *in vitro* growth of human CTLs. We therefore have used conditioned medium, i.e., supernatants from lectin- and allostimulated peripheral blood lymphocytes, as our source of T-cell growth factors (TCGFs) necessary for the long-term maintenance of CTL lines and clones.

Peripheral blood lymphocytes (PBLs) are obtained from plasmapheresis donors with approximately $(1–5) \times 10^9$ mononuclear cells obtained per donor. Cells from five different donors are pooled to minimize the possibility of "low IL-2-producers" as well as to maximize allostimulation. The cells are washed three times and cultured at 3×10^6 cells/ml. It is not necessary to remove contaminating erythrocytes.

We add mitogen and several cell cycle inhibitors to maximize TCGF yield. PHA-P (Difco) (0.15% v/v) is preferable to Con A or LPS in stimulating TCGF production by human PBLs. In addition, 2.8 μM indomethacin (Sigma) is added to inhibit prostaglandin synthesis by adherent cells. Hydroxyurea (50 μM) is added to prevent cells from entering S phase and thereby minimizes the absorption of IL-2 by proliferating cells (interleukin 2 is produced during late G_1).[7]

Cells are cultured in RPMI 1640 (M.A. Bioproducts) supplemented with 3% fetal calf serum, 2 mM L-glutamine (GIBCO), penicillin at 100 U/ml and streptomycin at 100 μg/ml (GIBCO), and 10 mM HEPES (M.A. Bioproducts) in 150-cm^2 flasks at 37°C in a 5% CO_2 humidified incubator for 72 hr. The supernatants are harvested and PHA and other additives are depleted by sequential precipitations at 50 and 75% ammonium sulfate saturation.[8] The precipitate at 50% saturation is discarded, and the precipitate at 75% saturation is suspended in one-tenth the original volume of RPMI 1640, and dialyzed against five changes of PBS and a final change of RPMI 1640. The final preparation is filtered and stored at 4°C or aliquoted and frozen at −20°C. The activity of each preparation is assessed by measuring proliferation ([^{3}H]thymidine incorporation) of an IL-2-dependent T-cell line such as HT-2.

2.2. Generation of CTL Lines and Clones

Cytolytic T lymphocytes (CTLs) are generated by stimulating PBLs with an Epstein–Barr virus (EBV)-transformed B-cell tumor of known HLA type. In general, 5 × 10^6 PBLs/ml are stimulated with 1 × 10^5 irradiated (10,000 rad) stimulator cells in 2-ml wells (Linbro). Cultures are restimulated at 7- to 10-day intervals and are cloned by limiting dilution at various times after primary stimulation. Limiting dilution methodology and theory have been described in detail elsewhere.[9] Cells are cloned in RPMI 1640, supplemented with 10% fetal calf serum, 2 mM L-glutamine, penicillin 100 U/ml, streptomycin 100 μg/ml, 25 μM 2-mercaptoethanol, and 10% conditioned medium. It should be noted that different lots of fetal calf serum vary significantly in their ability to support clonal growth. We therefore screen fetal calf serum by determining its influence on cloning efficiency. We have found that only about 10% of the lots support good clonal growth. Cells can be cloned in either round- or flat-bottom microtiter wells (Linbro), but we have found that the round-bottom wells yield slightly higher cloning efficiencies. Wells are seeded with 10, 1, 0.3, or 0.1 cells/well plus irradiated PBLs (2000 rad, 8 × 10^4 cells/well) or tumor cells (10,000 rad, 2 × 10^4 cells/well).

Colonies are visible after 1–3 weeks and are then split into flat-bottom microtiter wells containing 5 × 10^5 irradiated PBLs or 2 × 10^4 irradiated tumor cells. Colonies are then tested for cytotoxic activity, specificity, and phenotype. After cells are expanded to 4–8 wells, they are split into 2-ml wells (Linbro) containing 10^6 PBLs or 10^5 tumor cells. Allospecific human CTLs are assessed for specificity using panels of EBV B lymphoblasts as targets of known HLA types. Specificity is further confirmed by monoclonal antibody inhibition of specific cytolysis. Aliquots of each line are frozen (10% DMSO/90% fetal calf serum v/v) and stored in liquid nitrogen. Clones are subcloned by limiting dilution to ensure clonality.

3. Results and Discussion

3.1. The Use of CTL Lines and Clones to Define Allogeneic Target Molecules

For many years it was assumed that human allogeneic CTLs recognized only the HLA-A and -B antigens.[10] We and others have recently shown that CTLs can also recognize HLA-C,[11] HLA-DR,[12–16] DC,[17,18] and SB[19] target molecules.

The HLA-A and -B molecules induce the strongest allogeneic CTL response.[20] When peripheral blood lymphocytes are stimulated by cells expressing foreign class I (HLA-A, B, C) and class II (HLA-DR, DC, and SB) MHC antigens, CTLs of a variety of target specificities are generated.[21] After 3–4 weeks in culture the dominant target antigens recognized are the HLA-A and -B antigens.[12] If, however, class I MHC disparity between responding PBLs and stimulator cells is eliminated, class II-specific CTLs can be generated and propagated in long-term culture. For example, the system may be biased by using stimulator cells that are allogeneic at only some of the MHC loci. Albrechtsen *et al.*[22] and Feighery and Stastny[23] used this protocol to generate mixed lymphocyte cultures between HLA-A, B identical donors and showed that CTLs could recognize non-class I MHC molecules, presumably class II molecules. We used a different approach, in which peripheral blood lymphocytes were stimulated with cells that do not express certain MHC antigens. Daudi is an Epstein–Barr virus (EBV)-transformed lymphoblastoid cell line that does not express class I MHC antigens due to an inability to produce β_2-microglobulin. When peripheral blood lymphocytes were stimulated with a cell line (JY) that expresses both class I (HLA-A2, A2; B7, B7) and class II (HLA-DR4, 6; DC1, SB2, 4) antigens, the long-term CTL lines generated were specific for HLA-A2 and/or HLA-B7 determinants.[12] If, however, peripheral blood lymphocytes were stimulated with the JY cell line only once, followed by continued stimulation with the Daudi cell line (HLA-A$^-$, B$^-$, C$^-$, DR6; DC1; SB2), CTLs specific for HLA-DR6[12,13] or DC1[17] determinants were generated. Finally, Moretta *et al.*[24] derived largely OKT4$^+$, rather than OKT8$^+$, CTLs by cloning immediately after primary stimulation regardless of the MHC antigens expressed by the stimulator cells.[24]

Once the CTL lines have been generated, target specificity is determined by: (1) testing cytolysis of panels of EBV-transformed target cells expressing a variety of MHC antigens and (2) testing the ability of a panel of anti-MHC monoclonal antibodies to inhibit specific cytolysis.[12] Using such techniques, we and others have generated human allogeneic CTL lines and clones specific for HLA-A, B,[12,20] -C[11] and -DR,[12–16] SB,[19] and DC[17,18] MHC antigens.

At any point after primary stimulation, CTLs can be cloned by limiting dilution[9] or micromanipulation.[25] Clones of T cells arising from a single cell have been used to probe the variety of antigenic specificities recognized by T cells. Results from these studies have shown that CTLs may recognize a number of different determinants on a single molecule[26] and that T cells may recognize determinants other than those recognized serologicially, i.e., by antibodies.[27] CTL clones have also helped to define variants of MHC molecules.[28] For example, HLA-A2 was originally identified using alloantisera, and approximately 60% of North American Caucasians were found to be HLA-A2 positive.[29,30] Using CTL lines and clones as probes, however, subsets or "variants" of HLA-A2 have been demonstrated. Recent biochemical studies have identified the molecular and structural basis for these cell-mediated lympholysis-defined determinants.[31,32] In these ways, CTL lines and clones have provided important information regarding antigen recognition by lymphocytes.

3.2. Transfection of Cloned MHC Genes to Study Target Molecules

Advances in molecular biology have provided a new approach to the study of CTL specificity and recognition of target cell MHC antigens. Genes encoding various MHC antigens have been cloned and transfected into eukaryotic cells by DNA-mediated gene transfer, allowing analysis of the CTL interaction with individual gene products.[33] Murine L cells have been transfected with H-2 genes, but recently several groups have reported that human CTLs do not recognize HLA genes transfected and expressed in L cells.[34,35] When these same genes were transfected into human cells (an osteosarcoma and a rhabdomyosarcoma) allospecific human CTL clones could lyse the transfected cells.[36] It is unlikely that conformational changes induced by coexpression with murine β_2-microglobulin accounts for the lack of recognition.[35] Possible explanations include: (1) differences in species-specific posttranslational modification, (2) recognition of MHC + X, where X is missing from the transfected cells, and (3) lack of some critical cell surface molecule essential for cytolysis (see below).

3.3. Functional Studies of Cell Surface Antigens: The Importance of the OKT4 and OKT8 T-Cell Surface Molecules

Human T cells can be classified not only by function, but also by cell surface molecules defined by monoclonal antibodies, such as the OKT[37] and Leu[38] series of antibodies. All peripheral blood T cells bear the OKT3 (Leu-4) antigen. It was originally thought that OKT4 (Leu-3) antigen was exclusively found on the helper/inducer subset of T cells and the OKT5/OKT8 (Leu-2) antigens were specific for the suppressor/cytotoxic subset.[39] However, when CTLs specific for HLA-DR6 antigens were analyzed, they were found to express OKT4 and not OKT8[12]; thus, the CTLs expressed the phenotype thought specific for the helper/inducer subset and lacked the marker thought specific for CTLs. On the other hand, CTLs specific for HLA-A2 and -B7 antigens expressed OKT8 and not OKT4, as expected.[12] These findings raised the possibility that the OKT4 and OKT8 molecules are involved in the recognition of HLA-DR (class II) and HLA-A, B (class I) molecules, respectively, rather than defining the function of T-cell subsets.[12–16] This hypothesis was supported by numerous reports of OKT4$^+$ CTLs,[12–16] OKT8$^+$ helper cells,[40] and OKT4$^+$ suppressor cells.[41]

Although the hypothesis that OKT8 may be a receptor for class I MHC antigens (recognizing a monomorphic site on the MHC molecule) and that OKT4 is a receptor for class II MHC antigens is attractive, exceptions to this correlation have already been described. We have reported a DC1-specific CTL line that expresses OKT8 and not OKT4.[17] Similarly, other OKT8$^+$ HLA-DR-,[16,42] DC-,[18] and SB[19]-specific CTLs have been described.

To test whether these cell surface molecules were functionally involved in the CTL–target cell interaction, we examined the ability of anti-T-cell monoclonal antibodies to inhibit directly the CTL–target cell interaction. OKT3 (Leu-4) monoclonal antibody inhibits cytolysis by all the CTLs that we studied. Biddison *et al.*[43] and Moretta *et al.*,[44] however, have recently described OKT3$^+$ CTLs that are not inhibited by anti-OKT3 monoclonal antibodies. OKT4 (Leu-3a) monoclonal antibodies inhibited only the HLA-DR6 (OKT4$^+$)-specific CTLs, and OKT8 (Leu-2a) monoclonal antibodies inhibited only the HLA-A2 and -B7 (OKT8$^+$) CTLs.[13,45] Of particular note, neither OKT4 nor OKT8 monoclonal antibodies inhibited cytolysis by the OKT8$^+$, DC1-specific CTLs.[17] Frequently, when the OKT8-class I/OKT4-class II dichotomy does not hold, neither OKT4 nor OKT8 monoclonal antibodies block cytolysis.[45]

The ability of anti-T-cell antibodies to inhibit CTL–target cell conjugate formation has also been examined. Landegren *et al.*[46] and Tsoukas *et al.*[47] have shown that OKT8 (Leu-2) inhibits CTL–target cell conjugation, while OKT3 does not. We recently confirmed these results and also showed that anti-OKT4 monoclonal antibodies inhibit conjugation between an $OKT4^+$ CTL and its target.[48]

Thus the precise role of the OKT4 and OKT8 T-cell surface molecules remains unclear. Although they divide peripheral blood lymphocytes into two almost mutually exclusive subpopulations (there are rare $OKT4^+$, $OKT8^+$-peripheral blood lymphocytes), OKT4 and OKT8 are not simply associated with the helper/inducer and cytotoxic/suppressor functions as once thought. Neither are they strictly associated with either class I or class II MHC recognition.

3.4. Lymphocyte Function-Associated Antigens (LFA)-1, 2, and 3

To define other function-associated cell surface molecules, we generated a panel of anti-human CTL monoclonal antibodies and screened them for their ability to inhibit T-cell functions.[49] Springer and co-workers had previously used a similar protocol to identify functionally relevant epitopes on the murine cell surface molecules Lyt-2 (the homologue of OKT8) and lymphocyte function-associated antigen-1 (LFA-1).[50] We immunized mice with an $OKT4^+$, HLA-DR6-specific CTL line, and selected hybridomas for the ability to inhibit cytolysis by the immunizing cell line. Monoclonal antibodies specific for three different molecules, designated LFA-1, 2, and 3, inhibited cytolysis, suggesting that these cell surface structures participate in the CTL–target cell interaction.

Seven of the hybridomas produced antibodies that immunoprecipitated LFA-1 polypeptide chains of 177 and 95 kD from CTLs. One monoclonal antibody (TS1/18) recognizes the β chain (95 kD) of LFA-1, while all of the other monoclonal antibodies recognize the α chain (177 kD).[51] Three unique and three partially overlapping epitopes of human LFA-1 have been identified by competitive cross-inhibition binding assays using biosynthetically labeled anti-LFA-1 monoclonal antibodies.[50] Quantitative differences in the ability of different monoclonal antibodies to block cytolysis suggest distinct functional as well as antigenic epitopes.[50]

LFA-1 is expressed on 95% of peripheral blood lymphoctyes (PBLs), including both B and T lymphocytes, as well as the majority of thymocytes, phytohemagglutinin (PHA)-activated blasts, CTLs, granulocytes, monocytes, and one-third of bone marrow cells.[52] Immunoprecipitation and FACS analyses show quantitative differences in the expression of LFA-1 on various cell types: CTLs and PHA-activated cells >PBLs >thymocytes >B lymphoblastoid cells.[52] The broad distribution of LFA-1 on lymphoid cells prompted us to assess the ability of anti-LFA-1 monoclonal antibodies to block a variety of immune responses. Anti-LFA-1 monoclonal antibodies significantly inhibit: (1) cytolysis by $OKT8^+$, HLA-A, B-specific CTLs; $OKT4^+$, HLA-DR-specific CTLs; $OKT8^+$, DC1-specific CTLs, and NK cells[52]; and (2) proliferative responses to alloantigens (MLR), mitogens (PHA, Con A), and soluble antigens.[52] Complete blocking is achieved with 1–5 μg/ml of antibody.

Two other groups have recently reported monoclonal antibodies that also appear to recognize the LFA-1 molecule. Hildreth *et al.*[53] immunized mice with an EBV-transformed human lymphoblastoid cell line and generated two monoclonal antibodies, MHM23 and MHM24, which immunoprecipitate 180- and 95-kD polypeptide chains from both B and T lymphocytes. Both antibodies inhibit HLA-restricted lysis of influenza-infected and EBV-transformed target cells by binding to the effector cell.[53] Recently, Beatty *et al.*[54] described another monoclonal antibody, 60.3, which has similar properties. Further insight into the role of the LFA-1 molecule has recently been made possible by the discovery of immunodeficient patients who lack the LFA-1/Mol family of cell surface molecules (Refs. 45 and 55–60, and Springer and Anderson, this volume, Chapter 11). These patients have recurrent bacterial infections and impaired granulocyte phagocytosis. This group of patients offer a unique opportunity to study the functional role of the LFA-1 molecule.

We have studied three LFA-1-deficient patients, their families, and unrelated individuals. In all three cases, cells from the patients show decreased CTL-mediated cytotoxicity, NK-cell-mediated cytotoxicity, and proliferative responses to alloantigens and PHA.[45,56,60]

The broad cellular distribution of LFA-1 and its involvement in many immune functions suggest that, analogous to murine LFA-1, this molecule is involved in cell–cell adhesion. We therefore examined the effect of anti-LFA-1 on CTL–target cell conjugate formation. As expected, anti-LFA-1 blocked conjugate formation between CTLs and lymphoblastoid targets.[48]

The LFA-2 antigen is defined by two monoclonal antibodies that inhibit cytolysis and immunoprecipitate a diffuse band of 49 kD from thymocytes, PHA blasts, and CTLs, but not from granulocytes, monocytes, or B cells.[52] This antigen is expressed on PHA blasts >CTLs >thymocytes >PBLs, whereas OKT3 expression is similar on resting and activated T cells.[52] Further analysis showed that LFA-2 is identical to the "sheep erythrocyte receptor molecule," also recognized by OKT11,[61] Leu-5,[62] and monoclonal antibody 9.6.[63] The MAbs to this molecule inhibit the formation of spontaneous rosettes between T lymphocytes and sheep erythrocytes. This rosetting reaction has long been used to advantage by immunologists for the purification of human T lymphocytes on density gradients. All of these monoclonal antibodies inhibit cytolysis by HLA-A,B-, HLA-DR-, and DC-specific CTLs and block proliferative response to alloantigens, mitogens, and soluble antigens.[52] Only OKT11 completely modulates this molecule from the cell surface (anti-LFA-2, Leu-5, and 9.6 modulate 50–75% of the molecule from the cell surface). This indicates that complete modulation of the "sheep erythrocyte receptor molecule" is not necessary for functional inhibition.

Martin *et al.*[64] recently demonstrated that 9.6 and another monoclonal antibody, designated 35.1, recognize different epitopes in close proximity on the sheep erythrocyte receptor molecule, but that 9.6 inhibits E rosette formation and cell-mediated cytotoxicity, while 35.1 does not. Of note, these authors found that 9.6 also inhibits NK cell-mediated cytolysis.[64] In our system, anti-LFA-2 monoclonal antibodies (TS2/18, TS1/8) fail to inhibit NK-cell-mediated cytolysis.[52]

Anti-LFA-2 monoclonal antibody precipitates molecules of different molecular weights from T cells at different stages of activation and/or differentiation.[52] Since LFA-2 is a glycoprotein, this heterogeneity may be due to differences in either glycosylation or amino acid sequence. Because of the apparent similarity between the molecular weight of the putative T-cell receptor and the sheep erythrocyte receptor, LFA-2 was immunoprecipitated from a series of CTL clones and found to be of uniform molecular weight. In addition, preclearing experiments showed a lack of identity between the putative T-cell receptor and LFA-2. Lastly, comodulation experiments confirmed that OKT3 and Ti reciprocally comodulate, while OKT3 and LFA-2 do not.

Thus, the "sheep erythrocyte receptor" recognized by anti-LFA-2 and a number of other monoclonal antibodies is a T-cell function-associated molecule. It has a slightly broader cell distribution than OKT3.[52] We have shown that anti-LFA-2 monoclonal antibodies inhibit CTL–target cell conjugate formation.[48] Meuer *et al.*[65] have recently suggested that this cell surface antigen is involved in an "alternative" T-lymphocyte activation pathway separate from the OKT3 circuit.[65] The precise role of this T-cell function-associated molecule remains undefined.

LFA-3 (45–65 kD) is expressed on 40–60% of peripheral blood lymphocytes, including both B and T lymphocytes. It is also present on essentially all monocytes, granulocytes, CTLs, B-lymphoblastoid cell lines, platelets, vascular endothelial cells, smooth muscle, and fibroblasts.[52] Anti-LFA-3 monoclonal antibody blocks cytolysis by CTLs, but not NK cells, and inhibits all T-cell proliferative responses studied.[52]

To establish the locus of inhibition of anti-LFA monoclonal antibodies, effector or target cells were pretreated with anti-LFA-1, anti-LFA-2, or anti-LFA-3 monoclonal antibodies, and washed extensively, and inhibition of cytolysis was assessed in a standard ^{51}Cr-release assay. Both anti-LFA-1 and anti-LFA-2 monoclonal antibodies block cytolysis by binding to the effector cell, while anti-LFA-3 monoclonal antibody blocks cytolysis by binding to the target cells.[52]

In recent studies, we have shown that trypsin treatment of target cells removes LFA-3 but leaves LFA-1 and MHC molecules intact on the lymphoblastoid target cell surface.[66] Trypsin treatment of target cells results in increased blocking by anti-LFA-1 monoclonal antibodies, but a loss of inhibition by anti-LFA-3 monoclonal antibody. These findings confirm that LFA-3 is involved in the CTL–target cell interaction at the level of the target cell. Furthermore, they indicate that a trypsin-sensitive molecule (perhaps LFA-3) on the target cell is involved in the LFA-1–target cell interaction.

LFA-3 is a novel target molecule: It is present on all tissues studied and blocks function by binding to the target cell rather than the effector cell. Of note, immunoprecipitation of LFA-3 from lymphocytes, fibroblasts, and endothelial cells indicates a molecular weight heterogeneity from 50,000 to

60,000.[52] Studies to determine if this heterogeneity is due to carbohydrate or protein differences are in progress.

3.5. The Role of Cell Surface Antigens in the T-Lymphocyte–Mesenchymal Cell Interaction

The mechanism of CTL-mediated lysis has been largely studied using lymphoid and other bone marrow-derived target cells. Although the use of lymphoid target cells is experimentally convenient and has provided great insight into the CTL–target cell interaction, the pathophysiologically relevant targets in organ transplantation include other cells, such as vascular endothelium and stromal cells. It is possible that CTL recognition and lysis of these cell types proceeds through different mechanisms, perhaps involving different accessory molecules. We have shown that an HLA-DR6-specific CTL clone, generated against lymphoblastoid targets, can specifically recognize and lyse cultured human endothelial cells and fibroblasts that have been induced to express HLA-DR antigens by immune interferon.[67] We have used this system to show that the CTL–vascular endothelium and CTL–fibroblast interactions also involve at least OKT3, OKT4/OKT8, LFA-1, LFA-2, and LFA-3 molecules.[68]

4. Summary

A number of cell surface molecules have been identified that appear to be important in the human CTL–target cell interaction (Table I). The T3–Ti complex appears to be involved in antigen-specific T-cell interactions.[69] Meuer and his colleagues[69] defined the antigen-specific receptor (Ti) on T cells in man with a clonotypic (clone-specific) monoclonal antibody that blocks lymphocyte function. The T3 molecule is coprecipitated and comodulated with Ti. Monoclonal antibodies to T3 block all T-cell functions studied and are mitogenic.[69] Until recently, all monoclonal antibody blocking experiments indicated a requirement for OKT3. Moretta *et al.*[44] and Biddison *et al.*,[43] however, have described CTL clones that appear not to require the OKT3 molecule; cytolysis by these OKT3$^+$ CTLs is not inhibited by anti-OKT3 monoclonal antibodies. Thus, no single cell surface molecule has been shown to be "required" for lymphocyte function.

In addition to the antigen-specific receptor, other "accessory" (non-antigen-specific) molecules appear to be involved in the CTL-target cell interaction. These molecules appear to function, at least in part, by increasing the overall CTL–target cell affinity. High-affinity interaction between the T-cell receptor and antigen may be sufficient to allow cytolysis; alternately, low-affinity antigen–receptor interaction may require additional "accessory" molecules for cytolysis.

Martz *et al.* divided CTL-mediated cytolysis into two steps based on differing dependence on divalent cations.[70] The first step, requiring Mg^{+2} and

Table I. Human Cell Surface Molecules Associated with Lymphocyte Function

Molecule	Molecular weight	Cell distribution	Functions inhibited by monoclonal antibody		Monoclonal antibody inhibits by binding to	Proposed molecular function
			Cytotoxicity	Proliferation		
1. HLA-A, B, C	44,000, 12,000	All cells except red blood cells	+ (HLA-A, B, C-specific CTLs)	±[a]	Target	Class I MHC antigens
2. HLA-DR	34,000, 29,000	Macrophages, B cells, activated T cells, other "immune cells"	+ (HLA-DR-specific CTLs)	+	Target	Class II MHC antigens
3. SB (DP)	34,000, 29,000	Same as HLA-DR	+ (SB-specific CTLs)	+	Target	Class II MHC antigens
4. DC (DQ)	34,000, 29,000	Same as HLA-DR	+ (DC-specific CTLs)	+	Target	Class II MHC antigens
5. LFA-3	45,000, 65,000	Broad	+	+	Target	Target accessory molecule (? ligand)
6. Ti	49,000, 43,000	T Cells	+	+	Effector	Antigen receptor
7. OKT3 (Leu-4)	19,000	T Cells	+	+	Effector	Associated with Ti
8. OKT_4 (Leu-3a)	62,000	Sixty percent of T cells	+	+	Effector	HLA-DR-associated accessory molecule
9. OKT8 (Leu-2a)	43,000	Forty percent of T cells	+	+[a]	Effector	HLA-A, B, C-associated accessory molecule
10. LFA-1	177,000, 95,000	Leukocytes	+	+	Effector	Leukocyte accessory molecule (? adhesion)
11. LFA-2 (Leu-5, OKT11, E-rosette receptor)	49,000	T Cells	+	+	Effector	T-Cell accessory molecule

[a] Small subpopulation.

specific antigen recognition, involves adherence of the CTLs to the target. The studies that we have described suggest that OKT4 and OKT8 may be involved in recognition of monomorphic MHC determinants at this step. LFA-1, LFA-2, and LFA-3 similarly inhibit conjugate formation[48] and may be involved in some non-antigen-specific recognition process and/or adhesion. Once low-affinity, non-antigen-specific bonds form, the antigen-specific receptor may engage antigen. Then, depending on the avidity of the specific antigen–receptor interaction, other "stabilizing" interactions involving OKT4/OKT8, LFA-1, LFA-2, and/or LFA-3 may be required. A "lethal hit" is delivered in the second, Ca^{2+}-dependent step. Once the lethal hit occurs, the target cell is "programmed for lysis"; that is, lysis occurs even if the CTL–target conjugate is disrupted.[70] It is remarkable that the experimental methods described in this chapter have given rise only to monoclonal antibodies that recognize molecules that appear to be involved in the first step of the CTL–target cell interaction. It is possible that cell surface molecules are not involved after "triggering" of the cell, i.e., in delivery of the lethal hit.

5. Conclusion

Hybridoma technology and T-cell cloning have advanced our understanding of the molecules involved in the CTL–target cell interaction. Monoclonal antibodies selected for their ability to inhibit lymphocyte function have allowed us to define further the role of the OKT4 and OKT8 molecules and to define new lymphocyte function-associated antigens LFA-1, LFA-2, and LFA-3. These studies have demonstrated a series of accessory (not antigen-specific) molecular interactions which may be critical in the induction and stabilization of the CTL–target cell interaction. Such "accessory" molecules may be central to all cellular interactions.

Acknowledgments. We wish to thank Carolyn Gregory for her excellent secretarial assistance. This work was supported by NIH grant CA34129. S. J. B. and T. A. S. are recipients of American Cancer Society Research Faculty Awards.

References

1. Burakoff, S. J., Reiss, C. S., Finberg, R., and Mescher, M. F., 1980, Cell mediated immunity to viral glycoproteins, *Rev. Infect. Dis.* **2:**62–77.
2. Cerottini, J. C., and Brunner, K. T., 1974, Cell-mediated cytotoxicity, allograft rejection, and immunity, *Adv. Immunol.* **18:**67–132.
3. Herberman, R. B., 1974, Cell mediated immunity to tumor cells, *Adv. Cancer Res.* **19:**207–263.
4. Gillis, S., and Smith, K. A., 1977, Long-term culture of tumor-specific cytotoxic T cells, *Nature* **268:**154–156.
5. Bach, F. H., Inouge, H., Hank, J. A., and Alter, B. J., 1979, Human T lymphocyte clone reactive in primed lymphocyte typing and cytotoxicity, *Nature* **281:**307–309.

6. Kornbluth, J., and Dupont, B., 1980, Cloning and functional characterization of primary alloreactive T lymphocytes, *J. Exp. Med.* **152:**164s–181s.
7. Stadler, B. M., Doughterty, S. F., Farrar, J. J., and Oppenheim, J. J., 1981, Relationship of cell cycle to recovery of IL-2 activity from human mononuclear cells, human and mouse T cell lines, *J. Immunol.* **127:**1936–1940.
8. Mier, J. W., and Gallo, R. C., 1980, Purification and some characteristics of human T cell growth factor from phytohemagglutinin-stimulated lymphocyte conditioned media, *Proc. Natl. Acad. Sci. USA* **77:**6134–6138.
9. Lefkovits, I., 1979, Limiting dilution analysis, in *Immunological Methods,* Academic Press, New York, pp. 355–370.
10. Katz, D. S., and Benacerraf, B. (eds.), 1976, *The Role of Products of the Histocompatibility Gene Complex in Immune Response,* Academic Press, New York.
11. Malissen, B., Kristensen, T., Goridis, C., Madsen, M., and Mawas, C., 1981, Clones of human cytotoxic T lymphocytes derived from an allosensitized individual. HLA specificity and cell surface markers, *Scand. J. Immunol.* **14:**213–224.
12. Krensky, A. M., Reiss, C. S., Mier, J. W., Strominger, J. L., and Burakoff, S. J., 1982, Long-term human cytolytic T cell lines allospecific for HLA-DR6 antigen are OKT4$^+$, *Proc. Natl. Acad. Sci. USA* **79:**2365–2369.
13. Krensky, A. M., Clayberger, C., Reiss, C. S., Strominger, J. L., and Burakoff, S. J., 1982, Specificity of OKT4$^+$ cytotoxic T lymphocyte clones, *J. Immunol.* **129:**2001–2003.
14. Meuer, S. C., Schlossman, S. F., and Reinherz, E. L., 1982, Clonal analysis of human cytotoxic T lymphocytes; T4$^+$ and T8$^+$ effector T cells recognize products of different major histocompatibility complex regions, *Proc. Natl. Acad. Sci. USA* **79:**4395–4399.
15. Spits, H., Borst, J., Terhorst, C., and DeVries, J. E., 1982, The role of T cell differentiation markers in antigen specific and lectin-dependent cellular cytotoxicity mediated by T8$^+$ and T4$^+$ human cytotoxic T cell clones directed at class I and class II MHC antigens, *J. Immunol.* **129:**1563–1569.
16. Ball, E. J., and Stastny, P., 1982, Cell-mediated cytotoxicity against HLA-D region products expressed in monocytes and B lymphocytes. IV. Characterization of effector cells using monoclonal antibodies against human T cell subsets. *Immunogenetics* **16:**157–169.
17. Krensky, A. M., Clayberger, C., Greenstein, J., Crimmins, M., and Burakoff, S. J., 1983, A DC-specific cytolytic T lymphocyte line is OKT8$^+$, *J. Immunol.* **131:**2777–2780.
18. Spits, H. H., Yssl, H., Thompson, A., and DeVries, J. E., 1983, Human T4$^+$ and T8$^+$ cytotoxic T lymphocyte clones directed at products of different class II MHC loci, *J. Immunol.* **131:**678–683.
19. Biddison, W. E., Rao, P. E., Talle, M. A., Goldstein, G., and Shaw, J., 1982, Possible involvement of the OKT4 molecule in T cell recognition of class II antigen, *J. Exp. Med.* **156:**1065–1076.
20. Reiss, C. S., Hemler, M. E., Engelhard, V. H., Mier, J. W., Strominger, J. L., and Burakoff, S. J., 1980, Development and characterization of allospecific long-term human cytolytic T cell lines, *Proc. Natl. Acad. Sci. USA* **77:**5432–5436.
21. Krensky, A. M., Ault, K. A., Reiss, C. S., Strominger, J. L., and Burakoff, S. J., 1982, Generation of long-term human cytolytic cell lines with persistent natural killer activity, *J. Immunol.* **129:**1748–1751.
22. Albrechtsen, D., Arnesen, E., and Thorsby, E., 1979, Cell-mediated lymphocytotoxicity directed against HLA-D gene products, *Transplant.* **27:**338–341.
23. Feighery, C., and Stastny, P., 1979, HLA-D region-associated determinants serve as targets for human cell-mediated lysis, *J. Exp. Med.* **149:**485–494.
24. Moretta, L., Minyari, M. C., Sekaly, P. R., Moretta, A., Capuis, B., and Cerottini, J. C., 1981, Surface markers of cloned human T cells with various cytolytic activities, *J. Exp. Med.* **154:**569–574.
25. Zaguiry, D., Bernard, J., Thiemesse, N., Feldman, M., and Berke, G., 1975, Isolation and characterization of individual functionally reactive cytotoxic T lymphocytes, conjugation, killing, and recycling at the single cell level, *Eur. J. Immunol.* **5:**818–822.

26. Biddison, W. E., Ward, F. E., Shearer, G. M., and Shaw, S., 1980, The self determinants recognized by human virus-immune T cells can be distinguished from the serologically defined HLA antigens, *J. Immunol.* **124:**548–552.
27. Bach, F. H., Bunzendahl, H., Wee, S. L., Iwaki, J., and Segall, M., 1982, Cloning of T lymphocytes in man, in: *Isolation, Characterization, and Utilization of T Lymphocyte Clones* (C. G. Fathman and F. W. Fitch, eds.), Academic Press, New York, pp. 413–424.
28. Biddison, W. E., Krangel, M. S., Strominger, J. L., Ward, F. E., Shearer, G. M., and Shaw, S., 1980, Virus immune cytotoxic T cells recognize differences between serologically indistinguishable HLA-A2 molecules, *Hum. Immunol.* **3:**225–231.
29. Terasaki, P. I. (ed.), 1980, *Histocompatibility Testing*, UCLA Tissue Typing Laboratory, Los Angeles, California.
30. Biddison, W. E., Kostyn, D. D., Strominger, J. L., and Krangel, M. S., 1982, Delineation of immunologically and biochemically distinct HLA-A2 antigens, *J. Immunol.* **129:**730–734.
31. Krangel, M. S., Taketani, F., Biddison, W. E., and Strominger, J. L., 1983, Comparative structural analysis of HLA-A2 antigens distinguishable by cytotoxic T lymphocytes: Variants M7 and DRI, *Biochemistry* **21:**6313–6321.
32. Van der Poel, J. J., Molders, H., and Ploegh, H., 1983, Definition of four HLA-A2 subtypes by CML typing and biochemical analysis, *Immunogenetics* **17:**609–621.
33. Burakoff, S. J., Weinberger, O., Krensky, A. M., and Reiss, C. S., 1984, A molecular analysis of the cytotoxic T lymphocyte response, *Adv. Immunol.* **36:**45–85.
34. Bernabeu, C., Finlay, D., von de Rijn, M., Maziarz, R. T., Biro, P. A., Spits, H., deVries, J., and Terhorst, C. P., 1983, Expression of the major histocompatibility antigens HLA-A2 and HLA-B7 by DNA-mediated gene transfer, *J. Immunol.* **131:**2032–2037.
35. Bernabeu, C., Maziarz, R., Spits, H., deVries, J., Burakoff, S. J., and Terhorst, C., Coexpression of the human HLA-A2 and HLA-B7 heavy chain gene and human β_2-microglobulin gene in L cells, *J. Immunol.* **133:**3188–3194.
36. Barbosa, J. A., Mentzer, S., Strominger, J. L., Burakoff, S. J., and Biro, P. A., 1984, Functional recognition of human HLA-A2 and -B7 antigens following DNA-mediated gene transfer into human, monkey, and mouse cells, *Proc. Natl. Acad. Sci. USA* **81:**7549–7553.
37. Kung, P. C., Goldstein, G., Reinherz, E. L., and Schlossman, S. F., 1979, Monoclonal antibodies defining distinctive human T cell surface antigens, *Science* **206:**347–349.
38. Ledbetter, J. A., Evans, R. L., Lipinski, M., Cunningham-Rundles, C., Good, R. A., and Herzenberg, L. A., 1981, Evolutionary conservation of surface molecules that distinguish T lymphocyte helper/inducer and T cytotoxic/suppressor subpopulations in mouse and man, *J. Exp. Med.* **153:**310–323.
39. Reinherz, E. L., and Schlossman, S. F., 1980, Regulation of the immune response: Inducer and suppressor T lymphocyte subsets in human beings, *N. Engl. J. Med.* **303:**370–373.
40. Engleman, E. G., Benike, C. J., Grumet, F. C., and Evans, R. L., 1981, Activation of human T lymphocyte subsets; Helper and suppressor/cytotoxic T cells recognize and respond to distinct histocompatibility antigens, *J. Immunol.* **127:**2124–2129.
41. Thomas, Y. O., Rogozinski, L., Irigoyen, H., Shen, H. H., Talle, M. A., Goldstein, H., and Chess, L., 1982, Functional analysis of human T cell subsets defined by monoclonal antibodies. V. Suppressor cells within the activated OKT4$^+$ population belong to a distinct subset, *J. Immunol.* **128:**1386–1390.
42. Flomenberg, N., Duffy, E., Naito, K., and Dupont, B., 1983, Two distinct types of HLA-DR specific cytotoxic T-cell lines, *Immunogenetics* **17:**317–324.
43. Biddison, W. M., Rao, P. E., Talle, M. A., Goldstein, G., and Shaw, S., 1984, Possible involvement of the T4 molecule in T cell recognition of class II HLA antigens: Evidence from studies of CTL-target cell binding, *J. Exp. Med.* **159:**783–797.
44. Moretta, A., Pantaleo, G., Mingari, M. C., Moretta, L., and Cerottini, J. C., 1984, Clonal heterogeneity in the requirement for T3, T4, and T8 molecules in human cytolytic T lymphocyte function, *J. Exp. Med.* **159:**921–934.
45. Krensky, A. M., Clayberger, C., Greenstein, J. L., Collins, T., Pober, J. S., Robbins, E., Anderson, D., Springer, T. A., and Burakoff, S. J., 1984, Cell surface structures involved in the human

cytolytic T lymphocyte response, in: *Regulation of the Immune System*, Volume 18, Alan Liss, New York, pp. 209–219.

46. Landegren, U., Ramstedt, U., Axberg, I., Ullberg, M., Jondal, J., and Wigell, H., 1982, Selective inhibition of human T cell cytotoxicity at levels of target recognition or initiation of lysis by monoclonal OKT3 and Leu2a antibodies, *J. Exp. Med.* **155:**1579–1584.
47. Tsoukas, C. D., Carson, D. A., Fong, S., and Vaughan, J. H., 1982, Molecular interactions in human T cell mediated cytotoxicity to EBV. II. Monoclonal antibody OKT3 inhibits a post-killer-target recognition/adhesion step, *J. Immunol.* **129:**1421–1425.
48. Krensky, A. M., Robbins, E., Springer, T. A., and Burakoff, S. J., 1984, LFA-1, LFA-2, and LFA-3 antigens are involved in CTL-target cell conjugation, *J. Immunol.* **132:**2180–2812.
49. Sanchez-Madrid, F., Krensky, A. M., Ware, C. F., Robbins, E., Strominger, J. L., Burakoff, S. J., and Springer, T. A., 1982, Three distinct antigens associated with human T lymphocyte-mediated cytolysis: LFA-1, LFA-2, and LFA-3, *Proc. Natl. Acad. Sci. USA* **79:**7489–7493.
50. Ware, C. F., Sanchez-Madrid, F., Krensky, A. M., Burakoff, S. J., Strominger, J. L., and Springer, T. A., 1983, Human lymphocyte function-associated antigen-1 (LFA-1): Identification of multiple antigenic epitopes and their relationship to CTL-mediated cytotoxicity, *J. Immunol.* **131:**1182–1188.
51. Sanchez-Madrid, F., Nagy, J., Robbins, E., Simon, P., and Springer, T. A., 1983, A human leukocyte differentiation antigen family with distinct alpha subunits and a common beta subunit: The lymphocyte-function associated antigen (LFA-1), the C3bi complement receptor (OKM1/Mac-1), and the p150,95 molecule, *J. Exp. Med.* **158:**1785–1803.
52. Krensky, A. M., Sanchez-Madred, F., Robbins, E., Nagy, J., Springer, T. A., and Burakoff, S. J., 1983, The functional significance, distribution, and structure of LFA-1, LFA-2, and LFA-3: Cell surface antigens with the CTL-target interaction, *J. Immunol.* **131:**611–616.
53. Hildreth, J. E. K., Gotch, F. M., Hildreth, P. D. K., and McMichael, A. J., 1983, A human lymphocyte-associated antigen involved in cell-mediated lympholysis, *Eur. J. Immunol.* **13:**202–208.
54. Beatty, P. G., Ledbetter, J. A., Martin, P. J., Price, T. H., and Hansen, J. A., 1983, Definition of a common leukocyte cell surface antigen (Lgp95–150) associated with diverse cell-mediated immune functions, *J. Immunol.* **131:**2913–2918.
55. Springer, T. A., Thompson, W. S., Miller, L. J., Schmalstieg, F. C., and Anderson, D. C., 1984, Inherited deficiency of the Mac-1, LFA-1, p150,95 glycoprotein family and its molecular basis, *J. Exp. Med.* **160:**1901–1918.
56. Springer, T. A., Rothlein, R., Anderson, D. C., Burakoff, S. J., and Krensky, A. M., 1985, The function of LFA-1 in cell-mediated killing and adhesion: Studies on heritable LFA-1, Mac-1 deficiency and on lymphoid cell self-aggregation, in: *Mechanisms of Cell-Mediated Cytotoxicity II* (P. Henkart and E. Martz, eds.), Plenum Press, New York, in press.
57. Anderson, D. C., Schmalstieg, F. C., Kohl, S., Arnaout, M. A., Hughes, B. J., Tosi, M. F., Buffone, G. J., Brinkley, B. R., Dickey, W. D., Abramson, J. S., Springer, T. A., Boxer, L. A., Hollers, J. M., and Smith, C. W., 1984, Abnormalities of polymorphonuclear leukocyte function associated with a heritable deficiency of high molecular weight surface glycoproteins (GP138): Common relationship to diminished cell adherence, *J. Clin. Invest.* **74:**536–551.
58. Dana, N., Todd, R. F., III, Pitt, J., Springer, T. A., and Arnaout, M. A., 1984, Deficiency of a surface membrane glycoprotein (Mol) in man, *J. Clin. Invest.* **73:**153–159.
59. Beatty, P. G., Harlan, J. M., Rosen, H., Hansen, J. A., Ochs, H. D., Price, T. D., Taylor, R. F., and Klebanoff, S. J., 1984, Absence of a monoclonal-antibody-defined protein complex in a boy with abnormal leukocyte function, *Lancet* **I:**535–537.
60. Krensky, A. M., Mentzer, S. J., Clayberger, C, Anderson, D., Burakoff, S. J., Schmalstieg, F. C. and Springer, T. A., 1985, Heritable lymphocyte function-associated antigen-1 deficiency: Abnormalities of cytotoxicity and proliferation associated with abnormal expression of LFA-1, manuscript in preparation.
61. Palacios, R., and Martinez-Maza, J., 1982, Is the E receptor on human T lymphocytes a "negative signal receptor"?, *J. Immunol.* **129:**2479–2485.

62. Howard, F. D., Ledbetter, J. A., Wong, J., Bieber, C. P., Stinson, E. B., and Herzenberg, L. A., 1981, A human T lymphocyte differentiation marker defined by monoclonal antibodies that block E rosette formation, *J. Immunol.* **126:**2117–2122.
63. Kamoun, M. P., Martin, P. J., Hansen, J. A., Brown, M. A., Siadak, A. W., and Nowinski, R. C., 1981, Identification of a human T lymphocyte surface protein associated with the E rosette receptor, *J. Exp. Med.* **153:**207–212.
64. Martin, P. J., Longton, G., Ledbetter, J. A., Newman, W., Braun, M. P., Beatty, P. G., and Hansen, J. A., 1983, Identification and functional characterization of two distinct epitopes on the human T cell surface protein Tp50, *J. Immunol.* **131:**180–185.
65. Meuer, S. C., Hussey, R. E., Fabbi, M., Fox, D., Acuto, O., Fitzgerald, K. A., Hodgdon, J. C., Protentis, J., Schlossman, S. F., and Reinherz, E. L., 1984, An alternative pathway of T cell activation: A functional role of the 50 kd T11 sheep erythrocyte receptor protein, *Cell* **36:**897–906.
66. Gromkowski, S. H., Krensky, A. M., Martz, E., and Burakoff, S. J., 1985, Functional distinctions between the LFA-1, LFA-2, and LFA-3 membrane proteins on human CTL are revealed with trypsin pre-treated target cells, *J. Immunol.* **134:**244–249.
67. Pober, J. S., Collins, T., Gimbrone, M. A., Cotran, R. S., Gitlin, J., Fiers, W., Clayberger, C., Krensky, A. M., Burakoff, S. J., and Reiss, C. S., 1983, Lymphocytes recognize human vascular endothelial and dermal fibroblast Ia antigens induced by recombinant immune interferon, *Nature* **305:**726–729.
68. Collins, T., Krensky, A. M., Clayberger, C., Fiers, W., Gimbrone, M. A., Burakoff, S. J., and Pober, J. S., 1984, Human cytolytic T lymphocyte interactions with vascular endothelium and fibroblasts. Role of effector and target cell molecules, *J. Immunol.* **133:**1878–1884.
69. Meuer, S. C., Fitzgerald, K. A., Hussey, R. E., Hodgdon, J. C., Schlossman, S. F., and Reinherz, E. L., 1983, Clonotypic structures involved in antigen specific human T cell function, *J. Exp. Med.* **157:**705–719.
70. Martz, E., 1977, Mechanism of specific tumor cell lysis by alloimmune T lymphocytes. Resolution and characterization of discrete steps in cellular interaction, in: *Contemporary Topics in Immunobiology*, Volume 7, Plenum Press, New York, pp. 301–361.

Chapter 36

The Use of Mouse Lymphocyte Clones to Define T-Cell Gene Products and Analyze Lymphocyte Gene Activation

GARY J. NABEL

1. Introduction

Several systems have facilitated the study of gene activation in eukaryotic cells. Because they have been so well-characterized, mouse T lymphocytes have proven particularly useful for these studies. Many of the molecules expressed on the surface membranes of thymic-dependent lineages have been defined using monoclonal antibodies, biochemical purification, or identification of the genes encoding them.[1–5] This differentiation process has been characterized using gene products on cell surfaces to define the cellular stages of T-cell development.[6–9] More recently, the molecules that mediate biological functions of T cells have also become established. These include lymphokines, cell surface molecules involved in the recognition of antigen, and cell surface glycoproteins expressed during activation. The technology of T-cell cloning has facilitated the definition of these molecules. T-cell clones promise further to allow insight into the steps that lead to activation. This chapter will review several aspects of mouse T-cell clones. No attempt will be made to review completely the many contributions to this field. Attention will be devoted to the following topics: (1) What T cell clones can be grown *in vitro* and what are their properties? (2) What essential factors allow continuous propagation of T-cell clones? (3) How can these be used to understand gene activation in eukaryotic cells?

2. The Generation of T-Cell Clones

The complexity of T cells has been appreciated increasingly over the past 15 years. It has been possible to define T-cell subsets using antibodies directed

---

GARY J. NABEL • Department of Medicine, Brigham and Women's Hospital, and Harvard Medical School, Boston, Massachusetts 02115.

to cell surface glycoproteins since the early 1970s. To review briefly, the surface of T cells has been well-defined by antibodies to cell surface membrane glycoproteins of differentiation antigens. Many of the genes encoding these proteins have been precisely mapped. The sequential expression of these glycoproteins has served to define cells at progressive stages of T-cell differentiation. The TL,[5,9] Lyt-1, and Lyt-2 loci have been particularly useful in this regard. While the exact pathway of T-cell differentiation is yet unclear, the following observations have been made. Within the bone marrow, a group of cells, which can be distinguished from other hematopoietic precursor cells, is committed to migrate to the thymus.[10,11] These cells, termed prothymocytes, express neither TL, Lyt-1, nor Lyt-2 glycoproteins. Within the thymus, these prothymocytes proliferate and begin to express TL, Lyt-1, and Lyt-2 glycoproteins. These TL^+, Lyt-1^+2^+ thymocytes do not express mature T-cell function. Subsequent differentiation in the thymus allows the formation of at least three sublines of mature progeny T cells, which migrate to the bloodstream and lymphoid tissues. In the peripheral lymphoid tissues, the TL glycoprotein is lost and Thy-1 expression decreases. Three patterns of Ly expression can then be found. These include the Lyt-1^+2^-, Lyt-1^-2^+, and Lyt-1^+2^+ sets.

In the past, it had been difficult to define the roles of these cells and their products rigorously because homogenous populations were not available. Uncloned T-cell populations contain small numbers of cells that confound biochemical, genetic, and functional analyses. The precise definition of the events that result in T-cell differentiation and function is therefore difficult. Such an analysis requires a method to generate large numbers of cloned cells at defined stages of differentiation and identification of gene products synthesized exclusively by specialized, differentiated cells.

T-Cell clones had been generated as early as 1969 by Fibach,[12] and continuous T-cell lines were described subsequently by Morgan *et al.*[13] Gillis and Smith[14] later showed that clones of antigen-specific mouse cytolytic cells could be grown *in vitro*. While T-cell clones as well as T-cell hybridomas and viral-transformed T-cell lines had become available, the limits of that technology were unclear. Initially, the major question of this methodology was whether the cells that proliferated *in vitro* were representative of normal cells. It was unknown whether culture conditions might bias growth of particular types of cells; cloning efficiencies were not reported.

We had described a general method of producing cloned populations of cells at progressive stages of thymus-dependent differentiation. The procedure did not require hybridization to malignant cells, and cloned cells could be frozen for storage without loss of function upon thawing and regrowth. These T-cells clones expressed the surface glycoproteins and functions of cells at discrete stages of T-cell differentiation, and each clone could be expanded in culture to numbers $>10^8$.

The aim of our early work was to answer several questions. (1) What conditions were required to maintain cell division in continuous culture? (2) Did these cells maintain expression of T-cell-specific glycoproteins *in vitro*? Were

Table I. Immunofluorescent Analysis of Mouse T-Cell Clones[a]

Surface glycoprotein	Thy-1$^+$	Lyt-1$^+$2$^-$	Lyt-1$^+$2$^+$	Lyt-1$^-$2$^+$	Lyt-1$^-$2$^-$
Uncloned T cells, % positive	91.4	26	35	20	19
Cloned sublines, % positive	100	12.5	30	12.5	25

[a] Uncloned T cells were classified by indirect immunofluorescence as previously described.[18] Twenty-five T-cell clones derived from this T-cell population were classified similarly. T-Cell clones from each subset arose in frequencies comparable to their presence in the uncloned population, indicating that the cloning procedure did not select for the growth of a particular T-cell subset.

they representative of normal T cells? (3) What signals were required for proliferation? (4) Did these cells maintain immune function?

The first goal had been to optimize cloning efficiencies. These were calculated from the observed growth of cells that had been inoculated at different initial cell concentrations. Use of the Poisson distribution function applied to the frequency of negative wells made it possible to calculate cloning efficiencies.[15] Several lessons emerged from such an analysis. First, it was important to use a constant source of conditioned medium and to quantitative the amount of IL-2. Mouse T-cell clones required feeding every other day with a constant amount of IL-2. Second, the use of an irradiated monolayer as a source of "feeder" cells improved cloning efficiency up to 250-fold. Growth in liquid medium proved more efficient than in soft agar. Third, the selection of a source of nonmitogenic serum that supported cell growth at low density was necessary. Fourth, the activation of T cells prior to cloning improved cloning efficiencies and facilitated selection of antigen-specific lines. With the technique described in Section 4, we found that cloning efficiencies of 10–85% could be achieved, superior to the frequencies of viral transformation[16] or cell fusion,[17] which have yields of 10^{-5}–10^{-3}. This represents nearly a 10,000-fold improvement in cloning. Doubling times for these cells ranged from 24 to 48 hr, and normal karyotypes were observed after cloning.[18] In addition, these clones did not form tumors when injected into irradiated syngeneic recipients.

Table II. Immunologic Activity of Individual T-Cell Clones Correlates with Surface Glycoprotein Expression

		Immunologic function	
Surface glycoprotein profile	Total	Activation of Ig secretion,[a] number positive	Inhibition of Ig secretion,[b] number positive
Cl.Lyt-1$^+$2$^-$	8	8	0
Cl.Lyt-1$^+$2$^+$	7	0	3
Cl.Lyt-1$^-$2$^+$	3	0	3

[a] Mean stimulation of immunoglobin secretion was 11-fold above background production by B cells alone. The range of plaque-forming units per 10^5 B cells was 35–64.

[b] Mean inhibition of immunoglobin secretion was 106% (range 104–113%). One hundred percent suppression was defined as the ability to inhibit Ig secretion of cocultured B cells and Lyt-1$^+$ T cells to the level of the B-cell response alone.

Table III. Potential Uses of Mouse T-Cell Clones

1.	Definition of the precise cellular interactions in the immune response
2.	Source of cells to analyze cellular differentiation
3.	Definition and characterization of T-cell gene products
4.	Source of cell for bioassay of lymphokines
5.	Monoclonal source of lymphokines
6.	Monoclonal source of T-cell receptor for antigen and other cell surface glycoproteins
7.	Definition of determinants recognized by individual T cells
8.	Source of cellular material to analyze gene activation
9.	Source of cells for transfection of cloned gene products
10.	Definition of immunosuppressive reagents
11.	Source of cells to generate cDNA probes to define analogous human T-cell gene products

The cells generated under these conditions were representative of T cells at different stages of maturation. In general, the number of clones from each subset was equivalent to the distribution of these cells in the population prior to cloning (Table I), suggesting that culture conditions did not bias for the growth of a particular cell type. A central point emerged from the functional analyses of T-cell clones: the genetic "program" of each T-cell clone appeared to combine information coding for a unique pattern of cell surface glycoproteins and for a particular immunologic function. Individual T-cell clones mediated specific function according to the expression of unique surface membrane molecules (Table II), and these glycoprotein patterns correspond to those identified *in vivo*.[6,7,18]

T-cell clones divide continuously in culture, express characteristic cell surface glycoproteins, and may be activated to express differentiated function. These cells provide a source of cells to study a variety of processes, detailed in Table III. Because cells may be cloned from different T-cell subsets, they may be used to define the cellular interactions leading to activation of Ig secretion, cytotoxicity, or suppression. These cells may be used to define the soluble peptides that mediate these events, as well as the signals that cause the synthesis and secretion of these gene products. Several investigators have used T-cell clones to extend the understanding of T-cell gene products and the mechanism of their activation. An example of one such study, the definition of an inducer T-cell gene product, is summarized in the following section.

3. Definition of a T-Cell Gene Product in a T-Cell Clone

Inducer T cells play a major role in the initiation and maintenance of an immune response. These cells may stimulate a variety of functions,[19] including (1) the secretion of antibody,[6] (2) the generation of cytotoxic cells,[7] (3) the proliferation of mast cells,[20] and (4) the proliferation of bone marrow progenitors.[19,21] Because of their central role in this variety of processes and because specific cells can be activated to perform specialized function, inducer T-cell clones have been used to focus on the molecules released upon activation.

The signals required to activate inducer T cells are several. First, particular cell surface molecules including the antigen receptor must recognize determinants that are considered foreign as well as those of the host. Following cell surface recognition, the transmission of signal(s) from the cell surface to the nucleus leads to the expression of a new set of gene products.

The molecules activated in inducer T cells have not been fully defined. While complete definition of these molecules ultimately requires purification to homogeneity, one way to define the products responsible for inducer T-cell activities is to clone the cDNA encoding these molecules. This approach may provide additional material for biochemical analysis, and may also allow study of the events that regulate gene expression. In collaboration with several colleagues, we have used this approach to clone a mast cell growth factor (MCGF) cDNA from a T-cell clone, and it has been expressed in cultured monkey cells.[22] The MCGF cDNA was obtained from a library constructed in the pcD expression vector made with mRNA from the mouse T-cell clone Lyt-1^+2^-/9 after activation with Con A. Cloned plasmids were detected by their ability to anneal mRNA, which could be translated in *Xenopus laevis* oocytes to biologically active MCGF. Clones containing full-length cDNA directed the synthesis of MCGF production when transfected into COS 7 monkey cells.

Addition of this expressed cloned gene product to cultures of mouse bone marrow cells allowed the expansion of hematopoietic cells committed to multiple lineages; it supported the formation of burst-forming erythroid colonies, granulocyte/macrophage colonies, mast cell colonies, as well as colonies of multiple lineages, and sustained multipotential stem cells in liquid culture.[23] These biological activities, the homology between the deduced amino acid sequence of this cDNA[22] and interleukin 3 (IL-3),[24] as well as the nucleotide sequence homology,[25] support the conclusion that this clone encodes IL-3. The activities of this gene product are compared with two unrelated T-cell gene products in Table IV. These results suggest that T cells may play a role in the regulation of hematopoiesis. Myeloid cells, the production of which is stimulated by IL-3, are important in inflammatory reactions. Thus, inducer T cells may coordinate specific immune recognition with an effective inflammatory response, in part through the elaboration of this gene product. Further analysis of this factor may lend insight into the role of T lymphocytes in regulating the growth and differentiation of hematopoietic cells.

Preliminary studies have revealed a similar factor in man. This soluble factor appears to stimulate the expansion of bone marrow cells committed to multiple lineages. When human inducer T cells are activated, this gene product is also expressed coordinately with two unrelated and unlinked T-cell genes, interleukin 2 and interferon gamma. The expression of these genes can be repressed with corticosteroid or cyclosporin A *in vitro*. This system may allow definition of the molecular signals that govern human inducer T-cell gene

Table IV. Comparison of Biological Activities of COS-MCGF to Other Lymphokines

Lymphokine	Hematopoietic activity[a]	Mast cell proliferation	T-cell proliferation	B-cell proliferation	Antiviral activity	Fibroblast proliferation
COS-MCGF[22,23]	+	+	−	−	−	−
Interleukin 3[36,37]	+	+	−	−	−	−
Interleukin 2[14,32,33,38]	−	−	+	±	−	−
Interferon gamma[39–41]	−	−	−	−	+	−

[a] Hematopoietic activity is defined as the ability to stimulate the production of burst-forming units, granulocyte–macrophage colonies, and eosinophilic and lymphoblastoid colonies *in vitro*.[23]

expression and provide a source of large quantitites of T-cell gene products for clinical use.

4. Experimental Procedures

4.1. Introduction

The following section details a method for the growth of T-cell clones. While specific techniques utilized in our studies are described, other approaches have also been successful.[26–31] The key elements for the success of these techniques are (1) a constant source of T-cell growth factor, (2) a constant interval for feeding (every second day), and (3) maintenance of cells at the appropriate cell density.

4.2. Medium

"Modified DMEM" was prepared as follows: DMEM (4.5 g/liter) (GIBCO) was supplemented with 1% nonessential amino acids (100×) (Microbiologic Associates, MBA 13-114A), sodium pyruvate (MBA 13-115A), 1% essential amino acids (100×) (MBA 13-607C), arginine–HCl (0.116 g/liter) (GIBCO), asparagine–H_2O (0.036 g/liter) (GIBCO), folic acid (0.006 g/liter) (GIBCO), and $NaHCO_3$ (2 g/liter for 5% CO_2 incubators, or 3.7 g/liter for 10% CO_2). This medium was called modified DMEM and filtered before use.

4.3. Selection of Fetal Calf Serum

Ten batches of fetal calf serum (FCS) were screened to select an optimal source. Aliquots were heat-inactivated by incubation at 56°C for 30 min. Mitogenicity was assessed by incubation of female BALB/c spleen cells (5×10^6/ml) in modified DMEM with 10% FCS, 2 mM of fresh glutamine in the presence or absence of an optimal concentration of Con A (2 or 4 μg/ml; Calbiochem-Behring) for 45 hr in 0.2-ml Falcon plastic microtiter plates (#3040) before addition of [^{3}H]thymidine for 4 hr. Incorporation of [^{3}H]thymidine was measured by liquid scintillation after collection on glass filters using a Ph.D. cell harvester.[18] Supernatant was collected from Con A-stimulated cells and tested for IL-2 activity.[32,33] The HT-2 cell line was used as an indicator cell to measure IL-2 activity. Fetal calf serum, which yielded the highest titer IL-2 supernatant with the least mitogenicity in the absence of Con A, was selected for growth of T-cell clones.

4.4. Preparation of Conditioned Medium

Modified DMEM was further supplemented with 5×10^{-5} M 2-mercaptoethanol (2-ME), additional glutamine (2 mM), 4% heat-inactivated FCS, and an optimal concentration of Con A. BALB/c spleen cells (5×10^6/ml) were incubated in 40 ml of this medium (Falcon Plastics 3024) at 37°C for 45 hr in 10% CO_2. Following centrifugation at $300 \times g$ for 10 min, supernatant from these cultures was filtered (0.20-μm Nalgene filters), stored at −70°C in 40-ml aliquots until use, and designated conditioned medium (CM). Removal of residual Con A by absorption through G-50 did not affect the ability of CM to support growth on T-cell clones.

4.5. Preparation of Partially Purified Growth Factor

This procedure allows batch concentration of T-cell growth factor from CM. This preparation supports the growth of T cells, and may be used in place of conditioned medium. Purified preparation of growth factor may be helpful to generate antigen-specific cells. In general, cells should be maintained in either CM or partially purified IL-2, but do not grow well when changed from one source of IL-2 to another.

Using 10 g of DEAE for each liter of CM, we transferred DEAE-cellulose to a sintered glass funnel and washed for 15 min in 0.1 N HCl. After rinsing with deonized water, the resin was incubated with 0.1 N NaOH prior to rinsing with 3–4 volumes of deonized water.

Activated DEAE-cellulose was transferred to a 4-liter Ehrlenmeyer flask. After addition of CM, diluted with deonized water (1:3), the mixture was stirred for 1 hr at 4°C. This solution was transferred to a sintered glass funnel. Effluent was discarded. Adsorbed IL-2 was eluted with three volumes of 3 × PBS and vacuum dialyzed against 1 × PBS.

4.6. Cell Culture

Cells were grown in complete conditioned medium (CCM). An optimal concentration of CM (usually 25–50%) was combined with modified DMEM and further supplemented with 5×10^{-5} M 2-ME, fresh glutamine (2 mM) and additional FCS, 10% of the total volume. Cells were maintained at concentrations between 0.5 and 3×10^5 cells/ml, and cultures supplemented with fresh CCM (approximately 1:3) every other day. Cell cultures were maintained in the absence of antibiotics and checked periodically for mycoplasma contamination.[34]

4.7. Cloning

Cells were distributed into wells (Falcon plastic microtiter plates, #3040) at estimated final concentration of 100, 10, 1, and 0.3 cells/well in 0.1 ml of CCM. To each well, irradiated (1500 rad) spleen cells (final concentration of

8×10^5 cells/well) were added. Cultures were supplemented every 2 days with 30 μl CCM until colonies were visible (10–21 days).

Cloning efficiency (CE) was calculated according to a Poisson distribution[15] using at least 96 wells to calculate each CE. The fraction of negative wells was plotted as a function of the logarithm of initial cell number. Single-cell colonies arising at frequencies of <36% with Ce >5% were regrown twice after dilution of three cells per ten wells. Single cells, derived by micromanipulation, were also termed clones.

4.8. Preincubation

Cells may be preincubated in CCM for 7–10 days to improve CE. These cells were incubated at 10^6/ml for the first 2–3 days in CCM, and then maintained at concentrations of $(0.5–3) \times 10^6$/ml.

4.9. Clonal Expansion

Cloned cells were maintained in the absence of irradiated cell monolayers at concentrations of $(0.5–3) \times 10^5$ cells/ml in CCM. Clones were initially transferred to 2-ml wells (Linbro plates, Flow Labs), fed with 0.5 ml CCM, and maintained at $(0.5–3) \times 10^5$/ml. Cells were grown at this concentration in Linbro plates, Petri dishes (Falcon 1007, 1008, 3003), or tissue culture flasks (Falcon 3024), depending on cell volume. Adherent cells were grown in Petri dishes to facilitate recovery. Doubling times ranged from 18 to 48 hr for all cells. Cells could be expanded to numbers $>10^7$ and in some cases $>10^8$. At least 40 different cloned populations have been propagated for >8 months *in vitro*. The addition of irradiated monolayers facilitated expansion of cells during transfer to new plates, flasks, or dishes.

4.10. Cryopreservation

Cloned cells may be frozen in liquid N_2 and thawed with complete recovery of growth and function. Using a modification of the method of Lionetti,[35] we suspended cells (10^6/ml) in a 2-ml provial (Cooke 235-1) with 0.5 ml of cold FCS (4°C). An equal volume of medium containing cold FCS, 10% DMSO, and 12% hydroxyethyl starch was added dropwise to the provial immersed in ice. Cells were frozen in a controlled cooling chamber (Union Carbide Biological Freezer) at a rate of −1°C/min. At −50°C they were transferred to liquid N_2. To recover cells, provials were quickly thawed, transferred to test tubes on ice, diluted dropwise with cold modified DMEM and washed three times. Cells $[(1–2) \times 10^5]$ were then dispensed into wells of microtiter plates (Falcon 3040) containing 5×10^5 irradiated (1500 rad) spleen cells and 0.15 ml CCM. Medium was changed daily. When growth was observed (2–10 days) cells were expanded as described above.

ACKNOWLEDGMENT. The author would like to thank Patricia Al-Kotob for expert assistance in preparation of this manuscript.

References

1. Boyse, E. A., and Old, L. J., 1975, The immunogenetics of differentiation in the mouse, Harvey Lectures **71:**23–53.
2. McKenzie, I. F. C., and Potter, T., 1979, Murine lymphocyte surface antigens, *Adv. Immunol.* **27:**179–338.
3. Ledbetter, J., and Herzenberg, L. A., 1979, Xenogeneic monoclonal antibodies to mouse lymphoid differentiation antigens, *Immunol. Rev.* **47:**63–89.
4. Springer, T. A., Davignon, D., Ho, M. K., Kurzinger, K., Martz, E., and Sanchez-Madrid, F., 1982, LFA-1 and Lyt-2,3 molecules associated with T lymphocyte-mediated killing; and Mac-1, an LFA-1 homologue associated with complement receptor function, *Immunol. Rev.* **68:**171–195.
5. Boyse, E. A., Stockert, E., and Old, L. J., 1969, Properties of four antigens specified by the Tla locus. Similarities and differences, in: *International Convocation on Immunology* (N. R. Rose and F. Milgrom), eds. S. Karger, New York, pp. 353–357.
6. Cantor, H., and Boyse, E. A., 1975, Functional subclasses of T lymphocytes bearing different Ly antigens. I. The generation of functionally distinct T cell subclasses is a differentiative process independent of antigen, *J. Exp. Med.* **141:**1376–1389.
7. Cantor, H., and Boyse, E. A., 1975, Functional subclasses of T lymphocytes bearing different Ly antigens. II. Cooperation between subclasses of Ly^+ cells in the generation of killer activity, *J. Exp. Med.* **141:**1390–1399.
8. Cantor, H., and Weissman, I., 1976, Development and function of subpopulations of thymocytes and T-lymphocytes, *Prog. Allergy* **20:**1.
9. Cantor, H., and Boyse, E. A., 1977, Lymphocytes as models for the study of mammalian cellular differentiation, *Immunol. Rev.* **33:**105–124.
10. El-Arini, M. O., and Osoba, D., 1973, Differentiation of thymus-derived cells from precursors in mouse bone marrow, *J. Exp. Med.* **137:**821–837.
11. Komuro, K., Itakura, K., Boyse, E. A., and John, M., 1975, Ly 5: A new T-lymphocyte antigen system, *Immunogenetics* **1:**452–456.
12. Fibach, E., Gerassi, E., and Sachs, L., 1976, Induction of colony formation *in vitro* by human lymphocytes, *Nature* **259:**127–129.
13. Morgan, D. A., Ruscetti, F. W., and Gallo, R., 1976, Selective *in vitro* growth of T-lymphocytes from normal human bone marrows, *Science* **193:**1007–1008.
14. Gillis, S., and Smith, K. A., 1977, Long-term culture of tumour-specific cytotoxic T-cells, *Nature* **268:**154–156.
15. Quintans, J., and Lefkowits, I., 1973, Precursor cells specific to sheep red cells in nude mice. Estimation of frequency in the micro-culture system, *Eur. J. Immunol.* **3:**392–397.
16. Finn, O., Boniver, J., and Kaplan, H. S., 1979, Induction, establishment *in vitro*, and characterization of functional, antigen-specific, carrier-primed murine T-cell lymphomas, *Proc. Natl. Acad. Sci. USA* **76:**4033–4037.
17. Kappler, J. W., Skidmore, B., White, J., and Marrack, P., 1981, Antigen inducible, H-2 restricted, interleukin-2-producing T cell hybridomas. Lack of independent antigen and H-2 recognition, *J. Exp. Med.* **153:**1198–1214.
18. Nabel, G., Fresno, M., Chessman, A., and Cantor, H., 1981, Use of cloned populations of mouse lymphocytes to analyze cellular differentiation, *Cell* **23:**19–28.
19. Nabel, G., Greenberger, J. S., Sakakeeny, M. A., and Cantor, H., 1981, Multiple biologic activities of a cloned inducer T cell population, *Proc. Natl. Acad. Sci. USA* **78:**1157–1161.

20. Nabel, G., Galli, S. J., Dvorak, A. M., Dvorak, H. F., and Cantor, H., 1981, Inducer T lymphocytes synthesize a factor that stimulates proliferation of cloned mast cells, *Nature* **291**:332–334.
21. Nathan, D. G., Chess, L., Hillman, D. G., Clarke, B., Breard, J., Mesler, and Housman, D. E., 1978, Human erythroid burst-forming unit; T-cell requirement for proliferation *in vitro*, *J. Exp. Med.* **147**:324–339.
22. Yokota, T., Lee, F., Rennick, D., Hall, C., Arai, N., Mosmann, T., Nabel, G., Cantor, H., and Arai, K., 1984, Isolation and characterization of a mouse cDNA clone that expresses mast cell growth factor activity in monkey cells, *Proc. Natl. Acad. Sci. USA* **81**:1070–1074.
23. Rennick, D. M., Lee, F. D., Yokota, T., Arai, K., Cantor, H., and Nabel, G. J., 1985, A cloned MCGF cDNA encodes a multilineage hematopoietic growth factor: multiple activities of interleukin-3, *J. Immunol.* **134**:910–914.
24. Ihle, J., Keller, J., Henderson, L., Frederick, K., and Palaszynski, E., 1982, Procedures for the purification of interleukin-3 to homogeneity, *J. Immunol.* **129**:2431–2436.
25. Fung, M. C., Hapel, A. J., Ymer, S., Cohen, D. R., Johnson, R. M., Campbell, H. D., and Young, I. G., 1984, Molecular cloning of cDNA for murine interleukin-3, *Nature* **307**:233–237.
26. Watson, J. D., 1979, Continuous proliferation of murine antigen-specific helper T-lymphocytes in culture, *J. Exp. Med.* **150**:1510–1519.
27. Sredni, B., Tse, H. Y., and Schwartz, R. H., 1980, Direct cloning and extended culture of antigen-specific MHC-restricted, proliferating T-lymphocytes, *Nature* **283**:581–583.
28. Fathman, C. G., and Kimoto, M., 1980, Studies utilizing murine T cell clones. Ir genes, Ia antigens and MLR stimulating determinants, *Immunol. Rev.* **54**:55–80.
29. Glasebrook, A. L., Sarmiento, M., Loken, M. R., Dialynas, D. P., Quintans, J., Eisenberg, L., Lutz, C. T., Wild, D., and Fitch, F. W., 1981, Murine T lymphocyte clones with distinct immunologic functions, *Immunol. Rev.* **54**:225–266.
30. Von Boehmer, H., and Haas, W., 1981, H-2 restricted cytolytic and non-cytolytic T cell clones: Isolation, specificity and functional analysis, *Immunol. Rev.* **54**:27–56.
31. Nabholz, M., Conzelmann, A., Acusto, O., North, M., Haas, W., Pohlit, W., von Boehmer, H., Hengartner, H., Mach, J.-P., Engers, H., and Johnson, J. P., 1980, Established murine cytolitic T-cell lines as tools for a somatic cell genetic analysis of T-cell functions, *Immunol. Rev.* **51**:125–156.
32. Gillis, S., Fern, M., Oi, W., and Smith, K., 1978, T Cell growth factor; Parameters of production and quantitative microassay for activity, *J. Immunol.* **120**:2027–2032.
33. Watson, J., Gillis, S., Marbrook, J., Mochizuki, D., and Smith, K. A., 1979, Biochemical and biological characterization of lymphocyte regulatory molecules. I. Purification of a class of murine lymphokines, *J. Exp. Med.* **150**:849–861.
34. Hayflick, L., 1973, Screening cultures for mycoplasma infections, in *Tissue Culture, Methods and Applications* (P. Kruse and M. Patterson, eds.), Academic Press, New York, pp. 722–728.
35. Lionetti, F. J., Hunt, S. M., Mattaliano, R. J., and Valeri, C. R., 1978, in *vitro* studies of cryopreserved baboon granulocytes, *Transfusion* **18**:685–692.
36. Ihle, J. W., Keller, J., Oroszlan, S., Henderson, L., Copeland, T. D., Fitch, F., Prystowsky, M. B., Goldwasser, E., Schrader, J. W., Palaszynski, Dy. M., and Lebel, B., 1983, Biological properties of homogeneous interleukin-3. I. Demonstration of WEHI-3 growth factor activity, mast cell growth factor activity, colony-stimulating factor activity and histamine-producing cell-stimulating factor activity, *J. Immunol.* **131**:282–287.
37. Schrader, J. W., Clark-Lewis, I., Crapper, R. M., and Wong, G. W., 1983, P-Cell stimulating factor: Characterization, action on multiple lineages of bone-marrow-derived cells and role in oncogenesis, *Immunol. Rev.* **76**:79–104.
38. Smith, K. A., 1981, T-cell growth factor: present status and future implications, in: *Lymphokines, Volume 2* (E. Pick, ed.), Academic Press, New York, pp. 21–30.
39. Rubin, Y., and Gupta, S. L., 1980, Differential efficacies of human type I and type II interferons as antiviral and antiproliferative agents, *Proc. Natl. Acad. Sci. USA* **77**:5928–5937.
40. Hovanessian, A. G., La Bonnardiere, C., and Falcoff, E., 1980, Action of murine gamma (immune) interferon on beta (fibroblast)-interferon resistant L 1210 and embryonal carcinoma cells, *J. Interferon Res.* **1**:125–135.

41. Epstein, L. B., Weil, J., Lucas, D. O., Cox, D. R., and Epstein, C. J., 1981, The biology and properties of interferon-gamma; An overview, studies of production by T lymphocyte subsets, and analysis of peptide synthesis and antiviral effects in trisomy 21 and diploid human fibroblasts, in: *The Biology of the Interferon System* (E. De Maeyer, G. Galasso, and H. Schellekens, eds.), Elsevier, Amsterdam, pp. 247–256.

Chapter 37

Interleukin 1, Interferon Gamma, and the Modulation of Macrophage–T-Cell Interactions

DAVID I. BELLER

1. Introduction: Antigen Presentation

Activation of clones of T cells by the specific antigen to which they are reactive requires that the antigen be processed (i.e., metabolized and displayed on the cell surface) by antigen-presenting cells (APCs; reviewed in Ref. 1). While the macrophage has been the most thoroughly studied of APCs, over the past few years it has been determined that a variety of cell types may function in this capacity. We now know that dendritic cells, B cells, and endothelial and Langerhans cells are all capable of antigen presentation, although this may not be a *constitutive* property of each cell type.[1] The three basic properties that define the APCs are: (1) the ability to process antigen, usually by an endocytic route involving lysosomal function; (2) the expression of class II MHC products (the Ia glycoproteins), in association with which the processed antigenic determinant is recognized by the T-cell antigen receptor; and (3) the production of interleukin 1 (IL-1), which provides a requisite signal during T-cell activation. Antigen-induced activation is accompanied by a series of changes in the resting T cell, paramount among which is the induction of receptors for, and secretion of, interleukin 2 (IL-2). A variety of lymphokines that is important for immune function is also produced by the activated T cell, and one of them, interferon gamma (IFN-γ), plays a key role in macrophage activation. The end result of this antigen induced activation is the selective proliferation of the antigen-reactive T cells.

Two of the key mediators so far identified that regulate the interaction of macrophages and T cells are IL-1 and IFN-γ. During antigen presentation, IL-1 is necessary to allow the T cell to become competent to secrete IL-2. The IFN-γ secreted by T cells during this process can, in turn, induce the expression of Ia antigens on a variety of cell types, thus amplifying the potential

DAVID I. BELLER • Department of Pathology, Harvard Medical School, Boston, Massachusetts 02115.

complement of APC. While dendritic cells and B cells constitutively express Ia, macrophages and endothelial cells are predominantly Ia-negative until stimulated by IFN-γ.

2. Interleukin 1

2.1. Control of IL-1 Production

IL-1 is a protein with an apparent molecular weight of 15,000. It was originally identified by its capacity to stimulate proliferation of thymocytes but not mature lymphocytes, and to augment the thymocyte response to suboptimal concentrations of mitogens.[2] The most commonly studied sources of IL-1 are monocyte/macrophages derived from human peripheral blood or mouse peritoneal exudates, or the macrophage-like cell lines, such as the murine P388D1. There is also evidence for a similar, if not identical, mediator secreted by epidermal cells.[3]

Low levels of IL-1 are secreted by macrophages during the first 24–48 hr of culture. IL-1 production is not a constitutive property of the macrophage, as suggested by its transience in culture. This was further verified by Unanue and Kiely,[4] who showed that physical disruption of the macrophage revealed cytosolic IL-1 only after the macrophage had adhered in culture. Heightened secretion of IL-1 followed *in vitro* treatment with adjuvants (e.g., endotoxin) or by IFN-γ. Compounds such as $BeSO_4$ or silica at toxic or supratoxic concentrations have also been shown to enhance the secretion of IL-1.[5] A similar activation by endotoxin, latex particles, and immune complexes was noted for human monocytes.[6] The separate control over the biosynthesis and the release of IL-1 has been recently reviewed.[7]

2.2. Biochemistry of IL-1

IL-1 is traditionally characterized as a globular protein with a molecular weight of approximately 15,000. While higher molecular weight forms have been reported with mouse, rat, or human monocytes or from transformed cells such as P388D1, these have been variously interpreted as aggregation, precursors, or complexing with serum proteins of the molecular weight 15,000 form,[7] and only the latter has been thoroughly evaluated. Murine IL-1 is sensitive to certain proteases.[5] Other characteristics include a Stokes radius of 20 Å, a sedimentation coefficient of 2.0, a buoyant density of 1.30 g/cm^3, an isoelectric point of 4.8, and a calculated molecular weight of 16,400–19,600.[8] Antisera have been produced against highly purified IL-1.[9–11] Human IL-1 shows similar characteristics[12] and has been recently purified to homogeneity.[13] That the biologically active regions of the molecule will show little species variation is implicit in the finding that human IL-1 will stimulate mouse thymocytes. However, at least one difference has been reported: human IL-1 has a higher pI (6.8).[13]

2.3. Function of IL-1: Regulation of T-Cell Growth

As noted, IL-1 was first studied by evaluating its effects on thymocyte proliferation. It was found that IL-1 did not actually induce proliferation in resting thymocytes, but rather *maintained* the growth of spontaneously proliferating cells.[14] Upon isolation, murine thymocytes demonstrated significant proliferation (as assessed by [^{3}H]thymidine incorporation), but this terminated by 12–16 hr in culture. If IL-1-containing supernatants were added during the period of active cell cycling, then significant thymidine uptake could be detected over the next 3–4 days. If IL-1 was first added after 24 hr of culture (when there was no longer any basal thymidine incorporation), it would not trigger renewed proliferation. Brief exposure to lectins, even nonmitogenic lectins such as wheat-germ agglutinin, was able to restore the sensitivity of the "resting" thymocyte to IL-1.

The precise function of IL-1 appears to be the induction of IL-2 production and/or IL-2 receptors in the recently activated T cell. Thus, T cells that were rigorously depleted of APCs would not proliferate in response to IL-2. It had been reported that mitogen alone could induce IL-2 receptors but that triggering of IL-2 production required macrophages or IL-1.[15,16] More recent studies suggest that macrophages, and therefore possibly IL-1, are also required for the induction of IL-2 receptors by mitogen.[17]

We have recently used macrophages fixed in paraformaldehyde after a period of antigen processing as a means to assess IL-1 secretion independently from the process of antigen presentation. We found that antigen-pulsed, fixed macrophages presented antigen to T-cell clones or freshly isolated *in vivo*-primed T cells under conditions in which no soluble IL-1 release could be detected.[18] This finding raised the question of whether IL-1 was needed in all situations of T-cell stimulation, in particular, with continuously propagated T-cell lines. Subsequent studies resolved this question by showing that the fixed macrophage was competent to present antigen by virtue of a plasma membrane-associated IL-1.[19] The response to the fixed macrophages of antigen-specific clones as well as the D10.G4 clone (which requires IL-1 but not APCs in order to respond to Con A[20]) was blocked by anti-IL-1 antibodies. Thus, the concept that IL-1 is necessarily a soluble mediator now appears to be invalid. Why two forms of this important molecule exist is not yet clear, but we suspect that they may subserve different functions. For example, the membrane form might play a role in T cell/macrophage binding. Since membrane IL-1 can be induced independently of its soluble counterpart, no clear precursor–product relation exists between these two forms.

2.3.1. Effects of IL-1 on B Cells

Functional studies with IL-1 have not been limited to T cells. Calderon *et al.*[5] studied the effects of IL-1-containing media on B-cell differentiation. While spleen cells from recently primed mice showed a minimally enhanced response in the presence of exogenous IL-1, those cells from mice primed months earlier showed a markedly augmented response when IL-1 was added. The biological activity copurified on gel filtraton with thymocyte IL-1 activity. Using IL-1 purified to apparent homogeneity, Howard *et al.*[21] showed that IL-1 was necessary for the optimal activation of resting B cells by anti-immunoglobulin; there was no direct effect of IL-1 on the resting B cells.[21] Several reports have indicated a synergistic interaction between IL-1 and the B-cell differentiation stimulus, T-cell-replacing factor.[22,23] IL-1 also appears to function as an adjuvant *in vivo*.[24]

3. Interferon Gamma

3.1. IFN-γ Production

As noted, IFN-γ is produced by mitogen- or antigen-stimulated T cells, and by both helper and cytotoxic subsets.[25,26] The only cell type other than the T cell that has been reported as a source of IFN-γ is the NK cell.[27,28] However, this response appeared to require IL-2 and so was ultimately dependent on T-cell activation. Consistent with this was the finding by Farrar *et al.*[29] that IL-2 was necessary to allow cytotoxic T-cell precursors to differentiate and secrete IFN-γ. Thus, both cell types required exogenous IL-2 in order to maintain viability or attain a state of activation that would allow them to express their potential for IFN-γ production. We have noted IFN-γ production by spleen cells from athymic mice; these cells showed no proliferative response to Con A, as expected (D. I. Beller, unpublished results). Thus, either a cell type such as the NK was responsible for IFN production in this situation, or T-lineage stem cells in the athymic mouse may be able to secrete lymphokines such as IFN-γ, or IL-2, even though they have not matured sufficiently to proliferate in response to Con A.

3.2. Biochemistry of IFN-γ

One of the most salient characteristics of IFN-γ is its pH sensitivity: both antiviral and macrophage-activating activities are severely reduced after incubation at pH 2. The biological activities are resistant to pH 4 and heating to 56°C. IFN-γ is trypsin-sensitive and has a molecular weight of approximately 40,000 (as determined by gel filtration), a pI of 5.0–5.5, binds to poly U–Sepharose, and is recognized by antibodies against IFN-γ but not IFN-α, β.[30]

The genes for both mouse[23] and human[32] IFN-γ have been cloned and expressed in both bacterial and mammalian cells. The secreted, mature mouse protein contains 136 amino acids and the human IFN contains 146. The human and mouse proteins are only 40% homologous and display virtually no interspecies activity in either antiviral or macrophage-activation assays.

3.3 Function of IFN-γ in Ia Regulation

The first evidence for IFN controlling the expression of lymphoid MHC gene products was reported by Lindahl *et al.*[33] Steeg *et al.*[30] provided the first substantive evidence that the lymphokine that induced Ia on macrophages was IFN-γ. This molecule was also demonstrated to be the primary inducer of macrophage tumoricidal activity.[34,35] These reports on the copurification of the antiviral and macrophage-activating functions were substantiated by studies using IFN-γ derived by recombinant DNA technology.[36] IFN-γ has since been shown to induce Ia on a variety of cell types, including endothelium and mast cells.[1]

3.3.1. Mechanisms of Macrophage Ia Regulation *in Vivo* and *in Vitro*

As discussed previously, murine peritoneal macrophages are primarily Ia-negative. Those that are Ia-positive rapidly lose the capacity to synthesize and express Ia determinants *in vitro*, or, when the source of stem cells has been abrogated by irradiation, *in vivo* as well. This pattern appears to be unique for the Ia antigens, since Mac-1 and H-2 expression remain unperturbed under these conditions.[37,38] We interpret these findings as indicating that, like other parameters of macrophage activation, Ia expression is transient. The maintenance of an Ia-positive fraction in the exudate is based on a dynamic equilibrium between cells freshly derived from the circulation (of which a minority are Ia-positive) and those, resident in the peritoneum for a period of days, that have become Ia-negative. The half-life for Ia expression in the irradiated animal is approximately 2 days.[38]

The activation of T cells *in vivo* leads to the local induction of Ia expression,[39] and this is dependent upon lymphokine production by the T cell.[40] The available evidence argues against separate lineages for Ia-positive and Ia-negative macrophages: all Ia-positive macrophages become Ia-negative *in vitro*; and all macrophage stem cells (i.e., bone marrow-derived cells giving rise to growth factor-induced macrophage colonies), initially Ia-negative, produce progeny that will respond to IFN-γ by expressing Ia determinants.[41]

The kinetics of IFN-γ-induced Ia biosynthesis and expression is depicted in Fig. 1 (top panel). It can be seen that, even in the presence of IFN-γ, Ia was rapidly lost by the macrophages by the second day in culture (the high initial level of Ia reflects the elicitation of these macrophages by live *Listeria* bacteria). In the presence of IFN-γ, but not medium alone, Ia expression was subsequently induced in culture. The transition from Ia-positive to Ia-negative and (in the presence of IFN-γ) back to Ia-positive showed a clear temporal association with the pattern of Ia biosynthesis (Fig. 1, bottom panel). These data also revealed that relevant environmental stimuli (in this case, killed *Listeria* bacteria), while having no Ia inductive capacity of their own, could significantly augment the macrophage's response to IFN-γ. The data suggested that this "second signal" effect of bacteria might not itself be mediated via modulation of Ia biosynthesis. Finally, evaluation of Ia mRNA has indicated that Ia expression in response to

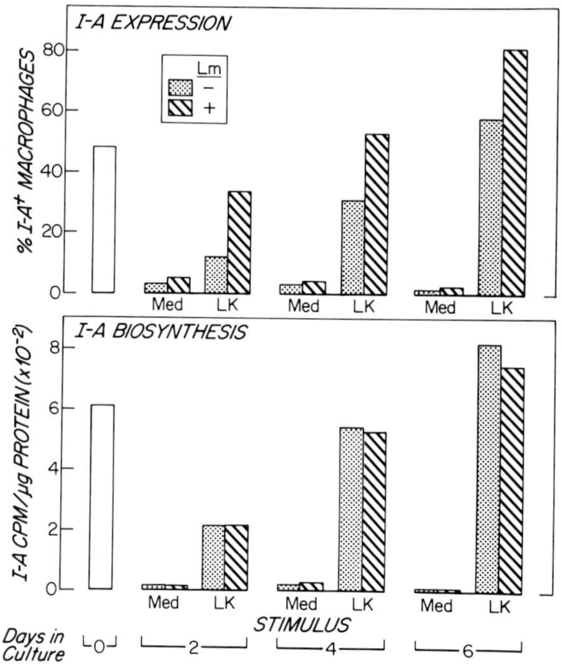

Figure 1. Kinetics of Ia expression and Ia biosynthesis. (Top) The percent of Ia-positive macrophages was determined by staining cells adherent to coverslips with fluorescein-labeled antibodies. PECs were elicited by injection (intraperitoneally) with live *Listeria* and were 48% Ia-positive when originally plated in culture. Macrophages were cultured in medium alone (Med) or IFN-γ-containing lymphokine (LK) for varying periods as indicated. Ia expression dropped dramatically by the second day of culture, whether or not the LK was present, but was thereafter induced in the presence of LK, so that by day 6 the macrophages were 56% Ia-positive. Moreover, if heat-killed *Listeria monocytogenes* (Lm) was added to cultures 16 hr before fixing and staining with the antibodies, there was a marked synergistic interaction with LK. Lm had no effect by itself on Ia levels. (Bottom) Macrophages were internally labeled with [^{3}H]leucine for 4 hr on the days indicated. The cells were detergent-extracted, and the counts specifically immunoprecipitated with anti-I-A^k monoclonal antibodies (determined after sizing by polyacrylamide gel electrophoresis) were expressed relative to the total cell protein in each experimental group (to control for cell number and viability). Ia biosynthesis followed a pattern very similar to that of Ia expression on the plasma membrane, except that Lm did not increase biosynthesis. It is thus possible that Lm may act posttranslationally.

IFN-γ appears to be transcriptionally controlled (Fig. 2). Ia mRNA was not detected in macrophages cultured in medium alone. However, significant hybridization of a cDNA probe for I-A_β to the RNA was noted after IFN-γ stimulation.

3.3.2. Functional Significance of Ia Regulation

The induction of Ia expression in Ia-negative macrophages[42] or macrophage-like cell lines[43] was associated with the acquisition of antigen-presenting capacity. In fact, as seen in Fig. 3, the extent of Ia expression was quantitatively related to the degree of antigen presentation[18] (as defined by antigen-induced T-cell proliferation). Because IL-1 expression is, like Ia, both transient and necessary for antigen presentation, IL-1 must also have been restimulated in these macrophages. In contrast to the lack of Ia induction by heat-killed bacteria, both IFN-γ and heat-killed bacteria were able to reinduce membrane IL-1 in the cultured macrophage (Ref. 19, and E. A. Kurt-Jones, unpublished observations). This indicates at least one difference in the control of these two proteins.

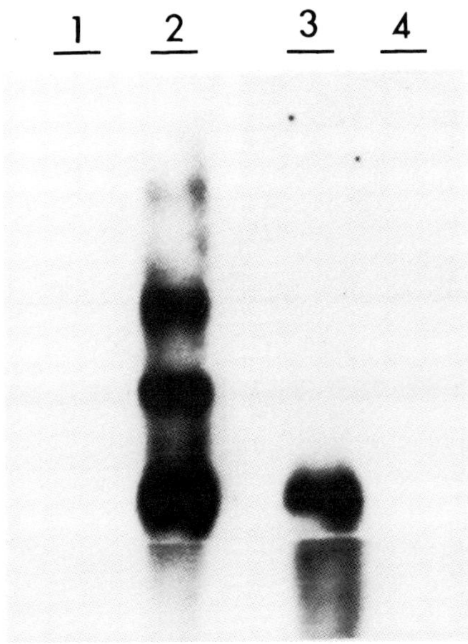

Figure 2. IFN-γ induces Ia mRNA. Peptone-elicited macrophages were cultured in medium with (lane 2) or without (lane 1) 1 ng/ml IFN-γ (derived from bacteria transfected with the gene for murine IFN-γ and purified to homogeneity by Genetech). Macrophages were lysed after 5 days in culture, and equivalent amounts of RNA were loaded into both lanes of a formaldehyde–agarose gel. (3) RNA from an Ia-positive B-cell tumor line; (4) an Ia-negative control. The results of standard Northern blotting procedures are indicated in the autoradiograph. It is clear that Ia mRNA is undetectable in macrophages maintained for 5 days in medium, even though there was no significant change in cell number, viability, or total RNA levels. Macrophages cultured in IFN-γ not only have substantial Ia mRNA, but also demonstrate higher molecular weight forms not seen in the B-cell tumor.

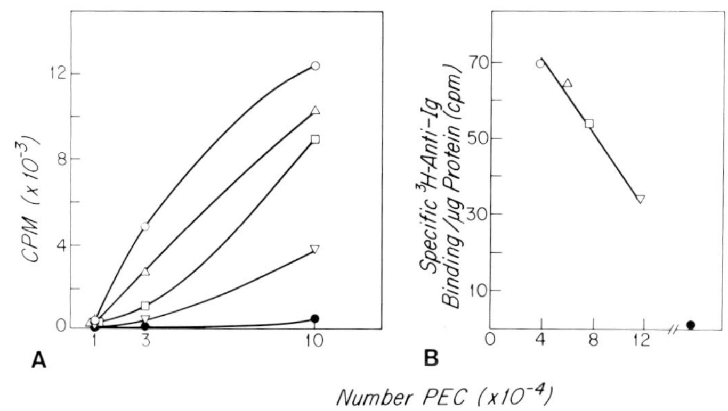

Figure 3. Quantitative relation of IFN-containing, lymphokine (LK)-induced Ia expression and function. (A) Peptone-elicited PECs were plated at the indicated numbers for 5 days in LK at (○) 5%, (△) 1%, (□) 0.2%, or (▽) 0.04% or (●) in medium without LK. On day 5, the cells were washed and T cells (clone A.11) added. Incorporation of [^{3}H]thymidine was determined at the end of a 3-day culture. (B) Duplicate trays of macrophages were also assessed on day 5 either for cell protein or for quantitation of Ia antigens by RIA. The latter consisted of binding monoclonal anti-I-A^k (or anti-I-A^d as control) followed by ^{3}H-labeled F(ab')$_2$ anti-Ig. The relative quantity of Ia per μg cell protein is plotted against the number of induced PECs required to stimulate half-maximal T-cell proliferation for each LK concentration (symbols as above). For macrophages cultured in 0.4% LK the latter value was obtained by extrapolation from part A; for macrophages maintained in medium, the response was too low to quantitate.

4. Summary

The findings discussed in this chapter concern two circuits of an amplification pathway for macrophage and T-cell interaction: production by activated T cells of IFN-γ, and IFN-induced Ia and IL-1 synthesis by macrophages. While Ia expression is critical for macrophage function as an antigen-presenting cell, macrophages in the peritoneum are primarily Ia-negative. We believe that inappropriate T-cell activation, e.g., autoimmune responsiveness coupled with subsequent delayed-type hypersensitivity, may be controlled in part by this limitation in the number of effective antigen-presenting cells (APCs). This type of control leads to a transient demand for increased numbers of APCs during challenge with antigen, and, in particular, during microbial infection. This need seems to be met by the rapid increase in the level of Ia-positive macrophages in response to IFN-γ. Since IL-1 production and membrane IL-1 are stimulated under the same conditions, it is clear that the activation of macrophages for antigen-presenting function is controlled by precisely that process that requires this specific change in macrophage physiology—T-cell activation. In this scheme, the low level of Ia-positive macrophages found even in non-overtly-stimulated mice might be important in the initial triggering of antigen-reactive T cells. It is also possible that other, constitutively Ia-positive APCs might be involved in this initial phase of the immune response.

References

1. Unanue, E. R., Beller, D. I., Lu, C. Y., and Allen, P. M., 1984, Antigen presentation: Comments on its regulation and mechanism, *J. Immunol.* **132:**1–5.
2. Gery, I., Gershon, R. K., and Waksman, B. H., 1972, Potentiation of the T-lymphocyte response to mitogens. I. The responding cell, *J. Exp. Med.* **135:**128–137.
3. Luger, T. A., Stadler, B. M., Luger, B. M., Mathieson, B. J., Mage, M., Schmidt, J. A., and Opperheim, J. J., 1982, Murine epidermal cell-derived thymocyte-activity factor resembles murine IL-1, *J. Immunol.* **128:**2147–2152.
4. Unanue, E. R., and Kiely, J.-M., 1977, Synthesis and secretion of a mitogenic protein by macrophages: Description of a superinduction phenomenon, *J. Immunol.* **119:**925–931.
5. Calderon, J., Kiely, J.-M., Lefko, J. L., and Unanue, E. R., 1975, The modulation of lymphocyte functions by molecules secreted by macrophages, *J. Exp. Med.* **142:**151–164.
6. Blyden, G., and Handschumacher, R. E., 1977, Purification and properties of human lymphocyte-activating factor (LAF), *J. Immunol.* **118:**1631–1638.
7. Gery, I., and Lepe-Zuniga, J. L., 1984, Interleukin 1: Uniqueness of its production and spectrum of activities, *Lymphokines* **9:**109–125.
8. Economou, J. S., and Shin, H. S., 1978, Lymphocyte-activating factor. I. Generation and physicochemical characterization, *J. Immunol.* **121:**1446–1452.
9. Mizel, S. B., and Mizel, D., 1981, Purification to apparent homogeneity of murine interleukin 1, *J. Immunol.* **126:**834–837.
10. Mizel, S. B., Dukovich, M., and Rothstein, J., 1983, Preparation of goat antibodies against interleukin 1: Use of an immunoadsorbent to purify interleukin 1, *J. Immunol.* **131:**1834–1837.
11. Dinarello, C. A., Renfer, L., and Wolff, S. M., 1977, Human leukocytic pyrogen: Purification and development of a radioimmunoassay, *Proc. Natl. Acad. Sci. USA* **74:**4624–4627.
12. Lachman, L. B., Page, S. O., and Metzger, R. S., 1980, Purification of human interleukin 1, *J. Supramol. Struct.* **13:**457–464.

13. Schmidt, J. A., 1984, Purification and partial biochemical characterization of normal human interleukin 1, *J. Exp. Med.* **160:**772–787.
14. Beller, D. I., and Unanue, E. R., 1979, Evidence that thymocytes require at least two distinct signals to proliferate, *J. Immunol.* **123:**2890–2893.
15. Larsson, E., and Coutinho, A., 1979, On the role of mitogenic lectins in T cell triggering, *Nature* **280:**239–241.
16. Smith, K. A., Lachman, L. B., Oppenheim, J. J., and Favata, M. F., 1980, The functional relationship of the interleukins, *J. Exp. Med.* **151:**1551–1560.
17. Hunig, T., Loos, M., and Schimpl, A., 1983, The role of accessory cells in polyclonal T cell activation. I. Both induction of interleukin 2 production and of interleukin 2 responsiveness by Con A are accessory cell dependent, *Eur. J. Immunol.* **13:**1–6.
18. Beller, D. I., 1984, Functional significance of the regulation of macrophage Ia expression, *Eur. J. Immunol.* **14:**138–143.
19. Kurt-Jones, E. A., Beller, D. I., Mizel, S. B., and Unanue, E. R., 1985, Identification of a surface-associated interleukin 1 in macrophages, *Proc. Natl. Acad. Sci. USA* **80:**1204–1208.
20. Kay, J., Porcelli, S., Tite, J., Jones, B., and Janeway, C. A., Jr., 1983, Both a monoclonal antibody and antisera specific for determinants unique to individual cloned helper T cell lines can substitute for antigen and antigen-presenting cells in the activation of T cells, *J. Exp. Med.* **158:**836–845.
21. Howard, M., Mizel, S. B., Lachman, L., Ansel, J., Johnson, B., and Paul, W. E., 1983, Role of interleukin 1 in anti-immunoglobulin-induced B cell proliferation, *J. Exp. Med.* **157:**1529–1543.
22. Farrar, J. J., Koopman, W. J., and Fuller-Bonan, J., 1977, Identification and partial purification of two synergistically acting helper mediators in human mixed leukocyte culture supernatants, *J. Immunol.* **119:**47–54.
23. Hoffman, M. K., and Watson, J., 1979, Helper T cell-replacing factors secreted by thymus-derived cells and macrophages: Cellular requirements for B cell activation and synergistic properties, *J. Immunol.* **122:**1371–1378.
24. Staruch, M. J., and Wood, D. D., 1983, The adjuvanticity of interleukin 1 *in vivo*, *J. Immunol.* **130:**2191–2194.
25. Prystowsky, M. B., Ely, J. M., Beller, D. I., Eisenberg, L., Goldman, J., Goldwasser, E., Ihle, J., Quintans, J., Remold, H., Vogel, S. N., and Fitch, F. W., 1982, Alloreactive cloned T cell lines. VI. Multiple lymphokine activities secreted by helper and cytolytic cloned T lymphocytes, *J. Immunol.* **129:**2337–2344.
26. Kelso, A., Glosebrook, A. L., Kanagawa, O., and Brunner, K. D., 1982, Production of macrophage-activating factor by T lymphocyte clones and correlation with other lymphokine activities, *J. Immunol.* **129:**550–556.
27. Honda, K., Suzuki, R., Matsui, H., Shimizu, Y., and Kumagai, K., 1983, Natural killer (NK) cells as a responder to interleukin 2 (IL-2). II. IL-2-induced interferon-gamma production, *J. Immunol.* **130:**988–992.
28. Kanase, I., Brooks, C. G., Kusibayashi, K., Olabuenagy, S., Newman, W., Gillis, S., and Henney, C. S., 1983, Interleukin 2 induces interferon-gamma production; Participation of macrophages and NK-like cells, *J. Immunol.* **131:**288–292.
29. Farrar, W. L., Johnson, H. M., and Farrar, J. J., 1981, Regulation of the production of immune interferon and cytotoxic T lymphocytes by interleukin 2, *J. Immunol.* **126:**1120–1125.
30. Steeg, P. S., Moore, R. N., Johnson, H. M., and Oppenheim, J. J., 1982, Regulation of murine macrophage Ia antigen expression by a lymphokine with immune interferon activity, *J. Exp. Med.* **156:**1780–1793.
31. Gray, P. W., and Goeddel, D. V., 1983, Cloning and expression of murine IFN-gamma cDNA, *Proc. Natl. Acad. Sci. USA* **80:**5842–5846.
32. Gray, P. W., and Goeddel, D. V., 1982, Structure of the human immune interferon gene, *Nature* **298:**859–863.
33. Lindahl, P., Leary, P., and Gresser, I., 1979, Enhancement of the expression of histocompatibility antigens of mouse lymphoid cells by interferon *in vitro*, *Eur. J. Immunol.* **4:**779–784.
34. Roberts, W. K., and Vasil, A., 1982, Evidence for the identity of murine gamma interferon and macrophage-activating factor, *J. Interferon Res.* **4:**519–528.

35. Schreiber, R. D., Pace, J. L., Russel, S. W., Altman, A., and Katz, D. H., 1983, Macrophage-activating factor produced by a T cell hybridoma: Physicochemical and biosynthetic resemblance to gamma interferon, *J. Immunol.* **131**:826–833.
36. King, D. P., and Jones, P. P., 1983, Induction of Ia and H-2 antigens on a macrophage cell line by immune interferon, *J. Immunol.* **131**:315–318.
37. Beller, D. I., and Unanue, E. R., 1981, Regulation of macrophage populations. II. Synthesis and expression of Ia antigens by peritoneal exudate macrophages is a transient event, *J. Immunol.* **126**:263–269.
38. Scher, M. G., Unanue, E. R., and Beller, D. I., 1982, Regulation of macrophage populations. III. The immunologic induction of exudates rich in Ia-bearing macrophages is a radiosensitive process, *J. Immunol.* **128**:447–450.
39. Beller, D. I., Kiely, J.-M., and Unanue, E. R., 1980, Regulation of macrophage populations. I. Preferential induction of Ia-rich peritoneal exudates by immunologic stimuli, *J. Immunol.* **124**:1426–1432.
40. Scher, M. G., Beller, D. I., and Unanue, E. R., 1980, Demonstration of a soluble mediator that induces exudates rich in Ia-positive macrophages, *J. Exp. Med.* **152**:1684–1698.
41. Calamai, E. G., Beller, D. I., and Unanue, E. R., 1982, Regulation of macrophage populations. IV. Modulation of Ia expression in bone marrow-derived macrophages, *J. Immunol.* **128**:1692–1694.
42. Beller, D. I., and Ho, K., 1982, Regulation of macrophage populations. V. Evaluation of the control of macrophage Ia expression *in vitro*, *J. Immunol.* **129**:971–976.
43. Walker, E. L., Lanier, L., and Warner, N., 1982, Concomitant induction of the cell surface expression of Ia determinants and accessory cell function by a murine macrophage tumor cell line, *J. Exp. Med.* **155**:269–272.

Index